Optum

Expert

HCPCS Level II

A resourceful compilation of HCPCS codes

Supports HIPAA compliance

2024

optumcoding.com

Publisher's Notice

The Optum *2024 HCPCS Level II* is designed to be an accurate and authoritative source of information about this government coding system. Every effort has been made to verify the accuracy of the listings, and all information is believed reliable at the time of publication. Absolute accuracy cannot be guaranteed, however. This publication is made available with the understanding that the publisher is not engaged in rendering legal or other services that require a professional license.

Our Commitment to Accuracy

Optum is committed to producing accurate and reliable materials.

To report corrections, please email customerassistance@optum.com. You can also reach customer service by calling 1.800.464.3649, option 1.

To view Optum updates/correction notices, please visit http://www.optumcoding.com/ProductUpdates/

Copyright

Acknowledgments

Denise M. Smith, RN, BSN, *Senior Product Manager*

Stacy Perry, *Manager, Desktop Publishing*

Elizabeth Leibold, RHIT, *Subject Matter Expert*

Jacqueline Petersen, RHIA, CHDA, CPC, *Subject Matter Expert*

Tracy Betzler, *Senior Desktop Publishing Specialist*

Hope M. Dunn, *Senior Desktop Publishing Specialist*

Katie Russell, *Desktop Publishing Specialist*

Lynn Speirs, *Editor*

Subject Matter Experts

Elizabeth Leibold, RHIT

Ms. Leibold has more than 30 years of experience in the health care profession. She has served in a variety of roles, ranging from patient registration to billing and collections, and has an extensive background in both physician and hospital outpatient coding and compliance. She has worked for large health care systems and health information management services companies, and has wide-ranging experience in facility and professional component coding, along with CPT expertise in interventional procedures, infusion services, emergency department, observation, and ambulatory surgery coding. Her areas of expertise include chart-to-claim coding audits and providing staff education to both tenured and new coding staff. She is an active member of the American Health Information Management Association (AHIMA) and Tennessee Health Information Management Association (THIMA).

Jacqueline Petersen, MHA, RHIA, CHDA, CPC

Ms. Petersen is a Registered Health Information Administrator with 30 years of experience in the healthcare profession. She has served as Senior Clinical Product Research Analyst with Optum developing business requirements for edits to support correct coding and reimbursement for claims processing applications. Her experience includes development of data-driven and system rules for both professional and facility claims and in-depth analysis of claims data inclusive of ICD-10-CM, CPT, HCPCS, and modifiers. Her background also includes consulting work for Optum, providing coding and reimbursement education to internal and external clients. Ms. Petersen is a member of the American Academy of Professional Coders (AAPC), and the American Health Information Management Association (AHIMA).

Contents

Introduction

Note: All data current as of November 15, 2023.

About HCPCS Codes

HCPCS Level II codes, except for the dental code series, are developed and maintained by a joint editorial panel consisting of the Centers for Medicare and Medicaid Services (CMS), the Blue Cross Blue Shield Association, and the Health Insurance Association of America. HCPCS Level II codes may be used throughout the United States in all Medicare regions. They consist of one alpha character (A through V) followed by four digits. Optum does not change the code descriptions other than correcting typographical errors. There are some codes that appear to be duplicates. CMS has indicated that each of the codes is used to report a specific condition or service. At press time, CMS had not provided further clarification regarding these codes. Additional information may be found on the CMS website, https://www.cms.gov/medicare/coding-billing/healthcare-common-procedure-system/release-information.

Any supplier or manufacturer can submit a request for coding modification to the HCPCS Level II National codes. A document explaining the HCPCS modification process, as well as a detailed format for submitting a recommendation for a modification to HCPCS Level II codes, is available on the HCPCS website at https://www.cms.gov/medicare/coding-billing/healthcare-common-procedure-system/coding-questions. Besides the information requested in this format, a requestor should also submit any additional descriptive material, including the manufacturer's product literature and information that is believed would be helpful in furthering CMS's understanding of the medical features of the item for which a coding modification is being recommended. The HCPCS coding review process is an ongoing, continuous process.

The dental (D) codes are not included in the official 2024 HCPCS Level II code set. The American Dental Association (ADA) holds the copyright on those codes and instructed CMS to remove them. As a result, Optum has removed them from this product; however, Optum has additional resources available for customers requiring the dental codes. Please visit www.optumcoding.com or call 1.800.464.3649.

Significant updates to this manual will be provided on our product updates page at Optumcoding.com, which can be accessed at the following: https://www.optumcoding.com/ProductUpdates/. Password: HCPCS24

Note: The expanded Medically Unlikely Edit (MUE) tables containing HCPCS/CPT codes, MUE values, MUE adjudication indicators, and MUE rationale are no longer published in this book. The tables are updated quarterly and can be found on the CMS website at https://www.cms.gov/medicare/coding-billing/national-correct-coding-initiative-ncci-edits/medicare-ncci-medically-unlikely-edits.

The table containing the Medicare national average payment (MAP) for services, supplies (DME, orthotics, prosthetics, etc.), drugs, biologicals, and nonphysician procedures using HCPCS Level II codes are available at www.optumcoding.com/2024MedAvPay. Password: OptumMAP24

How to Use HCPCS Level II

Coders should keep in mind that the insurance companies and government do not base payment solely on what was done for the patient. They need to know why the services were performed. In addition to using the HCPCS coding system for procedures and supplies, coders must also use the ICD-10-CM coding system to denote the diagnosis. This book will not discuss ICD-10-CM codes, which can be found in a current ICD-10-CM code book for diagnosis codes. To locate a HCPCS Level II code, follow these steps:

1. Identify the services or procedures that the patient received.

   Example:

   Patient administered PSA exam.

2. Look up the appropriate term in the index.

   Example:

   Screening
       prostate specific antigen test (PSA)

   Coding Tip: Coders who are unable to find the procedure or service in the index can look in the table of contents for the type of procedure or device to narrow the code choices. Also, coders should remember to check the unlisted procedure guidelines for additional choices.

3. Assign a tentative code.

   Example:

   Code G0103

Coding Tip: To the right of the terminology, there may be a single code or multiple codes, a cross-reference, or an indication that the code has been deleted. Tentatively assign all codes listed.

4. Locate the code or codes in the appropriate section. When multiple codes are listed in the index, be sure to read the narrative of all codes listed to find the appropriate code based on the service performed.

   Example:

G0103	Prostate cancer screening; prostate specific antigen test (PSA)

5. Check for color bars, symbols, notes, and references.

G0103	Prostate cancer screening; prostate specific antigen test (PSA) ♂ A

6. Review the appendixes for the reference definitions and other guidelines for coverage issues that apply.

7. Determine whether any modifiers should be appended.

8. Assign the code.

   Example:

   The code assigned is G0103.

Coding Standards

Levels of Use

Coders may find that the same procedure is coded at two or even three levels. Which code is correct? There are certain rules to follow if this should occur.

When both a CPT and a HCPCS Level II code have virtually identical narratives for a procedure or service, the CPT code should be used. If, however, the narratives are not identical (e.g., the CPT code narrative is generic, whereas the HCPCS Level II code is specific), the Level II code should be used.

Be sure to check for a national code when a CPT code description contains an instruction to include additional information, such as describing a specific medication. For example, when billing Medicare or Medicaid for supplies, avoid using CPT code 99070 Supplies and materials (except spectacles), provided by the physician over and above those usually included with the office visit or other services rendered (list drugs, trays, supplies, or materials provided). There are many HCPCS Level II codes that specify supplies in more detail.

Special Reports

Submit a special report with the claim when a new, unusual, or variable procedure is provided or a modifier is used. Include the following information:

- A copy of the appropriate report (e.g., operative, x-ray), explaining the nature, extent, and need for the procedure
- Documentation of the medical necessity of the procedure
- Documentation of the time and effort necessary to perform the procedure

How To Use Optum HCPCS Level II Books

Organization of Optum HCPCS Level II Expert

The Optum 2024 *HCPCS Level II* contains mandated changes and new codes for use as of January 1, 2024. Deleted codes have also been indicated and cross-referenced to active codes when possible. New codes have been added to the appropriate sections, eliminating the time-consuming step of looking in two places for a code. However, keep in mind that the information in this book is a reproduction of the 2024 HCPCS; additional information on coverage issues may have been provided to Medicare contractors after publication. All contractors periodically update their systems and records throughout the year. If this book does not agree with your contractor, it is either because of a mid-year update or correction, or a specific local or regional coverage policy.

HCPCS Code Index

Because HCPCS is organized by code number rather than by service or supply name, the index enables the coder to locate any code without looking through individual ranges of codes. Just look up the medical or surgical supply, service, orthotic, or prosthetic in question to find the appropriate codes. This index also refers to many of the brand names by which these items are known.

Appendixes

Appendix 1: Table of Drugs and Biologicals

The brand names of drugs and biologicals listed are examples only and may not include all products available for that type. The table lists HCPCS codes from any available section including A codes, C codes, J codes, S codes, and Q codes under brand and generic names with amount, route of administration, and code numbers. While every effort is made to make the table comprehensive, it is not all-inclusive.

Appendix 2: Modifiers

This appendix identifies current modifiers. A modifier is a two-position alpha or numeric code that is appended to a CPT or HCPCS code to clarify the services being reported. Modifiers provide a means by which a service can be altered without changing the procedure code. They add more information, such as anatomical site, to the code. In addition, they help eliminate the appearance of duplicate billing and unbundling. Modifiers are used to increase the accuracy in reimbursement and coding consistency, ease editing, and capture payment data.

Appendix 3: Abbreviations and Acronyms

This appendix contains a list of abbreviations and acronyms found throughout the HCPCS code set that may be helpful. It is not an all-inclusive list.

Appendix 4: Medicare Internet-only Manuals (IOMs)

Previously, this appendix contained a verbatim printout of the Medicare Internet-only Manual references pertaining to specific codes. This appendix now contains a link to the IOMs on the Centers for Medicare and Medicaid Services website. The IOM references to applicable to specific codes can still be found at the code level.

Appendix 5: New, Revised, and Deleted Codes

This appendix is a complete list of all new, revised, and deleted HCPCS codes for the current year. New and revised codes are listed along with their current code descriptors. Deleted codes are provided as a list of codes.

Appendix 6: Place of Service and Type of Service

This appendix contains lists of place-of-service codes that should be used on professional claims and type-of-service codes used by the Medicare Common Working File.

Appendix 7: Crosswalk of Deleted Codes

This appendix is a cross-reference from a deleted code to an active code when one is available. The deleted code cross-reference will also appear under the deleted code description in the tabular section of the book.

Appendix 8: Glossary

This appendix contains general terms and definitions that could be helpful for coding and reimbursement.

Appendix 9: Quality Payment Program (QPP)

Previously, this appendix contained lists of the numerators and denominators applicable to the Medicare PQRS. However, with the implementations of the Quality Payment Program (QPP) mandated by passage of the Medicare Access and Chip Reauthorization Act (MACRA) of 2015, the PQRS system will be obsolete. This appendix now contains information pertinent to that legislation as well as a brief overview of the proposed changes for the following year as available by date of this publication.

Color-coded Coverage Instructions

The Optum *HCPCS Level II* book provides colored symbols for each coverage and reimbursement instruction. A legend to these symbols is provided on the bottom of each two-page spread.

Green Color Bar—Special Coverage Instructions

A green bar for "special coverage instructions" over a code means that special coverage instructions apply to that code. These special instructions are also typically given in the form of Medicare Internet Only Manuals (IOM) reference numbers.

A4336	Incontinence supply, urethral insert, any type, each

Yellow Color Bar—Carrier Discretion

Issues that are left to "carrier discretion" are covered with a yellow bar. Contact the carrier for specific coverage information on those codes.

A9581	Injection, gadoxetate disodium, 1 ml

Pink Color Bar—Not Covered by or Invalid for Medicare

Codes that are not covered by or are invalid for Medicare are covered by a pink bar. The pertinent Medicare Internet-only Manuals (IOMs) reference numbers are also given explaining why a particular code is not covered. These numbers refer to the appendixes, where the Medicare references are listed.

A4264	Permanent implantable contraceptive intratubal occlusion device(s) and delivery system

Code Icons

Codes in the Optum *HCPCS Level II* follow the AMA CPT book conventions to indicate new, revised, and deleted codes.

A black circle (●) precedes a new code.

● J0391	Injection, artesunate, 1 mg

A black triangle (▲) precedes a code with revised terminology or rules.

▲ Q4225	AmnioBind or DermaBind TL, per sq cm

A circle (○) precedes a recycled/reinstated code.

○ Q4236	carePATCH, per sq cm

Codes deleted from the current active codes appear with a strike-out.

~~S0171~~	~~Injection, bumetanide, 0.5 mg~~

☑ Quantity Alert

Many codes in HCPCS report quantities that may not coincide with quantities available in the marketplace. For instance, a HCPCS code for an ostomy pouch with skin barrier reports each pouch, but the product is generally sold in a package of 10; "10" must be indicated in the quantity box on the CMS claim form to ensure proper reimbursement. This symbol indicates that care should be taken to verify quantities in this code. These quantity alerts do not represent Medicare Unlikely Edits (MUEs) and should not be used for MUEs.

☑ J0120	Injection, tetracycline, up to 250 mg

♀ Female Only

This icon identifies procedures that some payers may consider female only.

A4261	Cervical cap for contraceptive use	♀

♂ Male Only

This icon identifies procedures that some payers may consider male only.

A4326	Male external catheter with integral collection chamber, anytype, each	♂

Ⓐ Age Edit

This icon denotes codes intended for use with a specific age group, such as neonate, newborn, pediatric, and adult. Carefully review the code description to ensure that the code reported most appropriately reflects the patient's age.

Q2037	Influenza virus vaccine, split virus, when administered to individuals 3 years of age and older, for intramuscular use (FLUVIRIN)	Ⓐ

Ⓜ Maternity

This icon identifies procedures that by definition should only be used for maternity patients generally between 12 and 55 years of age.

H1001	Prenatal care, at-risk enhanced service; antepartum management	Ⓜ

🅐2–🅩3 ASC Payment Indicators

Codes designated as being paid by ASC groupings that were effective at the time of printing are denoted by the group number.

G0105	Colorectal cancer screening; colonoscopy on individual at high risk	🅐2

♿ DMEPOS

Use this icon to identify when to consult the CMS durable medical equipment, prosthetics, orthotics, and supplies (DMEPOS) for payment of this durable medical item. For modifiers NU, RR, and UE: These modifiers are for use when DME equipment is either new, used, or rented. The RR modifiers must also be used in conjunction with rental modifiers KH, KI, or KJ.

E0988	Manual wheelchair accessory, lever-activated, wheel drive, pair ♿

⃠ Skilled Nursing Facility (SNF)

Use this icon to identify certain items and services excluded from SNF consolidated billing. These items may be billed directly to the Medicare contractor by the provider or supplier of the service or item.

A4653	Peritoneal dialysis catheter anchoring device, belt, each ⃠

Drugs commonly reported with a code are listed underneath by brand or generic name.

C9254	Injection, lacosamide, 1 mg
	Use this code for VIMPAT.

CMS does not use consistent terminology when a code for a specific procedure is not listed. The code description may include any of the following terms: unlisted, not otherwise classified (NOC), unspecified, unclassified, other, and miscellaneous. If unsure there is no code for the service or supply provided or used, provide adequate documentation to the payer. Check with the payer for more information.

A0999	Unlisted ambulance service

CMS: This notation appears when instruction pertaining to a code appears in a CMS Internet-only Manual (IOM). Previously, appendix 4 contained a verbatim printout of the Medicare Internet-only Manual references pertaining to specific codes. This appendix now contains a link to the IOMs on the Centers for Medicare and Medicaid Services website. The IOM references applicable to specific codes can still be found at the code level.

A4618	Breathing circuits
	CMS: 100-04, 20, 100.2

AHA: American Hospital Association *Coding Clinic® for HCPCS* citations help in finding expanded information about specific codes and their usage. This includes citations for the current year and the preceding five years.

A2001	InnovaMatrix AC, per sq cm
	AHA: 1Q,22

Ⓐ-Ⓨ OPPS Status Indicators

Status indicators identify how individual HCPCS Level II codes are paid or not paid under the OPPS. The same status indicator is assigned to all the codes within an ambulatory payment classification (APC). Consult the payer or resource to learn which HCPCS codes fall within various APCs. **The OPSI contained in this publication were effective as of October 1, 2023. Once released by CMS, the table with data effective January 1, 2024, will be available on our product update page at www.optumcoding.com/ProductUpdates/.**

Ⓐ   Services furnished to a hospital outpatient that are paid under a fee schedule or payment system other than OPPS, for example:

- Ambulance Services
- Clinical Diagnostic Laboratory Services
- Non-Implantable Prosthetic and Orthotic Devices
- Physical, Occupational, and Speech Therapy
- Diagnostic Mammography
- Screening Mammography

Ⓑ   Codes that are not recognized by OPPS when submitted on an outpatient hospital Part B bill type (12x and 13x)

Ⓒ   Inpatient Procedures

Ⓔ   Items, Codes, and Services:

- Not covered by any Medicare outpatient benefit category
- Statutorily excluded by Medicare
- Not reasonable and necessary

Ⓕ   Corneal Tissue Acquisition; Certain CRNA Services and Hepatitis B Vaccines

Ⓖ   Pass-Through Drugs and Biologicals

Ⓗ   Pass-Through Device Categories

Ⓙ₁   Hospital Part B services paid through a comprehensive APC

Ⓚ   Nonpass-Through Drugs and Nonimplantable Biologicals, Including Therapeutic Radiopharmaceuticals

Ⓛ   Influenza Vaccine; Pneumococcal Pneumonia Vaccine

Ⓜ   Items and Services Not Billable to the MAC

Ⓝ   Items and Services Packaged into APC Rates

Ⓟ   Partial Hospitalization

Ⓠ₁   STVX-Packaged Codes

Ⓠ₂   T-Packaged Codes

Ⓠ₃   Codes That May Be Paid Through a Composite APC

Ⓠ₄   Conditionally Packaged Laboratory Tests

Ⓡ   Blood and Blood Products

Ⓢ   Significant Procedure, Not Discounted when Multiple

Ⓣ   Significant Procedure, Multiple Procedure Reduction Applies

Ⓤ   Brachytherapy Sources

Ⓥ   Clinic or Emergency Department Visit

Ⓨ   Nonimplantable Durable Medical Equipment

	Code	Description
Ⓐ	L8440	Prosthetic shrinker, below knee (BK), each
Ⓑ	Q4005	Cast supplies, long arm cast, adult (11 years +), plaster
Ⓒ	G0341	Percutaneous islet cell transplant, includes portal vein catheterization and infusion
Ⓔ	A0021	Ambulance service, outside state per mile, transport (Medicaid only)
Ⓕ	V2785	Processing, preserving and transporting corneal tissue
Ⓖ	C9460	Injection, cangrelor, 1 mg
Ⓗ	C2613	Lung biopsy plug with delivery system
Ⓚ	J1750	Injection, iron dextran, 50 mg
Ⓛ	Q2036	Influenza virus vaccine, split virus, when administered to individuals 3 years of age and older, for intramuscular use (FLULAVAL)
Ⓜ	G0333	Pharmacy dispensing fee for inhalation drug(s); initial 30-day supply as a beneficiary
Ⓝ	A4220	Refill kit for implantable infusion pump
Ⓟ	G0129	Occupational therapy services requiring the skills of a qualified occupational therapist, furnished as a component of a partial hospitalization treatment program, per session (45 minutes or more)
Ⓠ₃	C8935	Magnetic resonance angiography without contrast, upper extremity
Ⓡ	P9010	Blood (whole), for transfusion, per unit
Ⓢ	G0117	Glaucoma screening for high risk patients furnished by an optometrist or ophthalmologist
Ⓣ	C9727	Insertion of implants into the soft palate; minimum of three implants
Ⓤ	A9527	Iodine I-125, sodium iodide solution, therapeutic, per mCi
Ⓥ	G0101	Cervical or vaginal cancer screening; pelvic and clinical breast examination
Ⓨ	A5500	For diabetics only, fitting (including follow-up), custom preparation and supply of off-the-shelf depth-inlay shoe manufactured to accommodate multidensity insert(s), per shoe

A2–Z3 ASC Payment Indicators

This icon identifies the ASC status payment indicators. They indicate how the ASC payment rate was derived and/or how the procedure, item, or service is treated under the ASC payment system. For more information about these indicators and how they affect billing, consult Optum's *Revenue Cycle Pro*. **The ASC payment indicators contained in this publication were effective as of October 1, 2023. Once released by CMS, the table with data effective January 1, 2024, will be available on our product update page at www.optumcoding.com/ProductUpdates/.**

A2   Surgical procedure on ASC list in CY 2007 or later; payment based on OPPS relative payment weight

C5   Inpatient procedure

F4   Corneal tissue acquisition, hepatitis B vaccine; paid at reasonable cost

G2   Non-office-based surgical procedure added in CY 2008 or later; payment based on OPPS relative payment weight

H2   Brachytherapy source paid separately when provided integral to a surgical procedure on ASC list; payment based on OPPS rate

J7   OPPS pass-through device paid separately when provided integral to a surgical procedure on ASC list; payment based on OPPS rate

J8   Device-intensive procedure paid at adjusted rate

K2   Drugs and biologicals paid separately when provided integral to a surgical procedure on ASC list; payment based on OPPS rate

K7   Unclassified drugs and biologicals; payment contractor-priced

L1   Influenza vaccine; pneumococcal vaccine; packaged item/service; no separate payment made

L6   New Technology Intraocular Lens (NTIOL); special payment

N1   Packaged service/item; no separate payment made

P2   Office-based surgical procedure added to ASC list in CY 2008 or later with MPFS nonfacility PE RVUs; payment based on OPPS relative payment weight

P3   Office-based surgical procedure added to ASC list in CY 2008 or later with MPFS nonfacility PE RVUs; payment based on MPFS nonfacility PE RVUs

R2   Office-based surgical procedure added to ASC list in CY 2008 or later without MPFS nonfacility PE RVUs; payment based on OPPS relative payment weight

Z2   Radiology service paid separately when provided integral to a surgical procedure on ASC list; payment based on OPPS relative payment weight

Z3   Radiology service paid separately when provided integral to a surgical procedure on ASC list; payment based on MPFS nonfacility PE RVUs

F4	**V2785**	Processing, preserving and transporting corneal tissue
H2	**A9527**	Iodine I-125, sodium iodide solution, therapeutic per millicurie
J7	**C1052**	Hemostatic agent, gastrointestinal, topical
K2	**C9101**	Injection, oliceridine, 0.1 mg
K7	**C9399**	Unclassified drugs or biologicals
L1	**Q2037**	Influenza virus vaccine, split virus, when administered to individuals 3 years of age and older, for intramuscular use (FLUVIRIN)
N1	**C9353**	Microporous collagen implantable slit tube (NeuraWrap Nerve Protector), per cm length
Z3	**G0130**	Single energy x-ray absorptiometry (SEXA) bone density study, one or more sites; appendicular skeleton (peripheral) (e.g., radius, wrist, heel)
Z2	**C8911**	Magnetic resonance angiography without contrast followed by with contrast, chest (excluding myocardium)

Cogenex Flowable Amnion, Q4230
Coil, imaging, C1770
Cold fluid bottle/wrap, A9273
Collagen
    implant, urinary tract, L8603
    microporous nonhuman origin, C9352-C9353
    skin test, Q3031
    wound dressing, A6021-A6024, Q4164
Collar
    cervical
        contour (low, standard), L0120
        multiple post, L0180-L0200
        nonadjustable foam, L0120
        Philadelphia tracheotomy, L0172
        Philly one-piece extraction, L0150
        tracheotomy, L0172
        traction, E0856
        turtle neck safety, E0942
Collection
    physiologic data
        via remote patient monitoring, G0322
    specimen
        COVID-19
            self-administered, nonprescription, K1034
Coll-e-Derm, Q4193
Colonoscopy, G9659-G9661
    cancer screening
        patient at high risk, G0105
        patient not at high risk, G0121
    consultation, prescreening, S0285
Coloplast
    closed pouch, A5051
    drainable pouch, A5061
        closed, A5054
        small, A5063
    skin barrier
        4 x 4, A4362
        6 x 6, A5121
        8 x 8, A5122
    stoma cap, A5055
Colpopexy, vaginal, C9778
Coma stimulation, S9056
Combo-Seat universal raised toilet seat, E0244
Commode, E0160-E0171
    chair, E0163-E0165, E0170-E0171
    lift, E0172, E0625
    pail, E0167
    seat, wheelchair, E0968
Communication board, E1902
Community health integration services, G0019-G0022
Companion care, S5135-S5136
Complete AA, Q4303
Complete ACA, Q4302
Complete FT, Q4271
Complete SL, Q4270
Composite
    dressing, A6203-A6205
Compressed gas system, E0424-E0480
Compression
    bandage
        high, A6452
        light, A6448
        medium, A6451
    burn garment, A6501-A6512
    burn mask, A6513
    gradient garment
        accessory, A6593
        arm, A6522-A6523, A6576-A6578
        arm/glove combination, A6574-A6575
        bandage/bandaging supply, A6594-A6609
        bra, A6528-A6529
        full leg, A6526-A6527
        gauntlet, A6565, A6582
        genital area, A6570-A6571
        glove, A6520-A6521, A6579-A6581
        lower leg, A6524-A6525
        neck/head, A6566-A6567
        stocking, A6530-A6549, A6552-A6564, A6610
        toe caps, A6572-A6573

Compression — *continued*
    gradient garment — *continued*
        torso, A6568-A6569
        wrap, A6583-A6589
    nonpneumatic garment
        controller, E0680-E0681
        full arm, E0682
        full leg, E0678
        half leg, E0679
        trunk, E0677
    stockings, A6530-A6549
    wrap, A6545
Compressogrip prosthetic shrinker, L8440-L8465
Compressor, E0565, E0570, E0650-E0652, E0670, K0738
Computer aided detection
    breast MRI image, C8937
    echocardiography for heart failure, C9786
Concentrator
    oxygen, E1390-E1392
    rental, E1392
Condom
    female, A4268
    male, A4267
Conductive
    garment (for TENS), E0731
    paste or gel, A4558
Conductivity meter (for dialysis), E1550
Conference
    interdisciplinary team, G0175
Conforming bandage, A6442-A6447
Congenital torticollis orthotic, L0112
Congo red, blood, P2029
Consultation
    telehealth, G0406-G0408, G0425-G0427, G0508-G0509
Contact layer, A6206-A6208
Contact lens, S0500, S0512-S0514, V2500-V2599
Continent device, A5081, A5082
Continuous intraoperative neurophysiology monitoring, G0453
Continuous, monitor
    blood glucose
        adjunctive/nonimplanted, E2102
        invasive/nondurable
            receiver, A9278
            sensor, A9276
            transmitter, A9277
        nonadjunctive
            nonimplanted, A4239, E2103
            noninvasive, E0607, S1030-S1031
            lancet, A4258
            supply allowance, 1 month, A4238
            test strips, A4253, A4772
Continuous passive motion exercise device, E0936
Continuous positive airway pressure (CPAP) device, E0601
    chin strap, A7036
    face mask, A7030-A7031
    filter, A7038-A7039
    headgear, A7035
    intranasal resistance valve, A7049
    nasal application accessories, A7032-A7034
    oral interface, A7044
    tubing, A7037
Contraceptive
    cervical cap, A4261
    condom
        female, A4268
        male, A4267
    diaphragm, A4266
    etonogestrel, implant, J7307
    foam, A4269
    gel, A4269
    hormone patch, J7304
    implant, A4264, J7306-J7307
    intratubal occlusion device, A4264
    intrauterine
        copper contraceptive, J7300
        etonogestrel, J7307
        levonorgestrel-releasing, J7296-J7298, S4981
        other, S4989

Contraceptive — *continued*
    intrauterine — *continued*
        Progestasert, S4989
    Levonorgestrel, implants and supplies, J7296-J7298, J7301, J7306
    pills, S4993
    spermicide, A4269
    vaginal ring, J7294, J7295
Contracts, maintenance, ESRD, A4890
Contrast material
    high osmolar, Q9958-Q9964
    injection during MRI, A9575-A9579, Q9953
    low osmolar, Q9951, Q9965-Q9967
    nonradioactive NOC, A9698
    oral MRI, Q9954
Controlyte, enteral nutrition, B4155
Convalescent
    platelet rich plasma, C9507
Convulsive therapy, G2000
Coordinated care
    home monitoring, G9006
    initial rate, G9001
    maintenance rate, G9002
    physician oversight, G9008
    risk adjusted, G9003-G9005
    scheduled team conference, G9007
    specialty care
        psychosis, H2040-H2041
Copying fee, medical records, S9981-S9982
CoreCyte, Q4240
CoreText, Q4246
Corn, trim or remove, S0390
Corneal tissue processing, V2785
Coronary artery bypass surgery, direct
    with coronary arterial and venous grafts
        single, each, S2208
        two arterial and single venous, S2209
    with coronary arterial grafts, only
        single, S2205
        two grafts, S2206
    with coronary venous grafts, only
        single, S2207
Coronavirus (2019-nCoV) diagnostic panel, U0001-U0002
Corplex, Q4232
Corplex P, Q4231
Corset, spinal orthotic, L0970-L0976
Cough stimulation device, E0482
Counseling
    alcohol, G0443
    cardiovascular disease risk, G0446
    chaplain services, Q9001-Q9003
    end of life, S0257
    genetic, S0265
    lung cancer screening, G0296
    obesity, G0447
        group (2-10), G0473
    prevention
        sexually transmitted infection, G0445
    vaccine, G0310-G0313
        COVID-19, G0314-G0315
Coupling gel/paste, A4559
Cover, shower
    ventricular assist device, Q0501
Cover, wound
    alginate dressing, A6196-A6198
    foam dressing, A6209-A6214
    hydrocolloid dressing, A6234-A6239
    hydrogel dressing, A6242-A6248
    specialty absorptive dressing, A6251-A6256
COVID-19
    specimen collection
        self-administered, nonprescription, K1034
    vaccination administration, M0201
CPAP (continuous positive airway pressure) device, E0601
    chin strap, A7036
    exhalation port, A7045
    face mask, A7030-A7031
    headgear, A7035
    humidifier, E0561-E0562
    intranasal resistance valve, A7049
    nasal application accessories, A7032-A7034
    oral interface, A7044

CPAP (continuous positive airway pressure) device — *continued*
    supplies, E0470-E0472, E0561-E0562
    tubing, A7037
Cradle, bed, E0280
Cranial
    electrotherapy stimulation system, E0732
    supplies/accessories, A4596
Crisis intervention, H2011, S9484-S9485, T2034
Criticare HN, enteral nutrition, B4153
Crutch
    substitute
        lower leg platform, E0118
Crutches, E0110-E0116
    accessories, A4635-A4637, E2207
    aluminum, E0114
    articulating, spring assisted, E0117
    forearm, E0111
        Ortho-Ease, E0111
    underarm, other than wood, pair, E0114
        Quikfit Custom Pack, E0114
        Red Dot, E0114
    underarm, wood, single, E0113
        Ready-for-use, E0113
    wooden, E0112
Cryo-Cord, Q4237
Cryoprecipitate, each unit, P9012
    plasma, pathogen reduced, P9025
Cryoprecipitated fibrinogen complex
    pathogen reduced, P9026
CTLSO, L0700, L0710, L1000-L1120
Cuirass, E0457
Culture sensitivity study, P7001
Culture, urine, bacterial, P7001
Curasorb, alginate dressing, A6196-A6199
Cushion
    decubitus care, E0190
    Oral/Nasal, A7029
    positioning, E0190
    wheelchair
        AK addition, L5648
        BK addition, L5646
Custom
    DME, K0900
    wheelchair/base, K0008, K0013
Custom Masterhinge Hip Hinge 3, L2999
Customized item (in addition to code for basic item), S1002
Cyanocobalamin cobalt, A9546, A9559
Cycler
    disposable set, A4671
Cycler dialysis machine, E1594
Cygnus, Q4170, Q4199
Cygnus Dual, Q4282
Cylinder tank carrier, E2208
Cymetra, Q4112
Cystoscopy, blue light, C7554, C9738
    with biopsy(ies), C7550
Cystourethroscopy
    for ureteral calculi, S2070
    with adjunctive blue light cystoscopy, C7554
    with biopsy(ies), C7550
    with insertion of transprostatic implant; 1 to 3 implants, C9739
    with insertion of transprostatic implant; 4 or more implants, C9740
    with insertion temporary prostatic implant or stent, C9769
    with lithotripsy, C9761
Cytal, Q4166
Cytopathology, screening, G0123, G0124, G0141, G0143-G0148

D

Day care services, S5100-S5102, S5105
Debridement, bone
    with insertion drug delivery device, C7500, C7561
Decompression
    disc, S2348
    hip core, S2325
    lumbar
        percutaneous image guided (pild), G0276
    vertebral axial, S9090

Index

Drugs — Fluid Flow, Fluid GF

Drugs — *see* Table of Drugs — *continued*
infusion supplies, A4221, A4222, A4230-A4232
not otherwise classified, J3490, J7599, J7699, J7799, J8499, J8999, J9999
Part B drug CAP NOC, Q4082
Dry pressure pad/mattress, E0184, E0199
DSM IV criteria major depressive disorder, G9212-G9213
Dual Layer Impax Membrane, Q4262
Dunlap
heating pad, E0210
Duolock curved tail closures, A4421
Durable medical equipment (DME), E0100-E8002
Durr-Fillauer
cervical collar, L0140
Pavlik harness, L1620

E

Ear wax removal, G0268
Easy Care
folding walker, E0143
quad cane, E0105
ECG
initial Medicare ECG, G0403-G0405
Echocardiography
computer aided detection for heart failure, C9786
transesophageal, C8925-C8928
transthoracic, C8921-C8924, C8929-C8930
Echosclerotherapy, S2202
Economy knee splint, L1830
Edetate
calcium disodium, J0600
edetate disodium, J3520
Education
asthma, S9441
birthing, S9436-S9439, S9442
chronic kidney disease, G0420-G0421
diabetes, S9145
exercise, S9451
family planning
individualized programs, school based, T1018
nonmedical, H1010
infant safety, S9447
lactation, S9443
Lamaze, S9436
mental health problems, G0177
parenting, S9444
smoking cessation, S9453
stress management, S9454
weight management, S9449
Eggcrate dry pressure pad/mattress, E0184, E0199
E-Graft, Q4277
Elastic support stocking, A6530-A6549, A6552-A6564, A6610
Elbow
brace, universal rehabilitation, L3720
disarticulation, endoskeletal, L6450
Masterhinge Elbow Brace 3, L3999
orthotic
EO, E1800, L3702-L3740, L3760-L3762
EWHO, L3764-L3766
protector, E0191
Elbow, wrist, hand, finger orthotic (EWHFO), L8702
Elbow, wrist, hand orthotic (EWHO), L8701
Electric (electrical)
auricular acupuncture points, S8930
hand
adult, L7007
independently articulating digits, L6880
pediatric, L7008
heat pad for peritoneal dialysis, E0210
hook, L7009
impedance
esophageal mucosal integrity testing, C9777
stimulation device
disposable
replacement, A4560

Electric (electrical) — *continued*
stimulation device — *continued*
for cancer treatment, E0766
supplies, A4595, L8678
work
dialysis equipment, A4870
Electrode
Electrodes, per pair, A4556
Electrode/transducer, A4555
Electrodes, per pair, A4556
Electromagnetic therapy, G0295, G0329
Electron beam computed tomography, S8092
Electrophysiology
gastric mapping, C9787
Electrotherapy stimulation, cranial
supplies/accessories, A4596
Elevating leg rest, K0195
Elevator, air pressure, heel, E0370
Embolization, protection system, C1884
for tumor destruction, S2095
Embryo
cryopreserved transferred, S4037
monitor/store cryopreserved, S4040
storage, S4027
Emerge Matrix, Q4297
Emergency response system, S5160-S5162
EMG
biofeedback device, E0746
surface, S3900
Encounter, clinic, T1015
End of life care planning, S0257
Endarterectomy, chemical, M0300
Endoscope
colonoscope device (implantable), C1749
pulmonary, single use, C1601
sheath, A4270
upper GI, single use, C1748
urinary, single use, C1747
Endoscopic
outlet reduction
gastric pouch application, C9785
retrograde cholangiopancreatography (ERCP)
biopsy, C7542
calculi/debris removal, C7544
diagnostic, C7541
foreign body/stent removal, C7560
sphincterotomy/papillotomy, C7543
sleeve gastroplasty, C9784
Endoscopy
nasal, S2342
submucosal dissection (ESD), C9779
Endoskeletal system, addition, L5610-L5999
Endovascular, revascularization
femoral, popliteal artery(ies), C7531, C7534-C7535
intravascular lithotripsy, C9764, C9772
catheter, transluminal, C1761
with atherectomy, C9766, C9774
with atherectomy and stent placement, C9767, C9775
with stent placement, C9765, C9773
Enema
bag, reusable, A4458
barium, G0106
cancer screening, G0120
manual pump system, A4459
tube
replacement, any type, A4457
Enrich, enteral nutrition, B4150
Ensure, enteral nutrition, B4150
HN, B4150
Plus, B4152
Plus HN, B4152
powder, B4150
Enteral
administration services, feeding, S9340-S9343
digestive enzyme(s), B4105
feeding supply kit (syringe) (pump) (gravity), B4034-B4036, B4148
fiber or additive, B4104
formulae, B4150-B4162
electrolytes, B4102, B4103
for metabolic disease, B4157

Enteral — *continued*
formulae — *continued*
intact nutrients, B4149, B4150, B4152
pediatric, B4158-B4162
gastronomy tube, B4087-B4088
nutrition infusion pump, any type, B9002
supplies, not otherwise classified, B9998
Enterostomal therapy, S9474
Enverse, Q4258
Enzyme(s)
enteral feeding, B4105
Eosinophil count, S3630
EpiCord, Q4187
EpiEffect, Q4276
EpiFix (injectable), Q4145
EpiFix, Q4186
Equestrian/hippotherapy, S8940
ERCP, C7541-C7544
Esano A, Q4272
Esano AAA, Q4273
Esano AC, Q4274
Esano ACA, Q4275
ESD (endoscopic submucosal dissection), C9779
Esophageal mucosal integrity testing, C9777
ESRD End Stage Renal Disease — *see also* Dialysis
bundle demo/basic, G9013
expanded, G9014
documentation, G9231
ESRD facility
acute kidney injury without ESRD, G0491-G0492
machines and accessories, E1510-E1699
plumbing, A4870
supplies, A4651-A4913
Evaluation
comprehensive, multi-discipline, H2000
E/M, prolonged, G0316-G0318, G2212
for power mobility device, G0372
ocularist, S9150
remote, images/video, G2010
risk factors, G9298-G9299
self assessment, depression, S3005
team for handicapped, T1024
Eversion device, A9285
Exactech lancet device, A4258
Examination
breast, S0613
breast and pelvic, G0101
diabetic for LOPS, G0245-G0246
for college, S0622
initial Medicare, G0402
related to surgical procedure, S0260
Excellagen, Q4149
Exchange
biliary drainage catheter, C7545
nephrostomy catheter, C7548
Excision
deep cervical node(s), C7503
peripheral nerve neuroma, C7551
tissue localization, C1819
Exercise
class, S9451
continuous passive motion device, E0936
equipment, A9300
Exo-Static overdoor traction unit, E0860
Exsufflation belt, A4468
External
ambulatory infusion pump, E0781, E0784
counterpulsation, G0166
defibrillator
battery replacement, K0607
electrode replacement, K0609
garment replacement, K0608
power, battery components, L7360-L7499
power, elbow, L7191
urinary catheter for suction pump
disposable, A6590
nondisposable, A6591
Extracorporeal shock wave lithotripsy, S0400
Extrahepatic bile duct(s)
intraoperative
near-infrared fluorescence imaging, C9776

Extremity belt/harness, E0945
Eye
lens (contact) (spectacle), S0500-S0514, V2100-V2615
pad, A6410-A6411
patch, A6410-A6412
prosthetic, C1839, V2623-V2629
service (miscellaneous), V2700-V2799
E-Z Lite wheelchair, E1250
EZ-Derm, Q4136
E-ZJect disposable insulin syringes, up to 1 cc, per syringe, A4206
E-ZJect Lite Angle lancets, box of 100, A4259
E-Z-lets lancet device, A4258

F

Face tent, oxygen, A4619
Facility services
dental procedure requiring monitored anesthesia, G0330
Family stabilization, S9482
FDG, A9552
Fecal microbiota, preparation/instillation, G0455
Fee
coordinated care, G9001
pharmacy supply
anticancer oral antiemetic or immunosuppressive drug, Q0511-Q0512
HIV pre-exposure prophylaxis (PrEP), Q0516-Q0518
immunosuppressive drugs, Q0510
Fern test, Q0114
Fertility services
donor service (sperm or embryo), S4025
in vitro fertilization, S4013-S4022
ovulation induction, S4042
sperm procurement, S4026, S4030-S4031
Fertilization
in vitro, S4011
Fetal surgery, repair teratoma, S2405
Fetoscopic laser therapy, S2411
Filler
bone, C9359
wound
alginate, A6199
foam, A6215
hydrocolloid, A6240-A6241
hydrogel, A6248
not elsewhere classified, A6261-A6262
Film
dressing, A6257-A6259
Filter
aerosol compressor, A7013
carbon, A4680
CPAP device, A7038-A7039
dialysis carbon, A4680
ostomy, A4368
tracheostoma, A4481
ultrasonic generator, A7013
vena cava, C1880
ventricular assist device, Q0500
Financial management, self-directed, T2050
Finasteride, S0138
Finger
orthotic (FO), L3933-L3935
splint
baseball, A4570
fold-over, A4570
four-pronged, A4570
static, Q4049
Fisher&Paykel HC220, E0601
Fistula
cannulation set, A4730
Fitness club membership, S9970
Flashcast Elite casting material, A4590
Flex HD, Q4128
Flow rate meter, peak, A4614
FlowerAmnioFlo, Q4177
FlowerAmnioPatch, Q4148
FlowerDerm, Q4179
Flowmeter, E0440, E0555, E0580
Fluid barrier, dialysis, E1575
Fluid Flow, Fluid GF, Q4206

Management
advanced illness, S0311
chronic pain, G3002-G3003
disease, S0316-S0317
financial, self-directed, T2050

Mapping
topographic brain, S8040

Marker
tissue, A4648

Mask
burn compression, A6513
CPAP, A7027
oxygen, A4620
surgical, for dialysis, A4928

Mastectomy
bra, L8002
camisole, S8460
form, L8020
prosthesis, L8000-L8039, L8600
sleeve, L8010

Masterbrace 3, L2999
Masterfoot Walking Cast Sole, L3649
Masterhinge Adjustabrace 3, L2999
Masterhinge Elbow Brace 3, L3999
Masterhinge Hip Hinge 3, L2999
Masterhinge Shoulder Brace 3, L3999
Masters 2 step, S3904
Matrion, Q4201
MatriStem, Q4118
Matrix HD, Q4128

Mattress
air pressure, E0186, E0197
alternating pressure, E0277
    pad, Bio Flote, E0181
    pad, KoalaKair, E0181
AquaPedic Sectional, E0196
decubitus care, E0196
dry pressure, E0184
flotation, E0184
gel pressure, E0196
hospital bed, E0271, E0272
    non-powered, pressure reducing, E0373
Iris Preventix pressure relief/reduction, E0184
Overlay, E0371-E0372
pressure reducing, E0181
TenderFlo II, E0187
TenderGel II, E0196
water pressure, E0187, E0198
    powered, pressure reducing, E0277

MCCM, G9480
MCP, multi-axial rotation unit, L5986
MCT Oil, enteral nutrition, B4155
MDPP, G9873-G9891

Meals
adults in treatment, T1010
per diem NOS, S9977

Measurement
hepatic portosystemic pressure gradient, endoscopic, C9768

Mechanical
allergen particle barrier/inhalation filter nasal, topical, A7023
hand, L6708-L6709
hook, L6706-L6707
wound suction, A9272

Medialization material for vocal cord, C1878
Medical and surgical supplies, A4206-A6404
Medical conference, S0220-S0221
Medical food, S9435
Medical home program, S0280-S0281
Medical records copying fee, S9981-S9982
Medical visit, G0463, G9246-G9247
Medicare Care Choice Model (MCCM), G9480
Medicare Diabetes Prevention Program (MDPP), G9873-G9891

Medicare "welcome"
ECG, G0403-G0405
physical, G0402

Medication management device, T1505

Medication services
comprehensive, H2010
reminder, S5185

Medi-Jector injection device, A4210

MediSense 2 Pen blood glucose monitor, E0607
Mediskin, Q4135

Medralone
40, J1030
80, J1040

Membrane Graft, Membrane Wrap, Q4205
Membrane Wrap-Hydro, Q4290
MemoDerm, Q4126
Menotropins, S0122

Mental health
assessment, H0031
education, G0177
hospitalization, H0035
peer services, H0038
remote diagnosis, evaluation, treatment, C7900-C7902
self-help, H0038
service plan, H0032
services, NOS, H0046
supportive treatment, H0026-H0037
training, G0177

Meritene, enteral nutrition, B4150
    powder, B4150
MESA, S4028
Mesh, C1781
Metabolism error, food supplement, S9434
Metacarpophalangeal joint prosthesis, L8630
Metatarsal joint, prosthetic implant, L8641
Meter, bath conductivity, dialysis, E1550
Methylene blue injection, Q9968

Methylprednisolone
acetate, J1020-J1040
oral, J7509
sodium succinate, J2920, J2930

Microbiology test, P7001
Microcapillary tube, A4651
    sealant, A4652

Micro-Fine
disposable insulin syringes, up to 1 cc, per syringe, A4206
lancets, box of 100, A4259

Microinfusion
transcatheter therapy, C9759

Microlipids, enteral nutrition, B4155
Microlyte, A2005
Mileage, ambulance, A0380, A0390

Milk, breast
processing, T2101

Milwaukee spinal orthotic, L1000
Minerva, spinal orthotic, L0700, L0710
Mini-bus, nonemergency transportation, A0120

Minimed
3 cc syringe, A4232
506 insulin pump, E0784
insulin infusion set with bent needle wings, each, A4231
Sof-Set 24" insulin infusion set, each, A4230

Miro3D, A2025
Miroderm Biologic Wound Matrix, Q4175
Mirragen, A2002
Mitotic rate, G9292-G9294
MLG-Complete, Q4256
Mobilite hospital beds, E0293, E0295, E0297

Model/Modeling
CT angiography
    3D predictive model generation, C9793
therapeutic radiology simulation-aided field setting, C9794

Moderate sedation, G0500
Modular, enteral nutrition, B4155
Moisture exchanger for use with invasive mechanical ventilation, A4483
Moisturizer, skin, A6250

Molecular diagnostic test reader
nonprescription, K1035

Monitor
apnea, E0618
blood glucose
    device, continuous
        adjunctive/nonimplanted, E2102
        invasive/nondurable, receiver, A9278

Monitor — continued
blood glucose — continued
    device, continuous — continued
        invasive/nondurable — continued
            sensor, A9276
            transmitter, A9277
        nonadjunctive
            nonimplanted, A4239, E2103
        noninvasive, E0607, S1030-S1031
    lancet, A4258
    supply allowance, 1 month, A4238
    test strips, A4253, A4772
blood pressure, A4670
device, NOC, A9279
pacemaker, E0610, E0615
ultrafiltration, S9007

Monoclonal antibody therapy administration, M0220, M0221, M0222, M0223, M0240, M0241, M0243, M0244, M0245, M0246, M0247, M0248, M0249, M0250
Monoject disposable insulin syringes, up to 1 cc, per syringe, A4206
Monojector lancet device, A4258
Morcellator, C1782
Mouthpiece (for respiratory equipment), A4617
MRCP, S8037

MRI
cardiac
    strain imaging, C9762
    stress imaging, C9763
contrast material, A9576-A9579, Q9954
low field, S8042
with inhaled hyperpolarized xenon-129 contrast agent
    chest, C9791

Mucoadhesive, oral, A9156
Mucoprotein, blood, P2038
Mucus trap, S8210
Muenster Suspension, socket prosthesis, L6110
Multidisciplinary services, children, T1026
Multifetal pregnancy reduction, ultrasound guidance, S8055
Multiple post collar, cervical, L0180-L0200
Multipositional patient support system, E0636
Muscular dystrophy, genetic test, S3853
Myotonic muscular dystrophy, genetic test, S3853
MyOwn Skin, Q4226
Myringotomy, S2225

N

Nail trim, G0127, S0390
Narrowing device, wheelchair, E0969

Nasal
application device (for CPAP device), A7032-A7034
endoscopy, S2342
vaccine inhalation, J3530

Nasogastric tubing, B4081, B4082

Nebulizer, E0570-E0585
aerosol mask, A7015
aerosols, E0580
    Airlife Brand Misty-Neb, E0580
    Power-Mist, E0580
    Up-Draft Neb-U-Mist, E0580
    Up-Mist hand-held nebulizer, E0580
compressor, with, E0570
    Madamist II medication compressor/nebulizer, E0570
    Pulmo-Aide compressor/nebulizer, E0570
    Schuco Mist nebulizer system, E0570
corrugated tubing
    disposable, A7010, A7018
distilled water, A7018
filter
    disposable, A7013
    non-disposable, A7014
heater, E1372

Nebulizer — continued
large volume
    disposable, prefilled, A7008
    disposable, unfilled, A7007
not used with oxygen
    durable glass, A7017
pneumatic, administration set, A7003, A7005, A7006
pneumatic, nonfiltered, A7004
portable, E0570
small volume, E0574
spacer or nebulizer, S8100
    with mask, S8101
ultrasonic, dome and mouthpiece, A7016
ultrasonic, reservoir bottle
    nondisposable, A7009
water, A7018
water collection device large volume nebulizer, A7012
    distilled water, A7018

Needle, A4215
biopsy
    bone marrow, C1830
brachytherapy, C1715
non-coring, A4212
with syringe, A4206-A4209

Negative pressure wound therapy
dressing set, A6550
pump, E2402

NeoMatriX, A2021
NeoPatch, Q4176
NeoStim DL, Q4267
NeoStim Membrane, Q4266
NeoStim TL, A4265
Neox 100, Q4156
Neox 1K, Neox Cord 1K, Neox Cord RT, Q4148
Neox Flo, Q4155
NephrAmine, parenteral nutrition, B5000

Nephrostomy catheter
convert to nephroureteral catheter, C7547
exchange, C7548

Nephroureteral catheter
convert from nephrostomy catheter, C7547
removal and replacement, C7546

Neuroma
excision, C7551

Neurophysiology monitoring, G0453
Neuro-Pulse, E0720

Neurostimulator (Neuromuscular)
cranial electrotherapy (CES), A4596, K1002
diaphragm/phrenic nerve
    replacement, L8696
disposable
    replacement, A4560
electronic shock unit, E0745
functional transcutaneous, E0764, E0770
generator
    nonrechargeable, C1767, C1823, C1825, C1827
    with rechargeable battery/charging system, C1826
        high frequency, C1822
        nonhigh frequency, C1820
implantable
    antenna, L8696
    charging system, L8695
    electrode, L8680
    generator, C1826-C1827, L8679, L8685-L8688
    programmer, L8681
    radiofrequency
        receiver, L8682
        transmitter, L8683-L8684
    receiver, C1816, L8682
interferential current, S8130-S8131
lead, C1778
    adapter/extension, C1883
    sacral nerve test, A4290
    test kit, C1897
nausea/vomiting, E0765
patient programmer, C1787, L8681
peripheral nerve
    upper arm, K1023
receiver and/or transmitter, C1816, L8682
salivary reflex, E0755
scoliosis, E0744

Index

Skin substitute — Stimulation/Stimulators

Transportation Services Including Ambulance A0021-A0999

This code range includes ground and air ambulance, nonemergency transportation (taxi, bus, automobile, wheelchair van), and ancillary transportation-related fees.

HCPCS Level II codes for ambulance services must be reported with modifiers that indicate pick-up origins and destinations. The modifier describing the arrangement (QM, QN) is listed first. The modifiers describing the origin and destination are listed second. Origin and destination modifiers are created by combining two alpha characters from the following list. Each character, with the exception of X, represents either an origin or a destination. Each pair of alpha characters creates one modifier. The first position represents the origin and the second the destination. The modifiers most commonly used are:

D	Diagnostic or therapeutic site other than "P" or "H" when these are used as origin codes
E	Residential, domiciliary, custodial facility (other than 1819 facility)
G	Hospital-based ESRD facility
H	Hospital
I	Site of transfer (e.g., airport or helicopter pad) between modes of ambulance transport
J	Free standing ESRD facility
N	Skilled nursing facility (SNF)
P	Physician's office
R	Residence
S	Scene of accident or acute event
X	Intermediate stop at physician's office on way to hospital (destination code only)

Note: Modifier X can only be used as a destination code in the second position of a modifier. See S0215. For Medicaid, see T codes and T modifiers.

Ambulance Transport and Supplies

A0021   **Ambulance service, outside state per mile, transport (Medicaid only)**   EI
     CMS: 100-04,15,20.4

A0080   **Nonemergency transportation, per mile - vehicle provided by volunteer (individual or organization), with no vested interest**   EI
     CMS: 100-04,15,20.4

A0090   **Nonemergency transportation, per mile - vehicle provided by individual (family member, self, neighbor) with vested interest**   EI
     CMS: 100-04,15,20.4

A0100   **Nonemergency transportation; taxi**   EI
     CMS: 100-04,15,20.4

A0110   **Nonemergency transportation and bus, intra- or interstate carrier**   EI
     CMS: 100-04,15,20.4

A0120   **Nonemergency transportation: mini-bus, mountain area transports, or other transportation systems**   EI
     CMS: 100-04,15,20.4

A0130   **Nonemergency transportation: wheelchair van**   EI
     CMS: 100-04,15,20.4

A0140   **Nonemergency transportation and air travel (private or commercial) intra- or interstate**   EI
     CMS: 100-04,15,20.4

A0160   **Nonemergency transportation: per mile - caseworker or social worker**   EI
     CMS: 100-04,15,20.4

A0170   **Transportation ancillary: parking fees, tolls, other**   EI
     CMS: 100-04,15,20.4

A0180   **Nonemergency transportation: ancillary: lodging-recipient**   EI
     CMS: 100-04,15,20.4

A0190   **Nonemergency transportation: ancillary: meals, recipient**   EI
     CMS: 100-04,15,20.4

A0200   **Nonemergency transportation: ancillary: lodging, escort**   EI
     CMS: 100-04,15,20.4

A0210   **Nonemergency transportation: ancillary: meals, escort**   EI
     CMS: 100-04,15,20.4

A0225   **Ambulance service, neonatal transport, base rate, emergency transport, one way**   EI
     CMS: 100-02,10,10.1.2; 100-02,10,10.2.1; 100-02,10,30.1; 100-02,10,30.1.1; 100-04,15,20.4

A0380   **BLS mileage (per mile)**   EI ☑
     See code(s): A0425
     CMS: 100-02,10,10.1.2; 100-02,10,10.2.1; 100-02,10,10.3.3; 100-02,10,30.1; 100-02,10,30.1.1; 100-04,15,20.4; 100-04,15,30.2

A0382   **BLS routine disposable supplies**   EI
     CMS: 100-02,10,10.1.2; 100-02,10,10.2.1; 100-02,10,30.1; 100-02,10,30.1.1; 100-04,15,20.4

A0384   **BLS specialized service disposable supplies; defibrillation (used by ALS ambulances and BLS ambulances in jurisdictions where defibrillation is permitted in BLS ambulances)**   EI
     CMS: 100-02,10,10.1.2; 100-02,10,10.2.1; 100-02,10,30.1; 100-02,10,30.1.1; 100-04,15,20.4

A0390   **ALS mileage (per mile)**   EI ☑
     See code(s): A0425
     CMS: 100-02,10,10.1.2; 100-02,10,10.2.1; 100-02,10,10.3.3; 100-02,10,30.1; 100-02,10,30.1.1; 100-04,15,20.4; 100-04,15,30.2

A0392   **ALS specialized service disposable supplies; defibrillation (to be used only in jurisdictions where defibrillation cannot be performed in BLS ambulances)**   EI
     CMS: 100-02,10,10.1.2; 100-02,10,10.2.1; 100-02,10,30.1; 100-02,10,30.1.1; 100-04,15,20.4

A0394   **ALS specialized service disposable supplies; IV drug therapy**   EI
     CMS: 100-02,10,10.1.2; 100-02,10,10.2.1; 100-02,10,30.1; 100-02,10,30.1.1; 100-04,15,20.4

A0396   **ALS specialized service disposable supplies; esophageal intubation**   EI
     CMS: 100-02,10,10.1.2; 100-02,10,10.2.1; 100-02,10,30.1; 100-02,10,30.1.1; 100-04,15,20.4

A0398   **ALS routine disposable supplies**   EI
     CMS: 100-02,10,10.1.2; 100-02,10,10.2.1; 100-02,10,30.1; 100-02,10,30.1.1; 100-04,15,20.4

Waiting Time

Units	Time
1	1/2 to 1 hr.
2	1 to 1-1/2 hrs.
3	1-1/2 to 2 hrs.
4	2 to 2-1/2 hrs.
5	2-1/2 to 3 hrs.
6	3 to 3-1/2 hrs.
7	3-1/2 to 4 hrs.
8	4 to 4-1/2 hrs.
9	4-1/2 to 5 hrs.
10	5 to 5-1/2 hrs.

A0420   **Ambulance waiting time (ALS or BLS), one-half (1/2) hour increments**   EI
     CMS: 100-02,10,10.1.2; 100-02,10,10.2.1; 100-02,10,30.1; 100-02,10,30.1.1; 100-04,15,20.4

Special Coverage Instructions   Noncovered by Medicare   Carrier Discretion   ☑ Quantity Alert   ● New Code   ○ Recycled/Reinstated   ▲ Revised Code

© 2023 Optum360, LLC   A2-Z3 ASC Pmt   **CMS:** IOM   **AHA:** Coding Clinic   ❧ DMEPOS Paid   ⊘ SNF Excluded   **A Codes — 1**

Other Ambulance Services

A0422 Ambulance (ALS or BLS) oxygen and oxygen supplies, life sustaining situation 　[EI]
CMS: 100-02,10,10.1.2; 100-02,10,10.2.1; 100-02,10,30.1; 100-02,10,30.1.1; 100-04,15,20.4

A0424 Extra ambulance attendant, ground (ALS or BLS) or air (fixed or rotary winged); (requires medical review) 　[EI]
Pertinent documentation to evaluate medical appropriateness should be included when this code is reported.
CMS: 100-02,10,10.1.2; 100-02,10,10.2.1; 100-02,10,30.1; 100-02,10,30.1.1; 100-04,15,20.4; 100-04,15,30.2.1

A0425 Ground mileage, per statute mile 　[A] [✓]
CMS: 100-02,10,10.1.2; 100-02,10,10.2.1; 100-02,10,10.2.2; 100-02,10,10.3.3; 100-02,10,20; 100-02,10,30.1; 100-02,10,30.1.1; 100-02,10,20; 100-04,15,10.3; 100-04,15,20.1.4; 100-04,15,20.4; 100-04,15,20.6; 100-04,15,30; 100-04,15,30.1.2; 100-04,15,30.2.1; 100-04,15,40

A0426 Ambulance service, advanced life support, nonemergency transport, level 1 (ALS 1) 　[A]
CMS: 100-02,10,10.1.2; 100-02,10,10.2.1; 100-02,10,10.2.2; 100-02,10,10.3.3; 100-02,10,20; 100-02,10,30.1; 100-02,10,30.1.1; 100-02,10,20; 100-04,15,10.3; 100-04,15,20.1.4; 100-04,15,20.4; 100-04,15,30; 100-04,15,30.1.2; 100-04,15,30.2; 100-04,15,30.2.1; 100-04,15,40

A0427 Ambulance service, advanced life support, emergency transport, level 1 (ALS 1 - emergency) 　[A]
CMS: 100-02,10,10.1.2; 100-02,10,10.2.1; 100-02,10,10.2.2; 100-02,10,10.3.3; 100-02,10,20; 100-02,10,30.1; 100-02,10,30.1.1; 100-02,10,20; 100-04,15,10.3; 100-04,15,20.1.4; 100-04,15,20.4; 100-04,15,30; 100-04,15,30.1.2; 100-04,15,30.2; 100-04,15,30.2.1; 100-04,15,40

A0428 Ambulance service, basic life support, nonemergency transport, (BLS) 　[A]
CMS: 100-02,10,10.1.2; 100-02,10,10.2.1; 100-02,10,10.2.2; 100-02,10,10.3.3; 100-02,10,20; 100-02,10,30.1; 100-02,10,30.1.1; 100-02,10,20; 100-04,15,10.3; 100-04,15,20.1.4; 100-04,15,20.4; 100-04,15,20.6; 100-04,15,30; 100-04,15,30.1.2; 100-04,15,30.2; 100-04,15,30.2.1; 100-04,15,40

A0429 Ambulance service, basic life support, emergency transport (BLS, emergency) 　[A]
CMS: 100-02,10,10.1.2; 100-02,10,10.2.1; 100-02,10,10.2.2; 100-02,10,10.3.3; 100-02,10,20; 100-02,10,30.1; 100-02,10,30.1.1; 100-02,10,20; 100-04,15,10.3; 100-04,15,20.1.4; 100-04,15,20.4; 100-04,15,30; 100-04,15,30.1.2; 100-04,15,30.2; 100-04,15,30.2.1; 100-04,15,40

A0430 Ambulance service, conventional air services, transport, one way (fixed wing) 　[A]
CMS: 100-02,10,10.1.2; 100-02,10,10.2.1; 100-02,10,10.2.2; 100-02,10,10.3.3; 100-02,10,20; 100-02,10,30.1; 100-02,10,30.1.1; 100-02,10,20; 100-04,15,10.3; 100-04,15,20.1.4; 100-04,15,20.3; 100-04,15,20.4; 100-04,15,30; 100-04,15,30.1.2; 100-04,15,30.2; 100-04,15,30.2.1; 100-04,15,40

A0431 Ambulance service, conventional air services, transport, one way (rotary wing) 　[A]
CMS: 100-02,10,10.1.2; 100-02,10,10.2.1; 100-02,10,10.2.2; 100-02,10,10.3.3; 100-02,10,20; 100-02,10,30.1; 100-02,10,30.1.1; 100-02,10,20; 100-04,15,10.3; 100-04,15,20.1.4; 100-04,15,20.3; 100-04,15,20.4; 100-04,15,30; 100-04,15,30.1.2; 100-04,15,30.2; 100-04,15,30.2.1; 100-04,15,40

A0432 Paramedic intercept (PI), rural area, transport furnished by a volunteer ambulance company which is prohibited by state law from billing third-party payers 　[A]
CMS: 100-02,10,10.1.2; 100-02,10,10.2.1; 100-02,10,10.2.2; 100-02,10,10.3.3; 100-02,10,20; 100-02,10,30.1; 100-02,10,30.1.1; 100-02,10,20; 100-04,15,10.3; 100-04,15,20.1.4; 100-04,15,20.4; 100-04,15,30; 100-04,15,30.1.2; 100-04,15,30.2; 100-04,15,30.2.1; 100-04,15,40

A0433 Advanced life support, level 2 (ALS 2) 　[A]
CMS: 100-02,10,10.1.2; 100-02,10,10.2.1; 100-02,10,10.2.2; 100-02,10,10.3.3; 100-02,10,20; 100-02,10,30.1; 100-02,10,30.1.1; 100-02,10,20; 100-04,15,10.3; 100-04,15,20.1.4; 100-04,15,20.4; 100-04,15,30; 100-04,15,30.1.2; 100-04,15,30.2; 100-04,15,30.2.1; 100-04,15,40

A0434 Specialty care transport (SCT) 　[A]
CMS: 100-02,10,10.1.2; 100-02,10,10.2.1; 100-02,10,10.2.2; 100-02,10,10.3.3; 100-02,10,20; 100-02,10,30.1; 100-02,10,30.1.1; 100-02,10,20; 100-04,15,10.3; 100-04,15,20.1.4; 100-04,15,20.4; 100-04,15,30; 100-04,15,30.1.2; 100-04,15,30.2; 100-04,15,30.2.1; 100-04,15,40

A0435 Fixed wing air mileage, per statute mile 　[A]
CMS: 100-02,10,10.1.2; 100-02,10,10.2.1; 100-02,10,10.2.2; 100-02,10,10.3.3; 100-02,10,20; 100-02,10,30.1; 100-02,10,30.1.1; 100-02,10,20; 100-04,15,10.3; 100-04,15,20.1.4; 100-04,15,20.3; 100-04,15,20.4; 100-04,15,30; 100-04,15,30.1.2; 100-04,15,30.2; 100-04,15,30.2.1; 100-04,15,40

A0436 Rotary wing air mileage, per statute mile 　[A]
CMS: 100-02,10,10.1.2; 100-02,10,10.2.1; 100-02,10,10.2.2; 100-02,10,10.3.3; 100-02,10,20; 100-02,10,30.1; 100-02,10,30.1.1; 100-02,10,20; 100-04,15,10.3; 100-04,15,20.1.4; 100-04,15,20.3; 100-04,15,20.4; 100-04,15,30; 100-04,15,30.1.2; 100-04,15,30.2; 100-04,15,30.2.1; 100-04,15,40

A0888 Noncovered ambulance mileage, per mile (e.g., for miles traveled beyond closest appropriate facility) 　[EI]
CMS: 100-02,10,10.1.2; 100-02,10,10.2.1; 100-02,10,20; 100-02,10,30.1; 100-02,10,30.1.1; 100-04,15,20.4; 100-04,15,30.1.2; 100-04,15,30.2.4

A0998 Ambulance response and treatment, no transport 　[EI]
CMS: 100-02,10,10.1.2; 100-02,10,10.2.1; 100-02,10,30.1; 100-02,10,30.1.1; 100-04,15,20.4

A0999 Unlisted ambulance service 　[A]
CMS: 100-02,10,10.1; 100-02,10,10.1.2; 100-02,10,10.2.1; 100-02,10,20; 100-02,10,30.1; 100-02,10,30.1.1; 100-04,15,20.4

Medical and Surgical Supplies A2001-A9999

This section covers a wide variety of medical, surgical, and some durable medical equipment (DME) related supplies and accessories. DME-related supplies, accessories, maintenance, and repair required to ensure the proper functioning of this equipment is generally covered by Medicare under the prosthetic devices provision.

Skin Substitutes

A2001 InnovaMatrix AC, per sq cm 　[N1]
AHA: 1Q,22

A2002 Mirragen Advanced Wound Matrix, per sq cm 　[N1]
AHA: 1Q,22

A2004 XCelliStem, 1 mg 　[N1]
AHA: 1Q,22

A2005 Microlyte Matrix, per sq cm 　[N1]
AHA: 1Q,22

A2006 NovoSorb SynPath dermal matrix, per sq cm 　[N1]
AHA: 1Q,22

A2007 Restrata, per sq cm 　[N1]
AHA: 1Q,22

A2008 TheraGenesis, per sq cm 　[N1]
AHA: 1Q,22

A2009 Symphony, per sq cm 　[N1]
AHA: 1Q,22

A2010 Apis, per sq cm 　[N1]
AHA: 1Q,22

A2011 Supra SDRM, per sq cm 　[N1]
AHA: 2Q,22

Special Coverage Instructions　　Noncovered by Medicare　　Carrier Discretion　　☑ Quantity Alert　● New Code　　○ Recycled/Reinstated　▲ Revised Code

2 — A Codes　　[A] Age Edit　　[M] Maternity Edit　♀ Female Only　♂ Male Only　[A]-[Y] OPPS Status Indicators　　© 2023 Optum360, LLC

A2012	SUPRATHEL, per sq cm	N1
	AHA: 2Q,22	
A2013	InnovaMatrix FS, per sq cm	N1
	AHA: 2Q,22	
A2014	Omeza Collagen Matrix, per 100 mg	N1
	AHA: 4Q,22	
A2015	Phoenix Wound Matrix, per sq cm	N1
	AHA: 4Q,22	
A2016	PermeaDerm B, per sq cm	N1
	AHA: 4Q,22	
A2017	PermeaDerm Glove, each	N1
	AHA: 4Q,22	
A2018	PermeaDerm C, per sq cm	N1
	AHA: 4Q,22	
● A2019	Kerecis Omega3 MariGen Shield, per sq cm	N1
	AHA: 2Q,23	
● A2020	AC5 Advanced Wound System (AC5)	N1
	AHA: 2Q,23	
● A2021	NeoMatriX, per sq cm	N1
	AHA: 2Q,23	
● A2022	InnovaBurn or InnovaMatrix XL, per sq cm	N1
● A2023	InnovaMatrix PD, 1 mg	N1
● A2024	Resolve Matrix, per sq cm	N1
● A2025	Miro3D, per cu cm	N1
A4100	Skin substitute, FDA-cleared as a device, not otherwise specified	N1
	AHA: 2Q,22	

Injection Supplies

A4206	Syringe with needle, sterile, 1 cc or less, each	N ☑
A4207	Syringe with needle, sterile 2 cc, each	N ☑
A4208	Syringe with needle, sterile 3 cc, each	N ☑
A4209	Syringe with needle, sterile 5 cc or greater, each	N ☑
A4210	Needle-free injection device, each	EI ☑
	Sometimes covered by commercial payers with preauthorization and physician letter stating need (e.g., for insulin injection in young children).	
A4211	Supplies for self-administered injections	N
	When a drug that is usually injected by the patient (e.g., insulin or calcitonin) is injected by the physician, it is excluded from Medicare coverage unless administered in an emergency situation (e.g., diabetic coma).	
A4212	Noncoring needle or stylet with or without catheter	N
A4213	Syringe, sterile, 20 cc or greater, each	N ☑
A4215	Needle, sterile, any size, each	N
A4216	Sterile water, saline and/or dextrose, diluent/flush, 10 ml	N ☑ ዼ
A4217	Sterile water/saline, 500 ml	N ☑ ዼ (AU)
	CMS: 100-04,20,30.9	
A4218	Sterile saline or water, metered dose dispenser, 10 ml	N ☑
A4220	Refill kit for implantable infusion pump	N
A4221	Supplies for maintenance of noninsulin drug infusion catheter, per week (list drugs separately)	N ዼ
A4222	Infusion supplies for external drug infusion pump, per cassette or bag (list drugs separately)	N ዼ

A4223	Infusion supplies not used with external infusion pump, per cassette or bag (list drugs separately)	N ☑
A4224	Supplies for maintenance of insulin infusion catheter, per week	N ዼ
A4225	Supplies for external insulin infusion pump, syringe type cartridge, sterile, each	N ዼ
A4226	Supplies for maintenance of insulin infusion pump with dosage rate adjustment using therapeutic continuous glucose sensing, per week	
A4230	Infusion set for external insulin pump, nonneedle cannula type	N ☑
	Covered by some commercial payers as ongoing supply to preauthorized pump.	
A4231	Infusion set for external insulin pump, needle type	N ☑
	Covered by some commercial payers as ongoing supply to preauthorized pump.	
A4232	Syringe with needle for external insulin pump, sterile, 3 cc	EI ☑
	Covered by some commercial payers as ongoing supply to preauthorized pump.	

Batteries

A4233	Replacement battery, alkaline (other than J cell), for use with medically necessary home blood glucose monitor owned by patient, each	EI ☑ ዼ (NU)
A4234	Replacement battery, alkaline, J cell, for use with medically necessary home blood glucose monitor owned by patient, each	EI ☑ ዼ (NU)
A4235	Replacement battery, lithium, for use with medically necessary home blood glucose monitor owned by patient, each	EI ☑ ዼ (NU)
A4236	Replacement battery, silver oxide, for use with medically necessary home blood glucose monitor owned by patient, each	EI ☑ ዼ (NU)

Other Supplies

A4238	Supply allowance for adjunctive, nonimplanted continuous glucose monitor (CGM), includes all supplies and accessories, 1 month supply — 1 unit of service	(KF)
A4239	Supply allowance for nonadjunctive, nonimplanted continuous glucose monitor (CGM), includes all supplies and accessories, 1 month supply = 1 unit of service	(KF)
A4244	Alcohol or peroxide, per pint	N ☑
A4245	Alcohol wipes, per box	N ☑
A4246	Betadine or pHisoHex solution, per pint	N ☑
A4247	Betadine or iodine swabs/wipes, per box	N ☑
A4248	Chlorhexidine containing antiseptic, 1 ml	N ☑

Special Coverage Instructions   Noncovered by Medicare   Carrier Discretion   ☑ Quantity Alert   ● New Code   ○ Recycled/Reinstated   ▲ Revised Code

© 2023 Optum360, LLC   A2-Z3 ASC Pmt   CMS: IOM   AHA: Coding Clinic   ዼ DMEPOS Paid   ⊘ SNF Excluded   A Codes — 3

A4250 Urine test or reagent strips or tablets (100 tablets or strips) ☐ ☑
CMS: 100-02,15,110

Reference chart

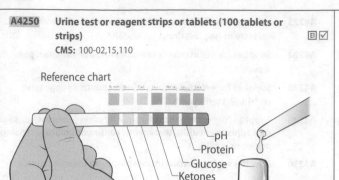

pH
Protein
Glucose
Ketones
Bilirubin
Hemoglobin
Nitrate

Tablet reagents turn specific colors when urine droplets are placed on them

Dipstick urinalysis: The strip is dipped and color-coded squares are read at timed intervals (e.g., pH immediately; ketones at 15 seconds, etc.). Results are compared against a reference chart

A4252 Blood ketone test or reagent strip, each ☐ ☑

A4253 Blood glucose test or reagent strips for home blood glucose monitor, per 50 strips ☐ ☑ ☐ (NU)
Medicare covers glucose strips for diabetic patients using home glucose monitoring devices prescribed by their physicians.

A4255 Platforms for home blood glucose monitor, 50 per box ☐ ☑ ☐
Some Medicare contractors cover monitor platforms for diabetic patients using home glucose monitoring devices prescribed by their physicians. Some commercial payers also provide this coverage to noninsulin dependent diabetics.

A4256 Normal, low, and high calibrator solution/chips ☐ ☐
Some Medicare contractors cover calibration solutions or chips for diabetic patients using home glucose monitoring devices prescribed by their physicians. Some commercial payers also provide this coverage to noninsulin dependent diabetics.

A4257 Replacement lens shield cartridge for use with laser skin piercing device, each ☐ ☑ ☐

A4258 Spring-powered device for lancet, each ☐ ☑ ☐
Some Medicare contractors cover lancing devices for diabetic patients using home glucose monitoring devices prescribed by their physicians. Medicare jurisdiction: DME regional contractor. Some commercial payers also provide this coverage to noninsulin dependent diabetics.

A4259 Lancets, per box of 100 ☐ ☑ ☐
Medicare covers lancets for diabetic patients using home glucose monitoring devices prescribed by their physicians. Medicare jurisdiction: DME regional contractor. Some commercial payers also provide this coverage to noninsulin dependent diabetics.

A4261 Cervical cap for contraceptive use ☐ ♀ ☐

A4262 Temporary, absorbable lacrimal duct implant, each ☐ ☑
Always report concurrent to the implant procedure.

A4263 Permanent, long-term, nondissolvable lacrimal duct implant, each ☐ ☑
Always report concurrent to the implant procedure.

A4264 Permanent implantable contraceptive intratubal occlusion device(s) and delivery system ☐ ♀ ☐ ☑

A4265 Paraffin, per pound ☐ ☑ ☐

A4266 Diaphragm for contraceptive use ☐ ♀ ☐

A4267 Contraceptive supply, condom, male, each ♂ ☐ ☑

A4268 Contraceptive supply, condom, female, each ☐ ♀ ☐ ☑

A4269 Contraceptive supply, spermicide (e.g., foam, gel), each ☐ ♀ ☐ ☑

A4270 Disposable endoscope sheath, each ☐ ☑

A4280 Adhesive skin support attachment for use with external breast prosthesis, each ☐ ☑ ☐

Two part prosthesis

Adhesive skin support (A4280)

Any of several breast prostheses fits over skin support

A4281 Tubing for breast pump, replacement ☐ ♀ ☐

A4282 Adapter for breast pump, replacement ☐ ♀ ☐

A4283 Cap for breast pump bottle, replacement ☐ ♀ ☐

A4284 Breast shield and splash protector for use with breast pump, replacement ☐ ♀ ☐

A4285 Polycarbonate bottle for use with breast pump, replacement ☐ ♀ ☐

A4286 Locking ring for breast pump, replacement ☐ ♀ ☐

● **A4287** Disposable collection and storage bag for breast milk, any size, any type, each

A4290 Sacral nerve stimulation test lead, each ☐ ☑
CMS: 100-04,32,40.1; 100-04,32,40.2.1; 100-04,32,40.4

Special Coverage Instructions Noncovered by Medicare Carrier Discretion ☑ Quantity Alert ● New Code ○ Recycled/Reinstated ▲ Revised Code

4 — A Codes ☐ Age Edit ☐ Maternity Edit ♀ Female Only ♂ Male Only ☐-☐ OPPS Status Indicators © 2023 Optum360, LLC

Vascular Catheters and Drug Delivery Systems

A4300 Implantable access catheter, (e.g., venous, arterial, epidural subarachnoid, or peritoneal, etc.) external access N

A4301

Needle access — Implanted reservoir under refill injection — Catheter — Body of reservoir and pump

Swan-Ganz catheter — Monitoring device — Tip with balloon — Detail of tapered tip and balloon

A4300 — Markings along catheter measure depth of insertion — Ports — Junction divider

A4301 Implantable access total catheter, port/reservoir (e.g., venous, arterial, epidural, subarachnoid, peritoneal, etc.) N

A4305 Disposable drug delivery system, flow rate of 50 ml or greater per hour N ☑

A4306 Disposable drug delivery system, flow rate of less than 50 ml per hour N ☑

Incontinence Appliances and Care Supplies

Covered by Medicare when the medical record indicates incontinence is permanent, or of long and indefinite duration.

A4310 Insertion tray without drainage bag and without catheter (accessories only) N &

A4311 Insertion tray without drainage bag with indwelling catheter, Foley type, two-way latex with coating (Teflon, silicone, silicone elastomer or hydrophilic, etc.) N &

A4312 Insertion tray without drainage bag with indwelling catheter, Foley type, two-way, all silicone N &

A4313 Insertion tray without drainage bag with indwelling catheter, Foley type, three-way, for continuous irrigation N &

A4314 Insertion tray with drainage bag with indwelling catheter, Foley type, two-way latex with coating (Teflon, silicone, silicone elastomer or hydrophilic, etc.) N &

A4315 Insertion tray with drainage bag with indwelling catheter, Foley type, two-way, all silicone N &

A4316 Insertion tray with drainage bag with indwelling catheter, Foley type, three-way, for continuous irrigation N &

A4320 Irrigation tray with bulb or piston syringe, any purpose N &

A4321 Therapeutic agent for urinary catheter irrigation N &

A4322 Irrigation syringe, bulb or piston, each N ☑ &

A4326 Male external catheter with integral collection chamber, any type, each ♂ N ☑ &

A4327 Female external urinary collection device; meatal cup, each ♀ N ☑ &

A4328 Female external urinary collection device; pouch, each A ♀ N ☑ &

A4330 Perianal fecal collection pouch with adhesive, each N ☑ &

A4331 Extension drainage tubing, any type, any length, with connector/adaptor, for use with urinary leg bag or urostomy pouch, each N ☑ &

A4332 Lubricant, individual sterile packet, each N ☑ &

A4333 Urinary catheter anchoring device, adhesive skin attachment, each N ☑ &

A4334 Urinary catheter anchoring device, leg strap, each N ☑ &

A4335 Incontinence supply; miscellaneous N

A4336 Incontinence supply, urethral insert, any type, each N ☑ &

A4337 Incontinence supply, rectal insert, any type, each N

A4338 Indwelling catheter; Foley type, two-way latex with coating (Teflon, silicone, silicone elastomer, or hydrophilic, etc.), each N ☑ &

A4340 Indwelling catheter; specialty type, (e.g., Coude, mushroom, wing, etc.), each N ☑ &

○ **A4341** Indwelling intraurethral drainage device with valve, patient inserted, replacement only, each
AHA: 2Q,23

○ **A4342** Accessories for patient inserted indwelling intraurethral drainage device with valve, replacement only, each
AHA: 2Q,23

▲ **A4344** Indwelling catheter, foley type, two-way, all silicone or polyurethane, each N M ☑ &

Special Coverage Instructions   Noncovered by Medicare   Carrier Discretion   ☑ Quantity Alert   ● New Code   ○ Recycled/Reinstated   ▲ Revised Code

© 2023 Optum360, LLC   A2-Z3 ASC Pmt   CMS: IOM   AHA: Coding Clinic   & DMEPOS Paid   ⊘ SNF Excluded   A Codes — 5

Medical and Surgical Supplies

A4346 — A4388

A4346 Indwelling catheter; Foley type, three-way for continuous irrigation, each �Ⓝ ☑ &

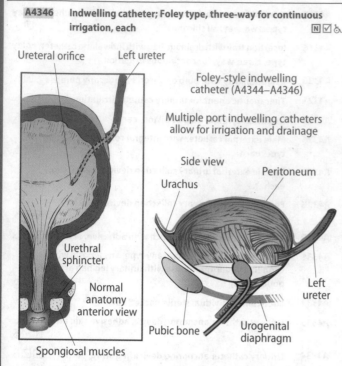

Foley-style indwelling catheter (A4344–A4346)

Multiple port indwelling catheters allow for irrigation and drainage

A4349 Male external catheter, with or without adhesive, disposable, each ♂ Ⓝ ☑ &

A4351 Intermittent urinary catheter; straight tip, with or without coating (Teflon, silicone, silicone elastomer, or hydrophilic, etc.), each Ⓝ ☑ &

A4352 Intermittent urinary catheter; Coude (curved) tip, with or without coating (Teflon, silicone, silicone elastomeric, or hydrophilic, etc.), each Ⓝ ☑ &

A4353 Intermittent urinary catheter, with insertion supplies Ⓝ &

A4354 Insertion tray with drainage bag but without catheter Ⓝ &

A4355 Irrigation tubing set for continuous bladder irrigation through a three-way indwelling Foley catheter, each Ⓝ ☑ &

A4356 External urethral clamp or compression device (not to be used for catheter clamp), each Ⓝ ☑ &

A4357 Bedside drainage bag, day or night, with or without antireflux device, with or without tube, each Ⓝ ☑ &

A4358 Urinary drainage bag, leg or abdomen, vinyl, with or without tube, with straps, each Ⓝ ☑ &

A4360 Disposable external urethral clamp or compression device, with pad and/or pouch, each Ⓝ ☑ &

Ostomy Supplies

A4361 Ostomy faceplate, each Ⓝ ☑ &

A4362 Skin barrier; solid, 4 x 4 or equivalent; each Ⓝ ☑ &

A4363 Ostomy clamp, any type, replacement only, each Ⓔ &

A4364 Adhesive, liquid or equal, any type, per oz Ⓝ ☑ &

A4366 Ostomy vent, any type, each Ⓝ ☑ &

A4367 Ostomy belt, each Ⓝ ☑ &

A4368 Ostomy filter, any type, each Ⓝ ☑ &

A4369 Ostomy skin barrier, liquid (spray, brush, etc.), per oz Ⓝ ☑ &

A4371 Ostomy skin barrier, powder, per oz Ⓝ ☑ &

A4372 Ostomy skin barrier, solid 4 x 4 or equivalent, standard wear, with built-in convexity, each Ⓝ ☑ &

A4373 Ostomy skin barrier, with flange (solid, flexible or accordion), with built-in convexity, any size, each Ⓝ ☑ &

Faceplate flange and skin barrier combination (A4373)

A4375 Ostomy pouch, drainable, with faceplate attached, plastic, each Ⓝ ☑ &

A4376 Ostomy pouch, drainable, with faceplate attached, rubber, each Ⓝ ☑ &

Colostomy pouch with faceplate and drain (A4376)

A4377 Ostomy pouch, drainable, for use on faceplate, plastic, each Ⓝ ☑ &

A4378 Ostomy pouch, drainable, for use on faceplate, rubber, each Ⓝ ☑ &

A4379 Ostomy pouch, urinary, with faceplate attached, plastic, each Ⓝ ☑ &

A4380 Ostomy pouch, urinary, with faceplate attached, rubber, each Ⓝ ☑ &

A4381 Ostomy pouch, urinary, for use on faceplate, plastic, each Ⓝ ☑ &

A4382 Ostomy pouch, urinary, for use on faceplate, heavy plastic, each Ⓝ ☑ &

A4383 Ostomy pouch, urinary, for use on faceplate, rubber, each Ⓝ ☑ &

A4384 Ostomy faceplate equivalent, silicone ring, each Ⓝ ☑ &

A4385 Ostomy skin barrier, solid 4 x 4 or equivalent, extended wear, without built-in convexity, each Ⓝ ☑ &

A4387 Ostomy pouch, closed, with barrier attached, with built-in convexity (one piece), each Ⓝ ☑ &

A4388 Ostomy pouch, drainable, with extended wear barrier attached, (one piece), each Ⓝ ☑ &

Special Coverage Instructions   Noncovered by Medicare   Carrier Discretion   ☑ Quantity Alert   ● New Code   ○ Recycled/Reinstated   ▲ Revised Code

Ⓐ Age Edit   Ⓜ Maternity Edit   ♀ Female Only   ♂ Male Only   Ⓐ-Ⓨ OPPS Status Indicators   © 2023 Optum360, LLC

A4389 Ostomy pouch, drainable, with barrier attached, with built-in convexity (one piece), each N ☑ &

A4390 Ostomy pouch, drainable, with extended wear barrier attached, with built-in convexity (one piece), each N ☑ &

A4391 Ostomy pouch, urinary, with extended wear barrier attached (one piece), each N ☑ &

A4392 Ostomy pouch, urinary, with standard wear barrier attached, with built-in convexity (one piece), each N ☑ &

A4393 Ostomy pouch, urinary, with extended wear barrier attached, with built-in convexity (one piece), each N ☑ &

A4394 Ostomy deodorant, with or without lubricant, for use in ostomy pouch, per fl oz N ☑ &

A4395 Ostomy deodorant for use in ostomy pouch, solid, per tablet N ☑ &

A4396 Ostomy belt with peristomal hernia support N &

A4398 Ostomy irrigation supply; bag, each N ☑ &

A4399 Ostomy irrigation supply; cone/catheter, with or without brush N &

A4400 Ostomy irrigation set N &

A4402 Lubricant, per oz N ☑ &

A4404 Ostomy ring, each N ☑ &

A4405 Ostomy skin barrier, nonpectin-based, paste, per oz N ☑ &

A4406 Ostomy skin barrier, pectin-based, paste, per oz N ☑ &

A4407 Ostomy skin barrier, with flange (solid, flexible, or accordion), extended wear, with built-in convexity, 4 x 4 in or smaller, each N ☑ &

A4408 Ostomy skin barrier, with flange (solid, flexible or accordion), extended wear, with built-in convexity, larger than 4 x 4 in, each N ☑ &

A4409 Ostomy skin barrier, with flange (solid, flexible or accordion), extended wear, without built-in convexity, 4 x 4 in or smaller, each N ☑ &

A4410 Ostomy skin barrier, with flange (solid, flexible or accordion), extended wear, without built-in convexity, larger than 4 x 4 in, each N ☑ &

A4411 Ostomy skin barrier, solid 4 x 4 or equivalent, extended wear, with built-in convexity, each N ☑ &

A4412 Ostomy pouch, drainable, high output, for use on a barrier with flange (two-piece system), without filter, each N ☑ &

A4413 Ostomy pouch, drainable, high output, for use on a barrier with flange (two-piece system), with filter, each N ☑ &

A4414 Ostomy skin barrier, with flange (solid, flexible or accordion), without built-in convexity, 4 x 4 in or smaller, each N ☑ &

A4415 Ostomy skin barrier, with flange (solid, flexible or accordion), without built-in convexity, larger than 4 x 4 in, each N ☑ &

A4416 Ostomy pouch, closed, with barrier attached, with filter (one piece), each N ☑ &

A4417 Ostomy pouch, closed, with barrier attached, with built-in convexity, with filter (one piece), each N ☑ &

A4418 Ostomy pouch, closed; without barrier attached, with filter (one piece), each N ☑ &

A4419 Ostomy pouch, closed; for use on barrier with nonlocking flange, with filter (two piece), each N ☑ &

A4420 Ostomy pouch, closed; for use on barrier with locking flange (two piece), each N ☑ &

A4421 Ostomy supply; miscellaneous N
Determine if an alternative HCPCS Level II or a CPT code better describes the service being reported. This code should be used only if a more specific code is unavailable.

A4422 Ostomy absorbent material (sheet/pad/crystal packet) for use in ostomy pouch to thicken liquid stomal output, each N ☑ &

A4423 Ostomy pouch, closed; for use on barrier with locking flange, with filter (two piece), each N ☑ &

A4424 Ostomy pouch, drainable, with barrier attached, with filter (one piece), each N ☑ &

A4425 Ostomy pouch, drainable; for use on barrier with nonlocking flange, with filter (two-piece system), each N ☑ &

A4426 Ostomy pouch, drainable; for use on barrier with locking flange (two-piece system), each N ☑ &

A4427 Ostomy pouch, drainable; for use on barrier with locking flange, with filter (two-piece system), each N ☑ &

A4428 Ostomy pouch, urinary, with extended wear barrier attached, with faucet-type tap with valve (one piece), each N ☑ &

A4429 Ostomy pouch, urinary, with barrier attached, with built-in convexity, with faucet-type tap with valve (one piece), each N ☑ &

A4430 Ostomy pouch, urinary, with extended wear barrier attached, with built-in convexity, with faucet-type tap with valve (one piece), each N ☑ &

A4431 Ostomy pouch, urinary; with barrier attached, with faucet-type tap with valve (one piece), each N ☑ &

A4432 Ostomy pouch, urinary; for use on barrier with nonlocking flange, with faucet-type tap with valve (two piece), each N ☑ &

A4433 Ostomy pouch, urinary; for use on barrier with locking flange (two piece), each N ☑ &

A4434 Ostomy pouch, urinary; for use on barrier with locking flange, with faucet-type tap with valve (two piece), each N ☑ &

A4435 Ostomy pouch, drainable, high output, with extended wear barrier (one-piece system), with or without filter, each N &

A4436 Irrigation supply; sleeve, reusable, per month

A4437 Irrigation supply; sleeve, disposable, per month

Miscellaneous Supplies

A4450 Tape, nonwaterproof, per 18 sq in N ☑ & (AU, AV, AW)
See also code A4452.
CMS: 100-04,20,30.9

A4452 Tape, waterproof, per 18 sq in N ☑ & (AU, AV, AW)
See also code A4450.
CMS: 100-04,20,30.9

A4453 Rectal catheter for use with the manual pump-operated enema system, replacement only

A4455 Adhesive remover or solvent (for tape, cement or other adhesive), per oz N ☑ &

A4456 Adhesive remover, wipes, any type, each N ☑ &

● **A4457** Enema tube, with or without adapter, any type, replacement only, each

A4458 Enema bag with tubing, reusable N

A4459 Manual pump-operated enema system, includes balloon, catheter and all accessories, reusable, any type N

A4461 Surgical dressing holder, nonreusable, each N ☑ &

A4463 Surgical dressing holder, reusable, each N ☑ &

Special Coverage Instructions Noncovered by Medicare Carrier Discretion ☑ Quantity Alert ● New Code ○ Recycled/Reinstated ▲ Revised Code

© 2023 Optum360, LLC A2-Z3 ASC Pmt **CMS:** IOM **AHA:** Coding Clinic & DMEPOS Paid ⊘ SNF Excluded A Codes — 7

Code	Description	Indicators
A4465	Nonelastic binder for extremity	N
A4467	Belt, strap, sleeve, garment, or covering, any type	EI
● A4468	Exsufflation belt, includes all supplies and accessories	
A4470	Gravlee jet washer	N
A4480	VABRA aspirator CMS: 100-03,230.6; 100-03,240.4	♀ N
A4481	Tracheostoma filter, any type, any size, each	N ☑ ⅄
A4483	Moisture exchanger, disposable, for use with invasive mechanical ventilation	N ⅄
A4490	Surgical stockings above knee length, each CMS: 100-02,15,110	EI ☑
A4495	Surgical stockings thigh length, each CMS: 100-02,15,110	EI ☑
A4500	Surgical stockings below knee length, each CMS: 100-02,15,110	EI ☑
A4510	Surgical stockings full-length, each CMS: 100-02,15,110	EI ☑
A4520	Incontinence garment, any type, (e.g., brief, diaper), each	EI ☑
● A4540	Distal transcutaneous electrical nerve stimulator, stimulates peripheral nerves of the upper arm	
● A4541	Monthly supplies for use of device coded at E0733	
● A4542	Supplies and accessories for external upper limb tremor stimulator of the peripheral nerves of the wrist	
A4550	Surgical trays CMS: 100-04,12,40.1	B
A4553	Nondisposable underpads, all sizes	EI
A4554	Disposable underpads, all sizes	EI ☑
A4555	Electrode/transducer for use with electrical stimulation device used for cancer treatment, replacement only	EI
A4556	Electrodes (e.g., apnea monitor), per pair If service is not separately payable, or incident to a physician's service, bill through the local carrier. If other, bill the DME MAC. Some payers only cover apnea monitors for newborn or pediatric use. Review specific carrier policy for apnea monitors and supplies.	N ☑ ⅄
A4557	Lead wires (e.g., apnea monitor), per pair If service is not separately payable, or incident to a physician's service, bill through the local carrier. If other, bill the DME MAC. Some payers only cover apnea monitors for newborn or pediatric use. Review specific carrier policy for apnea monitors and supplies.	N ☑ ⅄
A4558	Conductive gel or paste, for use with electrical device (e.g., TENS, NMES), per oz	N ☑ ⅄
A4559	Coupling gel or paste, for use with ultrasound device, per oz	N ☑ ⅄
○ A4560	Neuromuscular electrical stimulator (NMES), disposable, replacement only AHA: 2Q,23	
A4561	Pessary, rubber, any type	♀ N ⅄
A4562	Pessary, nonrubber, any type Medicare jurisdiction: DME regional contractor.	♀ N ⅄
A4563	Rectal control system for vaginal insertion, for long term use, includes pump and all supplies and accessories, any type each	
A4565	Slings	N ⅄
A4566	Shoulder sling or vest design, abduction restrainer, with or without swathe control, prefabricated, includes fitting and adjustment	EI
A4570	Splint Dressings applied by a physician are included as part of the professional service.	EI
A4575	Topical hyperbaric oxygen chamber, disposable	A
A4580	Cast supplies (e.g., plaster) See Q4001-Q4048.	EI
A4590	Special casting material (e.g., fiberglass) See Q4001-Q4048.	EI
A4595	Electrical stimulator supplies, 2 lead, per month, (e.g., TENS, NMES) CMS: 100-03,10.2	N ⅄
A4596	Cranial electrotherapy stimulation (CES) system supplies and accessories, per month AHA: 4Q,22	
A4600	Sleeve for intermittent limb compression device, replacement only, each	EI ☑
A4601	Lithium-ion battery, rechargeable, for nonprosthetic use, replacement	EI
A4602	Replacement battery for external infusion pump owned by patient, lithium, 1.5 volt, each	N ⅄ (NU)
A4604	Tubing with integrated heating element for use with positive airway pressure device CMS: 100-04,36,50.14	N ⅄ (NU)
A4605	Tracheal suction catheter, closed system, each	N ☑ ⅄ (NU)
A4606	Oxygen probe for use with oximeter device, replacement	N
A4608	Transtracheal oxygen catheter, each	N ☑ ⅄

Supplies for Oxygen and Related Respiratory Equipment

Code	Description	Indicators
A4611	Battery, heavy-duty; replacement for patient-owned ventilator	EI
A4612	Battery cables; replacement for patient-owned ventilator	EI
A4613	Battery charger; replacement for patient-owned ventilator	EI ☑
A4614	Peak expiratory flow rate meter, hand held	N ⅄
A4615	Cannula, nasal CMS: 100-04,20,100.2	N ⅄
A4616	Tubing (oxygen), per foot CMS: 100-04,20,100.2	N ☑ ⅄
A4617	Mouthpiece CMS: 100-04,20,100.2	N ⅄
A4618	Breathing circuits CMS: 100-04,20,100.2	N ⅄ (NU, RR, UE)
A4619	Face tent CMS: 100-04,20,100.2	N ⅄ (NU)
A4620	Variable concentration mask CMS: 100-04,20,100.2	N ⅄
A4623	Tracheostomy, inner cannula	N ⅄
A4624	Tracheal suction catheter, any type other than closed system, each	N ☑ ⅄ (NU)
A4625	Tracheostomy care kit for new tracheostomy	N ⅄
A4626	Tracheostomy cleaning brush, each	N ☑ ⅄
A4627	Spacer, bag or reservoir, with or without mask, for use with metered dose inhaler CMS: 100-02,15,110	EI
▲ A4628	Oral and/or oropharyngeal suction catheter, each AHA: 2Q,23	N ☑ ⅄ (NU)

Special Coverage Instructions	Noncovered by Medicare	Carrier Discretion	☑ Quantity Alert	● New Code	○ Recycled/Reinstated	▲ Revised Code

A Age Edit   M Maternity Edit   ♀ Female Only   ♂ Male Only   A-Y OPPS Status Indicators   © 2023 Optum360, LLC

A4629	Tracheostomy care kit for established tracheostomy	N ♿

Replacement Supplies for DME

A4630	Replacement batteries, medically necessary, transcutaneous electrical stimulator, owned by patient	EI ☑ ♿ (NU)
A4633	Replacement bulb/lamp for ultraviolet light therapy system, each	EI ☑ ♿ (NU)
A4634	Replacement bulb for therapeutic light box, tabletop model	N
A4635	Underarm pad, crutch, replacement, each	EI ☑ ♿ (NU, RR, UE)
A4636	Replacement, handgrip, cane, crutch, or walker, each CMS: 100-04,36,50.15	EI ☑ ♿ (NU, RR, UE)
A4637	Replacement, tip, cane, crutch, walker, each CMS: 100-04,36,50.15	EI ☑ ♿ (NU, RR, UE)
A4638	Replacement battery for patient-owned ear pulse generator, each	EI ☑ ♿ (NU, RR, UE)
A4639	Replacement pad for infrared heating pad system, each	EI ☑ ♿ (RR)
A4640	Replacement pad for use with medically necessary alternating pressure pad owned by patient	EI ♿ (NU, RR, UE)

Radiopharmaceuticals

A4641	Radiopharmaceutical, diagnostic, not otherwise classified CMS: 100-04,13,60.3; 100-04,13,60.3.2	N ☑
A4642	Indium In-111 satumomab pendetide, diagnostic, per study dose, up to 6 mCi Use this code for Oncoscint.	N ☑

Miscellaneous Supplies

A4648	Tissue marker, implantable, any type, each AHA: 2Q,18	N ☑ ⊘
A4649	Surgical supply; miscellaneous Determine if an alternative HCPCS Level II or a CPT code better describes the service being reported. This code should be used only if a more specific code is unavailable. AHA: 3Q,23	N
A4650	Implantable radiation dosimeter, each	N ☑ ⊘
A4651	Calibrated microcapillary tube, each	N ☑ ⊘
A4652	Microcapillary tube sealant	N ⊘

Dialysis Supplies

A4653	Peritoneal dialysis catheter anchoring device, belt, each	N ☑ ⊘
A4657	Syringe, with or without needle, each CMS: 100-04,8,60.2.1; 100-04,8,60.4.4; 100-04,8,60.4.6.3	N ☑ ⊘
A4660	Sphygmomanometer/blood pressure apparatus with cuff and stethoscope	N ⊘
A4663	Blood pressure cuff only	N ⊘
A4670	Automatic blood pressure monitor	EI
A4671	Disposable cycler set used with cycler dialysis machine, each	B ☑ ⊘
A4672	Drainage extension line, sterile, for dialysis, each	B ☑ ⊘
A4673	Extension line with easy lock connectors, used with dialysis	B
A4674	Chemicals/antiseptics solution used to clean/sterilize dialysis equipment, per 8 oz	B ☑ ⊘

A4680	Activated carbon filter for hemodialysis, each	N ☑ ⊘
A4690	Dialyzer (artificial kidneys), all types, all sizes, for hemodialysis, each	N ☑ ⊘
A4706	Bicarbonate concentrate, solution, for hemodialysis, per gallon	N ☑ ⊘
A4707	Bicarbonate concentrate, powder, for hemodialysis, per packet	N ☑ ⊘
A4708	Acetate concentrate solution, for hemodialysis, per gallon	N ☑ ⊘
A4709	Acid concentrate, solution, for hemodialysis, per gallon	N ☑ ⊘
A4714	Treated water (deionized, distilled, or reverse osmosis) for peritoneal dialysis, per gallon	N ☑ ⊘
A4719	"Y set" tubing for peritoneal dialysis	N ⊘
A4720	Dialysate solution, any concentration of dextrose, fluid volume greater than 249 cc, but less than or equal to 999 cc, for peritoneal dialysis	N ☑ ⊘
A4721	Dialysate solution, any concentration of dextrose, fluid volume greater than 999 cc but less than or equal to 1999 cc, for peritoneal dialysis	N ☑ ⊘
A4722	Dialysate solution, any concentration of dextrose, fluid volume greater than 1999 cc but less than or equal to 2999 cc, for peritoneal dialysis	N ☑ ⊘
A4723	Dialysate solution, any concentration of dextrose, fluid volume greater than 2999 cc but less than or equal to 3999 cc, for peritoneal dialysis	N ☑ ⊘
A4724	Dialysate solution, any concentration of dextrose, fluid volume greater than 3999 cc but less than or equal to 4999 cc, for peritoneal dialysis	N ☑ ⊘
A4725	Dialysate solution, any concentration of dextrose, fluid volume greater than 4999 cc but less than or equal to 5999 cc, for peritoneal dialysis	N ☑ ⊘
A4726	Dialysate solution, any concentration of dextrose, fluid volume greater than 5999 cc, for peritoneal dialysis	N ☑ ⊘
A4728	Dialysate solution, nondextrose containing, 500 ml	B ☑ ⊘
A4730	Fistula cannulation set for hemodialysis, each	N ☑ ⊘
A4736	Topical anesthetic, for dialysis, per g	N ☑ ⊘
A4737	Injectable anesthetic, for dialysis, per 10 ml	N ☑ ⊘
A4740	Shunt accessory, for hemodialysis, any type, each	N
A4750	Blood tubing, arterial or venous, for hemodialysis, each	N ☑ ⊘
A4755	Blood tubing, arterial and venous combined, for hemodialysis, each	N ☑ ⊘
A4760	Dialysate solution test kit, for peritoneal dialysis, any type, each	N ☑ ⊘
A4765	Dialysate concentrate, powder, additive for peritoneal dialysis, per packet	N ☑ ⊘
A4766	Dialysate concentrate, solution, additive for peritoneal dialysis, per 10 ml	N ☑ ⊘
A4770	Blood collection tube, vacuum, for dialysis, per 50	N ☑ ⊘
A4771	Serum clotting time tube, for dialysis, per 50	N ☑ ⊘
A4772	Blood glucose test strips, for dialysis, per 50	N ☑ ⊘
A4773	Occult blood test strips, for dialysis, per 50	N ☑ ⊘
A4774	Ammonia test strips, for dialysis, per 50	N ☑ ⊘

Special Coverage Instructions   Noncovered by Medicare   Carrier Discretion   ☑ Quantity Alert   ● New Code   ○ Recycled/Reinstated   ▲ Revised Code

© 2023 Optum360, LLC   A2-Z3 ASC Pmt   CMS: IOM   AHA: Coding Clinic   ♿ DMEPOS Paid   ⊘ SNF Excluded   A Codes — 9

A4802	Protamine sulfate, for hemodialysis, per 50 mg	N ☑ ⊘
A4860	Disposable catheter tips for peritoneal dialysis, per 10	N ☑ ⊘
A4870	Plumbing and/or electrical work for home hemodialysis equipment	N ⊘
A4890	Contracts, repair and maintenance, for hemodialysis equipment	N ⊘
A4911	Drain bag/bottle, for dialysis, each	N ☑ ⊘
A4913	Miscellaneous dialysis supplies, not otherwise specified	N ⊘

A4913 Pertinent documentation to evaluate medical appropriateness should be included when this code is reported. Determine if an alternative HCPCS Level II or a CPT code better describes the service being reported. This code should be used only if a more specific code is unavailable.
CMS: 100-04,8,20; 100-04,8,60.2.1

A4918	Venous pressure clamp, for hemodialysis, each	N ☑ ⊘
A4927	Gloves, nonsterile, per 100	N ☑ ⊘
A4928	Surgical mask, per 20	N ☑ ⊘
A4929	Tourniquet for dialysis, each	N ☑ ⊘
A4930	Gloves, sterile, per pair	N ☑ ⊘
A4931	Oral thermometer, reusable, any type, each	N ☑ ⊘
A4932	Rectal thermometer, reusable, any type, each	N ☑

Ostomy Pouches and Supplies

A5051	Ostomy pouch, closed; with barrier attached (one piece), each	N ☑ ᕧ
A5052	Ostomy pouch, closed; without barrier attached (one piece), each	N ☑ ᕧ
A5053	Ostomy pouch, closed; for use on faceplate, each	N ☑ ᕧ
A5054	Ostomy pouch, closed; for use on barrier with flange (two piece), each	N ☑ ᕧ
A5055	Stoma cap	N ᕧ
A5056	Ostomy pouch, drainable, with extended wear barrier attached, with filter, (one piece), each	N ☑ ᕧ
A5057	Ostomy pouch, drainable, with extended wear barrier attached, with built in convexity, with filter, (one piece), each	N ☑ ᕧ
A5061	Ostomy pouch, drainable; with barrier attached, (one piece), each	N ☑ ᕧ
A5062	Ostomy pouch, drainable; without barrier attached (one piece), each	N ☑ ᕧ
A5063	Ostomy pouch, drainable; for use on barrier with flange (two-piece system), each	N ☑ ᕧ
A5071	Ostomy pouch, urinary; with barrier attached (one piece), each	N ☑ ᕧ
A5072	Ostomy pouch, urinary; without barrier attached (one piece), each	N ☑ ᕧ
A5073	Ostomy pouch, urinary; for use on barrier with flange (two piece), each	N ☑ ᕧ
A5081	Stoma plug or seal, any type	N ᕧ
A5082	Continent device; catheter for continent stoma	N ᕧ
A5083	Continent device, stoma absorptive cover for continent stoma	N ᕧ
A5093	Ostomy accessory; convex insert	N ᕧ

Incontinence Supplies

| A5102 | Bedside drainage bottle with or without tubing, rigid or expandable, each | N ☑ ᕧ |

A5105	Urinary suspensory with leg bag, with or without tube, each	N ☑ ᕧ
A5112	Urinary drainage bag, leg or abdomen, latex, with or without tube, with straps, each	N ☑ ᕧ
A5113	Leg strap; latex, replacement only, per set	E ☑ ᕧ
A5114	Leg strap; foam or fabric, replacement only, per set	E ☑ ᕧ
A5120	Skin barrier, wipes or swabs, each	N ☑ ᕧ (AU, AV)
A5121	Skin barrier; solid, 6 x 6 or equivalent, each	N ☑ ᕧ
A5122	Skin barrier; solid, 8 x 8 or equivalent, each	N ☑ ᕧ
A5126	Adhesive or nonadhesive; disk or foam pad	N ᕧ
A5131	Appliance cleaner, incontinence and ostomy appliances, per 16 oz	N ☑ ᕧ
A5200	Percutaneous catheter/tube anchoring device, adhesive skin attachment	N ᕧ

Diabetic Shoes, Fitting, and Modifications

According to Medicare, documentation from the prescribing physician must certify the diabetic patient has one of the following conditions: peripheral neuropathy with evidence of callus formation; history of preulcerative calluses; history of ulceration; foot deformity; previous amputation; or poor circulation. The footwear must be fitted and furnished by a podiatrist, pedorthist, orthotist, or prosthetist.

A5500	For diabetics only, fitting (including follow-up), custom preparation and supply of off-the-shelf depth-inlay shoe manufactured to accommodate multidensity insert(s), per shoe	Y ☑ ᕧ
	CMS: 100-02,15,140	
A5501	For diabetics only, fitting (including follow-up), custom preparation and supply of shoe molded from cast(s) of patient's foot (custom molded shoe), per shoe	Y ☑ ᕧ
	CMS: 100-02,15,140	
A5503	For diabetics only, modification (including fitting) of off-the-shelf depth-inlay shoe or custom molded shoe with roller or rigid rocker bottom, per shoe	Y ☑ ᕧ
	CMS: 100-02,15,140	
A5504	For diabetics only, modification (including fitting) of off-the-shelf depth-inlay shoe or custom molded shoe with wedge(s), per shoe	Y ☑ ᕧ
	CMS: 100-02,15,140	
A5505	For diabetics only, modification (including fitting) of off-the-shelf depth-inlay shoe or custom molded shoe with metatarsal bar, per shoe	Y ☑ ᕧ
	CMS: 100-02,15,140	
A5506	For diabetics only, modification (including fitting) of off-the-shelf depth-inlay shoe or custom molded shoe with off-set heel(s), per shoe	Y ☑ ᕧ
	CMS: 100-02,15,140	
A5507	For diabetics only, not otherwise specified modification (including fitting) of off-the-shelf depth-inlay shoe or custom molded shoe, per shoe	Y ☑ ᕧ
	CMS: 100-02,15,140	
A5508	For diabetics only, deluxe feature of off-the-shelf depth-inlay shoe or custom molded shoe, per shoe	Y ☑
	CMS: 100-02,15,140	
A5510	For diabetics only, direct formed, compression molded to patient's foot without external heat source, multiple-density insert(s) prefabricated, per shoe	N ☑
	CMS: 100-02,15,140	

Special Coverage Instructions　　Noncovered by Medicare　　Carrier Discretion　　☑ Quantity Alert　● New Code　○ Recycled/Reinstated　▲ Revised Code

　　🅐 Age Edit　　🅜 Maternity Edit　　♀ Female Only　　♂ Male Only　　🅐-🅨 OPPS Status Indicators　　© 2023 Optum360, LLC

A5512	For diabetics only, multiple density insert, direct formed, molded to foot after external heat source of 230 degrees Fahrenheit or higher, total contact with patient's foot, including arch, base layer minimum of 1/4 inch material of Shore A 35 durometer or 3/16 inch material of Shore A 40 durometer (or higher), prefabricated, each Y ☑ &
A5513	For diabetics only, multiple density insert, custom molded from model of patient's foot, total contact with patient's foot, including arch, base layer minimum of 3/16 inch material of Shore A 35 durometer (or higher), includes arch filler and other shaping material, custom fabricated, each Y ☑ &
A5514	For diabetics only, multiple density insert, made by direct carving with CAM technology from a rectified CAD model created from a digitized scan of the patient, total contact with patient's foot, including arch, base layer minimum of 3/16 inch material of Shore A 35 durometer (or higher), includes arch filler and other shaping material, custom fabricated, each

Dressings

A6000	Noncontact wound-warming wound cover for use with the noncontact wound-warming device and warming card EI
A6010	Collagen based wound filler, dry form, sterile, per g of collagen N ☑ &
A6011	Collagen based wound filler, gel/paste, per g of collagen N ☑ &
A6021	Collagen dressing, sterile, size 16 sq in or less, each N ☑ &
A6022	Collagen dressing, sterile, size more than 16 sq in but less than or equal to 48 sq in, each N ☑ &
A6023	Collagen dressing, sterile, size more than 48 sq in, each N ☑ &
A6024	Collagen dressing wound filler, sterile, per 6 in N ☑ &
A6025	Gel sheet for dermal or epidermal application, (e.g., silicone, hydrogel, other), each N ☑
A6154	Wound pouch, each N ☑ &
A6196	Alginate or other fiber gelling dressing, wound cover, sterile, pad size 16 sq in or less, each dressing N ☑ &
A6197	Alginate or other fiber gelling dressing, wound cover, sterile, pad size more than 16 sq in but less than or equal to 48 sq in, each dressing N ☑ &
A6198	Alginate or other fiber gelling dressing, wound cover, sterile, pad size more than 48 sq in, each dressing N ☑
A6199	Alginate or other fiber gelling dressing, wound filler, sterile, per 6 in N ☑ &
A6203	Composite dressing, sterile, pad size 16 sq in or less, with any size adhesive border, each dressing N ☑ &
A6204	Composite dressing, sterile, pad size more than 16 sq in, but less than or equal to 48 sq in, with any size adhesive border, each dressing N ☑ &
A6205	Composite dressing, sterile, pad size more than 48 sq in, with any size adhesive border, each dressing N ☑
A6206	Contact layer, sterile, 16 sq in or less, each dressing N ☑
A6207	Contact layer, sterile, more than 16 sq in but less than or equal to 48 sq in, each dressing N ☑ &
A6208	Contact layer, sterile, more than 48 sq in, each dressing N ☑
A6209	Foam dressing, wound cover, sterile, pad size 16 sq in or less, without adhesive border, each dressing N ☑ &
A6210	Foam dressing, wound cover, sterile, pad size more than 16 sq in but less than or equal to 48 sq in, without adhesive border, each dressing N ☑ &

A6211	Foam dressing, wound cover, sterile, pad size more than 48 sq in, without adhesive border, each dressing N ☑ &
A6212	Foam dressing, wound cover, sterile, pad size 16 sq in or less, with any size adhesive border, each dressing N ☑ &
A6213	Foam dressing, wound cover, sterile, pad size more than 16 sq in but less than or equal to 48 sq in, with any size adhesive border, each dressing N ☑
A6214	Foam dressing, wound cover, sterile, pad size more than 48 sq in, with any size adhesive border, each dressing N ☑ &
A6215	Foam dressing, wound filler, sterile, per g N ☑
A6216	Gauze, nonimpregnated, nonsterile, pad size 16 sq in or less, without adhesive border, each dressing N ☑ &
A6217	Gauze, nonimpregnated, nonsterile, pad size more than 16 sq in but less than or equal to 48 sq in, without adhesive border, each dressing N ☑ &
A6218	Gauze, nonimpregnated, nonsterile, pad size more than 48 sq in, without adhesive border, each dressing N ☑
A6219	Gauze, nonimpregnated, sterile, pad size 16 sq in or less, with any size adhesive border, each dressing N ☑ &
A6220	Gauze, nonimpregnated, sterile, pad size more than 16 sq in but less than or equal to 48 sq in, with any size adhesive border, each dressing N ☑ &
A6221	Gauze, nonimpregnated, sterile, pad size more than 48 sq in, with any size adhesive border, each dressing N ☑
A6222	Gauze, impregnated with other than water, normal saline, or hydrogel, sterile, pad size 16 sq in or less, without adhesive border, each dressing N ☑ &
A6223	Gauze, impregnated with other than water, normal saline, or hydrogel, sterile, pad size more than 16 sq in but less than or equal to 48 sq in, without adhesive border, each dressing N ☑ &
A6224	Gauze, impregnated with other than water, normal saline, or hydrogel, sterile, pad size more than 48 sq in, without adhesive border, each dressing N ☑ &
A6228	Gauze, impregnated, water or normal saline, sterile, pad size 16 sq in or less, without adhesive border, each dressing N ☑
A6229	Gauze, impregnated, water or normal saline, sterile, pad size more than 16 sq in but less than or equal to 48 sq in, without adhesive border, each dressing N ☑ &
A6230	Gauze, impregnated, water or normal saline, sterile, pad size more than 48 sq in, without adhesive border, each dressing N ☑
A6231	Gauze, impregnated, hydrogel, for direct wound contact, sterile, pad size 16 sq in or less, each dressing N ☑ &
A6232	Gauze, impregnated, hydrogel, for direct wound contact, sterile, pad size greater than 16 sq in but less than or equal to 48 sq in, each dressing N ☑ &
A6233	Gauze, impregnated, hydrogel, for direct wound contact, sterile, pad size more than 48 sq in, each dressing N ☑ &
A6234	Hydrocolloid dressing, wound cover, sterile, pad size 16 sq in or less, without adhesive border, each dressing N ☑ &
A6235	Hydrocolloid dressing, wound cover, sterile, pad size more than 16 sq in but less than or equal to 48 sq in, without adhesive border, each dressing N ☑ &
A6236	Hydrocolloid dressing, wound cover, sterile, pad size more than 48 sq in, without adhesive border, each dressing N ☑ &
A6237	Hydrocolloid dressing, wound cover, sterile, pad size 16 sq in or less, with any size adhesive border, each dressing N ☑ &

Special Coverage Instructions Noncovered by Medicare Carrier Discretion ☑ Quantity Alert ● New Code ○ Recycled/Reinstated ▲ Revised Code

A6238 Hydrocolloid dressing, wound cover, sterile, pad size more than 16 sq in but less than or equal to 48 sq in, with any size adhesive border, each dressing　N ☑ &

A6239 Hydrocolloid dressing, wound cover, sterile, pad size more than 48 sq in, with any size adhesive border, each dressing　N ☑

A6240 Hydrocolloid dressing, wound filler, paste, sterile, per oz　N ☑ &

A6241 Hydrocolloid dressing, wound filler, dry form, sterile, per g　N ☑ &

A6242 Hydrogel dressing, wound cover, sterile, pad size 16 sq in or less, without adhesive border, each dressing　N ☑ &

A6243 Hydrogel dressing, wound cover, sterile, pad size more than 16 sq in but less than or equal to 48 sq in, without adhesive border, each dressing　N ☑ &

A6244 Hydrogel dressing, wound cover, sterile, pad size more than 48 sq in, without adhesive border, each dressing　N ☑ &

A6245 Hydrogel dressing, wound cover, sterile, pad size 16 sq in or less, with any size adhesive border, each dressing　N ☑ &

A6246 Hydrogel dressing, wound cover, sterile, pad size more than 16 sq in but less than or equal to 48 sq in, with any size adhesive border, each dressing　N ☑ &

A6247 Hydrogel dressing, wound cover, sterile, pad size more than 48 sq in, with any size adhesive border, each dressing　N ☑ &

A6248 Hydrogel dressing, wound filler, gel, per fl oz　N ☑ &

A6250 Skin sealants, protectants, moisturizers, ointments, any type, any size　N

Surgical dressings applied by a physician are included as part of the professional service. Surgical dressings obtained by the patient to perform homecare as prescribed by the physician are covered.

A6251 Specialty absorptive dressing, wound cover, sterile, pad size 16 sq in or less, without adhesive border, each dressing　N ☑ &

A6252 Specialty absorptive dressing, wound cover, sterile, pad size more than 16 sq in but less than or equal to 48 sq in, without adhesive border, each dressing　N ☑ &

A6253 Specialty absorptive dressing, wound cover, sterile, pad size more than 48 sq in, without adhesive border, each dressing　N ☑ &

A6254 Specialty absorptive dressing, wound cover, sterile, pad size 16 sq in or less, with any size adhesive border, each dressing　N ☑ &

A6255 Specialty absorptive dressing, wound cover, sterile, pad size more than 16 sq in but less than or equal to 48 sq in, with any size adhesive border, each dressing　N ☑ &

A6256 Specialty absorptive dressing, wound cover, sterile, pad size more than 48 sq in, with any size adhesive border, each dressing　N ☑

A6257 Transparent film, sterile, 16 sq in or less, each dressing　N ☑ &

Surgical dressings applied by a physician are included as part of the professional service. Surgical dressings obtained by the patient to perform homecare as prescribed by the physician are covered. Use this code for Polyskin, Tegaderm, and Tegaderm HP.

A6258 Transparent film, sterile, more than 16 sq in but less than or equal to 48 sq in, each dressing　N ☑ &

Surgical dressings applied by a physician are included as part of the professional service. Surgical dressings obtained by the patient to perform homecare as prescribed by the physician are covered.

A6259 Transparent film, sterile, more than 48 sq in, each dressing　N ☑ &

Surgical dressings applied by a physician are included as part of the professional service. Surgical dressings obtained by the patient to perform homecare as prescribed by the physician are covered.

A6260 Wound cleansers, any type, any size　N

Surgical dressings applied by a physician are included as part of the professional service. Surgical dressings obtained by the patient to perform homecare as prescribed by the physician are covered.

A6261 Wound filler, gel/paste, per fl oz, not otherwise specified　N ☑

Surgical dressings applied by a physician are included as part of the professional service. Surgical dressings obtained by the patient to perform homecare as prescribed by the physician are covered.

A6262 Wound filler, dry form, per g, not otherwise specified　N ☑

A6266 Gauze, impregnated, other than water, normal saline, or zinc paste, sterile, any width, per linear yd　N ☑ &

Surgical dressings applied by a physician are included as part of the professional service. Surgical dressings applied by a physician are included as part of the professional service. Surgical dressings obtained by the patient to perform homecare as prescribed by the physician are covered.

A6402 Gauze, nonimpregnated, sterile, pad size 16 sq in or less, without adhesive border, each dressing　N ☑ &

Surgical dressings applied by a physician are included as part of the professional service. Surgical dressings obtained by the patient to perform homecare as prescribed by the physician are covered.

A6403 Gauze, nonimpregnated, sterile, pad size more than 16 sq in but less than or equal to 48 sq in, without adhesive border, each dressing　N ☑ &

Surgical dressings applied by a physician are included as part of the professional service. Surgical dressings obtained by the patient to perform homecare as prescribed by the physician are covered.

A6404 Gauze, nonimpregnated, sterile, pad size more than 48 sq in, without adhesive border, each dressing　N ☑

A6407 Packing strips, nonimpregnated, sterile, up to 2 in in width, per linear yd　N ☑ &

A6410 Eye pad, sterile, each　N ☑ &

A6411 Eye pad, nonsterile, each　N ☑ &

A6412 Eye patch, occlusive, each　N ☑

A6413 Adhesive bandage, first aid type, any size, each　E ☑

A6441 Padding bandage, nonelastic, nonwoven/nonknitted, width greater than or equal to 3 in and less than 5 in, per yd　N ☑ &

A6442 Conforming bandage, nonelastic, knitted/woven, nonsterile, width less than 3 in, per yd　N ☑ &

A6443 Conforming bandage, nonelastic, knitted/woven, nonsterile, width greater than or equal to 3 in and less than 5 in, per yd　N ☑ &

A6444 Conforming bandage, nonelastic, knitted/woven, nonsterile, width greater than or equal to 5 in, per yd　N ☑ &

A6445 Conforming bandage, nonelastic, knitted/woven, sterile, width less than 3 in, per yd　N ☑ &

A6446 Conforming bandage, nonelastic, knitted/woven, sterile, width greater than or equal to 3 in and less than 5 in, per yd　N ☑ &

A6447 Conforming bandage, nonelastic, knitted/woven, sterile, width greater than or equal to 5 in, per yd　N ☑ &

A6448 Light compression bandage, elastic, knitted/woven, width less than 3 in, per yd　N ☑ &

A6449 Light compression bandage, elastic, knitted/woven, width greater than or equal to 3 in and less than 5 in, per yd　N ☑ &

A6450 Light compression bandage, elastic, knitted/woven, width greater than or equal to 5 in, per yd　N ☑ &

Special Coverage Instructions　　Noncovered by Medicare　　Carrier Discretion　　☑ Quantity Alert　● New Code　○ Recycled/Reinstated　▲ Revised Code

12 — A Codes　　A Age Edit　M Maternity Edit　♀ Female Only　♂ Male Only　A-Y OPPS Status Indicators　　© 2023 Optum360, LLC

| A6451 | Moderate compression bandage, elastic, knitted/woven, load resistance of 1.25 to 1.34 ft lbs at 50% maximum stretch, width greater than or equal to 3 in and less than 5 in, per yd N ☑ ᕚ |

| A6452 | High compression bandage, elastic, knitted/woven, load resistance greater than or equal to 1.35 ft lbs at 50% maximum stretch, width greater than or equal to 3 in and less than 5 in, per yd N ☑ ᕚ |

| A6453 | Self-adherent bandage, elastic, nonknitted/nonwoven, width less than 3 in, per yd N ☑ ᕚ |

| A6454 | Self-adherent bandage, elastic, nonknitted/nonwoven, width greater than or equal to 3 in and less than 5 in, per yd N ☑ ᕚ |

| A6455 | Self-adherent bandage, elastic, nonknitted/nonwoven, width greater than or equal to 5 in, per yd N ☑ ᕚ |

| A6456 | Zinc paste impregnated bandage, nonelastic, knitted/woven, width greater than or equal to 3 in and less than 5 in, per yd N ☑ ᕚ |

| A6457 | Tubular dressing with or without elastic, any width, per linear yd |

| A6460 | Synthetic resorbable wound dressing, sterile, pad size 16 sq in or less, without adhesive border, each dressing |

| A6461 | Synthetic resorbable wound dressing, sterile, pad size more than 16 sq in but less than or equal to 48 sq in, without adhesive border, each dressing |

Compression Garments

| A6501 | Compression burn garment, bodysuit (head to foot), custom fabricated N ᕚ |

| A6502 | Compression burn garment, chin strap, custom fabricated N ᕚ |

| A6503 | Compression burn garment, facial hood, custom fabricated N ᕚ |

| A6504 | Compression burn garment, glove to wrist, custom fabricated N ᕚ |

| A6505 | Compression burn garment, glove to elbow, custom fabricated N ᕚ |

| A6506 | Compression burn garment, glove to axilla, custom fabricated N ᕚ |

| A6507 | Compression burn garment, foot to knee length, custom fabricated N ᕚ |

| A6508 | Compression burn garment, foot to thigh length, custom fabricated N ᕚ |

| A6509 | Compression burn garment, upper trunk to waist including arm openings (vest), custom fabricated N ᕚ |

| A6510 | Compression burn garment, trunk, including arms down to leg openings (leotard), custom fabricated N ᕚ |

| A6511 | Compression burn garment, lower trunk including leg openings (panty), custom fabricated N ᕚ |

| A6512 | Compression burn garment, not otherwise classified N |

| A6513 | Compression burn mask, face and/or neck, plastic or equal, custom fabricated B ᕚ |

| ● A6520 | Gradient compression garment, glove, padded, for nighttime use, each |

| ● A6521 | Gradient compression garment, glove, padded, for nighttime use, custom, each |

| ● A6522 | Gradient compression garment, arm, padded, for nighttime use, each |

| ● A6523 | Gradient compression garment, arm, padded, for nighttime use, custom, each |

| ● A6524 | Gradient compression garment, lower leg and foot, padded, for nighttime use, each |

| ● A6525 | Gradient compression garment, lower leg and foot, padded, for nighttime use, custom, each |

| ● A6526 | Gradient compression garment, full leg and foot, padded, for nighttime use, each |

| ● A6527 | Gradient compression garment, full leg and foot, padded, for nighttime use, custom, each |

| ● A6528 | Gradient compression garment, bra, for nighttime use, each |

| ● A6529 | Gradient compression garment, bra, for nighttime use, custom, each |

| A6530 | Gradient compression stocking, below knee, 18-30 mm Hg, each EI ☑ |

| ▲ A6531 | Gradient compression stocking, below knee, 30-40 mm Hg, used as a surgical dressing, each N ☑ ᕚ (AW) |

| ▲ A6532 | Gradient compression stocking, below knee, 40-50 mm Hg, used as a surgical dressing, each N ☑ ᕚ (AW) |

| A6533 | Gradient compression stocking, thigh length, 18-30 mm Hg, each EI ☑ |

| A6534 | Gradient compression stocking, thigh length, 30-40 mm Hg, each EI ☑ |

| ▲ A6535 | Gradient compression stocking, thigh length, 40 mm Hg or greater, each EI ☑ |

| A6536 | Gradient compression stocking, full-length/chap style, 18-30 mm Hg, each EI ☑ |

| A6537 | Gradient compression stocking, full-length/chap style, 30-40 mm Hg, each EI ☑ |

| ▲ A6538 | Gradient compression stocking, full length/chap style, 40 mm Hg or greater, each EI ☑ |

| A6539 | Gradient compression stocking, waist length, 18-30 mm Hg, each EI ☑ |

| A6540 | Gradient compression stocking, waist length, 30-40 mm Hg, each EI ☑ |

| ▲ A6541 | Gradient compression stocking, waist length, 40 mm Hg or greater, each EI ☑ |

| A6544 | Gradient compression stocking, garter belt EI |

| ▲ A6545 | Gradient compression wrap, nonelastic, below knee, 30-50 mm Hg, used as a surgical dressing, each N ☑ ᕚ (AW) |

| ▲ A6549 | Gradient compression garment, not otherwise specified EI |

| A6550 | Wound care set, for negative pressure wound therapy electrical pump, includes all supplies and accessories N ☑ ᕚ
CMS: 100-02,7,40.1.2.8 |

| ● A6552 | Gradient compression stocking, below knee, 30-40 mm Hg, each |

| ● A6553 | Gradient compression stocking, below knee, 30-40 mm Hg, custom, each |

| ● A6554 | Gradient compression stocking, below knee, 40 mm Hg or greater, each |

| ● A6555 | Gradient compression stocking, below knee, 40 mm Hg or greater, custom, each |

| ● A6556 | Gradient compression stocking, thigh length, 18-30 mm Hg, custom, each |

| ● A6557 | Gradient compression stocking, thigh length, 30-40 mm Hg, custom, each |

| ● A6558 | Gradient compression stocking, thigh length, 40 mm Hg or greater, custom, each |

Special Coverage Instructions   Noncovered by Medicare   Carrier Discretion   ☑ Quantity Alert   ● New Code   ○ Recycled/Reinstated   ▲ Revised Code

© 2023 Optum360, LLC   A2-Z3 ASC Pmt   CMS: IOM   AHA: Coding Clinic   ᕚ DMEPOS Paid   ⊘ SNF Excluded   A Codes — 13

● A6559 Gradient compression stocking, full length/chap style, 18-30 mm Hg, custom, each

● A6560 Gradient compression stocking, full length/chap style, 30-40 mm Hg, custom, each

● A6561 Gradient compression stocking, full length/chap style, 40 mm Hg or greater, custom, each

● A6562 Gradient compression stocking, waist length, 18-30 mm Hg, custom, each

● A6563 Gradient compression stocking, waist length, 30-40 mm Hg, custom, each

● A6564 Gradient compression stocking, waist length, 40 mm Hg or greater, custom, each

● A6565 Gradient compression gauntlet, custom, each

● A6566 Gradient compression garment, neck/head, each

● A6567 Gradient compression garment, neck/head, custom, each

● A6568 Gradient compression garment, torso and shoulder, each

● A6569 Gradient compression garment, torso/shoulder, custom, each

● A6570 Gradient compression garment, genital region, each

● A6571 Gradient compression garment, genital region, custom, each

● A6572 Gradient compression garment, toe caps, each

● A6573 Gradient compression garment, toe caps, custom, each

● A6574 Gradient compression arm sleeve and glove combination, custom, each

● A6575 Gradient compression arm sleeve and glove combination, each

● A6576 Gradient compression arm sleeve, custom, medium weight, each

● A6577 Gradient compression arm sleeve, custom, heavy weight, each

● A6578 Gradient compression arm sleeve, each

● A6579 Gradient compression glove, custom, medium weight, each

● A6580 Gradient compression glove, custom, heavy weight, each

● A6581 Gradient compression glove, each

● A6582 Gradient compression gauntlet, each

● A6583 Gradient compression wrap with adjustable straps, below knee, 30-50 mm Hg, each

● A6584 Gradient compression wrap with adjustable straps, not otherwise specified

● A6585 Gradient pressure wrap with adjustable straps, above knee, each

● A6586 Gradient pressure wrap with adjustable straps, full leg, each

● A6587 Gradient pressure wrap with adjustable straps, foot, each

● A6588 Gradient pressure wrap with adjustable straps, arm, each

● A6589 Gradient pressure wrap with adjustable straps, bra, each

External Urinary Catheters

● A6590 External urinary catheters; disposable, with wicking material, for use with suction pump, per month
AHA: 2Q,23

● A6591 External urinary catheter; non-disposable, for use with suction pump, per month
AHA: 2Q,23

Gradient Compression Accessories/Supplies

● A6593 Accessory for gradient compression garment or wrap with adjustable straps, not otherwise specified

● A6594 Gradient compression bandaging supply, bandage liner, lower extremity, any size or length, each

● A6595 Gradient compression bandaging supply, bandage liner, upper extremity, any size or length, each

● A6596 Gradient compression bandaging supply, conforming gauze, per linear yd, any width, each

● A6597 Gradient compression bandage roll, elastic long stretch, linear yd, any width, each

● A6598 Gradient compression bandage roll, elastic medium stretch, per linear yd, any width, each

● A6599 Gradient compression bandage roll, inelastic short stretch, per linear yd, any width, each

● A6600 Gradient compression bandaging supply, high density foam sheet, per 250 sq cm, each

● A6601 Gradient compression bandaging supply, high density foam pad, any size or shape, each

● A6602 Gradient compression bandaging supply, high density foam roll for bandage, per linear yd, any width, each

● A6603 Gradient compression bandaging supply, low density channel foam sheet, per 250 sq cm, each

● A6604 Gradient compression bandaging supply, low density flat foam sheet, per 250 sq cm, each

● A6605 Gradient compression bandaging supply, padded foam, per linear yd, any width, each

● A6606 Gradient compression bandaging supply, padded textile, per linear yd, any width, each

● A6607 Gradient compression bandaging supply, tubular protective absorption layer, per linear yd, any width, each

● A6608 Gradient compression bandaging supply, tubular protective absorption padded layer, per linear yd, any width, each

● A6609 Gradient compression bandaging supply, not otherwise specified

● A6610 Gradient compression stocking, below knee, 18-30 mm Hg, custom, each

Respiratory Supplies

A7000 Canister, disposable, used with suction pump, each ☒ ☑ ⅚ (NU)

A7001 Canister, nondisposable, used with suction pump, each ☒ ☑ ⅚ (NU)

A7002 Tubing, used with suction pump, each ☒ ☑ ⅚ (NU)

A7003 Administration set, with small volume nonfiltered pneumatic nebulizer, disposable ☒ ⅚ (NU)

A7004 Small volume nonfiltered pneumatic nebulizer, disposable ☒ ⅚ (NU)

A7005 Administration set, with small volume nonfiltered pneumatic nebulizer, nondisposable ☒ ⅚ (NU)

A7006 Administration set, with small volume filtered pneumatic nebulizer ☒ ⅚ (NU)

A7007 Large volume nebulizer, disposable, unfilled, used with aerosol compressor ☒ ⅚ (NU)

A7008 Large volume nebulizer, disposable, prefilled, used with aerosol compressor ☒ ⅚ (NU)

A7009 Reservoir bottle, nondisposable, used with large volume ultrasonic nebulizer ☒ ⅚ (NU)

A7010 Corrugated tubing, disposable, used with large volume nebulizer, 100 ft ☒ ☑ ⅚ (NU)

Special Coverage Instructions   Noncovered by Medicare   Carrier Discretion   ☑ Quantity Alert ● New Code ○ Recycled/Reinstated ▲ Revised Code

14 — A Codes   🅐 Age Edit 🅜 Maternity Edit ♀ Female Only ♂ Male Only 🅐-🆈 OPPS Status Indicators   © 2023 Optum360, LLC

A7012	Water collection device, used with large volume nebulizer	Y ☐ (NU)
A7013	Filter, disposable, used with aerosol compressor or ultrasonic generator	Y ☐ (NU)
A7014	Filter, nondisposable, used with aerosol compressor or ultrasonic generator	Y ☐ (NU)
A7015	Aerosol mask, used with DME nebulizer	Y ☐ (NU)
A7016	Dome and mouthpiece, used with small volume ultrasonic nebulizer	Y ☐ (NU)
A7017	Nebulizer, durable, glass or autoclavable plastic, bottle type, not used with oxygen	Y ☐ (NU, RR, UE)
A7018	Water, distilled, used with large volume nebulizer, 1000 ml	Y ☑ ☐
A7020	Interface for cough stimulating device, includes all components, replacement only	Y ☐ (NU)
● **A7023**	Mechanical allergen particle barrier/inhalation filter, cream, nasal, topical	
A7025	High frequency chest wall oscillation system vest, replacement for use with patient-owned equipment, each	N ☑ ☐ (RR)
A7026	High frequency chest wall oscillation system hose, replacement for use with patient-owned equipment, each	Y ☑ ☐ (NU)
A7027	Combination oral/nasal mask, used with continuous positive airway pressure device, each	Y ☑ ☐ (NU)
A7028	Oral cushion for combination oral/nasal mask, replacement only, each	Y ☑ ☐ (NU)
A7029	Nasal pillows for combination oral/nasal mask, replacement only, pair	Y ☑ ☐ (NU)
A7030	Full face mask used with positive airway pressure device, each	Y ☑ ☐ (NU)
	CMS: 100-04,36,50.14	
A7031	Face mask interface, replacement for full face mask, each	Y ☑ ☐ (NU)
	CMS: 100-04,36,50.14	
A7032	Cushion for use on nasal mask interface, replacement only, each	Y ☑ ☐ (NU)
	CMS: 100-03,240.4; 100-04,36,50.14	
A7033	Pillow for use on nasal cannula type interface, replacement only, pair	Y ☑ ☐ (NU)
	CMS: 100-03,240.4; 100-04,36,50.14	
A7034	Nasal interface (mask or cannula type) used with positive airway pressure device, with or without head strap	Y ☐ (NU)
	CMS: 100-03,240.4; 100-04,36,50.14	
A7035	Headgear used with positive airway pressure device	Y ☐ (NU)
	CMS: 100-03,240.4; 100-04,36,50.14	
A7036	Chinstrap used with positive airway pressure device	Y ☐ (NU)
	CMS: 100-03,240.4; 100-04,36,50.14	
A7037	Tubing used with positive airway pressure device	Y ☐ (NU)
	CMS: 100-03,240.4; 100-04,36,50.14	
A7038	Filter, disposable, used with positive airway pressure device	Y ☐ (NU)
	CMS: 100-04,36,50.14	
A7039	Filter, nondisposable, used with positive airway pressure device	Y ☐ (NU)
	CMS: 100-04,36,50.14	
A7040	One way chest drain valve	N ☐
A7041	Water seal drainage container and tubing for use with implanted chest tube	N ☐

A7044	Oral interface used with positive airway pressure device, each	Y ☑ ☐ (NU)
	CMS: 100-03,240.4; 100-04,36,50.14	
A7045	Exhalation port with or without swivel used with accessories for positive airway devices, replacement only	Y ☐ (NU, RR, UE)
	CMS: 100-03,240.4; 100-04,36,50.14	
A7046	Water chamber for humidifier, used with positive airway pressure device, replacement, each	Y ☑ ☐ (NU)
	CMS: 100-04,36,50.14	
A7047	Oral interface used with respiratory suction pump, each	N ☑ ☐ (NU)
A7048	Vacuum drainage collection unit and tubing kit, including all supplies needed for collection unit change, for use with implanted catheter, each	N ☐
● **A7049**	Expiratory positive airway pressure intranasal resistance valve	
	AHA: 2Q,23	

Tracheostomy Supplies

A7501	Tracheostoma valve, including diaphragm, each	N ☑ ☐
A7502	Replacement diaphragm/faceplate for tracheostoma valve, each	N ☑ ☐
A7503	Filter holder or filter cap, reusable, for use in a tracheostoma heat and moisture exchange system, each	N ☑ ☐
A7504	Filter for use in a tracheostoma heat and moisture exchange system, each	N ☑ ☐
A7505	Housing, reusable without adhesive, for use in a heat and moisture exchange system and/or with a tracheostoma valve, each	N ☑ ☐
A7506	Adhesive disc for use in a heat and moisture exchange system and/or with tracheostoma valve, any type each	N ☑ ☐
A7507	Filter holder and integrated filter without adhesive, for use in a tracheostoma heat and moisture exchange system, each	N ☑ ☐
A7508	Housing and integrated adhesive, for use in a tracheostoma heat and moisture exchange system and/or with a tracheostoma valve, each	N ☑ ☐
A7509	Filter holder and integrated filter housing, and adhesive, for use as a tracheostoma heat and moisture exchange system, each	N ☑ ☐
A7520	Tracheostomy/laryngectomy tube, noncuffed, polyvinyl chloride (PVC), silicone or equal, each	N ☑ ☐
A7521	Tracheostomy/laryngectomy tube, cuffed, polyvinyl chloride (PVC), silicone or equal, each	N ☑ ☐
A7522	Tracheostomy/laryngectomy tube, stainless steel or equal (sterilizable and reusable), each	N ☑ ☐
A7523	Tracheostomy shower protector, each	N ☑
A7524	Tracheostoma stent/stud/button, each	N ☑ ☐
A7525	Tracheostomy mask, each	N ☑ ☐
A7526	Tracheostomy tube collar/holder, each	N ☑ ☐
A7527	Tracheostomy/laryngectomy tube plug/stop, each	N ☑ ☐

Protective Helmet

A8000	Helmet, protective, soft, prefabricated, includes all components and accessories	Y ☐ (NU, RR, UE)
A8001	Helmet, protective, hard, prefabricated, includes all components and accessories	Y ☐ (NU, RR, UE)

Special Coverage Instructions   Noncovered by Medicare   Carrier Discretion   ☑ Quantity Alert   ● New Code   ○ Recycled/Reinstated   ▲ Revised Code

© 2023 Optum360, LLC   A2-Z3 ASC Pmt   **CMS:** IOM   **AHA:** Coding Clinic   ☐ DMEPOS Paid   ○ SNF Excluded   **A Codes — 15**

A8002	Helmet, protective, soft, custom fabricated, includes all components and accessories	Y & (NU, RR, UE)
A8003	Helmet, protective, hard, custom fabricated, includes all components and accessories	Y & (NU, RR, UE)
A8004	Soft interface for helmet, replacement only	Y & (NU, RR, UE)

Other Supplies and Devices

A9150	Nonprescription drugs	B
A9152	Single vitamin/mineral/trace element, oral, per dose, not otherwise specified	EI ☑
A9153	Multiple vitamins, with or without minerals and trace elements, oral, per dose, not otherwise specified	EI ☑
A9155	Artificial saliva, 30 ml	B ☑
● A9156	Oral mucoadhesive, any type (liquid, gel, paste, etc.), per 1 ml	N1

Use this code for MuGard.

A9180	Pediculosis (lice infestation) treatment, topical, for administration by patient/caretaker	EI
● A9268	Programmer for transient, orally ingested capsule	
● A9269	Programmable, transient, orally ingested capsule, for use with external programmer, per month	
A9270	Noncovered item or service	EI

CMS: 100-04,11,100.1; 100-04,20,30.9; 100-04,23,20.9.1.1

A9272	Wound suction, disposable, includes dressing, all accessories and components, any type, each	EI ☑
A9273	Cold or hot fluid bottle, ice cap or collar, heat and/or cold wrap, any type	EI
A9274	External ambulatory insulin delivery system, disposable, each, includes all supplies and accessories	EI ☑
A9275	Home glucose disposable monitor, includes test strips	EI
A9276	Sensor; invasive (e.g., subcutaneous), disposable, for use with nondurable medical equipment interstitial continuous glucose monitoring system (CGM), one unit = 1 day supply	EI ☑
A9277	Transmitter; external, for use with nondurable medical equipment interstitial continuous glucose monitoring system (CGM)	EI
A9278	Receiver (monitor); external, for use with nondurable medical equipment interstitial continuous glucose monitoring system (CGM)	EI
A9279	Monitoring feature/device, stand-alone or integrated, any type, includes all accessories, components and electronics, not otherwise classified	EI
A9280	Alert or alarm device, not otherwise classified	EI
A9281	Reaching/grabbing device, any type, any length, each	EI ☑
A9282	Wig, any type, each	EI ☑
A9283	Foot pressure off loading/supportive device, any type, each	EI ☑
A9284	Spirometer, nonelectronic, includes all accessories	N
A9285	Inversion/eversion correction device	A
A9286	Hygienic item or device, disposable or nondisposable, any type, each	EI
A9291	Prescription digital cognitive and/or behavioral therapy, FDA-cleared, per course of treatment	

AHA: 4Q,22

● A9292	Prescription digital visual therapy, software-only, FDA cleared, per course of treatment	

A9300	Exercise equipment	EI

Radiopharmaceuticals

A9500	Technetium Tc-99m sestamibi, diagnostic, per study dose	N N1 ☑ ⊘

Use this code for Cardiolite.

A9501	Technetium Tc-99m teboroxime, diagnostic, per study dose	N N1 ☑ ⊘
A9502	Technetium Tc-99m tetrofosmin, diagnostic, per study dose	N N1 ☑ ⊘

Use this code for Myoview.

A9503	Technetium Tc-99m medronate, diagnostic, per study dose, up to 30 mCi	N N1 ☑ ⊘

Use this code for CIS-MDP, Draximage MDP-10, Draximage MDP-25, MDP-Bracco, Technetium Tc-99m MPI-MDP.

A9504	Technetium Tc-99m apcitide, diagnostic, per study dose, up to 20 mCi	N N1 ☑ ⊘

Use this code for Acutect.

A9505	Thallium Tl-201 thallous chloride, diagnostic, per mCi	N N1 ☑ ⊘

Use this code for MIBG, Thallous Chloride USP.

A9507	Indium In-111 capromab pendetide, diagnostic, per study dose, up to 10 millicuries	N N1 ☑ ⊘

Use this code for Prostascint.

A9508	Iodine I-131 iobenguane sulfate, diagnostic, per 0.5 mCi	N N1 ☑ ⊘

Use this code for MIBG.

A9509	Iodine I-123 sodium iodide, diagnostic, per mCi	N N1 ☑ ⊘
A9510	Technetium Tc-99m disofenin, diagnostic, per study dose, up to 15 mCi	N N1 ☑ ⊘

Use this code for Hepatolite.

A9512	Technetium Tc-99m pertechnetate, diagnostic, per mCi	N N1 ☑ ⊘

Use this code for Technelite, Ultra-Technekow.

A9513	Lutetium Lu 177, dotatate, therapeutic, 1 mCi	

Use this code for Lutathera.

AHA: 1Q,19

A9515	Choline C-11, diagnostic, per study dose up to 20 mCi	G N1 ☑
A9516	Iodine I-123 sodium iodide, diagnostic, per 100 mcCi, up to 999 mcCi	N N1 ☑ ⊘
A9517	Iodine I-131 sodium iodide capsule(s), therapeutic, per mCi	K ☑ ⊘
A9520	Technetium Tc-99m, tilmanocept, diagnostic, up to 0.5 mCi	N N1 ☑
A9521	Technetium Tc-99m exametazime, diagnostic, per study dose, up to 25 mCi	N N1 ☑ ⊘

Use this code for Ceretec.

A9524	Iodine I-131 iodinated serum albumin, diagnostic, per 5 mcCi	N N1 ☑ ⊘
A9526	Nitrogen N-13 ammonia, diagnostic, per study dose, up to 40 mCi	N N1 ☑ ⊘

CMS: 100-04,13,60.3; 100-04,13,60.3.2
AHA: 1Q,22

A9527	Iodine I-125, sodium iodide solution, therapeutic, per mCi	U H2 ☑ ⊘
A9528	Iodine I-131 sodium iodide capsule(s), diagnostic, per mCi	N N1 ☑ ⊘
A9529	Iodine I-131 sodium iodide solution, diagnostic, per mCi	N N1 ☑ ⊘

Special Coverage Instructions   Noncovered by Medicare   Carrier Discretion   ☑ Quantity Alert   ● New Code   ○ Recycled/Reinstated   ▲ Revised Code

16 — A Codes   A Age Edit   M Maternity Edit   ♀ Female Only   ♂ Male Only   A-Y OPPS Status Indicators   © 2023 Optum360, LLC

A9530	Iodine I-131 sodium iodide solution, therapeutic, per mCi	K ☑ ⊘
A9531	Iodine I-131 sodium iodide, diagnostic, per mcCi (up to 100 mcCi)	N N1 ☑ ⊘
A9532	Iodine I-125 serum albumin, diagnostic, per 5 mcCi	N N1 ☑ ⊘
A9536	Technetium Tc-99m depreotide, diagnostic, per study dose, up to 35 mCi	N N1 ☑ ⊘
A9537	Technetium Tc-99m mebrofenin, diagnostic, per study dose, up to 15 mCi	N N1 ☑ ⊘
A9538	Technetium Tc-99m pyrophosphate, diagnostic, per study dose, up to 25 mCi	N N1 ☑ ⊘
	Use this code for CIS-PYRO, Phosphotec, Technescan Pyp Kit.	
A9539	Technetium Tc-99m pentetate, diagnostic, per study dose, up to 25 mCi	N N1 ☑ ⊘
	Use this code for AN-DTPA, DTPA, MPI-DTPA Kit-Chelate, MPI Indium DTPA IN-111, Pentetate Calcium Trisodium, Pentate Zinc Trisodium.	
A9540	Technetium Tc-99m macroaggregated albumin, diagnostic, per study dose, up to 10 mCi	N N1 ☑ ⊘
A9541	Technetium Tc-99m sulfur colloid, diagnostic, per study dose, up to 20 mCi	N N1 ☑ ⊘
A9542	Indium In-111 ibritumomab tiuxetan, diagnostic, per study dose, up to 5 mCi	N N1 ☑ ⊘
	Use this code for Zevalin.	
A9543	Yttrium Y-90 ibritumomab tiuxetan, therapeutic, per treatment dose, up to 40 mCi	K ☑ ⊘
A9546	Cobalt Co-57/58, cyanocobalamin, diagnostic, per study dose, up to 1 mcCi	N N1 ☑ ⊘
A9547	Indium In-111 oxyquinoline, diagnostic, per 0.5 mCi	N N1 ☑ ⊘
A9548	Indium In-111 pentetate, diagnostic, per 0.5 mCi	N N1 ☑ ⊘
A9550	Technetium Tc-99m sodium gluceptate, diagnostic, per study dose, up to 25 mCi	N N1 ☑ ⊘
A9551	Technetium Tc-99m succimer, diagnostic, per study dose, up to 10 mCi	N N1 ☑ ⊘
	Use this code for MPI-DMSA Kidney Reagent.	
A9552	Fluorodeoxyglucose F-18 FDG, diagnostic, per study dose, up to 45 mCi	N N1 ☑ ⊘
	CMS: 100-03,220.6.13; 100-03,220.6.17; 100-04,13,60.15; 100-04,13,60.16; 100-04,13,60.3.2	
	AHA: 1Q,22	
A9553	Chromium Cr-51 sodium chromate, diagnostic, per study dose, up to 250 mcCi	N N1 ☑ ⊘
	Use this code for Chromitope Sodium.	
A9554	Iodine I-125 sodium iothalamate, diagnostic, per study dose, up to 10 mcCi	N N1 ☑ ⊘
	Use this code for Glofil-125.	
A9555	Rubidium Rb-82, diagnostic, per study dose, up to 60 mCi	N N1 ☑ ⊘
	Use this code for Cardiogen 82.	
	CMS: 100-03,220.6.1; 100-04,13,60.3.2	
	AHA: 1Q,22	
A9556	Gallium Ga-67 citrate, diagnostic, per mCi	N N1 ☑ ⊘
A9557	Technetium Tc-99m bicisate, diagnostic, per study dose, up to 25 mCi	N N1 ☑ ⊘
	Use this code for Neurolite.	
A9558	Xenon Xe-133 gas, diagnostic, per 10 mCi	N N1 ☑ ⊘
A9559	Cobalt Co-57 cyanocobalamin, oral, diagnostic, per study dose, up to 1 mcCi	N N1 ☑ ⊘
A9560	Technetium Tc-99m labeled red blood cells, diagnostic, per study dose, up to 30 mCi	N N1 ☑ ⊘
A9561	Technetium Tc-99m oxidronate, diagnostic, per study dose, up to 30 mCi	N N1 ☑ ⊘
	Use this code for TechneScan.	
A9562	Technetium Tc-99m mertiatide, diagnostic, per study dose, up to 15 mCi	N N1 ☑ ⊘
	Use this code for TechneScan MAG-3.	
A9563	Sodium phosphate P-32, therapeutic, per mCi	K ☑ ⊘
A9564	Chromic phosphate P-32 suspension, therapeutic, per mCi	E1 ☑ ⊘
	Use this code for Phosphocol (P32).	
A9566	Technetium Tc-99m fanolesomab, diagnostic, per study dose, up to 25 mCi	N N1 ☑ ⊘
A9567	Technetium Tc-99m pentetate, diagnostic, aerosol, per study dose, up to 75 mCi	N N1 ☑ ⊘
	Use this code for AN-DTPA, DTPA, MPI-DTPA Kit-Chelate, MPI Indium DTPA IN-111, Pentate Calcium Trisodium, Pentate Zinc Trisodium.	
A9568	Technetium Tc-99m arcitumomab, diagnostic, per study dose, up to 45 mCi	N N1 ☑ ⊘
	Use this code for CEA Scan.	
A9569	Technetium Tc-99m exametazime labeled autologous white blood cells, diagnostic, per study dose	N N1 ☑ ⊘
A9570	Indium In-111 labeled autologous white blood cells, diagnostic, per study dose	N N1 ☑ ⊘
A9571	Indium In-111 labeled autologous platelets, diagnostic, per study dose	N N1 ☑ ⊘
A9572	Indium In-111 pentetreotide, diagnostic, per study dose, up to 6 mCi	N N1 ☑ ⊘
	Use this code for Octreoscan.	
● **A9573**	Injection, gadopiclenol, 1 ml	N1
	Use this code for Vueway.	
A9575	Injection, gadoterate meglumine, 0.1 ml	N N1 ☑
	Use this code for Dotarem.	
A9576	Injection, gadoteridol, (ProHance multipack), per ml	N N1 ☑
A9577	Injection, gadobenate dimeglumine (MultiHance), per ml	N N1 ☑
A9578	Injection, gadobenate dimeglumine (MultiHance multipack), per ml	N N1 ☑
A9579	Injection, gadolinium-based magnetic resonance contrast agent, not otherwise specified (NOS), per ml	N N1 ☑
	Use this code for Omniscan, Magnevist.	
	CMS: 100-03,1,220.2	
A9580	Sodium fluoride F-18, diagnostic, per study dose, up to 30 mCi	N N1 ☑ ⊘
	CMS: 100-03,220.6.19; 100-04,13,60.18; 100-04,13,60.3.2	
A9581	Injection, gadoxetate disodium, 1 ml	N N1 ☑
	Use this code for Eovist.	
A9582	Iodine I-123 iobenguane, diagnostic, per study dose, up to 15 mCi	N N1 ☑
A9583	Injection, gadofosveset trisodium, 1 ml	N N1 ☑
	Use this code for Ablavar, Vasovist.	
A9584	Iodine I-123 ioflupane, diagnostic, per study dose, up to 5 mCi	N N1 ☑
	Use this code for DaTscan.	
A9585	Injection, gadobutrol, 0.1 ml	N N1 ☑
	Use this code for Gadavist.	

Special Coverage Instructions   Noncovered by Medicare   Carrier Discretion   ☑ Quantity Alert   ● New Code   ○ Recycled/Reinstated   ▲ Revised Code

© 2023 Optum360, LLC   A2-A3 ASC Pmt   **CMS:** IOM   **AHA:** Coding Clinic   ⅙ DMEPOS Paid   ⊘ SNF Excluded   **A Codes — 17**

A9586	Florbetapir F18, diagnostic, per study dose, up to 10 mCi	N N1 ☑
	Use this code for Amyvid.	
	CMS: 100-04,13,60.12; 100-04,17, 80.12; 100-04,32,60.12	

A9587	Gallium Ga-68, dotatate, diagnostic, 0.1 mCi	G N1 ☑
	Use this code for Netspot.	
	CMS: 100-04,13,60.3.2	

A9588	Fluciclovine F-18, diagnostic, 1 mCi	G N1 ☑
	Use this code for Axumin.	
	CMS: 100-04,13,60.3.2	

A9589	Instillation, hexaminolevulinate HCl, 100 mg	
	Use this code for Cysview.	
	CMS: 100-04,13,60.3.2	
	AHA: 1Q,19	

A9590	Iodine I-131, iobenguane, 1 mCi	K2
	Use this code for Azedra.	
	CMS: 100-04,13,60.3.2	

A9591	Fluoroestradiol F-18, diagnostic, 1 mCi	N1
	Use this code for Cerianna.	
	CMS: 100-04,13,60.3.2	
	AHA: 1Q,21	

A9592	Copper Cu-64, dotatate, diagnostic, 1 mCi	K2
	Use this code for Detectnet.	
	CMS: 100-04,13,60.3.2	
	AHA: 1Q,21	

A9593	Gallium Ga-68 PSMA-11, diagnostic, (UCSF), 1 mCi	K2
	CMS: 100-04,13,60.3.2	
	AHA: 3Q,21	

A9594	Gallium Ga-68 PSMA-11, diagnostic, (UCLA), 1 mCi	K2
	CMS: 100-04,13,60.3.2	
	AHA: 3Q,21	

A9595	Piflufolastat F-18, diagnostic, 1 mCi	K2
	Use this code for Pylarify.	
	CMS: 100-04,13,60.3.2	
	AHA: 1Q,22	

A9596	Gallium Ga-68 gozetotide, diagnostic, (Illuccix), 1 mCi	K2
	CMS: 100-04,13,60.3.2	
	AHA: 3Q,22	

| A9597 | Positron emission tomography radiopharmaceutical, diagnostic, for tumor identification, not otherwise classified | N N1 ☑ |
| | CMS: 100-04,13,60.3.2 | |

| A9598 | Positron emission tomography radiopharmaceutical, diagnostic, for nontumor identification, not otherwise classified | N N1 ☑ |
| | CMS: 100-04,13,60.3.2 | |

| A9600 | Strontium Sr-89 chloride, therapeutic, per mCi | K ☑ ⊘ |
| | Use this code for Metastron. | |

A9601	Flortaucipir F 18 injection, diagnostic, 1 mCi	
	Use this code for Tauvid.	
	AHA: 3Q,22	

| A9602 | Fluorodopa F-18, diagnostic, per mCi | K2 |
| | AHA: 4Q,22 | |

| ○ A9603 | Injection, pafolacianine, 0.1 mg | N1 |
| | Use this code for Cytalux. | |

| A9604 | Samarium Sm-153 lexidronam, therapeutic, per treatment dose, up to 150 mCi | K ☑ |
| | Use this code for Quadramet. | |

| A9606 | Radium RA-223 dichloride, therapeutic, per UCI | K ☑ |
| | Use this code for Xofigo. | |

A9607	Lutetium Lu 177 vipivotide tetraxetan, therapeutic, 1 mCi	
	Use this code for Pluvicto.	
	AHA: 4Q,22	

| ● A9608 | Flotufolastat F18, diagnostic, 1 mCi | |
| | Use this code for Posluma. | |

| ● A9609 | Fludeoxyglucose F18, up to 15 mCi | |

| ● A9697 | Injection, carboxydextran-coated superparamagnetic iron oxide, per study dose | N1 |
| | Use this code for Magtrace. | |

| A9698 | Nonradioactive contrast imaging material, not otherwise classified, per study | N N1 ☑ ⊘ |

| A9699 | Radiopharmaceutical, therapeutic, not otherwise classified | N ☑ ⊘ |

| A9700 | Supply of injectable contrast material for use in echocardiography, per study | N N1 |

| A9800 | Gallium Ga-68 gozetotide, diagnostic, (Locametz), 1 mCi | K2 |
| | AHA: 4Q,22 | |

Miscellaneous

| A9900 | Miscellaneous DME supply, accessory, and/or service component of another HCPCS code | Y |

| A9901 | DME delivery, set up, and/or dispensing service component of another HCPCS code | A |

| A9999 | Miscellaneous DME supply or accessory, not otherwise specified | Y |

Special Coverage Instructions   Noncovered by Medicare   Carrier Discretion   ☑ Quantity Alert   ● New Code   ○ Recycled/Reinstated   ▲ Revised Code

18 — A Codes   A Age Edit   M Maternity Edit   ♀ Female Only   ♂ Male Only   A–Y OPPS Status Indicators   © 2023 Optum360, LLC

Enteral and Parenteral Therapy B4034-B9999

This section includes codes for supplies, formulae, nutritional solutions, and infusion pumps.

Enteral Formulae and Enteral Medical Supplies

B4034 Enteral feeding supply kit; syringe fed, per day, includes but not limited to feeding/flushing syringe, administration set tubing, dressings, tape ☑ ☑
CMS: 100-03,180.2; 100-04,20,160.2

B4035 Enteral feeding supply kit; pump fed, per day, includes but not limited to feeding/flushing syringe, administration set tubing, dressings, tape ☑ ☑
CMS: 100-03,180.2; 100-04,20,160.2

B4036 Enteral feeding supply kit; gravity fed, per day, includes but not limited to feeding/flushing syringe, administration set tubing, dressings, tape ☑ ☑
CMS: 100-03,180.2; 100-04,20,160.2

B4081 Nasogastric tubing with stylet ☑
CMS: 100-03,180.2; 100-04,20,160.2

Many types of stylets are used. Some may be fitted with lights or optics. Others are used as guides

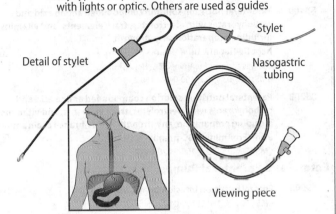

B4082 Nasogastric tubing without stylet ☑
CMS: 100-03,180.2; 100-04,20,160.2

B4083 Stomach tube - Levine type ☑
CMS: 100-03,180.2; 100-04,20,160.2

B4087 Gastrostomy/jejunostomy tube, standard, any material, any type, each ☑ ☑
CMS: 100-03,180.2

B4088 Gastrostomy/jejunostomy tube, low-profile, any material, any type, each ☑ ☑
CMS: 100-03,180.2

B4100 Food thickener, administered orally, per oz ☑ ☑
CMS: 100-03,180.2

B4102 Enteral formula, for adults, used to replace fluids and electrolytes (e.g., clear liquids), 500 ml = 1 unit ☑ ☑
CMS: 100-03,180.2

B4103 Enteral formula, for pediatrics, used to replace fluids and electrolytes (e.g., clear liquids), 500 ml = 1 unit ☑ ☑
CMS: 100-03,180.2

B4104 Additive for enteral formula (e.g., fiber) ☑
CMS: 100-03,180.2

B4105 In-line cartridge containing digestive enzyme(s) for enteral feeding, each
CMS: 100-03,180.2

● B4148 Enteral feeding supply kit; elastomeric control fed, per day, includes but not limited to feeding/flushing syringe, administration set tubing, dressings, tape
CMS: 100-03,180.2

B4149 Enteral formula, manufactured blenderized natural foods with intact nutrients, includes proteins, fats, carbohydrates, vitamins and minerals, may include fiber, administered through an enteral feeding tube, 100 calories = 1 unit ☑ ☑
CMS: 100-03,180.2

B4150 Enteral formula, nutritionally complete with intact nutrients, includes proteins, fats, carbohydrates, vitamins and minerals, may include fiber, administered through an enteral feeding tube, 100 calories = 1 unit
Use this code for Enrich, Ensure, Ensure HN, Ensure Powder, Isocal, Lonalac Powder, Meritene, Meritene Powder, Osmolite, Osmolite HN, Portagen Powder, Sustacal, Renu, Sustagen Powder, Travasorb.
CMS: 100-03,180.2; 100-04,20,160.2

B4152 Enteral formula, nutritionally complete, calorically dense (equal to or greater than 1.5 kcal/ml) with intact nutrients, includes proteins, fats, carbohydrates, vitamins and minerals, may include fiber, administered through an enteral feeding tube, 100 calories = 1 unit ☑ ☑
Use this code for Magnacal, Isocal HCN, Sustacal HC, Ensure Plus, Ensure Plus HN.
CMS: 100-03,180.2; 100-04,20,160.2

B4153 Enteral formula, nutritionally complete, hydrolyzed proteins (amino acids and peptide chain), includes fats, carbohydrates, vitamins and minerals, may include fiber, administered through an enteral feeding tube, 100 calories = 1 unit ☑ ☑
Use this code for Criticare HN, Vivonex t.e.n. (Total Enteral Nutrition), Vivonex HN, Vital (Vital HN), Travasorb HN, Isotein HN, Precision HN, Precision Isotonic.
CMS: 100-03,180.2; 100-04,20,160.2

B4154 Enteral formula, nutritionally complete, for special metabolic needs, excludes inherited disease of metabolism, includes altered composition of proteins, fats, carbohydrates, vitamins and/or minerals, may include fiber, administered through an enteral feeding tube, 100 calories = 1 unit ☑ ☑
Use this code for Hepatic-aid, Travasorb Hepatic, Travasorb MCT, Travasorb Renal, Traum-aid, Tramacal, Aminald.
CMS: 100-03,180.2; 100-04,20,160.2

B4155 Enteral formula, nutritionally incomplete/modular nutrients, includes specific nutrients, carbohydrates (e.g., glucose polymers), proteins/amino acids (e.g., glutamine, arginine), fat (e.g., medium chain triglycerides) or combination, administered through an enteral feeding tube, 100 calories = 1 unit ☑ ☑
Use this code for Propac, Gevral Protein, Promix, Casec, Moducal, Controlyte, Polycose Liquid or Powder, Sumacal, Microlipids, MCT Oil, Nutri-source.
CMS: 100-03,180.2; 100-04,20,160.2

B4157 Enteral formula, nutritionally complete, for special metabolic needs for inherited disease of metabolism, includes proteins, fats, carbohydrates, vitamins and minerals, may include fiber, administered through an enteral feeding tube, 100 calories = 1 unit ☑ ☑
CMS: 100-03,180.2

B4158 Enteral formula, for pediatrics, nutritionally complete with intact nutrients, includes proteins, fats, carbohydrates, vitamins and minerals, may include fiber and/or iron, administered through an enteral feeding tube, 100 calories = 1 unit ☑ ☑
CMS: 100-03,180.2

Special Coverage Instructions   Noncovered by Medicare   Carrier Discretion   ☑ Quantity Alert   ● New Code   ○ Recycled/Reinstated   ▲ Revised Code

© 2023 Optum360, LLC   A2-Z3 ASC Pmt   CMS: IOM   AHA: Coding Clinic   DMEPOS Paid   SNF Excluded   B Codes — 19

Enteral and Parenteral Therapy

B4159 — B9999

B4159 Enteral formula, for pediatrics, nutritionally complete soy based with intact nutrients, includes proteins, fats, carbohydrates, vitamins and minerals, may include fiber and/or iron, administered through an enteral feeding tube, 100 calories = 1 unit Y ☑
CMS: 100-03,180.2

B4160 Enteral formula, for pediatrics, nutritionally complete calorically dense (equal to or greater than 0.7 kcal/ml) with intact nutrients, includes proteins, fats, carbohydrates, vitamins and minerals, may include fiber, administered through an enteral feeding tube, 100 calories = 1 unit Y ☑
CMS: 100-03,180.2

B4161 Enteral formula, for pediatrics, hydrolyzed/amino acids and peptide chain proteins, includes fats, carbohydrates, vitamins and minerals, may include fiber, administered through an enteral feeding tube, 100 calories = 1 unit Y ☑
CMS: 100-03,180.2

B4162 Enteral formula, for pediatrics, special metabolic needs for inherited disease of metabolism, includes proteins, fats, carbohydrates, vitamins and minerals, may include fiber, administered through an enteral feeding tube, 100 calories = 1 unit Y ☑
CMS: 100-03,180.2

Parenteral Nutrition Solutions and Supplies

B4164 Parenteral nutrition solution: carbohydrates (dextrose), 50% or less (500 ml = 1 unit), home mix Y ☑
CMS: 100-03,180.2; 100-04,20,160.2

B4168 Parenteral nutrition solution; amino acid, 3.5%, (500 ml = 1 unit) - home mix Y ☑
CMS: 100-03,180.2; 100-04,20,160.2

B4172 Parenteral nutrition solution; amino acid, 5.5% through 7%, (500 ml = 1 unit) - home mix Y ☑
CMS: 100-03,180.2; 100-04,20,160.2

B4176 Parenteral nutrition solution; amino acid, 7% through 8.5%, (500 ml = 1 unit) - home mix Y ☑
CMS: 100-03,180.2; 100-04,20,160.2

B4178 Parenteral nutrition solution: amino acid, greater than 8.5% (500 ml = 1 unit) - home mix Y ☑
CMS: 100-03,180.2; 100-04,20,160.2

B4180 Parenteral nutrition solution: carbohydrates (dextrose), greater than 50% (500 ml = 1 unit), home mix Y ☑
CMS: 100-03,180.2; 100-04,20,160.2

B4185 Parenteral nutrition solution, not otherwise specified, 10 g lipids B ☑
CMS: 100-03,180.2

B4187 Omegaven, 10 g lipids
CMS: 100-03,180.2

B4189 Parenteral nutrition solution: compounded amino acid and carbohydrates with electrolytes, trace elements, and vitamins, including preparation, any strength, 10 to 51 g of protein, premix Y ☑
CMS: 100-03,180.2; 100-04,20,160.2

B4193 Parenteral nutrition solution: compounded amino acid and carbohydrates with electrolytes, trace elements, and vitamins, including preparation, any strength, 52 to 73 g of protein, premix Y ☑
CMS: 100-03,180.2; 100-04,20,160.2

B4197 Parenteral nutrition solution; compounded amino acid and carbohydrates with electrolytes, trace elements and vitamins, including preparation, any strength, 74 to 100 g of protein - premix Y ☑
CMS: 100-03,180.2; 100-04,20,160.2

B4199 Parenteral nutrition solution; compounded amino acid and carbohydrates with electrolytes, trace elements and vitamins, including preparation, any strength, over 100 g of protein - premix Y ☑
CMS: 100-03,180.2; 100-04,20,160.2

B4216 Parenteral nutrition; additives (vitamins, trace elements, Heparin, electrolytes), home mix, per day Y
CMS: 100-03,180.2; 100-04,20,160.2

B4220 Parenteral nutrition supply kit; premix, per day Y
CMS: 100-03,180.2; 100-04,20,160.2

B4222 Parenteral nutrition supply kit; home mix, per day Y
CMS: 100-03,180.2; 100-04,20,160.2

B4224 Parenteral nutrition administration kit, per day Y
CMS: 100-03,180.2; 100-04,20,160.2

B5000 Parenteral nutrition solution: compounded amino acid and carbohydrates with electrolytes, trace elements, and vitamins, including preparation, any strength, renal - Amirosyn RF, NephrAmine, RenAmine - premix Y
Use this code for Amirosyn-RF, NephrAmine, RenAmin.
CMS: 100-03,180.2; 100-04,20,160.2

B5100 Parenteral nutrition solution compounded amino acid and carbohydrates with electrolytes, trace elements, and vitamins, including preparation, any strength, hepatic-HepatAmine-premix Y
Use this code for FreAmine HBC, HepatAmine.
CMS: 100-03,180.2; 100-04,20,160.2

B5200 Parenteral nutrition solution compounded amino acid and carbohydrates with electrolytes, trace elements, and vitamins, including preparation, any strength, stress-branch chain amino acids-FreAmine-HBC-premix Y
CMS: 100-03,180.2; 100-04,20,160.2

Enteral and Parenteral Pumps

B9002 Enteral nutrition infusion pump, any type Y
CMS: 100-03,180.2; 100-04,20,160.2

B9004 Parenteral nutrition infusion pump, portable Y
CMS: 100-03,180.2; 100-04,20,160.2

B9006 Parenteral nutrition infusion pump, stationary Y
CMS: 100-03,180.2; 100-04,20,160.2

B9998 NOC for enteral supplies Y
CMS: 100-03,180.2

B9999 NOC for parenteral supplies Y
Determine if an alternative HCPCS Level II or a CPT code better describes the service being reported. This code should be used only if a more specific code is unavailable.
CMS: 100-03,180.2

Special Coverage Instructions Noncovered by Medicare Carrier Discretion ☑ Quantity Alert ● New Code ○ Recycled/Reinstated ▲ Revised Code

A Age Edit M Maternity Edit ♀ Female Only ♂ Male Only A-Y OPPS Status Indicators © 2023 Optum360, LLC

Outpatient PPS C1052-C9899

This section reports drug, biological, and device codes that must be used by OPPS hospitals. Non-OPPS hospitals, Critical Access Hospitals (CAHs), Indian Health Service Hospitals (HIS), hospitals located in American Samoa, Guam, Saipan, or the Virgin Islands, and Maryland waiver hospitals may report these codes at their discretion. The codes can only be reported for facility (technical) services.

The C series of HCPCS may include device categories, new technology procedures, and drugs, biologicals and radiopharmaceuticals that do not have other HCPCS codes assigned. Some of these items and services are eligible for transitional pass-through payments for OPPS hospitals, have separate APC payments, or are items that are packaged. Hospitals are encouraged to report all appropriate C codes regardless of payment status.

C1052 Hemostatic agent, gastrointestinal, topical [J7]
CMS: 100-04,4,60.4.2

C1062 Intravertebral body fracture augmentation with implant (e.g., metal, polymer) [J7]
CMS: 100-04,4,60.4.2

● **C1600** Catheter, transluminal intravascular lesion preparation device, bladed, sheathed (insertable)

● **C1601** Endoscope, single-use (i.e., disposable), pulmonary, imaging/illumination device (insertable)

● **C1602** Orthopedic/device/drug matrix/absorbable bone void filler, antimicrobial-eluting (implantable)

● **C1603** Retrieval device, insertable, laser (used to retrieve intravascular Inferior vena cava filter)

● **C1604** Graft, transmural transvenous arterial bypass (implantable), with all delivery system components

C1713 Anchor/screw for opposing bone-to-bone or soft tissue-to-bone (implantable) [N][N1]
CMS: 100-04,4,60.4.2; 100-04,4,60.4.3
AHA: 4Q,22; 3Q,22; 2Q,21; 1Q,21; 4Q,20; 2Q,18; 1Q,18

C1714 Catheter, transluminal atherectomy, directional [N][N1]
CMS: 100-04,4,60.4.2

C1715 Brachytherapy needle [N][N1]⊘
CMS: 100-04,4,60.4.2

C1716 Brachytherapy source, nonstranded, gold-198, per source [U][H2]☑⊘
CMS: 100-04,4,60.4.2

C1717 Brachytherapy source, nonstranded, high dose rate iridium-192, per source [U][H2]☑⊘
CMS: 100-04,4,60.4.2

C1719 Brachytherapy source, nonstranded, nonhigh dose rate iridium-192, per source [U][H2]☑⊘
CMS: 100-04,4,60.4.2

C1721 Cardioverter-defibrillator, dual chamber (implantable) [N][N1]
CMS: 100-04,14,40.8; 100-04,4,60.4.2

C1722 Cardioverter-defibrillator, single chamber (implantable) [N][N1]
CMS: 100-04,14,40.8; 100-04,4,60.4.2

C1724 Catheter, transluminal atherectomy, rotational [N][N1]
CMS: 100-04,4,60.4.1; 100-04,4,60.4.2

C1725 Catheter, transluminal angioplasty, nonlaser (may include guidance, infusion/perfusion capability) [N][N1]
To appropriately report drug-coated transluminal angioplasty catheters, use HCPCS code C2623.
CMS: 100-04,4,60.4.2; 100-04,4,60.4.3

C1726 Catheter, balloon dilatation, nonvascular [N][N1]
CMS: 100-04,4,60.4.2; 100-04,4,60.4.3

C1727 Catheter, balloon tissue dissector, nonvascular (insertable) [N][N1]
CMS: 100-04,4,60.4.2; 100-04,4,60.4.3

C1728 Catheter, brachytherapy seed administration [N][N1]⊘
CMS: 100-04,4,60.4.2

C1729 Catheter, drainage [N][N1]
CMS: 100-04,4,60.4.2; 100-04,4,60.4.3

C1730 Catheter, electrophysiology, diagnostic, other than 3D mapping (19 or fewer electrodes) [N][N1]
CMS: 100-04,4,60.4.2; 100-04,4,60.4.3

C1731 Catheter, electrophysiology, diagnostic, other than 3D mapping (20 or more electrodes) [N][N1]
CMS: 100-04,4,60.4.2; 100-04,4,60.4.3

C1732 Catheter, electrophysiology, diagnostic/ablation, 3D or vector mapping [N][N1]
CMS: 100-04,4,60.4.2; 100-04,4,60.4.3

C1733 Catheter, electrophysiology, diagnostic/ablation, other than 3D or vector mapping, other than cool-tip [N][N1]
CMS: 100-04,4,60.4.2; 100-04,4,60.4.3

C1734 Orthopedic/device/drug matrix for opposing bone-to-bone or soft tissue-to bone (implantable) [J7]
CMS: 100-04,4,60.4.2
AHA: 1Q,20

C1747 Endoscope, single-use (i.e., disposable), urinary tract, imaging/illumination device (insertable) [J7]
AHA: 3Q,23; 1Q,23

C1748 Endoscope, single-use (i.e. disposable), upper GI, imaging/illumination device (insertable) [N1]
CMS: 100-04,4,60.4.2
AHA: 3Q,23; 2Q,20

C1749 Endoscope, retrograde imaging/illumination colonoscope device (implantable) [N][N1]
CMS: 100-04,4,60.4.2

C1750 Catheter, hemodialysis/peritoneal, long-term [N][N1]
CMS: 100-04,4,60.4.2

C1751 Catheter, infusion, inserted peripherally, centrally or midline (other than hemodialysis) [N][N1]
CMS: 100-04,4,60.4.1; 100-04,4,60.4.2
AHA: 2Q,19

C1752 Catheter, hemodialysis/peritoneal, short-term [N][N1]
CMS: 100-04,4,60.4.2

C1753 Catheter, intravascular ultrasound [N][N1]
CMS: 100-04,4,60.4.2

C1754 Catheter, intradiscal [N][N1]
CMS: 100-04,4,60.4.2

C1755 Catheter, intraspinal [N][N1]
CMS: 100-04,4,60.4.2

C1756 Catheter, pacing, transesophageal [N][N1]
CMS: 100-04,4,60.4.2

C1757 Catheter, thrombectomy/embolectomy [N][N1]
CMS: 100-04,4,60.4.2

C1758 Catheter, ureteral [N][N1]

C1759 Catheter, intracardiac echocardiography [N][N1]
CMS: 100-04,4,60.4.2

C1760 Closure device, vascular (implantable/insertable) [N][N1]
CMS: 100-04,4,60.4.2; 100-04,4,60.4.3

C1761 Catheter, transluminal intravascular lithotripsy, coronary [J7]
CMS: 100-04,4,60.4.2
AHA: 2Q,23; 4Q,21; 3Q,21

C1762 Connective tissue, human (includes fascia lata) [N][N1]
CMS: 100-04,4,60.4.2; 100-04,4,60.4.3

Special Coverage Instructions   Noncovered by Medicare   Carrier Discretion   ☑ Quantity Alert   ● New Code   ○ Recycled/Reinstated   ▲ Revised Code

Outpatient PPS

C1763 — C1827

C1763 Connective tissue, nonhuman (includes synthetic) N N1
CMS: 100-04,4,60.4.2; 100-04,4,60.4.3
AHA: 4Q,22

C1764 Event recorder, cardiac (implantable) N N1
CMS: 100-04,14,40.8; 100-04,4,60.4.2

C1765 Adhesion barrier N N1
CMS: 100-04,4,60.4.2; 100-04,4,60.4.3

C1766 Introducer/sheath, guiding, intracardiac electrophysiological, steerable, other than peel-away N N1
CMS: 100-04,4,60.4.2

C1767 Generator, neurostimulator (implantable), nonrechargeable N N1
CMS: 100-04,14,40.8; 100-04,32,40.1; 100-04,32,40.2.1; 100-04,32,40.2.4; 100-04,32,40.4; 100-04,4,60.4.2
AHA: 1Q,21

C1768 Graft, vascular N N1
CMS: 100-04,4,60.4.2

C1769 Guide wire N N1
CMS: 100-04,4,60.4.2
AHA: 1Q,22; 3Q,19; 2Q,19

C1770 Imaging coil, magnetic resonance (insertable) N N1
CMS: 100-04,4,60.4.2

C1771 Repair device, urinary, incontinence, with sling graft N N1
CMS: 100-04,14,40.8; 100-04,4,60.4.2; 100-04,4,60.4.3

C1772 Infusion pump, programmable (implantable) N N1
CMS: 100-04,14,40.8; 100-04,4,60.4.2

C1773 Retrieval device, insertable (used to retrieve fractured medical devices) N N1
CMS: 100-04,4,60.4.2; 100-04,4,60.4.3

C1776 Joint device (implantable) N N1
CMS: 100-04,14,40.8; 100-04,4,60.4.2; 100-04,4,60.4.3
AHA: 3Q,21; 1Q,20; 3Q,18

C1777 Lead, cardioverter-defibrillator, endocardial single coil (implantable) N N1
CMS: 100-04,4,60.4.2

C1778 Lead, neurostimulator (implantable) N N1
CMS: 100-04,14,40.8; 100-04,32,40.1; 100-04,32,40.2.1; 100-04,32,40.2.4; 100-04,32,40.4; 100-04,4,60.4.2
AHA: 4Q,22; 1Q,21; 3Q,19; 1Q,19

C1779 Lead, pacemaker, transvenous VDD single pass N N1
CMS: 100-04,14,40.8; 100-04,4,60.4.2; 100-04,4,60.4.3

C1780 Lens, intraocular (new technology) N N1
CMS: 100-04,4,60.4.2; 100-04,4,60.4.3

C1781 Mesh (implantable) N N1
Use this code for OrthADAPT Bioimplant.
CMS: 100-04,4,60.4.2; 100-04,4,60.4.3
AHA: 4Q,22; 1Q,19

C1782 Morcellator N N1
CMS: 100-04,4,60.4.2; 100-04,4,60.4.3

C1783 Ocular implant, aqueous drainage assist device N N1
CMS: 100-04,4,60.4.2

C1784 Ocular device, intraoperative, detached retina N N1
CMS: 100-04,4,60.4.2; 100-04,4,60.4.3

C1785 Pacemaker, dual chamber, rate-responsive (implantable) N N1
CMS: 100-04,14,40.8; 100-04,21,320.4.7; 100-04,32,320.4.1; 100-04,32,320.4.2; 100-04,32,320.4.4; 100-04,32,320.4.6; 100-04,32,320.4.7; 100-04,4,60.4.2

C1786 Pacemaker, single chamber, rate-responsive (implantable) N N1
CMS: 100-04,14,40.8; 100-04,21,320.4.7; 100-04,32,320.4.1; 100-04,32,320.4.2; 100-04,32,320.4.4; 100-04,32,320.4.6; 100-04,32,320.4.7; 100-04,4,60.4.2

C1787 Patient programmer, neurostimulator N N1
CMS: 100-04,4,60.4.2; 100-04,4,60.4.3

C1788 Port, indwelling (implantable) N N1
CMS: 100-04,4,60.4.2
AHA: 2Q,19

C1789 Prosthesis, breast (implantable) N N1
CMS: 100-04,4,60.4.2

C1813 Prosthesis, penile, inflatable N N1
CMS: 100-04,14,40.8; 100-04,4,60.4.2

C1814 Retinal tamponade device, silicone oil N N1
CMS: 100-04,4,60.4.2; 100-04,4,60.4.3

C1815 Prosthesis, urinary sphincter (implantable) N N1
CMS: 100-04,14,40.8; 100-04,4,60.4.2

C1816 Receiver and/or transmitter, neurostimulator (implantable) N N1
CMS: 100-04,4,60.4.2
AHA: 4Q,22

C1817 Septal defect implant system, intracardiac N N1
CMS: 100-04,4,60.4.2; 100-04,4,60.4.3

C1818 Integrated keratoprosthesis N N1
CMS: 100-04,4,60.4.2; 100-04,4,60.4.3

C1819 Surgical tissue localization and excision device (implantable) N N1
CMS: 100-04,4,60.4.2

C1820 Generator, neurostimulator (implantable), with rechargeable battery and charging system N N1
Use to report neurostimulator generators that are not high frequency.
CMS: 100-04,14,40.8; 100-04,32,40.2.1; 100-04,32,40.2.4; 100-04,32,40.4; 100-04,4,10.12; 100-04,4,60.4.2

C1821 Interspinous process distraction device (implantable) N N1
CMS: 100-04,4,60.4.2

C1822 Generator, neurostimulator (implantable), high frequency, with rechargeable battery and charging system N N1
Use to report neurostimulator generators that are high frequency.
CMS: 100-04,4,60.4.2

C1823 Generator, neurostimulator (implantable), nonrechargeable, with transvenous sensing and stimulation leads N1
CMS: 100-04,4,260.1; 100-04,4,260.1.1; 100-04,4,60.4.2
AHA: 1Q,23; 1Q,19

C1824 Generator, cardiac contractility modulation (implantable) J7
CMS: 100-04,4,60.4.2
AHA: 1Q,20

C1825 Generator, neurostimulator (implantable), nonrechargeable with carotid sinus baroreceptor stimulation lead(s) J7
CMS: 100-04,4,60.4.2

C1826 Generator, neurostimulator (implantable), includes closed feedback loop leads and all implantable components, with rechargeable battery and charging system J7
AHA: 1Q,23

C1827 Generator, neurostimulator (implantable), nonrechargeable, with implantable stimulation lead and external paired stimulation controller J7
AHA: 1Q,23

Special Coverage Instructions   Noncovered by Medicare   Carrier Discretion   ☑ Quantity Alert ● New Code ○ Recycled/Reinstated ▲ Revised Code

🅐 Age Edit   🅜 Maternity Edit   ♀ Female Only   ♂ Male Only   🅐-🅨 OPPS Status Indicators   © 2023 Optum360, LLC

C1830	**Powered bone marrow biopsy needle** [N] [N1]
	CMS: 100-04,4,60.4.2
C1831	**Interbody cage, anterior, lateral or posterior, personalized (implantable)** [N1]
	CMS: 100-04,4,60.4.2
	AHA: 1Q,23; 1Q,22; 4Q,21
C1832	**Autograft suspension, including cell processing and application, and all system components** [J7]
	CMS: 100-04,4,60.4.2
	AHA: 1Q,22
C1833	**Monitor, cardiac, including intracardiac lead and all system components (implantable)** [J7]
	CMS: 100-04,4,60.4.2
	AHA: 1Q,22
C1834	~~Pressure sensor system, includes all components (e.g., introducer, sensor), intramuscular (implantable), excludes mobile (wireless) software application~~
C1839	**Iris prosthesis** [J7]
	CMS: 100-04,4,60.4.2
	AHA: 1Q,20
C1840	**Lens, intraocular (telescopic)** [N] [N1]
	CMS: 100-04,4,60.4.2
C1874	**Stent, coated/covered, with delivery system** [N] [N1]
	CMS: 100-04,4,60.4.2; 100-04,4,60.4.3
	AHA: 2Q,23
C1875	**Stent, coated/covered, without delivery system** [N] [N1]
	CMS: 100-04,4,60.4.2; 100-04,4,60.4.3
	AHA: 2Q,23; 2Q,20
C1876	**Stent, noncoated/noncovered, with delivery system** [N] [N1]
	CMS: 100-04,4,60.4.2; 100-04,4,60.4.3
C1877	**Stent, noncoated/noncovered, without delivery system** [N] [N1]
	CMS: 100-04,4,60.4.2
C1878	**Material for vocal cord medialization, synthetic (implantable)** [N] [N1]
	CMS: 100-04,4,60.4.2; 100-04,4,60.4.3
C1880	**Vena cava filter** [N] [N1]
	CMS: 100-04,4,60.4.2
C1881	**Dialysis access system (implantable)** [N] [N1]
	CMS: 100-04,14,40.8; 100-04,4,60.4.2
C1882	**Cardioverter-defibrillator, other than single or dual chamber (implantable)** [N] [N1]
	CMS: 100-04,14,40.8; 100-04,4,60.4.2; 100-04,4,60.4.3
C1883	**Adaptor/extension, pacing lead or neurostimulator lead (implantable)** [N] [N1]
	CMS: 100-04,32,40.1; 100-04,32,40.2.1; 100-04,32,40.2.4; 100-04,32,40.4; 100-04,4,60.4.2; 100-04,4,60.4.3
C1884	**Embolization protective system** [N] [N1]
	CMS: 100-04,4,60.4.2; 100-04,4,60.4.3
C1885	**Catheter, transluminal angioplasty, laser** [N] [N1]
	CMS: 100-04,4,60.4.2; 100-04,4,60.4.3
C1886	**Catheter, extravascular tissue ablation, any modality (insertable)** [N] [N1]
	CMS: 100-04,4,60.4.2
C1887	**Catheter, guiding (may include infusion/perfusion capability)** [N] [N1]
	CMS: 100-04,4,60.4.2; 100-04,4,60.4.3
C1888	**Catheter, ablation, noncardiac, endovascular (implantable)** [N] [N1]
	CMS: 100-04,4,60.4.2; 100-04,4,60.4.3

C1889	**Implantable/insertable device, not otherwise classified** [N] [N1]
C1890	**No implantable/insertable device used with device-intensive procedures** [J7]
	CMS: 100-04,4,260.1; 100-04,4,260.1.1
	AHA: 1Q,19
C1891	**Infusion pump, nonprogrammable, permanent (implantable)** [N] [N1]
	CMS: 100-04,14,40.8; 100-04,4,60.4.2
C1892	**Introducer/sheath, guiding, intracardiac electrophysiological, fixed-curve, peel-away** [N] [N1]
	CMS: 100-04,4,60.4.2; 100-04,4,60.4.3
C1893	**Introducer/sheath, guiding, intracardiac electrophysiological, fixed-curve, other than peel-away** [N] [N1]
	CMS: 100-04,4,60.4.2
C1894	**Introducer/sheath, other than guiding, other than intracardiac electrophysiological, nonlaser** [N] [N1]
	CMS: 100-04,4,60.4.1; 100-04,4,60.4.2
	AHA: 2Q,19
C1895	**Lead, cardioverter-defibrillator, endocardial dual coil (implantable)** [N] [N1]
	CMS: 100-04,4,60.4.2
C1896	**Lead, cardioverter-defibrillator, other than endocardial single or dual coil (implantable)** [N] [N1]
	CMS: 100-04,4,60.4.2
C1897	**Lead, neurostimulator test kit (implantable)** [N] [N1]
	CMS: 100-04,14,40.8; 100-04,32,40.1; 100-04,32,40.2.1; 100-04,32,40.2.4; 100-04,32,40.4; 100-04,4,60.4.2
C1898	**Lead, pacemaker, other than transvenous VDD single pass** [N] [N1]
	CMS: 100-04,14,40.8; 100-04,4,60.4.2
C1899	**Lead, pacemaker/cardioverter-defibrillator combination (implantable)** [N] [N1]
	CMS: 100-04,4,60.4.2
C1900	**Lead, left ventricular coronary venous system** [N] [N1]
	CMS: 100-04,14,40.8; 100-04,4,60.4.2; 100-04,4,60.4.3
C1982	**Catheter, pressure generating, one-way valve, intermittently occlusive** [J7]
	CMS: 100-04,4,60.4.2
	AHA: 1Q,20
C2596	**Probe, image guided, robotic, waterjet ablation** [J7]
	CMS: 100-04,4,60.4.2
	AHA: 1Q,20
C2613	**Lung biopsy plug with delivery system** [N] [N1]
	CMS: 100-04,4,60.4.2
C2614	**Probe, percutaneous lumbar discectomy** [N] [N1]
	CMS: 100-04,4,60.4.2
C2615	**Sealant, pulmonary, liquid** [N] [N1]
	CMS: 100-04,4,60.4.2; 100-04,4,60.4.3
C2616	**Brachytherapy source, nonstranded, yttrium-90, per source** [U] [H2] ☑ ⊘
	CMS: 100-04,4,60.4.2
C2617	**Stent, noncoronary, temporary, without delivery system** [N] [N1]
	CMS: 100-04,4,60.4.2; 100-04,4,60.4.3
	AHA: 1Q,18
C2618	**Probe/needle, cryoablation** [N] [N1]
	CMS: 100-04,4,60.4.2

C1830 — C2618

Special Coverage Instructions	Noncovered by Medicare	Carrier Discretion	☑ Quantity Alert	● New Code	○ Recycled/Reinstated	▲ Revised Code

© 2023 Optum360, LLC [A2]-[Z3] ASC Pmt **CMS:** IOM **AHA:** Coding Clinic ⚲ DMEPOS Paid ⊘ SNF Excluded **C Codes — 23**

C2619 Pacemaker, dual chamber, nonrate-responsive (implantable) N N1
CMS: 100-04,14,40.8; 100-04,21,320.4.7; 100-04,32,320.4.1; 100-04,32,320.4.2; 100-04,32,320.4.4; 100-04,32,320.4.6; 100-04,32,320.4.7; 100-04,4,60.4.2

C2620 Pacemaker, single chamber, nonrate-responsive (implantable) N N1
CMS: 100-04,14,40.8; 100-04,21,320.4.7; 100-04,32,320.4.1; 100-04,32,320.4.2; 100-04,32,320.4.4; 100-04,32,320.4.6; 100-04,32,320.4.7; 100-04,4,60.4.2

C2621 Pacemaker, other than single or dual chamber (implantable) N N1
CMS: 100-04,14,40.8; 100-04,4,60.4.2; 100-04,4,60.4.3

C2622 Prosthesis, penile, noninflatable N N1
CMS: 100-04,14,40.8; 100-04,4,60.4.2

C2623 Catheter, transluminal angioplasty, drug-coated, nonlaser N N1
CMS: 100-04,4,60.4.2

C2624 Implantable wireless pulmonary artery pressure sensor with delivery catheter, including all system components N N1
CMS: 100-04,4,60.4.2

C2625 Stent, noncoronary, temporary, with delivery system N N1
CMS: 100-04,4,60.4.2; 100-04,4,60.4.3

C2626 Infusion pump, nonprogrammable, temporary (implantable) N N1
CMS: 100-04,14,40.8; 100-04,4,60.4.2; 100-04,4,60.4.3

C2627 Catheter, suprapubic/cystoscopic N N1
CMS: 100-04,4,60.4.2

C2628 Catheter, occlusion N N1
CMS: 100-04,4,60.4.2

C2629 Introducer/sheath, other than guiding, other than intracardiac electrophysiological, laser N N1
CMS: 100-04,4,60.4.2

C2630 Catheter, electrophysiology, diagnostic/ablation, other than 3D or vector mapping, cool-tip N N1
CMS: 100-04,4,60.4.2; 100-04,4,60.4.3

C2631 Repair device, urinary, incontinence, without sling graft N N1
CMS: 100-04,14,40.8; 100-04,4,60.4.2; 100-04,4,60.4.3

C2634 Brachytherapy source, nonstranded, high activity, iodine-125, greater than 1.01 mCi (NIST), per source U H2 ☑ ⊘

C2635 Brachytherapy source, nonstranded, high activity, palladium-103, greater than 2.2 mCi (NIST), per source U H2 ☑ ⊘

C2636 Brachytherapy linear source, nonstranded, palladium-103, per 1 mm U H2 ☑ ⊘

C2637 Brachytherapy source, nonstranded, ytterbium-169, per source B ☑ ⊘

C2638 Brachytherapy source, stranded, iodine-125, per source U H2 ☑

C2639 Brachytherapy source, nonstranded, iodine-125, per source U H2 ☑ ⊘

C2640 Brachytherapy source, stranded, palladium-103, per source U H2 ☑

C2641 Brachytherapy source, nonstranded, palladium-103, per source U H2 ☑ ⊘

C2642 Brachytherapy source, stranded, cesium-131, per source U H2 ☑

C2643 Brachytherapy source, nonstranded, cesium-131, per source U H2 ☑ ⊘

C2644 Brachytherapy source, cesium-131 chloride solution, per mCi U ☑

C2645 Brachytherapy planar source, palladium-103, per sq mm U H2 ☑

C2698 Brachytherapy source, stranded, not otherwise specified, per source U H2 ☑

C2699 Brachytherapy source, nonstranded, not otherwise specified, per source U H2 ☑

C5271 Application of low cost skin substitute graft to trunk, arms, legs, total wound surface area up to 100 sq cm; first 25 sq cm or less wound surface area T G2 ☑

C5272 Application of low cost skin substitute graft to trunk, arms, legs, total wound surface area up to 100 sq cm; each additional 25 sq cm wound surface area, or part thereof (list separately in addition to code for primary procedure) N N1 ☑

C5273 Application of low cost skin substitute graft to trunk, arms, legs, total wound surface area greater than or equal to 100 sq cm; first 100 sq cm wound surface area, or 1% of body area of infants and children T G2 ☑

C5274 Application of low cost skin substitute graft to trunk, arms, legs, total wound surface area greater than or equal to 100 sq cm; each additional 100 sq cm wound surface area, or part thereof, or each additional 1% of body area of infants and children, or part thereof (list separately in addition to code for primary procedure) N N1 ☑

C5275 Application of low cost skin substitute graft to face, scalp, eyelids, mouth, neck, ears, orbits, genitalia, hands, feet, and/or multiple digits, total wound surface area up to 100 sq cm; first 25 sq cm or less wound surface area T G2 ☑

C5276 Application of low cost skin substitute graft to face, scalp, eyelids, mouth, neck, ears, orbits, genitalia, hands, feet, and/or multiple digits, total wound surface area up to 100 sq cm; each additional 25 sq cm wound surface area, or part thereof (list separately in addition to code for primary procedure) N N1 ☑

C5277 Application of low cost skin substitute graft to face, scalp, eyelids, mouth, neck, ears, orbits, genitalia, hands, feet, and/or multiple digits, total wound surface area greater than or equal to 100 sq cm; first 100 sq cm wound surface area, or 1% of body area of infants and children T G2 ☑

C5278 Application of low cost skin substitute graft to face, scalp, eyelids, mouth, neck, ears, orbits, genitalia, hands, feet, and/or multiple digits, total wound surface area greater than or equal to 100 sq cm; each additional 100 sq cm wound surface area, or part thereof, or each additional 1% of body area of infants and children, or part thereof (list separately in addition to code for primary procedure) N N1 ☑

C7500 Debridement, bone including epidermis, dermis, subcutaneous tissue, muscle and/or fascia, if performed, first 20 sq cm or less with manual preparation and insertion of deep (e.g., subfascial) drug-delivery device(s) G2
AHA: 1Q,23

C7501 Percutaneous breast biopsies using stereotactic guidance, with placement of breast localization device(s) (e.g., clip, metallic pellet), when performed, and imaging of the biopsy specimen, when performed, all lesions unilateral and bilateral (for single lesion biopsy, use appropriate code) G2
AHA: 1Q,23

Special Coverage Instructions   Noncovered by Medicare   Carrier Discretion   ☑ Quantity Alert ● New Code   ○ Recycled/Reinstated   ▲ Revised Code

24 — C Codes   A Age Edit   M Maternity Edit   ♀ Female Only   ♂ Male Only   A-Y OPPS Status Indicators   © 2023 Optum360, LLC

C7502 Percutaneous breast biopsies using magnetic resonance guidance, with placement of breast localization device(s) (e.g., clip, metallic pellet), when performed, and imaging of the biopsy specimen, when performed, all lesions unilateral or bilateral (for single lesion biopsy, use appropriate code) G2
AHA: 1Q,23

C7503 Open biopsy or excision of deep cervical node(s) with intraoperative identification (e.g., mapping) of sentinel lymph node(s) including injection of nonradioactive dye when performed G2
AHA: 1Q,23

C7504 Percutaneous vertebroplasties (bone biopsies included when performed), first cervicothoracic and any additional cervicothoracic or lumbosacral vertebral bodies, unilateral or bilateral injection, inclusive of all imaging guidance G2
AHA: 1Q,23

C7505 Percutaneous vertebroplasties (bone biopsies included when performed), first lumbosacral and any additional cervicothoracic or lumbosacral vertebral bodies, unilateral or bilateral injection, inclusive of all imaging guidance G2
AHA: 1Q,23

C7506 Arthrodesis, interphalangeal joints, with or without internal fixation G2
AHA: 1Q,23

C7507 Percutaneous vertebral augmentations, first thoracic and any additional thoracic or lumbar vertebral bodies, including cavity creations (fracture reductions and bone biopsies included when performed) using mechanical device (e.g., kyphoplasty), unilateral or bilateral cannulations, inclusive of all imaging guidance G2
AHA: 1Q,23

C7508 Percutaneous vertebral augmentations, first lumbar and any additional thoracic or lumbar vertebral bodies, including cavity creations (fracture reductions and bone biopsies included when performed) using mechanical device (e.g., kyphoplasty), unilateral or bilateral cannulations, inclusive of all imaging guidance G2
AHA: 1Q,23

C7509 Bronchoscopy, rigid or flexible, diagnostic with cell washing(s) when performed, with computer-assisted image-guided navigation, including fluoroscopic guidance when performed G2
AHA: 1Q,23

C7510 Bronchoscopy, rigid or flexible, with bronchial alveolar lavage(s), with computer-assisted image-guided navigation, including fluoroscopic guidance when performed G2
AHA: 1Q,23

C7511 Bronchoscopy, rigid or flexible, with single or multiple bronchial or endobronchial biopsy(ies), single or multiple sites, with computer-assisted image-guided navigation, including fluoroscopic guidance when performed G2
AHA: 1Q,23

C7512 Bronchoscopy, rigid or flexible, with single or multiple bronchial or endobronchial biopsy(ies), single or multiple sites, with transendoscopic endobronchial ultrasound (EBUS) during bronchoscopic diagnostic or therapeutic intervention(s) for peripheral lesion(s), including fluoroscopic guidance when performed G2
AHA: 1Q,23

C7513 Dialysis circuit, introduction of needle(s) and/or catheter(s), with diagnostic angiography of the dialysis circuit, including all direct puncture(s) and catheter placement(s), injection(s) of contrast, all necessary imaging from the arterial anastomosis and adjacent artery through entire venous outflow including the inferior or superior vena cava, fluoroscopic guidance, with transluminal balloon angioplasty of central dialysis segment, performed through dialysis circuit, including all required imaging, radiological supervision and interpretation, image documentation and report R2
AHA: 1Q,23

C7514 Dialysis circuit, introduction of needle(s) and/or catheter(s), with diagnostic angiography of the dialysis circuit, including all direct puncture(s) and catheter placement(s), injection(s) of contrast, all necessary imaging from the arterial anastomosis and adjacent artery through entire venous outflow including the inferior or superior vena cava, fluoroscopic guidance, with all angioplasty in the central dialysis segment, and transcatheter placement of intravascular stent(s), central dialysis segment, performed through dialysis circuit, including all required imaging, radiological supervision and interpretation, image documentation and report R2
AHA: 1Q,23

C7515 Dialysis circuit, introduction of needle(s) and/or catheter(s), with diagnostic angiography of the dialysis circuit, including all direct puncture(s) and catheter placement(s), injection(s) of contrast, all necessary imaging from the arterial anastomosis and adjacent artery through entire venous outflow including the inferior or superior vena cava, fluoroscopic guidance, with dialysis circuit permanent endovascular embolization or occlusion of main circuit or any accessory veins, including all required imaging, radiological supervision and interpretation, image documentation and report R2
AHA: 1Q,23

C7516 Catheter placement in coronary artery(s) for coronary angiography, including intraprocedural injection(s) for coronary angiography, with endoluminal imaging of initial coronary vessel or graft using intravascular ultrasound (IVUS) or optical coherence tomography (OCT) during diagnostic evaluation and/or therapeutic intervention including imaging supervision, interpretation and report G2
AHA: 1Q,23

C7517 Catheter placement in coronary artery(s) for coronary angiography, including intraprocedural injection(s) for coronary angiography, with iliac and/or femoral artery angiography, nonselective, bilateral or ipsilateral to catheter insertion, performed at the same time as cardiac catheterization and/or coronary angiography, includes positioning or placement of the catheter in the distal aorta or ipsilateral femoral or iliac artery, injection of dye, production of permanent images, and radiologic supervision and interpretation G2
AHA: 1Q,23

C7518 Catheter placement in coronary artery(ies) for coronary angiography, including intraprocedural injection(s) for coronary angiography, imaging supervision and interpretation, with catheter placement(s) in bypass graft(s) (internal mammary, free arterial, venous grafts) including intraprocedural injection(s) for bypass graft angiography with endoluminal imaging of initial coronary vessel or graft using intravascular ultrasound (IVUS) or optical coherence tomography (OCT) during diagnostic evaluation and/or therapeutic intervention including imaging, supervision, interpretation and report G2
AHA: 1Q,23

Special Coverage Instructions   Noncovered by Medicare   Carrier Discretion   ☑ Quantity Alert ● New Code   ○ Recycled/Reinstated   ▲ Revised Code

© 2023 Optum360, LLC   A2-Z3 ASC Pmt   **CMS:** IOM   **AHA:** Coding Clinic   ⅄ DMEPOS Paid   ⊘ SNF Excluded   **C Codes — 25**

C7519 Catheter placement in coronary artery(ies) for coronary angiography, including intraprocedural injection(s) for coronary angiography, imaging supervision and interpretation, with catheter placement(s) in bypass graft(s) (internal mammary, free arterial, venous grafts) including intraprocedural injection(s) for bypass graft angiography with intravascular doppler velocity and/or pressure derived coronary flow reserve measurement (initial coronary vessel or graft) during coronary angiography including pharmacologically induced stress [G2]
AHA: 1Q,23

C7520 Catheter placement in coronary artery(ies) for coronary angiography, including intraprocedural injection(s) for coronary angiography, imaging supervision and interpretation, with catheter placement(s) in bypass graft(s) (internal mammary, free arterial, venous grafts) includes intraprocedural injection(s) for bypass graft angiography with iliac and/or femoral artery angiography, nonselective, bilateral or ipsilateral to catheter insertion, performed at the same time as cardiac catheterization and/or coronary angiography, includes positioning or placement of the catheter in the distal aorta or ipsilateral femoral or iliac artery, injection of dye, production of permanent images, and radiologic supervision and interpretation [G2]
AHA: 1Q,23

C7521 Catheter placement in coronary artery(ies) for coronary angiography, including intraprocedural injection(s) for coronary angiography with right heart catheterization with endoluminal imaging of initial coronary vessel or graft using intravascular ultrasound (IVUS) or optical coherence tomography (OCT) during diagnostic evaluation and/or therapeutic intervention including imaging supervision, interpretation and report [G2]
AHA: 1Q,23

C7522 Catheter placement in coronary artery(ies) for coronary angiography, including intraprocedural injection(s) for coronary angiography, imaging supervision and interpretation with right heart catheterization, with intravascular doppler velocity and/or pressure derived coronary flow reserve measurement (initial coronary vessel or graft) during coronary angiography including pharmacologically induced stress [G2]
AHA: 1Q,23

C7523 Catheter placement in coronary artery(ies) for coronary angiography, including intraprocedural injection(s) for coronary angiography, imaging supervision and interpretation, with left heart catheterization including intraprocedural injection(s) for left ventriculography, when performed, with endoluminal imaging of initial coronary vessel or graft using intravascular ultrasound (IVUS) or optical coherence tomography (OCT) during diagnostic evaluation and/or therapeutic intervention including imaging supervision, interpretation and report [G2]
AHA: 1Q,23

C7524 Catheter placement in coronary artery(ies) for coronary angiography, including intraprocedural injection(s) for coronary angiography, imaging supervision and interpretation, with left heart catheterization including intraprocedural injection(s) for left ventriculography, when performed, with intravascular doppler velocity and/or pressure derived coronary flow reserve measurement (initial coronary vessel or graft) during coronary angiography including pharmacologically induced stress [G2]
AHA: 1Q,23

C7525 Catheter placement in coronary artery(ies) for coronary angiography, including intraprocedural injection(s) for coronary angiography, imaging supervision and interpretation, with left heart catheterization including intraprocedural injection(s) for left ventriculography, when performed, catheter placement(s) in bypass graft(s) (internal mammary, free arterial, venous grafts) with bypass graft angiography with endoluminal imaging of initial coronary vessel or graft using intravascular ultrasound (IVUS) or optical coherence tomography (OCT) during diagnostic evaluation and/or therapeutic intervention including imaging supervision, interpretation and report [G2]
AHA: 1Q,23

C7526 Catheter placement in coronary artery(ies) for coronary angiography, including intraprocedural injection(s) for coronary angiography, imaging supervision and interpretation, with left heart catheterization including intraprocedural injection(s) for left ventriculography, when performed, catheter placement(s) in bypass graft(s) (internal mammary, free arterial, venous grafts) with bypass graft angiography with intravascular doppler velocity and/or pressure derived coronary flow reserve measurement (initial coronary vessel or graft) during coronary angiography including pharmacologically induced stress [G2]
AHA: 1Q,23

C7527 Catheter placement in coronary artery(ies) for coronary angiography, including intraprocedural injection(s) for coronary angiography, imaging supervision and interpretation, with right and left heart catheterization including intraprocedural injection(s) for left ventriculography, when performed, with endoluminal imaging of initial coronary vessel or graft using intravascular ultrasound (IVUS) or optical coherence tomography (OCT) during diagnostic evaluation and/or therapeutic intervention including imaging supervision, interpretation and report [G2]
AHA: 1Q,23

C7528 Catheter placement in coronary artery(ies) for coronary angiography, including intraprocedural injection(s) for coronary angiography, imaging supervision and interpretation, with right and left heart catheterization including intraprocedural injection(s) for left ventriculography, when performed, with intravascular doppler velocity and/or pressure derived coronary flow reserve measurement (initial coronary vessel or graft) during coronary angiography including pharmacologically induced stress [G2]
AHA: 1Q,23

C7529 Catheter placement in coronary artery(ies) for coronary angiography, including intraprocedural injection(s) for coronary angiography, imaging supervision and interpretation, with right and left heart catheterization including intraprocedural injection(s) for left ventriculography, when performed, catheter placement(s) in bypass graft(s) (internal mammary, free arterial, venous grafts) with bypass graft angiography with intravascular doppler velocity and/or pressure derived coronary flow reserve measurement (initial coronary vessel or graft) during coronary angiography including pharmacologically induced stress [G2]
AHA: 1Q,23

Special Coverage Instructions   Noncovered by Medicare   Carrier Discretion   ☑ Quantity Alert ● New Code   ○ Recycled/Reinstated   ▲ Revised Code

26 — C Codes   Ⓐ Age Edit   Ⓜ Maternity Edit   ♀ Female Only   ♂ Male Only   Ⓐ-Ⓨ OPPS Status Indicators   © 2023 Optum360, LLC

C7530 Dialysis circuit, introduction of needle(s) and/or catheter(s), with diagnostic angiography of the dialysis circuit, including all direct puncture(s) and catheter placement(s), injection(s) of contrast, all necessary imaging from the arterial anastomosis and adjacent artery through entire venous outflow including the inferior or superior vena cava, fluoroscopic guidance, with transluminal balloon angioplasty, peripheral dialysis segment, including all imaging and radiological supervision and interpretation necessary to perform the angioplasty and all angioplasty in the central dialysis segment, with transcatheter placement of intravascular stent(s), central dialysis segment, performed through dialysis circuit, including all imaging, radiological supervision and interpretation, documentation and report ▣
AHA: 1Q,23

C7531 Revascularization, endovascular, open or percutaneous, femoral, popliteal artery(ies), unilateral, with transluminal angioplasty with intravascular ultrasound (initial noncoronary vessel) during diagnostic evaluation and/or therapeutic Intervention, including radiological supervision and interpretation ▣
AHA: 1Q,23

C7532 Transluminal balloon angioplasty (except lower extremity artery(ies) for occlusive disease, intracranial, coronary, pulmonary, or dialysis circuit), Initial artery, open or percutaneous, including all imaging and radiological supervision and interpretation necessary to perform the angioplasty within the same artery, with intravascular ultrasound (initial noncoronary vessel) during diagnostic evaluation and/or therapeutic intervention, including radiological supervision and interpretation ▣
AHA: 1Q,23

C7533 Percutaneous transluminal coronary angioplasty, single major coronary artery or branch with transcatheter placement of radiation delivery device for subsequent coronary intravascular brachytherapy ▣
AHA: 1Q,23

C7534 Revascularization, endovascular, open or percutaneous, femoral, popliteal artery(ies), unilateral, with atherectomy, Includes angioplasty within the same vessel, when performed with intravascular ultrasound (initial noncoronary vessel) during diagnostic evaluation and/or therapeutic intervention, including radiological supervision and interpretation ▣
AHA: 1Q,23

C7535 Revascularization, endovascular, open or percutaneous, femoral, popliteal artery(ies), unilateral, with transluminal stent placement(s), includes angioplasty within the same vessel, when performed, with intravascular ultrasound (initial noncoronary vessel) during diagnostic evaluation and/or therapeutic intervention, including radiological supervision and interpretation ▣
AHA: 1Q,23

C7537 Insertion of new or replacement of permanent pacemaker with atrial transvenous electrode(s), with insertion of pacing electrode, cardiac venous system, for left ventricular pacing, at time of insertion of implantable defibrillator or pacemaker pulse generator (e.g., for upgrade to dual chamber system) ▣
AHA: 1Q,23

C7538 Insertion of new or replacement of permanent pacemaker with ventricular transvenous electrode(s), with insertion of pacing electrode, cardiac venous system, for left ventricular pacing, at time of insertion of implantable defibrillator or pacemaker pulse generator (e.g., for upgrade to dual chamber system) ▣
AHA: 1Q,23

C7539 Insertion of new or replacement of permanent pacemaker with atrial and ventricular transvenous electrode(s), with insertion of pacing electrode, cardiac venous system, for left ventricular pacing, at time of insertion of implantable defibrillator or pacemaker pulse generator (e.g., for upgrade to dual chamber system) ▣
AHA: 1Q,23

C7540 Removal of permanent pacemaker pulse generator with replacement of pacemaker pulse generator, dual lead system, with insertion of pacing electrode, cardiac venous system, for left ventricular pacing, at time of insertion of implantable defibrillator or pacemaker pulse generator (e.g., for upgrade to dual chamber system) ▣
AHA: 1Q,23

C7541 Diagnostic endoscopic retrograde cholangiopancreatography (ERCP), including collection of specimen(s) by brushing or washing, when performed, with endoscopic cannulation of papilla with direct visualization of pancreatic/common bile ducts(s) ▣
AHA: 1Q,23

C7542 Endoscopic retrograde cholangiopancreatography (ERCP) with biopsy, single or multiple, with endoscopic cannulation of papilla with direct visualization of pancreatic/common bile ducts(s) ▣
AHA: 1Q,23

C7543 Endoscopic retrograde cholangiopancreatography (ERCP) with sphincterotomy/papillotomy, with endoscopic cannulation of papilla with direct visualization of pancreatic/common bile ducts(s) ▣
AHA: 1Q,23

C7544 Endoscopic retrograde cholangiopancreatography (ERCP) with removal of calculi/debris from biliary/pancreatic duct(s), with endoscopic cannulation of papilla with direct visualization of pancreatic/common bile ducts(s) ▣
AHA: 1Q,23

C7545 Percutaneous exchange of biliary drainage catheter (e.g., external, internal-external, or conversion of internal-external to external only), with removal of calculi/debris from biliary duct(s) and/or gallbladder, including destruction of calculi by any method (e.g., mechanical, electrohydraulic, lithotripsy) when performed, including diagnostic cholangiography(ies) when performed, imaging guidance (e.g., fluoroscopy), and all associated radiological supervision and interpretation ▣
AHA: 1Q,23

C7546 Removal and replacement of externally accessible nephroureteral catheter (e.g., external/internal stent) requiring fluoroscopic guidance, with ureteral stricture balloon dilation, including imaging guidance and all associated radiological supervision and interpretation ▣
AHA: 1Q,23

C7547 Convert nephrostomy catheter to nephroureteral catheter, percutaneous via pre-existing nephrostomy tract, with ureteral stricture balloon dilation, including diagnostic nephrostogram and/or ureterogram when performed, imaging guidance (e.g., ultrasound and/or fluoroscopy) and all associated radiological supervision and interpretation ▣
AHA: 1Q,23

C7548 Exchange nephrostomy catheter, percutaneous, with ureteral stricture balloon dilation, including diagnostic nephrostogram and/or ureterogram when performed, imaging guidance (e.g., ultrasound and/or fluoroscopy) and all associated radiological supervision and interpretation ▣
AHA: 1Q,23

Special Coverage Instructions   Noncovered by Medicare   Carrier Discretion   ☑ Quantity Alert   ● New Code   ○ Recycled/Reinstated   ▲ Revised Code

Outpatient PPS

C7549 — C8908

C7549 Change of ureterostomy tube or externally accessible ureteral stent via ileal conduit with ureteral stricture balloon dilation, including imaging guidance (e.g., ultrasound and/or fluoroscopy) and all associated radiological supervision and interpretation [G2]
AHA: 1Q,23

C7550 Cystourethroscopy, with biopsy(ies) with adjunctive blue light cystoscopy with fluorescent imaging agent [G2]
AHA: 1Q,23

C7551 Excision of major peripheral nerve neuroma, except sciatic, with implantation of nerve end into bone or muscle [G2]
AHA: 1Q,23

C7552 Catheter placement in coronary artery(s) for coronary angiography, including intraprocedural injection(s) for coronary angiography, imaging supervision and interpretation; with catheter placement(s) in bypass graft(s) (internal mammary, free arterial, venous grafts) including intraprocedural injection(s) for bypass graft angiography and right heart catheterization with intravascular doppler velocity and/or pressure derived coronary flow reserve measurement (coronary vessel or graft) during coronary angiography including pharmacologically induced stress, initial vessel [G2]
AHA: 1Q,23

C7553 Catheter placement in coronary artery(s) for coronary angiography, including intraprocedural injection(s) for coronary angiography, imaging supervision and interpretation; with right and left heart catheterization including intraprocedural injection(s) for left ventriculography, when performed, catheter placement(s) in bypass graft(s) (internal mammary, free arterial, venous grafts) with bypass graft angiography with pharmacologic agent administration (e.g., inhaled nitric oxide, intravenous infusion of nitroprusside, dobutamine, milrinone, or other agent) including assessing hemodynamic measurements before, during, after and repeat pharmacologic agent administration, when performed [G2]
AHA: 1Q,23

C7554 Cystourethroscopy with adjunctive blue light cystoscopy with fluorescent imaging agent [G2]
AHA: 1Q,23

C7555 Thyroidectomy, total or complete with parathyroid autotransplantation [G2]
AHA: 1Q,23

● **C7556** Bronchoscopy, rigid or flexible, with bronchial alveolar lavage and transendoscopic endobronchial ultrasound (EBUS) during bronchoscopic diagnostic or therapeutic intervention(s) for peripheral lesion(s), including fluoroscopic guidance, when performed

● **C7557** Catheter placement in coronary artery(s) for coronary angiography, including intraprocedural injection(s) for coronary angiography, imaging supervision and interpretation with left heart catheterization including intraprocedural injection(s) for left ventriculography, when performed and intraprocedural coronary fractional flow reserve (FFR) with 3D functional mapping of color-coded FFR values for the coronary tree, derived from coronary angiogram data, for real-time review and interpretation of possible atherosclerotic stenosis(es) intervention

● **C7558** Catheter placement in coronary artery(s) for coronary angiography, including intraprocedural injection(s) for coronary angiography, imaging supervision and interpretation with right and left heart catheterization including intraprocedural injection(s) for left ventriculography, when performed, catheter placement(s) in bypass graft(s) (internal mammary, free arterial, venous grafts) with bypass graft angiography with pharmacologic agent administration (eg, inhaled nitric oxide, intravenous infusion of nitroprusside, dobutamine, milrinone, or other agent) including assessing hemodynamic measurements before, during, after and repeat pharmacologic agent administration, when performed

● **C7560** Endoscopic retrograde cholangiopancreatography (ERCP) with removal of foreign body(ies) or stent(s) from biliary/pancreatic duct(s) and endoscopic cannulation of papilla with direct visualization of pancreatic/common bile duct(s)

● **C7561** Debridement, bone (includes epidermis, dermis, subcutaneous tissue, muscle and/or fascia, if performed); first 20 sq cm or less with manual preparation and insertion of drug-delivery device(s), deep (e.g., subfascial)

C7900 Service for diagnosis, evaluation, or treatment of a mental health or substance use disorder, initial 15-29 minutes, provided remotely by hospital staff who are licensed to provide mental health services under applicable state law(s), when the patient is in their home, and there is no associated professional service
AHA: 1Q,23

C7901 Service for diagnosis, evaluation, or treatment of a mental health or substance use disorder, initial 30-60 minutes, provided remotely by hospital staff who are licensed to provided mental health services under applicable state law(s), when the patient is in their home, and there is no associated professional service
AHA: 1Q,23

C7902 Service for diagnosis, evaluation, or treatment of a mental health or substance use disorder, each additional 15 minutes, provided remotely by hospital staff who are licensed to provide mental health services under applicable state law(s), when the patient is in their home, and there is no associated professional service (list separately in addition to code for primary service)
AHA: 1Q,23

● **C7903** Group psychotherapy service for diagnosis, evaluation, or treatment of a mental health or substance use disorder provided remotely by hospital staff who are licensed to provide mental health services under applicable state law(s), when the patient is in their home, and there is no associated professional service

C8900 Magnetic resonance angiography with contrast, abdomen [Q3] [Z2] ⊘
CMS: 100-04,13,40.1.1; 100-04,13,40.1.2

C8901 Magnetic resonance angiography without contrast, abdomen [Q3] [Z2] ⊘
CMS: 100-04,13,40.1.1; 100-04,13,40.1.2

C8902 Magnetic resonance angiography without contrast followed by with contrast, abdomen [Q3] [Z2] ⊘
CMS: 100-04,13,40.1.1; 100-04,13,40.1.2

C8903 Magnetic resonance imaging with contrast, breast; unilateral [Q3] [Z2] ⊘

C8905 Magnetic resonance imaging without contrast followed by with contrast, breast; unilateral [Q3] [Z2] ⊘

C8906 Magnetic resonance imaging with contrast, breast; bilateral [Q3] [Z2] ⊘

C8908 Magnetic resonance imaging without contrast followed by with contrast, breast; bilateral [Q3] [Z2] ⊘

Special Coverage Instructions   Noncovered by Medicare   Carrier Discretion   ☑ Quantity Alert ● New Code   ○ Recycled/Reinstated   ▲ Revised Code

28 — C Codes   Ⓐ Age Edit   Ⓜ Maternity Edit   ♀ Female Only   ♂ Male Only   Ⓐ-Ⓨ OPPS Status Indicators   © 2023 Optum360, LLC

C8909 Magnetic resonance angiography with contrast, chest (excluding myocardium) 03 Z2 ⊘
CMS: 100-04,13,40.1.1; 100-04,13,40.1.2

C8910 Magnetic resonance angiography without contrast, chest (excluding myocardium) 03 Z2 ⊘
CMS: 100-04,13,40.1.1; 100-04,13,40.1.2

C8911 Magnetic resonance angiography without contrast followed by with contrast, chest (excluding myocardium) 03 Z2 ⊘
CMS: 100-04,13,40.1.1; 100-04,13,40.1.2

C8912 Magnetic resonance angiography with contrast, lower extremity 03 Z2 ⊘
CMS: 100-04,13,40.1.1; 100-04,13,40.1.2

C8913 Magnetic resonance angiography without contrast, lower extremity 03 Z2 ⊘
CMS: 100-04,13,40.1.1; 100-04,13,40.1.2

C8914 Magnetic resonance angiography without contrast followed by with contrast, lower extremity 03 Z2 ⊘
CMS: 100-04,13,40.1.1; 100-04,13,40.1.2

C8918 Magnetic resonance angiography with contrast, pelvis 03 Z2 ⊘
CMS: 100-04,13,40.1.1; 100-04,13,40.1.2

C8919 Magnetic resonance angiography without contrast, pelvis 03 Z2 ⊘
CMS: 100-04,13,40.1.1; 100-04,13,40.1.2

C8920 Magnetic resonance angiography without contrast followed by with contrast, pelvis 03 Z2 ⊘
CMS: 100-04,13,40.1.1; 100-04,13,40.1.2

C8921 Transthoracic echocardiography (TTE) with contrast, or without contrast followed by with contrast, for congenital cardiac anomalies, complete S
CMS: 100-04,4,200.7.2

C8922 Transthoracic echocardiography (TTE) with contrast, or without contrast followed by with contrast, for congenital cardiac anomalies; follow-up or limited study S

C8923 Transthoracic echocardiography (TTE) with contrast, or without contrast followed by with contrast, real-time with image documentation (2D), includes M-mode recording, when performed, complete, without spectral or color doppler echocardiography 0

C8924 Transthoracic echocardiography (TTE) with contrast, or without contrast followed by with contrast, real-time with image documentation (2D), includes M-mode recording when performed, follow-up or limited study S

C8925 Transesophageal echocardiography (TEE) with contrast, or without contrast followed by with contrast, real time with image documentation (2D) (with or without M-mode recording); including probe placement, image acquisition, interpretation and report S

C8926 Transesophageal echocardiography (TEE) with contrast, or without contrast followed by with contrast, for congenital cardiac anomalies; including probe placement, image acquisition, interpretation and report S

C8927 Transesophageal echocardiography (TEE) with contrast, or without contrast followed by with contrast, for monitoring purposes, including probe placement, real time (2D) image acquisition and interpretation leading to ongoing (continuous) assessment of (dynamically changing) cardiac pumping function and to therapeutic measures on an immediate time basis S

C8928 Transthoracic echocardiography (TTE) with contrast, or without contrast followed by with contrast, real-time with image documentation (2D), includes M-mode recording, when performed, during rest and cardiovascular stress test using treadmill, bicycle exercise and/or pharmacologically induced stress, with interpretation and report S

C8929 Transthoracic echocardiography (TTE) with contrast, or without contrast followed by with contrast, real-time with image documentation (2D), includes M-mode recording, when performed, complete, with spectral doppler echocardiography, and with color flow doppler echocardiography S

C8930 Transthoracic echocardiography (TTE) with contrast, or without contrast followed by with contrast, real-time with image documentation (2D), includes M-mode recording, when performed, during rest and cardiovascular stress test using treadmill, bicycle exercise and/or pharmacologically induced stress, with interpretation and report; including performance of continuous electrocardiographic monitoring, with physician supervision S

C8931 Magnetic resonance angiography with contrast, spinal canal and contents 03 Z2

C8932 Magnetic resonance angiography without contrast, spinal canal and contents 03 Z2

C8933 Magnetic resonance angiography without contrast followed by with contrast, spinal canal and contents 03 Z2

C8934 Magnetic resonance angiography with contrast, upper extremity 03 Z2

C8935 Magnetic resonance angiography without contrast, upper extremity 03 Z2

C8936 Magnetic resonance angiography without contrast followed by with contrast, upper extremity 03 Z2

C8937 Computer-aided detection, including computer algorithm analysis of breast MRI image data for lesion detection/characterization, pharmacokinetic analysis, with further physician review for interpretation (list separately in addition to code for primary procedure)

C8957 Intravenous infusion for therapy/diagnosis; initiation of prolonged infusion (more than 8 hours), requiring use of portable or implantable pump S
CMS: 100-04,4,230.2

C9046 Cocaine HCl nasal solution for topical administration, 1 mg N1
Use this code for Goprelto.
AHA: 1Q,23; 2Q,19

C9047 Injection, caplacizumab-yhdp, 1 mg K2
Use this code for Cablivi.
AHA: 3Q,19

C9067 Gallium Ga-68, Dotatoc, diagnostic, 0.01 mCi N1
AHA: 4Q,20

C9088 Instillation, bupivacaine and meloxicam, 1 mg/0.03 mg K2
Use this code for Zynrelef.
AHA: 1Q,22

C9089 Bupivacaine, collagen-matrix implant, 1 mg K2
Use this code for Xaracoll.
AHA: 1Q,22

C9101 Injection, oliceridine, 0.1 mg K2
Use this code for Olinvyk.
AHA: 4Q,22

C9113 Injection, pantoprazole sodium, per vial N N1 ☑
Use this code for Protonix.

Special Coverage Instructions   Noncovered by Medicare   Carrier Discretion   ☑ Quantity Alert   ● New Code   ○ Recycled/Reinstated   ▲ Revised Code

© 2023 Optum360, LLC   A2-Z3 ASC Pmt   CMS: IOM   AHA: Coding Clinic   ⅃ DMEPOS Paid   ⊘ SNF Excluded   C Codes — 29

C9143 Cocaine HCl nasal solution (Numbrino), 1 mg
Use this code for cocaine HCl (Numbrino) manufactured by Lannett.
AHA: 1Q,23

C9144 Injection, bupivacaine (Posimir), 1 mg ☒K2
AHA: 1Q,23

● **C9145** Injection, aprepitant, (Aponvie), 1 mg ☒K2
Use this code for Aponvie.
AHA: 2Q,23

~~C9146~~ ~~Injection, mirvetuximab soravtansine-gynx, 1 mg~~

~~C9147~~ ~~Injection, tremelimumab-actl, 1 mg~~

~~C9148~~ ~~Injection, teclistamab-cqyv, 0.5 mg~~

~~C9149~~ ~~Injection, teplizumab-mzwv, 5 mcg~~

● **C9150** Xenon Xe-129 hyperpolarized gas, diagnostic, per study dose
Use this code for Xenoview.
AHA: 3Q,23

~~C9151~~ ~~Injection, pegcetacoplan, 1 mg~~
To report, see ~J2781

~~C9152~~ ~~Injection, aripiprazole, (Abilify Asimtufii), 1 mg~~
To report, see ~J0402

~~C9153~~ ~~Injection, amisulpride, 1 mg~~
To report, see ~J0184

~~C9154~~ ~~Injection, buprenorphine extended-release (Brixadi), 1 mg~~
To report, see ~J0576

~~C9155~~ ~~Injection, epcoritamab-bysp, 0.16 mg~~
To report, see ~J9321

~~C9156~~ ~~Flotufolastat F-18, diagnostic, 1 mCi~~
To report, see ~A9608

~~C9157~~ ~~Injection, tofersen, 1 mg~~
To report, see ~J1304

~~C9158~~ ~~Injection, risperidone, (Uzedy), 1 mg~~
To report, see ~J2799

● **C9159** Injection, prothrombin complex concentrate (human), Balfaxar, per IU of Factor IX activity

● **C9160** Injection, daxibotulinumtoxina-lanm, 1 unit
Use this code for Daxxify.

● **C9161** Injection, aflibercept HD, 1 mg
Use this code for Eylea HD.

● **C9162** Injection, avacincaptad pegol, 0.1 mg
Use this code for Izervay.

● **C9163** Injection, talquetamab-tgvs, 0.25 mg
Use this code for Talvey.

● **C9164** Cantharidin for topical administration, 0.7%, single unit dose applicator (3.2 mg)
Use this code for Ycanth.

● **C9165** Injection, elranatamab-bcmm, 1 mg
Use this code for Elrexfio.

C9248 Injection, clevidipine butyrate, 1 mg ☒N ☒K2 ☑
Use this code for Cleviprex.

C9254 Injection, lacosamide, 1 mg ☒N ☒N1 ☑
Use this code for VIMPAT.

C9257 Injection, bevacizumab, 0.25 mg ☒K ☒K2 ☑
Use this code for Avastin.
CMS: 100-03,110.17

C9285 Lidocaine 70 mg/tetracaine 70 mg, per patch ☒N ☒N1 ☑
Use this code for SYNERA.

C9290 Injection, bupivacaine liposome, 1 mg ☒N ☒K2 ☑
Use this code for EXPAREL.
AHA: 1Q,23

C9293 Injection, glucarpidase, 10 units ☒K ☑
Use this code for Voraxaze.

C9352 Microporous collagen implantable tube (NeuraGen Nerve Guide), per cm length ☒N ☒N1 ☑

Damaged nerve

Healthy nerve

Artificial nerve conduit

A synthetic "bridge" is affixed to each end of a severed nerve with sutures. This procedure is performed using an operating microscope

C9353 Microporous collagen implantable slit tube (NeuraWrap Nerve Protector), per cm length ☒N ☒N1 ☑

C9354 Acellular pericardial tissue matrix of nonhuman origin (Veritas), per sq cm ☒N ☒N1 ☑

C9355 Collagen nerve cuff (NeuroMatrix), per 0.5 cm length ☒N ☒N1 ☑

C9356 Tendon, porous matrix of cross-linked collagen and glycosaminoglycan matrix (TenoGlide Tendon Protector Sheet), per sq cm ☒N ☒N1 ☑

C9358 Dermal substitute, native, nondenatured collagen, fetal bovine origin (SurgiMend Collagen Matrix), per 0.5 sq cm ☒N ☒N1 ☑

C9361 Collagen matrix nerve wrap (NeuroMend Collagen Nerve Wrap), per 0.5 cm length ☒N ☒N1 ☑

C9362 Porous purified collagen matrix bone void filler (Integra Mozaik Osteoconductive Scaffold Strip), per 0.5 cc ☒N ☒N1 ☑

C9363 Skin substitute (Integra Meshed Bilayer Wound Matrix), per sq cm ☒N ☒N1 ☑
CMS: 100-04,4,260.1; 100-04,4,260.1.1

C9364 Porcine implant, Permacol, per sq cm ☒N ☒N1 ☑

C9399 Unclassified drugs or biologicals ☒A ☒K7
CMS: 100-02,15,50.5; 100-04,17,90.3; 100-04,32,400; 100-04,32,400.1; 100-04,32,400.2; 100-04,32,400.2.1; 100-04,32,400.2.2; 100-04,32,400.2.3; 100-04,32,400.2.3.1; 100-04,32,400.2.4; 100-04,32,400.2.5; 100-04,32,400.3; 100-04,32,400.4; 100-04,4,260.1; 100-04,4,260.1.1
AHA: 3Q,23; 1Q,17

Special Coverage Instructions   Noncovered by Medicare   Carrier Discretion   ☑ Quantity Alert ● New Code ○ Recycled/Reinstated ▲ Revised Code

30 — C Codes   ☒A Age Edit   ☒M Maternity Edit   ♀ Female Only   ♂ Male Only   ☒A-Y OPPS Status Indicators   © 2023 Optum360, LLC

C9460	**Injection, cangrelor, 1 mg**	G K2 ☑

Use this code for Kengreal.

C9462	**Injection, delafloxacin, 1 mg**	G

Use this code for Baxdela.
AHA: 2Q,18

C9482	**Injection, sotalol HCl, 1 mg**	G K2 ☑

C9488	**Injection, conivaptan HCl, 1 mg**	G K2 ☑

Use this code for Vaprisol.

C9507	**Fresh frozen plasma, high titer COVID-19 convalescent, frozen within 8 hours of collection, each unit**	

AHA: 2Q,22

C9600	**Percutaneous transcatheter placement of drug eluting intracoronary stent(s), with coronary angioplasty when performed; single major coronary artery or branch**	J J8

AHA: 2Q,23; 4Q,21

C9601	**Percutaneous transcatheter placement of drug-eluting intracoronary stent(s), with coronary angioplasty when performed; each additional branch of a major coronary artery (list separately in addition to code for primary procedure)**	N N1

AHA: 2Q,23

C9602	**Percutaneous transluminal coronary atherectomy, with drug eluting intracoronary stent, with coronary angioplasty when performed; single major coronary artery or branch**	J

AHA: 2Q,23; 4Q,21

C9603	**Percutaneous transluminal coronary atherectomy, with drug-eluting intracoronary stent, with coronary angioplasty when performed; each additional branch of a major coronary artery (list separately in addition to code for primary procedure)**	N

AHA: 2Q,23

C9604	**Percutaneous transluminal revascularization of or through coronary artery bypass graft (internal mammary, free arterial, venous), any combination of drug-eluting intracoronary stent, atherectomy and angioplasty, including distal protection when performed; single vessel**	J

AHA: 2Q,23

C9605	**Percutaneous transluminal revascularization of or through coronary artery bypass graft (internal mammary, free arterial, venous), any combination of drug-eluting intracoronary stent, atherectomy and angioplasty, including distal protection when performed; each additional branch subtended by the bypass graft (list separately in addition to code for primary procedure)**	N

AHA: 2Q,23

C9606	**Percutaneous transluminal revascularization of acute total/subtotal occlusion during acute myocardial infarction, coronary artery or coronary artery bypass graft, any combination of drug-eluting intracoronary stent, atherectomy and angioplasty, including aspiration thrombectomy when performed, single vessel**	J

CMS: 100-04,4,260.1; 100-04,4,260.1.1
AHA: 2Q,23; 1Q,19

C9607	**Percutaneous transluminal revascularization of chronic total occlusion, coronary artery, coronary artery branch, or coronary artery bypass graft, any combination of drug-eluting intracoronary stent, atherectomy and angioplasty; single vessel**	J

AHA: 2Q,23; 4Q,21

C9608	**Percutaneous transluminal revascularization of chronic total occlusion, coronary artery, coronary artery branch, or coronary artery bypass graft, any combination of drug-eluting intracoronary stent, atherectomy and angioplasty; each additional coronary artery, coronary artery branch, or bypass graft (list separately in addition to code for primary procedure)**	N

AHA: 2Q,23

C9725	**Placement of endorectal intracavitary applicator for high intensity brachytherapy**	T G2 ⊘

C9726	**Placement and removal (if performed) of applicator into breast for intraoperative radiation therapy, add-on to primary breast procedure**	N N1

C9727	**Insertion of implants into the soft palate; minimum of three implants**	T G2 ☑

C9728	**Placement of interstitial device(s) for radiation therapy/surgery guidance (e.g., fiducial markers, dosimeter), for other than the following sites (any approach): abdomen, pelvis, prostate, retroperitoneum, thorax, single or multiple**	S J8

AHA: 2Q,18

C9733	**Nonophthalmic fluorescent vascular angiography**	Q2

AHA: 1Q,23

C9734	**Focused ultrasound ablation/therapeutic intervention, other than uterine leiomyomata, with magnetic resonance (MR) guidance**	J

C9738	**Adjunctive blue light cystoscopy with fluorescent imaging agent (list separately in addition to code for primary procedure)**	N N1

C9739	**Cystourethroscopy, with insertion of transprostatic implant; one to three implants**	♂ J J8

C9740	**Cystourethroscopy, with insertion of transprostatic implant; four or more implants**	♂ J J8

C9751	**Bronchoscopy, rigid or flexible, transbronchial ablation of lesion(s) by microwave energy, including fluoroscopic guidance, when performed, with computed tomography acquisition(s) and 3D rendering, computer-assisted, image-guided navigation, and endobronchial ultrasound (EBUS) guided transtracheal and/or transbronchial sampling (e.g., aspiration[s]/biopsy[ies]) and all mediastinal and/or hilar lymph node stations or structures and therapeutic intervention(s)**	

CMS: 100-04,4,260.1; 100-04,4,260.1.1
AHA: 1Q,19

C9756	**Intraoperative near-infrared fluorescence lymphatic mapping of lymph node(s) (sentinel or tumor draining) with administration of indocyanine green (ICG) (List separately in addition to code for primary procedure)**	

AHA: 1Q,21; 3Q,19

C9757	**Laminotomy (hemilaminectomy), with decompression of nerve root(s), including partial facetectomy, foraminotomy and excision of herniated intervertebral disc, and repair of annular defect with implantation of bone anchored annular closure device, including annular defect measurement, alignment and sizing assessment, and image guidance; 1 interspace, lumbar**	J8

AHA: 1Q,20

C9758	**Blind procedure for NYHA Class III/IV heart failure; transcatheter implantation of interatrial shunt including right heart catheterization, transesophageal echocardiography (TEE)/intracardiac echocardiography (ICE), and all imaging with or without guidance (e.g., ultrasound, fluoroscopy), performed in an approved investigational device exemption (IDE) study**	

Special Coverage Instructions   Noncovered by Medicare   Carrier Discretion   ☑ Quantity Alert ● New Code   ○ Recycled/Reinstated ▲ Revised Code

© 2023 Optum360, LLC   A2–Z3 ASC Pmt   CMS: IOM   AHA: Coding Clinic   ⅏ DMEPOS Paid   ⊘ SNF Excluded   C Codes — 31

C9759 Transcatheter intraoperative blood vessel microinfusion(s) (e.g., intraluminal, vascular wall and/or perivascular) therapy, any vessel, including radiological supervision and interpretation, when performed N1
AHA: 2Q,20

C9760 Nonrandomized, nonblinded procedure for NYHA Class II, III, IV heart failure; transcatheter implantation of interatrial shunt, including right and left heart catheterization, transseptal puncture, transesophageal echocardiography (TEE)/intracardiac echocardiography (ICE), and all imaging with or without guidance (e.g., ultrasound, fluoroscopy), performed in an approved investigational device exemption (IDE) study
AHA: 2Q,20

C9761 Cystourethroscopy, with ureteroscopy and/or pyeloscopy, with lithotripsy, and ureteral catheterization for steerable vacuum aspiration of the kidney, collecting system, ureter, bladder, and urethra if applicable (must use a steerable ureteral catheter) G2
AHA: 1Q,23; 2Q,21; 4Q,20

C9762 Cardiac magnetic resonance imaging for morphology and function, quantification of segmental dysfunction; with strain imaging Z2
AHA: 2Q,20

C9763 Cardiac magnetic resonance imaging for morphology and function, quantification of segmental dysfunction; with stress imaging Z2
AHA: 2Q,20

C9764 Revascularization, endovascular, open or percutaneous, lower extremity artery(ies), except tibial/peroneal; with intravascular lithotripsy, includes angioplasty within the same vessel(s), when performed J8
AHA: 2Q,20

C9765 Revascularization, endovascular, open or percutaneous, lower extremity artery(ies), except tibial/peroneal; with intravascular lithotripsy, and transluminal stent placement(s), includes angioplasty within the same vessel(s), when performed J8
AHA: 2Q,20

C9766 Revascularization, endovascular, open or percutaneous, lower extremity artery(ies), except tibial/peroneal; with intravascular lithotripsy and atherectomy, includes angioplasty within the same vessel(s), when performed J8
AHA: 2Q,20

C9767 Revascularization, endovascular, open or percutaneous, lower extremity artery(ies), except tibial/peroneal; with intravascular lithotripsy and transluminal stent placement(s), and atherectomy, includes angioplasty within the same vessel(s), when performed J8
AHA: 2Q,20

C9768 Endoscopic ultrasound-guided direct measurement of hepatic portosystemic pressure gradient by any method (list separately in addition to code for primary procedure)
AHA: 2Q,23; 4Q,20

C9769 Cystourethroscopy, with insertion of temporary prostatic implant/stent with fixation/anchor and incisional struts ♂ J8
AHA: 4Q,20

C9770 Vitrectomy, mechanical, pars plana approach, with subretinal injection of pharmacologic/biologic agent

C9771 Nasal/sinus endoscopy, cryoablation nasal tissue(s) and/or nerve(s), unilateral or bilateral

C9772 Revascularization, endovascular, open or percutaneous, tibial/peroneal artery(ies), with intravascular lithotripsy, includes angioplasty within the same vessel(s), when performed J8
AHA: 1Q,21

C9773 Revascularization, endovascular, open or percutaneous, tibial/peroneal artery(ies); with intravascular lithotripsy, and transluminal stent placement(s), includes angioplasty within the same vessel(s), when performed J8
AHA: 1Q,21

C9775 Revascularization, endovascular, open or percutaneous, tibial/peroneal artery(ies); with intravascular lithotripsy and transluminal stent placement(s), and atherectomy, includes angioplasty within the same vessel(s), when performed J8
AHA: 1Q,21

C9776 Intraoperative near-infrared fluorescence imaging of major extra-hepatic bile duct(s) (e.g., cystic duct, common bile duct and common hepatic duct) with intravenous administration of indocyanine green (ICG) (list separately in addition to code for primary procedure) N1
AHA: 2Q,23; 1Q,22; 2Q,21

C9777 Esophageal mucosal integrity testing by electrical impedance, transoral, includes esophagoscopy or esophagogastroduodenoscopy J8
AHA: 2Q,21

C9779 Endoscopic submucosal dissection (ESD), including endoscopy or colonoscopy, mucosal closure, when performed
AHA: 3Q,23; 4Q,21

C9780 Insertion of central venous catheter through central venous occlusion via inferior and superior approaches (e.g., inside-out technique), including imaging guidance
AHA: 4Q,21

C9781 Arthroscopy, shoulder, surgical; with implantation of subacromial spacer (e.g., balloon), includes debridement (e.g., limited or extensive), subacromial decompression, acromioplasty, and biceps tenodesis when performed J8
AHA: 2Q,22

C9782 Blinded procedure for New York Heart Association (NYHA) Class II or III heart failure, or Canadian Cardiovascular Society (CCS) Class III or IV chronic refractory angina; transcatheter intramyocardial transplantation of autologous bone marrow cells (e.g., mononuclear) or placebo control, autologous bone marrow harvesting and preparation for transplantation, left heart catheterization including ventriculography, all laboratory services, and all imaging with or without guidance (e.g., transthoracic echocardiography, ultrasound, fluoroscopy), performed in an approved investigational device exemption (IDE) study
AHA: 2Q,22

C9783 Blinded procedure for transcatheter implantation of coronary sinus reduction device or placebo control, including vascular access and closure, right heart catherization, venous and coronary sinus angiography, imaging guidance and supervision and interpretation when performed in an approved investigational device exemption (IDE) study
AHA: 2Q,22

● **C9784** Gastric restrictive procedure, endoscopic sleeve gastroplasty, with esophagogastroduodenoscopy and intraluminal tube insertion, if performed, including all system and tissue anchoring components
AHA: 3Q,23

● **C9785** Endoscopic outlet reduction, gastric pouch application, with endoscopy and intraluminal tube insertion, if performed, including all system and tissue anchoring components
AHA: 3Q,23

● **C9786** Echocardiography image post processing for computer aided detection of heart failure with preserved ejection fraction, including interpretation and report
AHA: 3Q,23

Special Coverage Instructions   Noncovered by Medicare   Carrier Discretion   ☑ Quantity Alert ● New Code   ○ Recycled/Reinstated   ▲ Revised Code

32 — C Codes   A Age Edit   M Maternity Edit   ♀ Female Only   ♂ Male Only   A-Y OPPS Status Indicators   © 2023 Optum360, LLC

● **C9787** **Gastric electrophysiology mapping with simultaneous patient symptom profiling**
AHA: 3Q,23

~~C9788~~ ~~Opto-acoustic imaging, breast (including axilla when performed), unilateral, with image documentation, analysis and report, obtained with ultrasound examination~~

● **C9789** **Instillation of antineoplastic pharmacologic/biologic agent into renal pelvis, any method, including all imaging guidance, including volumetric measurement if performed** G2

● **C9790** **Histotripsy (i.e., nonthermal ablation via acoustic energy delivery) of malignant renal tissue, including image guidance** G2

● **C9791** **Magnetic resonance imaging with inhaled hyperpolarized xenon-129 contrast agent, chest, including preparation and administration of agent**

● **C9792** **Blinded or nonblinded procedure for symptomatic New York Heart Association (NYHA) Class II, III, IVA heart failure; transcatheter implantation of left atrial to coronary sinus shunt using jugular vein access, including all imaging necessary to intra procedurally map the coronary sinus for optimal shunt placement (e.g., transesophageal echocardiography (TTE), intracardiac echocardiography (ICE), fluoroscopy), performed under general anesthesia in an approved investigational device exemption (IDE) study**

● **C9793** **3D predictive model generation for preplanning of a cardiac procedure, using data from cardiac computed tomographic angiography with report**

● **C9794** **Therapeutic radiology simulation-aided field setting; complex, including acquisition of PET and CT imaging data required for radiopharmaceutical-directed radiation therapy treatment planning (i.e., modeling)**

● **C9795** **Stereotactic body radiation therapy, treatment delivery, per fraction to 1 or more lesions, including image guidance and real-time positron emissions-based delivery adjustments to 1 or more lesions, entire course not to exceed 5 fractions**

~~C9803~~ ~~Hospital outpatient clinic visit specimen collection for severe acute respiratory syndrome coronavirus 2 (SARS-CoV-2) (coronavirus disease [COVID-19]), any specimen source~~

C9898 **Radiolabeled product provided during a hospital inpatient stay** N
CMS: 100-04,4,260.1; 100-04,4,260.1.1

C9899 **Implanted prosthetic device, payable only for inpatients who do not have inpatient coverage** A

Special Coverage Instructions   Noncovered by Medicare   Carrier Discretion   ☑ Quantity Alert   ● New Code   ○ Recycled/Reinstated   ▲ Revised Code

© 2023 Optum360, LLC   A2-Z3 ASC Pmt   CMS: IOM   AHA: Coding Clinic   ⅃ DMEPOS Paid   ⊘ SNF Excluded   C Codes — 33

Durable Medical Equipment E0100-E8002

E codes include durable medical equipment such as canes, crutches, walkers, commodes, decubitus care, bath and toilet aids, hospital beds, oxygen and related respiratory equipment, monitoring equipment, pacemakers, patient lifts, safety equipment, restraints, traction equipment, fracture frames, wheelchairs, and artificial kidney machines.

Canes

E0100   **Cane, includes canes of all materials, adjustable or fixed, with tip**   Y & (NU, RR, UE)
White canes for the blind are not covered under Medicare.

E0105   **Cane, quad or three-prong, includes canes of all materials, adjustable or fixed, with tips**   Y & (NU, RR, UE)

Crutches

E0110   **Crutches, forearm, includes crutches of various materials, adjustable or fixed, pair, complete with tips and handgrips**   Y ☑ & (NU, RR, UE)

Forearm cuff

Axilla pad

Standard underarm crutch (E0112-E0117)

Hand grip

Hand grip

Adjustment

Standard forearm crutch (L0110–L0111)

E0111   **Crutch, forearm, includes crutches of various materials, adjustable or fixed, each, with tip and handgrips**   Y ☑ & (NU, RR, UE)

E0112   **Crutches, underarm, wood, adjustable or fixed, pair, with pads, tips, and handgrips**   Y ☑ & (NU, RR, UE)

E0113   **Crutch, underarm, wood, adjustable or fixed, each, with pad, tip, and handgrip**   Y ☑ & (NU, RR, UE)

E0114   **Crutches, underarm, other than wood, adjustable or fixed, pair, with pads, tips, and handgrips**   Y ☑ & (NU, RR, UE)

E0116   **Crutch, underarm, other than wood, adjustable or fixed, with pad, tip, handgrip, with or without shock absorber, each**   Y ☑ & (NU, RR, UE)

E0117   **Crutch, underarm, articulating, spring assisted, each**   Y ☑ & (RR)

E0118   **Crutch substitute, lower leg platform, with or without wheels, each**   E ☑
Medicare covers walkers if patient's ambulation is impaired.

Walkers

E0130   **Walker, rigid (pickup), adjustable or fixed height**   Y & (NU, RR, UE)
CMS: 100-04,36,50.15

E0135   **Walker, folding (pickup), adjustable or fixed height**   Y & (NU, RR, UE)
Medicare covers walkers if patient's ambulation is impaired.
CMS: 100-04,36,50.15

E0140   **Walker, with trunk support, adjustable or fixed height, any type**   Y & (RR)
CMS: 100-04,36,50.15

E0141   **Walker, rigid, wheeled, adjustable or fixed height**   Y & (NU, RR, UE)
Medicare covers walkers if patient's ambulation is impaired.
CMS: 100-04,36,50.15

E0143   **Walker, folding, wheeled, adjustable or fixed height**   Y & (NU, RR, UE)
Medicare covers walkers if patient's ambulation is impaired.
CMS: 100-04,36,50.15

E0144   **Walker, enclosed, four-sided framed, rigid or folding, wheeled with posterior seat**   Y & (RR)
CMS: 100-04,36,50.15

E0147   **Walker, heavy-duty, multiple braking system, variable wheel resistance**   Y & (NU, RR, UE)
Medicare covers safety roller walkers only in patients with severe neurological disorders or restricted use of one hand. In some cases, coverage will be extended to patients with a weight exceeding the limits of a standard wheeled walker.
CMS: 100-04,36,50.15

E0148   **Walker, heavy-duty, without wheels, rigid or folding, any type, each**   Y ☑ & (NU, RR, UE)
CMS: 100-04,36,50.15

E0149   **Walker, heavy-duty, wheeled, rigid or folding, any type**   Y & (RR)
CMS: 100-04,36,50.15

Attachments

E0153   **Platform attachment, forearm crutch, each**   Y ☑ & (NU, RR, UE)

E0154   **Platform attachment, walker, each**   Y ☑ & (NU, RR, UE)
CMS: 100-04,36,50.14; 100-04,36,50.15

E0155   **Wheel attachment, rigid pick-up walker, per pair**   Y ☑ & (NU, RR, UE)
CMS: 100-04,36,50.15

E0156   **Seat attachment, walker**   Y & (NU, RR, UE)
CMS: 100-04,36,50.14; 100-04,36,50.15

E0157   **Crutch attachment, walker, each**   Y ☑ & (NU, RR, UE)
CMS: 100-04,36,50.14; 100-04,36,50.15

E0158   **Leg extensions for walker, per set of four**   Y ☑ & (NU, RR, UE)
CMS: 100-04,36,50.14; 100-04,36,50.15

E0159   **Brake attachment for wheeled walker, replacement, each**   Y ☑ & (NU, RR, UE)
CMS: 100-04,36,50.15

Commodes

E0160   **Sitz type bath or equipment, portable, used with or without commode**   Y & (NU, RR, UE)
Medicare covers sitz baths if medical record indicates that the patient has an infection or injury of the perineal area and the sitz bath is prescribed by the physician.

E0161   **Sitz type bath or equipment, portable, used with or without commode, with faucet attachment(s)**   Y & (NU, RR, UE)
Medicare covers sitz baths if medical record indicates that the patient has an infection or injury of the perineal area and the sitz bath is prescribed by the physician.

Special Coverage Instructions   Noncovered by Medicare   Carrier Discretion   ☑ Quantity Alert   ● New Code   ○ Recycled/Reinstated   ▲ Revised Code

© 2023 Optum360, LLC   A2-Z3 ASC Pmt   CMS: IOM   AHA: Coding Clinic   & DMEPOS Paid   ○ SNF Excluded   E Codes — 35

Durable Medical Equipment

E0162 — E0240

E0162 Sitz bath chair ☑ ﭑ (NU, RR, UE)
Medicare covers sitz baths if medical record indicates that the patient has an infection or injury of the perineal area and the sitz bath is prescribed by the physician.

E0163 Commode chair, mobile or stationary, with fixed arms ☑ ﭑ (NU, RR, UE)
Medicare covers commodes for patients confined to their beds or rooms, for patients without indoor bathroom facilities, and to patients who cannot climb or descend the stairs necessary to reach the bathrooms in their homes.

E0165 Commode chair, mobile or stationary, with detachable arms ☑ ﭑ (RR)
Medicare covers commodes for patients confined to their beds or rooms, for patients without indoor bathroom facilities, and to patients who cannot climb or descend the stairs necessary to reach the bathrooms in their homes.

E0167 Pail or pan for use with commode chair, replacement only ☑ ﭑ (NU, RR, UE)
Medicare covers commodes for patients confined to their beds or rooms, for patients without indoor bathroom facilities, and to patients who cannot climb or descend the stairs necessary to reach the bathrooms in their homes.

E0168 Commode chair, extra wide and/or heavy-duty, stationary or mobile, with or without arms, any type, each ☑ ☑ ﭑ (NU, RR, UE)

E0170 Commode chair with integrated seat lift mechanism, electric, any type ☑ ﭑ (RR)

E0171 Commode chair with integrated seat lift mechanism, nonelectric, any type ☑ ﭑ (RR)

E0172 Seat lift mechanism placed over or on top of toilet, any type ☑

E0175 Footrest, for use with commode chair, each ☑ ☑ ﭑ (NU, RR, UE)

Decubitus Care Equipment

E0181 Powered pressure reducing mattress overlay/pad, alternating, with pump, includes heavy-duty ☑ ﭑ (RR)
For Medicare coverage, a detailed written order must be received by the supplier before a claim is submitted.

E0182 Pump for alternating pressure pad, for replacement only ☑ ﭑ (RR)
For Medicare coverage, a detailed written order must be received by the supplier before a claim is submitted.

E0183 Powered pressure reducing underlay/pad, alternating, with pump, includes heavy duty (RR)

E0184 Dry pressure mattress ☑ ﭑ (NU, RR, UE)
For Medicare coverage, a detailed written order must be received by the supplier before a claim is submitted.

E0185 Gel or gel-like pressure pad for mattress, standard mattress length and width ☑ ﭑ (NU, RR, UE)
For Medicare coverage, a detailed written order must be received by the supplier before a claim is submitted.

E0186 Air pressure mattress ☑ ﭑ (RR)
For Medicare coverage, a detailed written order must be received by the supplier before a claim is submitted.

E0187 Water pressure mattress ☑ ﭑ (RR)
For Medicare coverage, a detailed written order must be received by the supplier before a claim is submitted.

E0188 Synthetic sheepskin pad ☑ ﭑ (NU, RR, UE)
For Medicare coverage, a detailed written order must be received by the supplier before a claim is submitted.

E0189 Lambswool sheepskin pad, any size ☑ ﭑ (NU, RR, UE)
For Medicare coverage, a detailed written order must be received by the supplier before a claim is submitted.

E0190 Positioning cushion/pillow/wedge, any shape or size, includes all components and accessories ☑

E0191 Heel or elbow protector, each ☑ ☑ ﭑ (NU, RR, UE)

E0193 Powered air flotation bed (low air loss therapy) ☑ ﭑ (RR)

E0194 Air fluidized bed ☑ ﭑ (RR)
An air fluidized bed is covered by Medicare if the patient has a stage 3 or stage 4 pressure sore and, without the bed, would require institutionalization. For Medicare coverage, a detailed written order must be received by the supplier before a claim is submitted.

E0196 Gel pressure mattress ☑ ﭑ (RR)
Medicare covers pads if physicians supervise their use in patients who have decubitus ulcers or susceptibility to them. For Medicare coverage, a detailed written order must be received by the supplier before a claim is submitted.

E0197 Air pressure pad for mattress, standard mattress length and width ☑ ﭑ (RR)
Medicare covers pads if physicians supervise their use in patients who have decubitus ulcers or susceptibility to them. For Medicare coverage, a detailed written order must be received by the supplier before a claim is submitted.

E0198 Water pressure pad for mattress, standard mattress length and width ☑ ﭑ (RR)
Medicare covers pads if physicians supervise their use in patients who have decubitus ulcers or susceptibility to them. For Medicare coverage, a detailed written order must be received by the supplier before a claim is submitted.

E0199 Dry pressure pad for mattress, standard mattress length and width ☑ ﭑ (NU, RR, UE)
Medicare covers pads if physicians supervise their use in patients who have decubitus ulcers or susceptibility to them. For Medicare coverage, a detailed written order must be received by the supplier before a claim is submitted.

Heat/Cold Application

E0200 Heat lamp, without stand (table model), includes bulb, or infrared element ☑ ﭑ (NU, RR, UE)

E0202 Phototherapy (bilirubin) light with photometer ☑ ﭑ (RR)

E0203 Therapeutic lightbox, minimum 10,000 lux, table top model ☑

E0205 Heat lamp, with stand, includes bulb, or infrared element ☑ ﭑ (NU, RR, UE)

E0210 Electric heat pad, standard ☑ ﭑ (NU, RR, UE)

E0215 Electric heat pad, moist ☑ ﭑ (NU, RR, UE)

E0217 Water circulating heat pad with pump ☑ ﭑ (NU, RR, UE)

E0218 Fluid circulating cold pad with pump, any type ☑

E0221 Infrared heating pad system ☑

E0225 Hydrocollator unit, includes pads ☑ ﭑ (NU, RR, UE)

E0231 Noncontact wound-warming device (temperature control unit, AC adapter and power cord) for use with warming card and wound cover ☑

E0232 Warming card for use with the noncontact wound-warming device and noncontact wound-warming wound cover ☑

E0235 Paraffin bath unit, portable (see medical supply code A4265 for paraffin) ☑ ﭑ (RR)

E0236 Pump for water circulating pad ☑ ﭑ (RR)

E0239 Hydrocollator unit, portable ☑ ﭑ (NU, RR, UE)

Bath and Toilet Aids

E0240 Bath/shower chair, with or without wheels, any size ☑

Special Coverage Instructions   Noncovered by Medicare   Carrier Discretion   ☑ Quantity Alert ● New Code   ○ Recycled/Reinstated ▲ Revised Code

36 — E Codes   Ⓐ Age Edit   Ⓜ Maternity Edit   ♀ Female Only   ♂ Male Only   Ⓐ-Ⓨ OPPS Status Indicators   © 2023 Optum360, LLC

E0241	Bathtub wall rail, each	☒ ☑
E0242	Bathtub rail, floor base	☒
E0243	Toilet rail, each	☒ ☑
E0244	Raised toilet seat	☒
E0245	Tub stool or bench	☒
E0246	Transfer tub rail attachment	☒
E0247	Transfer bench for tub or toilet with or without commode opening	☒
E0248	Transfer bench, heavy-duty, for tub or toilet with or without commode opening	☒
E0249	Pad for water circulating heat unit, for replacement only	Ⓨ ♿ (NU, RR, UE)

Hospital Beds and Accessories

E0250	Hospital bed, fixed height, with any type side rails, with mattress	Ⓨ ♿ (RR)
E0251	Hospital bed, fixed height, with any type side rails, without mattress	Ⓨ ♿ (RR)
E0255	Hospital bed, variable height, hi-lo, with any type side rails, with mattress	Ⓨ ♿ (RR)
E0256	Hospital bed, variable height, hi-lo, with any type side rails, without mattress	Ⓨ ♿ (RR)
E0260	Hospital bed, semi-electric (head and foot adjustment), with any type side rails, with mattress	Ⓨ ♿ (RR)
E0261	Hospital bed, semi-electric (head and foot adjustment), with any type side rails, without mattress	Ⓨ ♿ (RR)
E0265	Hospital bed, total electric (head, foot, and height adjustments), with any type side rails, with mattress	Ⓨ ♿ (RR)
E0266	Hospital bed, total electric (head, foot, and height adjustments), with any type side rails, without mattress	Ⓨ ♿ (RR)
E0270	Hospital bed, institutional type includes: oscillating, circulating and Stryker frame, with mattress	☒
E0271	Mattress, innerspring **CMS:** 100-04,36,50.14	Ⓨ ♿ (NU, RR, UE)
E0272	Mattress, foam rubber **CMS:** 100-04,36,50.14	Ⓨ ♿ (NU, RR, UE)
E0273	Bed board	☒
E0274	Over-bed table	☒
E0275	Bed pan, standard, metal or plastic Reusable, autoclavable bedpans are covered by Medicare for bed-confined patients.	Ⓨ ♿ (NU, RR, UE)
E0276	Bed pan, fracture, metal or plastic Reusable, autoclavable bedpans are covered by Medicare for bed-confined patients.	Ⓨ ♿ (NU, RR, UE)
E0277	Powered pressure-reducing air mattress	Ⓨ ♿ (RR)
E0280	Bed cradle, any type **CMS:** 100-04,36,50.14	Ⓨ ♿ (NU, RR, UE)
E0290	Hospital bed, fixed height, without side rails, with mattress	Ⓨ ♿ (RR)
E0291	Hospital bed, fixed height, without side rails, without mattress	Ⓨ ♿ (RR)
E0292	Hospital bed, variable height, hi-lo, without side rails, with mattress	Ⓨ ♿ (RR)
E0293	Hospital bed, variable height, hi-lo, without side rails, without mattress	Ⓨ ♿ (RR)

E0294	Hospital bed, semi-electric (head and foot adjustment), without side rails, with mattress	Ⓨ ♿ (RR)
E0295	Hospital bed, semi-electric (head and foot adjustment), without side rails, without mattress	Ⓨ ♿ (RR)
E0296	Hospital bed, total electric (head, foot, and height adjustments), without side rails, with mattress	Ⓨ ♿ (RR)
E0297	Hospital bed, total electric (head, foot, and height adjustments), without side rails, without mattress	Ⓨ ♿ (RR)
E0300	Pediatric crib, hospital grade, fully enclosed, with or without top enclosure	Ⓨ ♿ (RR)
E0301	Hospital bed, heavy-duty, extra wide, with weight capacity greater than 350 pounds, but less than or equal to 600 pounds, with any type side rails, without mattress	Ⓨ ♿ (RR)
E0302	Hospital bed, extra heavy-duty, extra wide, with weight capacity greater than 600 pounds, with any type side rails, without mattress	Ⓨ ♿ (RR)
E0303	Hospital bed, heavy-duty, extra wide, with weight capacity greater than 350 pounds, but less than or equal to 600 pounds, with any type side rails, with mattress	Ⓨ ♿ (RR)
E0304	Hospital bed, extra heavy-duty, extra wide, with weight capacity greater than 600 pounds, with any type side rails, with mattress	Ⓨ ♿ (RR)
E0305	Bedside rails, half-length	Ⓨ ♿ (RR)
E0310	Bedside rails, full-length **CMS:** 100-04,36,50.14	Ⓨ ♿ (NU, RR, UE)
E0315	Bed accessory: board, table, or support device, any type	☒
E0316	Safety enclosure frame/canopy for use with hospital bed, any type	Ⓨ ♿ (RR)
E0325	Urinal; male, jug-type, any material	♂ Ⓨ ♿ (NU, RR, UE)
E0326	Urinal; female, jug-type, any material	Ⓐ ♀ Ⓨ ♿ (NU, RR, UE)
E0328	Hospital bed, pediatric, manual, 360 degree side enclosures, top of headboard, footboard and side rails up to 24 in above the spring, includes mattress	Ⓨ
E0329	Hospital bed, pediatric, electric or semi-electric, 360 degree side enclosures, top of headboard, footboard and side rails up to 24 in above the spring, includes mattress	Ⓨ
E0350	Control unit for electronic bowel irrigation/evacuation system	☒
E0352	Disposable pack (water reservoir bag, speculum, valving mechanism, and collection bag/box) for use with the electronic bowel irrigation/evacuation system	☒
E0370	Air pressure elevator for heel	☒
E0371	Nonpowered advanced pressure reducing overlay for mattress, standard mattress length and width	Ⓨ ♿ (RR)
E0372	Powered air overlay for mattress, standard mattress length and width	Ⓨ ♿ (RR)
E0373	Nonpowered advanced pressure reducing mattress	Ⓨ ♿ (RR)

Special Coverage Instructions   Noncovered by Medicare   Carrier Discretion   ☑ Quantity Alert   ● New Code   ○ Recycled/Reinstated   ▲ Revised Code

Durable Medical Equipment

E0424 — E0493

Oxygen and Related Respiratory Equipment

E0424 Stationary compressed gaseous oxygen system, rental; includes container, contents, regulator, flowmeter, humidifier, nebulizer, cannula or mask, and tubing Ⓨ ♿ (RR)

For the first claim filed for home oxygen equipment or therapy, submit a certificate of medical necessity that includes the oxygen flow rate, anticipated frequency and duration of oxygen therapy, and physician signature. Medicare accepts oxygen therapy as medically necessary in cases documenting any of the following: erythocythemia with a hematocrit greater than 56 percent; a P pulmonale on EKG; or dependent edema consistent with congestive heart failure.
CMS: 100-04,20,130.6; 100-04,20,30.6

E0425 Stationary compressed gas system, purchase; includes regulator, flowmeter, humidifier, nebulizer, cannula or mask, and tubing ⒺⒾ

E0430 Portable gaseous oxygen system, purchase; includes regulator, flowmeter, humidifier, cannula or mask, and tubing ⒺⒾ

E0431 Portable gaseous oxygen system, rental; includes portable container, regulator, flowmeter, humidifier, cannula or mask, and tubing Ⓨ ♿ (RR)
CMS: 100-04,20,130.6

E0433 Portable liquid oxygen system, rental; home liquefier used to fill portable liquid oxygen containers, includes portable containers, regulator, flowmeter, humidifier, cannula or mask and tubing, with or without supply reservoir and contents gauge Ⓨ ♿ (RR)
CMS: 100-04,20,130.6

E0434 Portable liquid oxygen system, rental; includes portable container, supply reservoir, humidifier, flowmeter, refill adaptor, contents gauge, cannula or mask, and tubing Ⓨ ♿ (RR)
CMS: 100-04,20,130.6

E0435 Portable liquid oxygen system, purchase; includes portable container, supply reservoir, flowmeter, humidifier, contents gauge, cannula or mask, tubing and refill adaptor ⒺⒾ

E0439 Stationary liquid oxygen system, rental; includes container, contents, regulator, flowmeter, humidifier, nebulizer, cannula or mask, & tubing Ⓨ ♿ (RR)
CMS: 100-04,20,130.6

E0440 Stationary liquid oxygen system, purchase; includes use of reservoir, contents indicator, regulator, flowmeter, humidifier, nebulizer, cannula or mask, and tubing ⒺⒾ

E0441 Stationary oxygen contents, gaseous, 1 month's supply = 1 unit Ⓨ ☑ ♿
CMS: 100-04,20,30.6

E0442 Stationary oxygen contents, liquid, 1 month's supply = 1 unit Ⓨ ☑ ♿

E0443 Portable oxygen contents, gaseous, 1 month's supply = 1 unit Ⓨ ☑ ♿
CMS: 100-04,20,30.6

E0444 Portable oxygen contents, liquid, 1 month's supply = 1 unit Ⓨ ☑ ♿

E0445 Oximeter device for measuring blood oxygen levels noninvasively Ⓝ

E0446 Topical oxygen delivery system, not otherwise specified, includes all supplies and accessories Ⓐ

E0447 Portable oxygen contents, liquid, 1 month's supply = 1 unit, prescribed amount at rest or nighttime exceeds 4 liters per minute (LPM)

E0455 Oxygen tent, excluding croup or pediatric tents Ⓨ

E0457 Chest shell (cuirass) ⒺⒾ

E0459 Chest wrap ⒺⒾ

E0462 Rocking bed, with or without side rails Ⓨ ♿ (RR)

E0465 Home ventilator, any type, used with invasive interface, (e.g., tracheostomy tube) Ⓨ ♿ (RR)

E0466 Home ventilator, any type, used with noninvasive interface, (e.g., mask, chest shell) Ⓨ ♿ (RR)

E0467 Home ventilator, multi-function respiratory device, also performs any or all of the additional functions of oxygen concentration, drug nebulization, aspiration, and cough stimulation, includes all accessories, components and supplies for all functions (RR)

E0470 Respiratory assist device, bi-level pressure capability, without backup rate feature, used with noninvasive interface, e.g., nasal or facial mask (intermittent assist device with continuous positive airway pressure device) Ⓨ ♿ (RR)
CMS: 100-03,240.4

E0471 Respiratory assist device, bi-level pressure capability, with back-up rate feature, used with noninvasive interface, e.g., nasal or facial mask (intermittent assist device with continuous positive airway pressure device) Ⓨ ♿ (RR)
CMS: 100-03,240.4

E0472 Respiratory assist device, bi-level pressure capability, with backup rate feature, used with invasive interface, e.g., tracheostomy tube (intermittent assist device with continuous positive airway pressure device) Ⓨ ♿ (RR)
CMS: 100-03,240.4

E0480 Percussor, electric or pneumatic, home model Ⓨ ♿ (RR)

E0481 Intrapulmonary percussive ventilation system and related accessories ⒺⒾ

E0482 Cough stimulating device, alternating positive and negative airway pressure Ⓨ ♿ (RR)

E0483 High frequency chest wall oscillation system, with full anterior and/or posterior thoracic region receiving simultaneous external oscillation, includes all accessories and supplies, each Ⓨ ☑ ♿ (RR)
AHA: 4Q,22

E0484 Oscillatory positive expiratory pressure device, nonelectric, any type, each Ⓨ ☑ ♿ (NU, RR, UE)

E0485 Oral device/appliance used to reduce upper airway collapsibility, adjustable or nonadjustable, prefabricated, includes fitting and adjustment Ⓨ ♿ (NU, RR, UE)

E0486 Oral device/appliance used to reduce upper airway collapsibility, adjustable or nonadjustable, custom fabricated, includes fitting and adjustment Ⓨ ♿ (NU, RR, UE)

E0487 Spirometer, electronic, includes all accessories Ⓝ

Oral Devices

● **E0490** Power source and control electronics unit for oral device/appliance for neuromuscular electrical stimulation of the tongue muscle, controlled by hardware remote (RR)

● **E0491** Oral device/appliance for neuromuscular electrical stimulation of the tongue muscle, used in conjunction with the power source and control electronics unit, controlled by hardware remote, 90-day supply

● **E0492** Power source and control electronics unit for oral device/appliance for neuromuscular electrical stimulation of the tongue muscle, controlled by phone application

● **E0493** Oral device/appliance for neuromuscular electrical stimulation of the tongue muscle, used in conjunction with the power source and control electronics unit, controlled by phone application, 90-day supply

---

■ Special Coverage Instructions   ■ Noncovered by Medicare   ■ Carrier Discretion   ☑ Quantity Alert   ● New Code   ○ Recycled/Reinstated   ▲ Revised Code

38 — E Codes   Ⓐ Age Edit   Ⓜ Maternity Edit   ♀ Female Only   ♂ Male Only   Ⓐ-Ⓨ OPPS Status Indicators   © 2023 Optum360, LLC

IPPB Machines

E0500 IPPB machine, all types, with built-in nebulization; manual or automatic valves; internal or external power source ☑ & (RR)

Intermittent Positive Pressure Breathing (IPPB) devices

Battery pack and controls

Nebulizer

Nebulizer reservoir

Oxygen supply tube

IPPB unit in use

Obstructive Sleep Apnea Treatment

● **E0530** Electronic positional obstructive sleep apnea treatment, with sensor, includes all components and accessories, any type

Humidifiers/Compressors/Nebulizers

E0550 Humidifier, durable for extensive supplemental humidification during IPPB treatments or oxygen delivery ☑ & (RR)

E0555 Humidifier, durable, glass or autoclavable plastic bottle type, for use with regulator or flowmeter ☑

E0560 Humidifier, durable for supplemental humidification during IPPB treatment or oxygen delivery ☑ & (NU, RR, UE)

E0561 Humidifier, nonheated, used with positive airway pressure device ☑ & (NU, RR, UE)
CMS: 100-03,240.4; 100-04,36,50.14

E0562 Humidifier, heated, used with positive airway pressure device ☑ & (NU, RR, UE)
CMS: 100-03,240.4; 100-04,36,50.14

E0565 Compressor, air power source for equipment which is not self-contained or cylinder driven ☑ & (RR)

E0570 Nebulizer, with compressor ☑ & (RR)

E0572 Aerosol compressor, adjustable pressure, light duty for intermittent use ☑ & (RR)

E0574 Ultrasonic/electronic aerosol generator with small volume nebulizer ☑ & (RR)

E0575 Nebulizer, ultrasonic, large volume ☑ & (RR)

E0580 Nebulizer, durable, glass or autoclavable plastic, bottle type, for use with regulator or flowmeter ☑ & (NU, RR, UE)

E0585 Nebulizer, with compressor and heater ☑ & (RR)

Pumps and Vaporizers

E0600 Respiratory suction pump, home model, portable or stationary, electric ☑ & (RR)

E0601 Continuous positive airway pressure (CPAP) device ☑ & (RR)
CMS: 100-03,240.4

E0602 Breast pump, manual, any type Ⓜ ♀ ☑ & (NU, RR, UE)

E0603 Breast pump, electric (AC and/or DC), any type Ⓜ ♀ Ⓝ

E0604 Breast pump, hospital grade, electric (AC and/or DC), any type Ⓜ ♀ Ⓐ

E0605 Vaporizer, room type ☑ & (NU, RR, UE)

E0606 Postural drainage board ☑ & (RR)

Monitoring Devices

E0607 Home blood glucose monitor ☑ & (NU, RR, UE)
Medicare covers home blood testing devices for diabetic patients when the devices are prescribed by the patients' physicians. Many commercial payers provide this coverage to noninsulin dependent diabetics as well.

E0610 Pacemaker monitor, self-contained, (checks battery depletion, includes audible and visible check systems) ☑ & (NU, RR, UE)

E0615 Pacemaker monitor, self-contained, checks battery depletion and other pacemaker components, includes digital/visible check systems ☑ & (NU, RR, UE)

E0616 Implantable cardiac event recorder with memory, activator, and programmer Ⓝ

E0617 External defibrillator with integrated electrocardiogram analysis ☑ & (RR)

E0618 Apnea monitor, without recording feature ☑ & (RR)

E0619 Apnea monitor, with recording feature ☑ & (RR)

E0620 Skin piercing device for collection of capillary blood, laser, each ☑ & (RR)

Patient Lifts

E0621 Sling or seat, patient lift, canvas or nylon ☑ & (NU, RR, UE)

E0625 Patient lift, bathroom or toilet, not otherwise classified Ⓔ

E0627 Seat lift mechanism, electric, any type ☑ & (NU, RR, UE)
CMS: 100-04,20,100; 100-04,20,130.2; 100-04,20,130.3; 100-04,20,130.4; 100-04,20,130.5

E0629 Seat lift mechanism, nonelectric, any type ☑ & (NU, RR, UE)
CMS: 100-04,20,100; 100-04,20,130.2; 100-04,20,130.3; 100-04,20,130.4; 100-04,20,130.5

E0630 Patient lift, hydraulic or mechanical, includes any seat, sling, strap(s), or pad(s) ☑ & (RR)

E0635 Patient lift, electric, with seat or sling ☑ & (RR)

E0636 Multipositional patient support system, with integrated lift, patient accessible controls ☑ & (RR)

E0637 Combination sit-to-stand frame/table system, any size including pediatric, with seat lift feature, with or without wheels Ⓔ

E0638 Standing frame/table system, one position (e.g., upright, supine or prone stander), any size including pediatric, with or without wheels Ⓔ

E0639 Patient lift, moveable from room to room with disassembly and reassembly, includes all components/accessories Ⓔ & (RR)

E0640 Patient lift, fixed system, includes all components/accessories Ⓔ & (RR)

Special Coverage Instructions   Noncovered by Medicare   Carrier Discretion   ☑ Quantity Alert   ● New Code   ○ Recycled/Reinstated   ▲ Revised Code

© 2023 Optum360, LLC   Ⓐ²-Ⓩ³ ASC Pmt   CMS: IOM   AHA: Coding Clinic   & DMEPOS Paid   ⊘ SNF Excluded   E Codes — 39

Durable Medical Equipment

E0641 — E0730

E0641 Standing frame/table system, multi-position (e.g., 3-way stander), any size including pediatric, with or without wheels ▢EI

E0642 Standing frame/table system, mobile (dynamic stander), any size including pediatric ▢EI

Compression Devices

E0650 Pneumatic compressor, nonsegmental home model ▢Y ✧ (NU, RR, UE)

E0651 Pneumatic compressor, segmental home model without calibrated gradient pressure ▢Y ✧ (NU, RR, UE)

E0652 Pneumatic compressor, segmental home model with calibrated gradient pressure ▢Y ✧ (NU, RR, UE)

E0655 Nonsegmental pneumatic appliance for use with pneumatic compressor, half arm ▢Y ✧ (NU, RR, UE)

E0656 Segmental pneumatic appliance for use with pneumatic compressor, trunk ▢Y ✧ (RR)

E0657 Segmental pneumatic appliance for use with pneumatic compressor, chest ▢Y ✧ (RR)

E0660 Nonsegmental pneumatic appliance for use with pneumatic compressor, full leg ▢Y ✧ (NU, RR, UE)

E0665 Nonsegmental pneumatic appliance for use with pneumatic compressor, full arm ▢Y ✧ (NU, RR, UE)

E0666 Nonsegmental pneumatic appliance for use with pneumatic compressor, half leg ▢Y ✧ (NU, RR, UE)

E0667 Segmental pneumatic appliance for use with pneumatic compressor, full leg ▢Y ✧ (NU, RR, UE)

E0668 Segmental pneumatic appliance for use with pneumatic compressor, full arm ▢Y ✧ (NU, RR, UE)

E0669 Segmental pneumatic appliance for use with pneumatic compressor, half leg ▢Y ✧ (NU, RR, UE)

E0670 Segmental pneumatic appliance for use with pneumatic compressor, integrated, two full legs and trunk ▢Y ✧ (NU, RR, UE)

E0671 Segmental gradient pressure pneumatic appliance, full leg ▢Y ✧ (NU, RR, UE)

E0672 Segmental gradient pressure pneumatic appliance, full arm ▢Y ✧ (NU, RR, UE)

E0673 Segmental gradient pressure pneumatic appliance, half leg ▢Y ✧ (NU, RR, UE)

E0675 Pneumatic compression device, high pressure, rapid inflation/deflation cycle, for arterial insufficiency (unilateral or bilateral system) ▢Y ✧ (RR)

E0676 Intermittent limb compression device (includes all accessories), not otherwise specified ▢Y

● **E0677** Nonpneumatic sequential compression garment, trunk (RR)
AHA: 2Q,23

● **E0678** Nonpneumatic sequential compression garment, full leg

● **E0679** Nonpneumatic sequential compression garment, half leg

● **E0680** Nonpneumatic compression controller with sequential calibrated gradient pressure

● **E0681** Nonpneumatic compression controller without calibrated gradient pressure

● **E0682** Nonpneumatic sequential compression garment, full arm

Ultraviolet Light

E0691 Ultraviolet light therapy system, includes bulbs/lamps, timer and eye protection; treatment area 2 sq ft or less ▢Y ✧ (NU, RR, UE)

E0692 Ultraviolet light therapy system panel, includes bulbs/lamps, timer and eye protection, 4 ft panel ▢Y ✧ (NU, RR, UE)

E0693 Ultraviolet light therapy system panel, includes bulbs/lamps, timer and eye protection, 6 ft panel ▢Y ✧ (NU, RR, UE)

E0694 Ultraviolet multidirectional light therapy system in 6 ft cabinet, includes bulbs/lamps, timer, and eye protection ▢Y ✧ (NU, RR, UE)

Safety Equipment

E0700 Safety equipment, device or accessory, any type ▢EI

Restraints (E0710)

Fabric wrist restraint

Padded leather restraints may feature a locking device

Body restraint

Fabric gait belt for assistance in walking (E0700)

E0705 Transfer device, any type, each ▢B ☑ ✧ (NU, RR, UE)

E0710 Restraints, any type (body, chest, wrist, or ankle) ▢EI

● **E0711** Upper extremity medical tubing/lines enclosure or covering device, restricts elbow range of motion
AHA: 2Q,23

Nerve Stimulators and Devices

E0720 Transcutaneous electrical nerve stimulation (TENS) device, two-lead, localized stimulation ▢Y ✧ (NU)
A Certificate of Medical Necessity is required for the purchase of a TENS. It is not required for rentals.
CMS: 100-03,10.2; 100-03,160.27; 100-03,160.7.1; 100-04,20,30.1.2

E0730 Transcutaneous electrical nerve stimulation (TENS) device, four or more leads, for multiple nerve stimulation ▢Y ✧ (NU)
A Certificate of Medical Necessity is required for the purchase of a TENS. It is not required for rentals.
CMS: 100-03,10.2; 100-03,160.27; 100-03,160.7.1; 100-04,20,30.1.2

Special Coverage Instructions   Noncovered by Medicare   Carrier Discretion   ☑ Quantity Alert ● New Code   ○ Recycled/Reinstated   ▲ Revised Code

40 — E Codes   Ⓐ Age Edit   Ⓜ Maternity Edit   ♀ Female Only   ♂ Male Only   Ⓐ-Ⓨ OPPS Status Indicators   © 2023 Optum360, LLC

E0731 Form-fitting conductive garment for delivery of TENS or NMES (with conductive fibers separated from the patient's skin by layers of fabric) ☒ ⅋ (NU)
CMS: 100-03,10.2; 100-03,160.13

● **E0732** Cranial electrotherapy stimulation (CES) system, any type

● **E0733** Transcutaneous electrical nerve stimulator for electrical stimulation of the trigeminal nerve

● **E0734** External upper limb tremor stimulator of the peripheral nerves of the wrist

● **E0735** Noninvasive vagus nerve stimulator

E0740 Nonimplanted pelvic floor electrical stimulator, complete system ☒ ⅋ (RR)

E0744 Neuromuscular stimulator for scoliosis ☒ ⅋ (RR)

E0745 Neuromuscular stimulator, electronic shock unit ☒ ⅋ (RR)

E0746 Electromyography (EMG), biofeedback device ☒
Biofeedback therapy is covered by Medicare only for re-education of specific muscles or for treatment of incapacitating muscle spasm or weakness.

E0747 Osteogenesis stimulator, electrical, noninvasive, other than spinal applications ☒ (NU, RR, UE)
Medicare covers noninvasive osteogenic stimulation for nonunion of long bone fractures, failed fusion, or congenital pseudoarthroses.

E0748 Osteogenesis stimulator, electrical, noninvasive, spinal applications ☒ (NU, RR, UE)
Medicare covers noninvasive osteogenic stimulation as an adjunct to spinal fusion surgery for patients at high risk of pseudoarthroses due to previously failed spinal fusion, or for those undergoing fusion of three or more vertebrae.

E0749 Osteogenesis stimulator, electrical, surgically implanted ☒ (RR)
Medicare covers invasive osteogenic stimulation for nonunion of long bone fractures or as an adjunct to spinal fusion surgery for patients at high risk of pseudoarthroses due to previously failed spinal fusion, or for those undergoing fusion of three or more vertebrae.
CMS: 100-04,4,190

E0755 Electronic salivary reflex stimulator (intraoral/noninvasive) ☒

E0760 Osteogenesis stimulator, low intensity ultrasound, noninvasive ☒ (NU, RR, UE)
CMS: 100-04,32,110.5

E0761 Nonthermal pulsed high frequency radiowaves, high peak power electromagnetic energy treatment device ☒

E0762 Transcutaneous electrical joint stimulation device system, includes all accessories ☒ ⅋ (RR)

E0764 Functional neuromuscular stimulation, transcutaneous stimulation of sequential muscle groups of ambulation with computer control, used for walking by spinal cord injured, entire system, after completion of training program ☒ (RR)

E0765 FDA approved nerve stimulator, with replaceable batteries, for treatment of nausea and vomiting ☒ ⅋ (NU, RR, UE)

E0766 Electrical stimulation device used for cancer treatment, includes all accessories, any type ☒ (RR)

E0769 Electrical stimulation or electromagnetic wound treatment device, not otherwise classified ☒
CMS: 100-04,32,11.1

E0770 Functional electrical stimulator, transcutaneous stimulation of nerve and/or muscle groups, any type, complete system, not otherwise specified ☒

Infusion Supplies

E0776 IV pole ☒ ⅋ (NU, RR, UE)

E0779 Ambulatory infusion pump, mechanical, reusable, for infusion 8 hours or greater ☒ ⅋ (RR)

E0780 Ambulatory infusion pump, mechanical, reusable, for infusion less than 8 hours ☒ ⅋ (NU)

E0781 Ambulatory infusion pump, single or multiple channels, electric or battery operated, with administrative equipment, worn by patient ☒ ⅋ (RR)

E0782 Infusion pump, implantable, nonprogrammable (includes all components, e.g., pump, catheter, connectors, etc.) ☒ (NU, RR, UE)
CMS: 100-04,4,190

E0783 Infusion pump system, implantable, programmable (includes all components, e.g., pump, catheter, connectors, etc.) ☒ (NU, RR, UE)
CMS: 100-04,4,190

E0784 External ambulatory infusion pump, insulin ☒ ⅋ (RR)
Covered by some commercial payers with preauthorization.

E0785 Implantable intraspinal (epidural/intrathecal) catheter used with implantable infusion pump, replacement ☒ ⅋ (KF)
CMS: 100-04,4,190

E0786 Implantable programmable infusion pump, replacement (excludes implantable intraspinal catheter) ☒ (NU, RR, UE)

E0787 External ambulatory infusion pump, insulin, dosage rate adjustment using therapeutic continuous glucose sensing

E0791 Parenteral infusion pump, stationary, single, or multichannel ☒ ⅋ (RR)

Traction Equipment

E0830 Ambulatory traction device, all types, each ☒

E0840 Traction frame, attached to headboard, cervical traction ☒ ⅋ (NU, RR, UE)

E0849 Traction equipment, cervical, free-standing stand/frame, pneumatic, applying traction force to other than mandible ☒ ⅋ (RR)

E0850 Traction stand, freestanding, cervical traction ☒ ⅋ (NU, RR, UE)

E0855 Cervical traction equipment not requiring additional stand or frame ☒ ⅋ (RR)

E0856 Cervical traction device, with inflatable air bladder(s) ☒ ⅋ (RR)

E0860 Traction equipment, overdoor, cervical ☒ ⅋ (NU, RR, UE)

E0870 Traction frame, attached to footboard, extremity traction (e.g., Buck's) ☒ ⅋ (NU, RR, UE)

E0890 Traction frame, attached to footboard, pelvic traction ☒ ⅋ (NU, RR, UE)

E0900 Traction stand, freestanding, pelvic traction (e.g., Buck's) ☒ ⅋ (NU, RR, UE)

Orthopedic Devices

E0910 Trapeze bars, also known as Patient Helper, attached to bed, with grab bar ☒ ⅋ (RR)

E0911 Trapeze bar, heavy-duty, for patient weight capacity greater than 250 pounds, attached to bed, with grab bar ☒ ⅋ (RR)

E0912 Trapeze bar, heavy-duty, for patient weight capacity greater than 250 pounds, freestanding, complete with grab bar ☒ ⅋ (RR)

E0920 Fracture frame, attached to bed, includes weights ☒ ⅋ (RR)

E0930 Fracture frame, freestanding, includes weights ☒ ⅋ (RR)

E0935 Continuous passive motion exercise device for use on knee only ☒ ⅋ (RR)

Special Coverage Instructions   Noncovered by Medicare   Carrier Discretion   ☑ Quantity Alert   ● New Code   ○ Recycled/Reinstated   ▲ Revised Code

© 2023 Optum360, LLC   A2-Z3 ASC Pmt   CMS: IOM   AHA: Coding Clinic   ⅋ DMEPOS Paid   ⊘ SNF Excluded   E Codes — 41

Durable Medical Equipment

E0936 — E1020

Code	Description	
E0936	Continuous passive motion exercise device for use other than knee	Ⓔ
E0940	Trapeze bar, freestanding, complete with grab bar	Ⓨ ♿ (RR)
E0941	Gravity assisted traction device, any type	Ⓨ ♿ (RR)
E0942	Cervical head harness/halter	Ⓨ ♿ (NU, RR, UE)
E0944	Pelvic belt/harness/boot	Ⓨ ♿ (NU, RR, UE)
E0945	Extremity belt/harness	Ⓨ ♿ (NU, RR, UE)
E0946	Fracture, frame, dual with cross bars, attached to bed, (e.g., Balkan, four-poster)	Ⓨ ♿ (RR)
E0947	Fracture frame, attachments for complex pelvic traction	♿ (NU, RR, UE)
E0948	Fracture frame, attachments for complex cervical traction	♿ (NU, RR, UE)

Wheelchair Accessories

Code	Description	
E0950	Wheelchair accessory, tray, each	Ⓨ ☑ ♿ (NU, RR, UE)
E0951	Heel loop/holder, any type, with or without ankle strap, each	Ⓨ ☑ ♿ (NU, RR, UE)
E0952	Toe loop/holder, any type, each	Ⓨ ☑ ♿ (NU, RR, UE)
E0953	Wheelchair accessory, lateral thigh or knee support, any type including fixed mounting hardware, each	Ⓨ ♿ (NU, RR, UE)
E0954	Wheelchair accessory, foot box, any type, includes attachment and mounting hardware, each foot	Ⓨ ♿ (NU, RR, UE)
E0955	Wheelchair accessory, headrest, cushioned, any type, including fixed mounting hardware, each	Ⓨ ☑ ♿ (RR)
E0956	Wheelchair accessory, lateral trunk or hip support, any type, including fixed mounting hardware, each	Ⓨ ☑ ♿ (NU, RR, UE)
E0957	Wheelchair accessory, medial thigh support, any type, including fixed mounting hardware, each	Ⓨ ☑ ♿ (NU, RR, UE)
E0958	Manual wheelchair accessory, one-arm drive attachment, each	Ⓨ ☑ ♿ (RR)
E0959	Manual wheelchair accessory, adapter for amputee, each	Ⓑ ♿ (NU, RR, UE)
E0960	Wheelchair accessory, shoulder harness/straps or chest strap, including any type mounting hardware	Ⓨ ♿ (NU, RR, UE)
E0961	Manual wheelchair accessory, wheel lock brake extension (handle), each	Ⓑ ☑ ♿ (NU, RR, UE)
E0966	Manual wheelchair accessory, headrest extension, each	Ⓑ ☑ ♿ (NU, RR, UE)
E0967	Manual wheelchair accessory, hand rim with projections, any type, replacement only, each	Ⓨ ☑ ♿ (NU, RR, UE)
E0968	Commode seat, wheelchair	Ⓨ ♿ (RR)
E0969	Narrowing device, wheelchair	Ⓨ ♿ (NU, RR, UE)
E0970	No. 2 footplates, except for elevating legrest	Ⓔ
	See code(s): K0037, K0042	
E0971	Manual wheelchair accessory, antitipping device, each	Ⓑ ♿ (NU, RR, UE)
E0973	Wheelchair accessory, adjustable height, detachable armrest, complete assembly, each	Ⓑ ☑ ♿ (NU, RR, UE)
E0974	Manual wheelchair accessory, antirollback device, each	Ⓑ ☑ ♿ (NU, RR, UE)
E0978	Wheelchair accessory, positioning belt/safety belt/pelvic strap, each	Ⓑ ☑ ♿ (NU, RR, UE)
E0980	Safety vest, wheelchair	Ⓨ ♿ (NU, RR, UE)
E0981	Wheelchair accessory, seat upholstery, replacement only, each	Ⓨ ☑ ♿ (NU, RR, UE)
E0982	Wheelchair accessory, back upholstery, replacement only, each	Ⓨ ☑ ♿ (NU, RR, UE)
E0983	Manual wheelchair accessory, power add-on to convert manual wheelchair to motorized wheelchair, joystick control	Ⓨ ♿ (RR)
E0984	Manual wheelchair accessory, power add-on to convert manual wheelchair to motorized wheelchair, tiller control	Ⓨ ♿ (RR)
E0985	Wheelchair accessory, seat lift mechanism	Ⓨ ♿ (RR)
E0986	Manual wheelchair accessory, push-rim activated power assist system	Ⓨ ☑ ♿ (RR)
E0988	Manual wheelchair accessory, lever-activated, wheel drive, pair	Ⓨ ☑ ♿ (RR)
E0990	Wheelchair accessory, elevating legrest, complete assembly, each	Ⓑ ☑ ♿ (NU, RR, UE)
E0992	Manual wheelchair accessory, solid seat insert	Ⓑ ♿ (NU, RR, UE)
E0994	Armrest, each	Ⓨ ☑ ♿ (NU, RR, UE)
E0995	Wheelchair accessory, calf rest/pad, replacement only, each	Ⓑ ☑ ♿ (NU, RR, UE)
E1002	Wheelchair accessory, power seating system, tilt only	Ⓨ ♿ (RR)
E1003	Wheelchair accessory, power seating system, recline only, without shear reduction	Ⓨ ♿ (RR)
E1004	Wheelchair accessory, power seating system, recline only, with mechanical shear reduction	Ⓨ ♿ (RR)
E1005	Wheelchair accessory, power seating system, recline only, with power shear reduction	Ⓨ ♿ (RR)
E1006	Wheelchair accessory, power seating system, combination tilt and recline, without shear reduction	Ⓨ ♿ (RR)
E1007	Wheelchair accessory, power seating system, combination tilt and recline, with mechanical shear reduction	Ⓨ ♿ (RR)
E1008	Wheelchair accessory, power seating system, combination tilt and recline, with power shear reduction	Ⓨ ♿ (RR)
E1009	Wheelchair accessory, addition to power seating system, mechanically linked leg elevation system, including pushrod and legrest, each	Ⓨ ☑ ♿ (NU, RR, UE)
E1010	Wheelchair accessory, addition to power seating system, power leg elevation system, including legrest, pair	Ⓨ ☑ ♿ (RR)
E1011	Modification to pediatric size wheelchair, width adjustment package (not to be dispensed with initial chair)	Ⓨ ♿ (NU, RR, UE)
E1012	Wheelchair accessory, addition to power seating system, center mount power elevating leg rest/platform, complete system, any type, each	Ⓨ ♿ (RR)
E1014	Reclining back, addition to pediatric size wheelchair	Ⓨ ♿ (RR)
E1015	Shock absorber for manual wheelchair, each	Ⓨ ☑ ♿ (NU, RR, UE)
E1016	Shock absorber for power wheelchair, each	Ⓨ ☑ ♿ (NU, RR, UE)
E1017	Heavy-duty shock absorber for heavy-duty or extra heavy-duty manual wheelchair, each	Ⓨ ☑ ♿ (NU, RR, UE)
E1018	Heavy-duty shock absorber for heavy-duty or extra heavy-duty power wheelchair, each	Ⓨ ☑ ♿ (NU, RR, UE)
E1020	Residual limb support system for wheelchair, any type	Ⓨ ♿ (RR)

Special Coverage Instructions   Noncovered by Medicare   Carrier Discretion   ☑ Quantity Alert ● New Code   ○ Recycled/Reinstated   ▲ Revised Code

E1028	Wheelchair accessory, manual swingaway, retractable or removable mounting hardware for joystick, other control interface or positioning accessory Y �& (RR)
E1029	Wheelchair accessory, ventilator tray, fixed Y �& (RR)
E1030	Wheelchair accessory, ventilator tray, gimbaled Y �& (RR)
E1031	Rollabout chair, any and all types with castors 5 in or greater Y �& (RR)
E1035	Multi-positional patient transfer system, with integrated seat, operated by care giver, patient weight capacity up to and including 300 lbs Y �& (RR) **CMS:** 100-02,15,110
E1036	Multi-positional patient transfer system, extra-wide, with integrated seat, operated by caregiver, patient weight capacity greater than 300 lbs Y �& (RR)
E1037	Transport chair, pediatric size Y �& (RR)
E1038	Transport chair, adult size, patient weight capacity up to and including 300 pounds Y �& (RR)
E1039	Transport chair, adult size, heavy-duty, patient weight capacity greater than 300 pounds Y ᆼ (RR)

Wheelchairs

E1050	Fully-reclining wheelchair, fixed full-length arms, swing-away detachable elevating legrests Y ᆼ (RR)
E1060	Fully-reclining wheelchair, detachable arms, desk or full-length, swing-away detachable elevating legrests Y ᆼ (RR)
E1070	Fully-reclining wheelchair, detachable arms (desk or full-length) swing-away detachable footrest Y ᆼ (RR)
E1083	Hemi-wheelchair, fixed full-length arms, swing-away detachable elevating legrest Y ᆼ (RR)
E1084	Hemi-wheelchair, detachable arms desk or full-length arms, swing-away detachable elevating legrests Y ᆼ (RR)
E1085	Hemi-wheelchair, fixed full-length arms, swing-away detachable footrests EI See code(s): K0002
E1086	Hemi-wheelchair, detachable arms, desk or full-length, swing-away detachable footrests EI See code(s): K0002
E1087	High strength lightweight wheelchair, fixed full-length arms, swing-away detachable elevating legrests Y ᆼ (RR)
E1088	High strength lightweight wheelchair, detachable arms desk or full-length, swing-away detachable elevating legrests Y ᆼ (RR)
E1089	High-strength lightweight wheelchair, fixed-length arms, swing-away detachable footrest EI See code(s): K0004
E1090	High-strength lightweight wheelchair, detachable arms, desk or full-length, swing-away detachable footrests EI See code(s): K0004
E1092	Wide heavy-duty wheel chair, detachable arms (desk or full-length), swing-away detachable elevating legrests Y ᆼ (RR)
E1093	Wide heavy-duty wheelchair, detachable arms, desk or full-length arms, swing-away detachable footrests Y ᆼ (RR)
E1100	Semi-reclining wheelchair, fixed full-length arms, swing-away detachable elevating legrests Y ᆼ (RR)
E1110	Semi-reclining wheelchair, detachable arms (desk or full-length) elevating legrest Y ᆼ (RR)
E1130	Standard wheelchair, fixed full-length arms, fixed or swing-away detachable footrests EI See code(s): K0001
E1140	Wheelchair, detachable arms, desk or full-length, swing-away detachable footrests EI See code(s): K0001
E1150	Wheelchair, detachable arms, desk or full-length swing-away detachable elevating legrests Y ᆼ (RR)
E1160	Wheelchair, fixed full-length arms, swing-away detachable elevating legrests Y ᆼ (RR)
E1161	Manual adult size wheelchair, includes tilt in space Y ᆼ (RR)
E1170	Amputee wheelchair, fixed full-length arms, swing-away detachable elevating legrests Y ᆼ (RR)
E1171	Amputee wheelchair, fixed full-length arms, without footrests or legrest Y ᆼ (RR)
E1172	Amputee wheelchair, detachable arms (desk or full-length) without footrests or legrest Y ᆼ (RR)
E1180	Amputee wheelchair, detachable arms (desk or full-length) swing-away detachable footrests Y ᆼ (RR)
E1190	Amputee wheelchair, detachable arms (desk or full-length) swing-away detachable elevating legrests Y ᆼ (RR)
E1195	Heavy-duty wheelchair, fixed full-length arms, swing-away detachable elevating legrests Y ᆼ (RR)
E1200	Amputee wheelchair, fixed full-length arms, swing-away detachable footrest Y ᆼ (RR)
E1220	Wheelchair; specially sized or constructed, (indicate brand name, model number, if any) and justification Y
E1221	Wheelchair with fixed arm, footrests Y ᆼ (RR)
E1222	Wheelchair with fixed arm, elevating legrests Y ᆼ (RR)
E1223	Wheelchair with detachable arms, footrests Y ᆼ (RR)
E1224	Wheelchair with detachable arms, elevating legrests Y ᆼ (RR)
E1225	Wheelchair accessory, manual semi-reclining back, (recline greater than 15 degrees, but less than 80 degrees), each Y ☑ ᆼ (RR)
E1226	Wheelchair accessory, manual fully reclining back, (recline greater than 80 degrees), each B ☑ ᆼ (NU, RR, UE) See also K0028
E1227	Special height arms for wheelchair Y ᆼ (NU, RR, UE)
E1228	Special back height for wheelchair Y ᆼ (RR)
E1229	Wheelchair, pediatric size, not otherwise specified Y
E1230	Power operated vehicle (three- or four-wheel nonhighway), specify brand name and model number Y ᆼ (NU, RR, UE) Prior authorization is required by Medicare for this item.
E1231	Wheelchair, pediatric size, tilt-in-space, rigid, adjustable, with seating system Y ᆼ (NU, RR, UE)
E1232	Wheelchair, pediatric size, tilt-in-space, folding, adjustable, with seating system Y ᆼ (RR)
E1233	Wheelchair, pediatric size, tilt-in-space, rigid, adjustable, without seating system Y ᆼ (RR)
E1234	Wheelchair, pediatric size, tilt-in-space, folding, adjustable, without seating system Y ᆼ (RR)
E1235	Wheelchair, pediatric size, rigid, adjustable, with seating system Y ᆼ (RR)
E1236	Wheelchair, pediatric size, folding, adjustable, with seating system Y ᆼ (RR)

Special Coverage Instructions   Noncovered by Medicare   Carrier Discretion   ☑ Quantity Alert   ● New Code   ○ Recycled/Reinstated   ▲ Revised Code

E1237	Wheelchair, pediatric size, rigid, adjustable, without seating system	Y & (RR)
E1238	Wheelchair, pediatric size, folding, adjustable, without seating system	Y & (RR)
E1239	Power wheelchair, pediatric size, not otherwise specified	Y
E1240	Lightweight wheelchair, detachable arms, (desk or full-length) swing-away detachable, elevating legrest	Y & (RR)
E1250	Lightweight wheelchair, fixed full-length arms, swing-away detachable footrest See code(s): K0003	EI
E1260	Lightweight wheelchair, detachable arms (desk or full-length) swing-away detachable footrest See code(s): K0003	EI
E1270	Lightweight wheelchair, fixed full-length arms, swing-away detachable elevating legrests	Y & (RR)
E1280	Heavy-duty wheelchair, detachable arms (desk or full-length) elevating legrests	Y & (RR)
E1285	Heavy-duty wheelchair, fixed full-length arms, swing-away detachable footrest See code(s): K0006	EI
E1290	Heavy-duty wheelchair, detachable arms (desk or full-length) swing-away detachable footrest See code(s): K0006	EI
E1295	Heavy-duty wheelchair, fixed full-length arms, elevating legrest	Y & (RR)
E1296	Special wheelchair seat height from floor	Y & (NU, RR, UE)
E1297	Special wheelchair seat depth, by upholstery	Y & (NU, RR, UE)
E1298	Special wheelchair seat depth and/or width, by construction	Y & (NU, RR, UE)

Whirlpool - Equipment

E1300	Whirlpool, portable (overtub type)	EI
● E1301	Whirlpool tub, walk-in, portable	
E1310	Whirlpool, nonportable (built-in type)	Y & (NU, RR, UE)

Additional Oxygen Related Equipment

E1352	Oxygen accessory, flow regulator capable of positive inspiratory pressure	Y
E1353	Regulator	Y &
E1354	Oxygen accessory, wheeled cart for portable cylinder or portable concentrator, any type, replacement only, each	Y ☑
E1355	Stand/rack	Y &
E1356	Oxygen accessory, battery pack/cartridge for portable concentrator, any type, replacement only, each	Y ☑
E1357	Oxygen accessory, battery charger for portable concentrator, any type, replacement only, each	Y ☑
E1358	Oxygen accessory, DC power adapter for portable concentrator, any type, replacement only, each	Y ☑
E1372	Immersion external heater for nebulizer	Y & (NU, RR, UE)
E1390	Oxygen concentrator, single delivery port, capable of delivering 85 percent or greater oxygen concentration at the prescribed flow rate CMS: 100-04,20,130.6	Y & (RR)
E1391	Oxygen concentrator, dual delivery port, capable of delivering 85 percent or greater oxygen concentration at the prescribed flow rate, each CMS: 100-04,20,130.6	Y ☑ & (RR)

E1392	Portable oxygen concentrator, rental CMS: 100-04,20,130.6	Y & (RR)
E1399	Durable medical equipment, miscellaneous CMS: 100-04,20,30.9; 100-04,32,110.5	Y
E1405	Oxygen and water vapor enriching system with heated delivery CMS: 100-04,20,20; 100-04,20,20.4	Y & (RR)
E1406	Oxygen and water vapor enriching system without heated delivery CMS: 100-04,20,20; 100-04,20,20.4	Y & (RR)

Artificial Kidney Machines and Accessories

E1500	Centrifuge, for dialysis	A ⊘
E1510	Kidney, dialysate delivery system kidney machine, pump recirculating, air removal system, flowrate meter, power off, heater and temperature control with alarm, IV poles, pressure gauge, concentrate container	A ⊘
E1520	Heparin infusion pump for hemodialysis	A ⊘
E1530	Air bubble detector for hemodialysis, each, replacement	A ☑ ⊘
E1540	Pressure alarm for hemodialysis, each, replacement	A ☑ ⊘
E1550	Bath conductivity meter for hemodialysis, each	A ☑ ⊘
E1560	Blood leak detector for hemodialysis, each, replacement	A ☑ ⊘
E1570	Adjustable chair, for ESRD patients	A ⊘
E1575	Transducer protectors/fluid barriers, for hemodialysis, any size, per 10	A ☑ ⊘
E1580	Unipuncture control system for hemodialysis	A ⊘
E1590	Hemodialysis machine	A ⊘
E1592	Automatic intermittent peritoneal dialysis system	A ⊘
E1594	Cycler dialysis machine for peritoneal dialysis	A ⊘
E1600	Delivery and/or installation charges for hemodialysis equipment	A ⊘
E1610	Reverse osmosis water purification system, for hemodialysis	A ⊘
E1615	Deionizer water purification system, for hemodialysis	A ⊘
E1620	Blood pump for hemodialysis, replacement	A ⊘
E1625	Water softening system, for hemodialysis	A ⊘
E1629	Tablo hemodialysis system for the billable dialysis service	
E1630	Reciprocating peritoneal dialysis system	A ⊘
E1632	Wearable artificial kidney, each	A ☑ ⊘
E1634	Peritoneal dialysis clamps, each	B ☑
E1635	Compact (portable) travel hemodialyzer system	A ⊘
E1636	Sorbent cartridges, for hemodialysis, per 10	A ☑ ⊘
E1637	Hemostats, each	A ☑ ⊘
E1639	Scale, each	A ☑ ⊘
E1699	Dialysis equipment, not otherwise specified CMS: 100-04,8,20	A ⊘

Jaw Motion Rehabilitation System and Accessories

| E1700 | Jaw motion rehabilitation system
Medicare jurisdiction: local contractor. | Y & (RR) |

Special Coverage Instructions   Noncovered by Medicare   Carrier Discretion   ☑ Quantity Alert   ● New Code   ○ Recycled/Reinstated   ▲ Revised Code

44 — E Codes   A Age Edit   M Maternity Edit   ♀ Female Only   ♂ Male Only   A-Y OPPS Status Indicators   © 2023 Optum360, LLC

E1701 Replacement cushions for jaw motion rehabilitation system, package of 6 ☑ ☑ &
Medicare jurisdiction: local contractor.

E1702 Replacement measuring scales for jaw motion rehabilitation system, package of 200 ☑ ☑ &
Medicare jurisdiction: local contractor.

Flexion/Extension Device

E1800 Dynamic adjustable elbow extension/flexion device, includes soft interface material ☑ & (RR)

E1801 Static progressive stretch elbow device, extension and/or flexion, with or without range of motion adjustment, includes all components and accessories ☑ & (RR)

E1802 Dynamic adjustable forearm pronation/supination device, includes soft interface material ☑ & (RR)

E1805 Dynamic adjustable wrist extension/flexion device, includes soft interface material ☑ & (RR)

E1806 Static progressive stretch wrist device, flexion and/or extension, with or without range of motion adjustment, includes all components and accessories ☑ & (RR)

E1810 Dynamic adjustable knee extension/flexion device, includes soft interface material ☑ & (RR)

E1811 Static progressive stretch knee device, extension and/or flexion, with or without range of motion adjustment, includes all components and accessories ☑ & (RR)

E1812 Dynamic knee, extension/flexion device with active resistance control ☑ & (RR)

E1815 Dynamic adjustable ankle extension/flexion device, includes soft interface material ☑ & (RR)

E1816 Static progressive stretch ankle device, flexion and/or extension, with or without range of motion adjustment, includes all components and accessories ☑ & (RR)

E1818 Static progressive stretch forearm pronation/supination device, with or without range of motion adjustment, includes all components and accessories ☑ & (RR)

E1820 Replacement soft interface material, dynamic adjustable extension/flexion device ☑ & (NU, RR, UE)

E1821 Replacement soft interface material/cuffs for bi-directional static progressive stretch device ☑ & (NU, RR, UE)

E1825 Dynamic adjustable finger extension/flexion device, includes soft interface material ☑ & (RR)

E1830 Dynamic adjustable toe extension/flexion device, includes soft interface material ☑ & (RR)

E1831 Static progressive stretch toe device, extension and/or flexion, with or without range of motion adjustment, includes all components and accessories ☑ & (RR)

E1840 Dynamic adjustable shoulder flexion/abduction/rotation device, includes soft interface material ☑ & (RR)

E1841 Static progressive stretch shoulder device, with or without range of motion adjustment, includes all components and accessories ☑ & (RR)

Other Devices

E1902 Communication board, nonelectronic augmentative or alternative communication device ☑

● **E1905** Virtual reality cognitive behavioral therapy device (CBT), including preprogrammed therapy software (RR)
AHA: 2Q,23

E2000 Gastric suction pump, home model, portable or stationary, electric ☑ & (RR)

● **E2001** Suction pump, home model, portable or stationary, electric, any type, for use with external urine management system

E2100 Blood glucose monitor with integrated voice synthesizer ☑ & (NU, RR, UE)

E2101 Blood glucose monitor with integrated lancing/blood sample ☑ & (NU, RR, UE)

E2102 Adjunctive, nonimplanted continuous glucose monitor (CGM) or receiver (NU, RR, UE)

E2103 Nonadjunctive, nonimplanted continuous glucose monitor (CGM) or receiver (NU, RR, UE)

E2120 Pulse generator system for tympanic treatment of inner ear endolymphatic fluid ☑ & (RR)

DME Wheelchair Accessory

E2201 Manual wheelchair accessory, nonstandard seat frame, width greater than or equal to 20 in and less than 24 in ☑ ☑ & (NU, RR, UE)

E2202 Manual wheelchair accessory, nonstandard seat frame width, 24-27 in ☑ ☑ & (NU, RR, UE)

E2203 Manual wheelchair accessory, nonstandard seat frame depth, 20 to less than 22 in ☑ ☑ & (NU, RR, UE)

E2204 Manual wheelchair accessory, nonstandard seat frame depth, 22 to 25 in ☑ ☑ & (NU, RR, UE)

E2205 Manual wheelchair accessory, handrim without projections (includes ergonomic or contoured), any type, replacement only, each ☑ ☑ & (NU, RR, UE)

E2206 Manual wheelchair accessory, wheel lock assembly, complete, replacement only, each ☑ ☑ & (NU, RR, UE)

E2207 Wheelchair accessory, crutch and cane holder, each ☑ ☑ & (NU, RR, UE)

E2208 Wheelchair accessory, cylinder tank carrier, each ☑ ☑ & (NU, RR, UE)

E2209 Accessory, arm trough, with or without hand support, each ☑ ☑ & (NU, RR, UE)

E2210 Wheelchair accessory, bearings, any type, replacement only, each ☑ ☑ & (NU, RR, UE)

E2211 Manual wheelchair accessory, pneumatic propulsion tire, any size, each ☑ ☑ & (NU, RR, UE)

E2212 Manual wheelchair accessory, tube for pneumatic propulsion tire, any size, each ☑ ☑ & (NU, RR, UE)

E2213 Manual wheelchair accessory, insert for pneumatic propulsion tire (removable), any type, any size, each ☑ ☑ & (NU, RR, UE)

E2214 Manual wheelchair accessory, pneumatic caster tire, any size, each ☑ ☑ & (NU, RR, UE)

E2215 Manual wheelchair accessory, tube for pneumatic caster tire, any size, each ☑ ☑ & (NU, RR, UE)

E2216 Manual wheelchair accessory, foam filled propulsion tire, any size, each ☑ ☑ & (NU, RR, UE)

E2217 Manual wheelchair accessory, foam filled caster tire, any size, each ☑ ☑ & (NU, RR, UE)

E2218 Manual wheelchair accessory, foam propulsion tire, any size, each ☑ ☑ & (NU, RR, UE)

E2219 Manual wheelchair accessory, foam caster tire, any size, each ☑ ☑ & (NU, RR, UE)

E2220 Manual wheelchair accessory, solid (rubber/plastic) propulsion tire, any size, replacement only, each ☑ ☑ & (NU, RR, UE)

Special Coverage Instructions   Noncovered by Medicare   Carrier Discretion   ☑ Quantity Alert ● New Code   ○ Recycled/Reinstated ▲ Revised Code

© 2023 Optum360, LLC   A2-Z3 ASC Pmt   **CMS:** IOM   **AHA:** Coding Clinic   & DMEPOS Paid   ⊘ SNF Excluded   **E Codes — 45**

E2221 Manual wheelchair accessory, solid (rubber/plastic) caster tire (removable), any size, replacement only, each Y ☑ (NU, RR, UE)

E2222 Manual wheelchair accessory, solid (rubber/plastic) caster tire with integrated wheel, any size, replacement only, each Y ☑ ᴋ (NU, RR, UE)

E2224 Manual wheelchair accessory, propulsion wheel excludes tire, any size, replacement only, each Y ☑ ᴋ (NU, RR, UE)

E2225 Manual wheelchair accessory, caster wheel excludes tire, any size, replacement only, each Y ☑ ᴋ (NU, RR, UE)

E2226 Manual wheelchair accessory, caster fork, any size, replacement only, each Y ☑ ᴋ (NU, RR, UE)

E2227 Manual wheelchair accessory, gear reduction drive wheel, each Y ☑ ᴋ (RR)

E2228 Manual wheelchair accessory, wheel braking system and lock, complete, each Y ☑ ᴋ (RR)

E2230 Manual wheelchair accessory, manual standing system Y

E2231 Manual wheelchair accessory, solid seat support base (replaces sling seat), includes any type mounting hardware Y ᴋ (NU, RR, UE)

E2291 Back, planar, for pediatric size wheelchair including fixed attaching hardware Y

E2292 Seat, planar, for pediatric size wheelchair including fixed attaching hardware Y

E2293 Back, contoured, for pediatric size wheelchair including fixed attaching hardware Y

E2294 Seat, contoured, for pediatric size wheelchair including fixed attaching hardware Y

E2295 Manual wheelchair accessory, for pediatric size wheelchair, dynamic seating frame, allows coordinated movement of multiple positioning features Y

E2300 Wheelchair accessory, power seat elevation system, any type Y
CMS: 100-04,20,30.9

E2301 Wheelchair accessory, power standing system, any type Y

E2310 Power wheelchair accessory, electronic connection between wheelchair controller and one power seating system motor, including all related electronics, indicator feature, mechanical function selection switch, and fixed mounting hardware Y ᴋ (RR)

E2311 Power wheelchair accessory, electronic connection between wheelchair controller and 2 or more power seating system motors, including all related electronics, indicator feature, mechanical function selection switch, and fixed mounting hardware Y ᴋ (RR)

E2312 Power wheelchair accessory, hand or chin control interface, mini-proportional remote joystick, proportional, including fixed mounting hardware Y ᴋ (RR)

E2313 Power wheelchair accessory, harness for upgrade to expandable controller, including all fasteners, connectors and mounting hardware, each Y ☑ ᴋ (RR)

E2321 Power wheelchair accessory, hand control interface, remote joystick, nonproportional, including all related electronics, mechanical stop switch, and fixed mounting hardware Y ᴋ (RR)

E2322 Power wheelchair accessory, hand control interface, multiple mechanical switches, nonproportional, including all related electronics, mechanical stop switch, and fixed mounting hardware Y ᴋ (RR)

E2323 Power wheelchair accessory, specialty joystick handle for hand control interface, prefabricated Y ᴋ (NU, RR, UE)

E2324 Power wheelchair accessory, chin cup for chin control interface Y ᴋ (NU, RR, UE)

E2325 Power wheelchair accessory, sip and puff interface, nonproportional, including all related electronics, mechanical stop switch, and manual swingaway mounting hardware Y ᴋ (RR)

E2326 Power wheelchair accessory, breath tube kit for sip and puff interface Y ᴋ (RR)

E2327 Power wheelchair accessory, head control interface, mechanical, proportional, including all related electronics, mechanical direction change switch, and fixed mounting hardware Y ᴋ (RR)

E2328 Power wheelchair accessory, head control or extremity control interface, electronic, proportional, including all related electronics and fixed mounting hardware Y ᴋ (RR)

E2329 Power wheelchair accessory, head control interface, contact switch mechanism, nonproportional, including all related electronics, mechanical stop switch, mechanical direction change switch, head array, and fixed mounting hardware Y ᴋ (RR)

E2330 Power wheelchair accessory, head control interface, proximity switch mechanism, nonproportional, including all related electronics, mechanical stop switch, mechanical direction change switch, head array, and fixed mounting hardware Y ᴋ (RR)

E2331 Power wheelchair accessory, attendant control, proportional, including all related electronics and fixed mounting hardware Y

E2340 Power wheelchair accessory, nonstandard seat frame width, 20-23 in Y ☑ ᴋ (NU, RR, UE)

E2341 Power wheelchair accessory, nonstandard seat frame width, 24-27 in Y ☑ ᴋ (NU, RR, UE)

E2342 Power wheelchair accessory, nonstandard seat frame depth, 20 or 21 in Y ☑ ᴋ (NU, RR, UE)

E2343 Power wheelchair accessory, nonstandard seat frame depth, 22-25 in Y ☑ ᴋ (NU, RR, UE)

E2351 Power wheelchair accessory, electronic interface to operate speech generating device using power wheelchair control interface Y ᴋ (NU, RR, UE)

E2358 Power wheelchair accessory, group 34 nonsealed lead acid battery, each Y ☑

E2359 Power wheelchair accessory, group 34 sealed lead acid battery, each (e.g., gel cell, absorbed glass mat) Y ᴋ (NU, RR, UE)

E2360 Power wheelchair accessory, 22 NF nonsealed lead acid battery, each Y ☑ ᴋ (NU, RR, UE)

E2361 Power wheelchair accessory, 22 NF sealed lead acid battery, each (e.g., gel cell, absorbed glassmat) Y ☑ ᴋ (NU, RR, UE)

E2362 Power wheelchair accessory, group 24 nonsealed lead acid battery, each Y ☑ ᴋ (NU, RR, UE)

E2363 Power wheelchair accessory, group 24 sealed lead acid battery, each (e.g., gel cell, absorbed glassmat) Y ☑ ᴋ (NU, RR, UE)

E2364 Power wheelchair accessory, U-1 nonsealed lead acid battery, each Y ☑ ᴋ (NU, RR, UE)

E2365 Power wheelchair accessory, U-1 sealed lead acid battery, each (e.g., gel cell, absorbed glassmat) Y ☑ ᴋ (NU, RR, UE)

E2366 Power wheelchair accessory, battery charger, single mode, for use with only one battery type, sealed or nonsealed, each Y ☑ ᴋ (NU, RR, UE)

Special Coverage Instructions   Noncovered by Medicare   Carrier Discretion   ☑ Quantity Alert ● New Code ○ Recycled/Reinstated ▲ Revised Code

46 — E Codes   Ⓐ Age Edit   Ⓜ Maternity Edit   ♀ Female Only   ♂ Male Only   Ⓐ-Ⓨ OPPS Status Indicators   © 2023 Optum360, LLC

Durable Medical Equipment

E2367   Power wheelchair accessory, battery charger, dual mode, for use with either battery type, sealed or nonsealed, each ☑ ☒ ঙ (NU, RR, UE)

E2368   Power wheelchair component, drive wheel motor, replacement only ☑ ঙ (RR)

E2369   Power wheelchair component, drive wheel gear box, replacement only ☑ ঙ (RR)

E2370   Power wheelchair component, integrated drive wheel motor and gear box combination, replacement only ☑ ঙ (RR)

E2371   Power wheelchair accessory, group 27 sealed lead acid battery, (e.g., gel cell, absorbed glassmat), each ☑ ☒ ঙ (NU, RR, UE)

E2372   Power wheelchair accessory, group 27 nonsealed lead acid battery, each ☑ ☒ ঙ (NU, RR, UE)

E2373   Power wheelchair accessory, hand or chin control interface, compact remote joystick, proportional, including fixed mounting hardware ☑ ঙ (RR)

E2374   Power wheelchair accessory, hand or chin control interface, standard remote joystick (not including controller), proportional, including all related electronics and fixed mounting hardware, replacement only ☑ ঙ (RR)

E2375   Power wheelchair accessory, nonexpandable controller, including all related electronics and mounting hardware, replacement only ☑ ঙ (RR)

E2376   Power wheelchair accessory, expandable controller, including all related electronics and mounting hardware, replacement only ☑ ঙ (RR)

E2377   Power wheelchair accessory, expandable controller, including all related electronics and mounting hardware, upgrade provided at initial issue ☑ ঙ (RR)

E2378   Power wheelchair component, actuator, replacement only ☑ ঙ (RR)

E2381   Power wheelchair accessory, pneumatic drive wheel tire, any size, replacement only, each ☑ ☒ ঙ (NU, RR, UE)

E2382   Power wheelchair accessory, tube for pneumatic drive wheel tire, any size, replacement only, each ☑ ☒ ঙ (NU, RR, UE)

E2383   Power wheelchair accessory, insert for pneumatic drive wheel tire (removable), any type, any size, replacement only, each ☑ ☒ ঙ (NU, RR, UE)

E2384   Power wheelchair accessory, pneumatic caster tire, any size, replacement only, each ☑ ☒ ঙ (NU, RR, UE)

E2385   Power wheelchair accessory, tube for pneumatic caster tire, any size, replacement only, each ☑ ☒ ঙ (NU, RR, UE)

E2386   Power wheelchair accessory, foam filled drive wheel tire, any size, replacement only, each ☑ ☒ ঙ (NU, RR, UE)

E2387   Power wheelchair accessory, foam filled caster tire, any size, replacement only, each ☑ ☒ ঙ (NU, RR, UE)

E2388   Power wheelchair accessory, foam drive wheel tire, any size, replacement only, each ☑ ☒ ঙ (NU, RR, UE)

E2389   Power wheelchair accessory, foam caster tire, any size, replacement only, each ☑ ☒ ঙ (NU, RR, UE)

E2390   Power wheelchair accessory, solid (rubber/plastic) drive wheel tire, any size, replacement only, each ☑ ☒ ঙ (NU, RR, UE)

E2391   Power wheelchair accessory, solid (rubber/plastic) caster tire (removable), any size, replacement only, each ☑ ☒ ঙ (NU, RR, UE)

E2392   Power wheelchair accessory, solid (rubber/plastic) caster tire with integrated wheel, any size, replacement only, each ☑ ☒ ঙ (NU, RR, UE)

E2394   Power wheelchair accessory, drive wheel excludes tire, any size, replacement only, each ☑ ☒ ঙ (NU, RR, UE)

E2395   Power wheelchair accessory, caster wheel excludes tire, any size, replacement only, each ☑ ☒ ঙ (NU, RR, UE)

E2396   Power wheelchair accessory, caster fork, any size, replacement only, each ☑ ☒ ঙ (NU, RR, UE)

E2397   Power wheelchair accessory, lithium-based battery, each ☑ ☒ ঙ (NU, RR, UE)

E2398   Wheelchair accessory, dynamic positioning hardware for back

Wound Therapy

E2402   Negative pressure wound therapy electrical pump, stationary or portable ☑ ঙ (RR)
CMS: 100-02,7,40.1.2.8

Speech Generating Device

E2500   Speech generating device, digitized speech, using prerecorded messages, less than or equal to eight minutes recording time ☑ ☒ ঙ (NU, RR, UE)

E2502   Speech generating device, digitized speech, using prerecorded messages, greater than eight minutes but less than or equal to 20 minutes recording time ☑ ☒ ঙ (NU, RR, UE)

E2504   Speech generating device, digitized speech, using prerecorded messages, greater than 20 minutes but less than or equal to 40 minutes recording time ☑ ☒ ঙ (NU, RR, UE)

E2506   Speech generating device, digitized speech, using prerecorded messages, greater than 40 minutes recording time ☑ ☒ ঙ (NU, RR, UE)

E2508   Speech generating device, synthesized speech, requiring message formulation by spelling and access by physical contact with the device ☑ ঙ (NU, RR, UE)

E2510   Speech generating device, synthesized speech, permitting multiple methods of message formulation and multiple methods of device access ☑ ঙ (NU, RR, UE)

E2511   Speech generating software program, for personal computer or personal digital assistant ☑ ঙ (NU, RR, UE)

E2512   Accessory for speech generating device, mounting system ☑ ঙ (NU, RR, UE)

E2599   Accessory for speech generating device, not otherwise classified ☑

Wheelchair Cushion

E2601   General use wheelchair seat cushion, width less than 22 in, any depth ☑ ঙ (NU, RR, UE)

E2602   General use wheelchair seat cushion, width 22 in or greater, any depth ☑ ঙ (NU, RR, UE)

E2603   Skin protection wheelchair seat cushion, width less than 22 in, any depth ☑ ঙ (NU, RR, UE)

E2604   Skin protection wheelchair seat cushion, width 22 in or greater, any depth ☑ ঙ (NU, RR, UE)

E2605   Positioning wheelchair seat cushion, width less than 22 in, any depth ☑ ঙ (NU, RR, UE)

E2606   Positioning wheelchair seat cushion, width 22 in or greater, any depth ☑ ঙ (NU, RR, UE)

E2607   Skin protection and positioning wheelchair seat cushion, width less than 22 in, any depth ☑ ঙ (NU, RR, UE)

E2608   Skin protection and positioning wheelchair seat cushion, width 22 in or greater, any depth ☑ ঙ (NU, RR, UE)

E2609   Custom fabricated wheelchair seat cushion, any size ☑

Special Coverage Instructions   Noncovered by Medicare   Carrier Discretion   ☑ Quantity Alert   ● New Code   ○ Recycled/Reinstated   ▲ Revised Code

Durable Medical Equipment

E2610 — E8002

E2610	Wheelchair seat cushion, powered ▫B
E2611	General use wheelchair back cushion, width less than 22 in, any height, including any type mounting hardware ▫Y & (NU, RR, UE)
E2612	General use wheelchair back cushion, width 22 in or greater, any height, including any type mounting hardware ▫Y & (NU, RR, UE)
E2613	Positioning wheelchair back cushion, posterior, width less than 22 in, any height, including any type mounting hardware ▫Y & (NU, RR, UE)
E2614	Positioning wheelchair back cushion, posterior, width 22 in or greater, any height, including any type mounting hardware ▫Y & (NU, RR, UE)
E2615	Positioning wheelchair back cushion, posterior-lateral, width less than 22 in, any height, including any type mounting hardware ▫Y & (NU, RR, UE)
E2616	Positioning wheelchair back cushion, posterior-lateral, width 22 in or greater, any height, including any type mounting hardware ▫Y & (NU, RR, UE)
E2617	Custom fabricated wheelchair back cushion, any size, including any type mounting hardware ▫Y
E2619	Replacement cover for wheelchair seat cushion or back cushion, each ▫Y ☑ & (NU, RR, UE)
E2620	Positioning wheelchair back cushion, planar back with lateral supports, width less than 22 in, any height, including any type mounting hardware ▫Y & (NU, RR, UE)
E2621	Positioning wheelchair back cushion, planar back with lateral supports, width 22 in or greater, any height, including any type mounting hardware ▫Y & (NU, RR, UE)
E2622	Skin protection wheelchair seat cushion, adjustable, width less than 22 in, any depth ▫Y & (NU, RR, UE)
E2623	Skin protection wheelchair seat cushion, adjustable, width 22 in or greater, any depth ▫Y & (NU, RR, UE)
E2624	Skin protection and positioning wheelchair seat cushion, adjustable, width less than 22 in, any depth ▫Y & (NU, RR, UE)
E2625	Skin protection and positioning wheelchair seat cushion, adjustable, width 22 in or greater, any depth ▫Y & (NU, RR, UE)

Wheelchair Arm Support

E2626	Wheelchair accessory, shoulder elbow, mobile arm support attached to wheelchair, balanced, adjustable ▫Y & (NU, RR, UE)
E2627	Wheelchair accessory, shoulder elbow, mobile arm support attached to wheelchair, balanced, adjustable Rancho type ▫Y & (NU, RR, UE)
E2628	Wheelchair accessory, shoulder elbow, mobile arm support attached to wheelchair, balanced, reclining ▫Y & (NU, RR, UE)
E2629	Wheelchair accessory, shoulder elbow, mobile arm support attached to wheelchair, balanced, friction arm support (friction dampening to proximal and distal joints) ▫Y & (NU, RR, UE)
E2630	Wheelchair accessory, shoulder elbow, mobile arm support, monosuspension arm and hand support, overhead elbow forearm hand sling support, yoke type suspension support ▫Y & (NU, RR, UE)
E2631	Wheelchair accessory, addition to mobile arm support, elevating proximal arm ▫Y & (NU, RR, UE)
E2632	Wheelchair accessory, addition to mobile arm support, offset or lateral rocker arm with elastic balance control ▫Y & (NU, RR, UE)
E2633	Wheelchair accessory, addition to mobile arm support, supinator ▫Y & (NU, RR, UE)

Speech Volume Modulation System

● **E3000**	Speech volume modulation system, any type, including all components and accessories

Gait Trainer

E8000	Gait trainer, pediatric size, posterior support, includes all accessories and components ▫E
E8001	Gait trainer, pediatric size, upright support, includes all accessories and components ▫E
E8002	Gait trainer, pediatric size, anterior support, includes all accessories and components ▫E

Special Coverage Instructions   Noncovered by Medicare   Carrier Discretion   ☑ Quantity Alert ● New Code   ○ Recycled/Reinstated   ▲ Revised Code

48 — E Codes   🄰 Age Edit   🄼 Maternity Edit   ♀ Female Only   ♂ Male Only   🄰-🅈 OPPS Status Indicators   © 2023 Optum360, LLC

Procedures/Professional Services (Temporary) G0008-G9999

The G codes are used to identify professional health care procedures and services that would otherwise be coded in CPT but for which there are no CPT codes. Please refer to your CPT book for possible alternate code(s).

Immunization Administration

G0008   **Administration of influenza virus vaccine**   S
CMS: 100-02,12,40.11; 100-02,13,220; 100-02,13,220.1; 100-02,13,220.3; 100-02,15,50.4.4.2; 100-04,18,1.2; 100-04,18,10.2; 100-04,18,10.2.1; 100-04,18,10.2.2.1; 100-04,18,10.2.5.2; 100-04,18,10.3.1.1; 100-04,18,10.4; 100-04,18,10.4.1; 100-04,18,10.4.2; 100-04,18,10.4.3; 100-04,18,140.8; 1004-04,13,220.1
AHA: 3Q,18

G0009   **Administration of pneumococcal vaccine**   S
CMS: 100-02,12,40.11; 100-02,13,220; 100-02,13,220.1; 100-02,13,220.3; 100-02,15,50.4.4.2; 100-04,18,1.2; 100-04,18,10.2.1; 100-04,18,10.2.2.1; 100-04,18,10.2.5.2; 100-04,18,10.3.1.1; 100-04,18,10.4; 100-04,18,10.4.1; 100-04,18,10.4.2; 100-04,18,10.4.3; 100-04,18,140.8; 1004-04,13,220.1
AHA: 3Q,18

G0010   **Administration of hepatitis B vaccine**   S
CMS: 100-02,12,40.11; 100-02,13,220; 100-02,13,220.1; 100-02,13,220.3; 100-02,15,50.4.4.2; 100-04,18,1.2; 100-04,18,10.2.1; 100-04,18,10.2.2.1; 100-04,18,10.2.5.2; 100-04,18,10.3.1.1; 100-04,18,140.8; 1004-04,13,220.1
AHA: 3Q,18

Pre-exposure Prophylaxis

● **G0011**   **Individual counseling for pre-exposure prophylaxis (PrEP) by physician or qualified health care professional (QHP) to prevent human immunodeficiency virus (HIV), includes HIV risk assessment (initial or continued assessment of risk HIV risk reduction and medication adherence, 15 to 30 minutes**

● **G0012**   **Injection of pre-exposure prophylaxis (PrEP) drug for HIV prevention, under skin or into muscle**

● **G0013**   **Individual counseling for pre-exposure prophylaxis (PrEP) by clinical staff to prevent human immunodeficiency virus (HIV), includes: HIV risk assessment (initial or continued assessment of risk), HIV risk reduction and medication adherence**

Psychotherapy Services

● **G0017**   **Psychotherapy for crisis furnished in an applicable site of service (any place of service at which the nonfacility rate for psychotherapy for crisis services applies, other than the office setting); first 60 minutes**

● **G0018**   **Psychotherapy for crisis furnished in an applicable site of service (any place of service at which the nonfacility rate for psychotherapy for crisis services applies, other than the office setting); each additional 30 minutes (list separately in addition to code for primary service)**

Community Health Integration Services

● **G0019**   **Community health integration services performed by certified or trained auxiliary personnel, including a community health worker, under the direction of a physician or other practitioner, 60 minutes per calendar month, in the following activities to address social determinants of health (SDOH) need(s) that are significantly limiting the ability to diagnose or treat problem(s) addressed in an initiating visit:**
— person-centered assessment, performed to better understand the individualized context of the intersection between the SDOH need(s) and the problem(s) addressed in the initiating visit;
— conducting a person-centered assessment to understand patient's life story, strengths, needs, goals, preferences and desired outcomes, including understanding cultural and linguistic factors and including unmet SDOH needs (that are not separately billed);
— facilitating patient-driven goal-setting and establishing an action plan;
— providing tailored support to the patient as needed to accomplish the practitioner's treatment plan;
— practitioner, home-, and community-based care coordination;
— coordinating receipt of needed services from health care practitioners, providers, and facilities, and from home- and community-based service providers, social service providers, and caregiver (if applicable);
— communication with practitioners, home- and community-based service providers, hospitals, and skilled nursing facilities (or other health care facilities) regarding the patient's psychosocial strengths and needs, functional deficits, goals, preferences, and desired outcomes, including cultural and linguistic factors;
— coordination of care transitions between and among health care practitioners and settings, including transitions involving referral to other clinicians;
— follow-up after an emergency department visit, or follow-up after discharges from hospitals, skilled nursing facilities or other health care facilities;
— facilitating access to community-based social services (e.g., housing, utilities, transportation, food assistance) to address the SDOH need(s),
— health education-helping the patient contextualize health education provided by the patient's treatment team with the patient's individual needs, goals, and preferences, in the context of the SDOH need(s), and educating the patient on how to best participate in medical decision-making;
— building patient self-advocacy skills, so that the patient can interact with members of the health care team and related community-based services addressing the SDOH need(s), in ways that are more likely to promote personalized and effective diagnosis or treatment;
— health care access/health system navigation; helping the patient access health care, including identifying appropriate practitioners or providers for clinical care and helping secure appointments with them;
— facilitating behavioral change as necessary for meeting diagnosis and treatment goals, including promoting patient motivation to participate in care and reach person-centered diagnosis or treatment goals;
— facilitating and providing social and emotional support to help the patient cope with the problem(s) addressed in the initiating visit, the SDOH need(s), and adjust daily routines to better meet diagnosis and treatment goals;
— leveraging lived experience when applicable to provide support, mentorship, or inspiration to meet treatment goals

● **G0022**   **Community health integration services, each additional 30 minutes per calendar month (list separately in addition to G0019)**

Special Coverage Instructions   Noncovered by Medicare   Carrier Discretion   ☑ Quantity Alert   ● New Code   ○ Recycled/Reinstated   ▲ Revised Code

© 2023 Optum360, LLC   A2-Z3 ASC Pmt   CMS: IOM   AHA: Coding Clinic   ⅃ DMEPOS Paid   ⊘ SNF Excluded   G Codes — 49

Principle Illness Navigation Services

● **G0023**　**Principal illness navigation services by certified or trained auxiliary personnel under the direction of a physician or other practitioner, including a patient navigator, 60 minutes per calendar month, in the following activities:**
— person-centered assessment, performed to better understand the individual context of the serious, high-risk condition;
— conducting a person-centered assessment to understand the patient's life story, strengths, needs, goals, preferences, and desired outcomes, including understanding cultural and linguistic factors and including unmet SDOH needs (that are not separately billed);
— facilitating patient-driven goal setting and establishing an action plan; providing tailored support as needed to accomplish the practitioner's treatment plan;
— identifying or referring patient (and caregiver or family, if applicable) to appropriate supportive services; practitioner, home, and community-based care coordination;
— coordinating receipt of needed services from health care practitioners, providers, and facilities, home- and community-based service providers, and caregiver (if applicable);
— communication with practitioners, home-, and community-based service providers, hospitals, and skilled nursing facilities (or other health care facilities) regarding the patient's psychosocial strengths and needs, functional deficits, goals, preferences, and desired outcomes, including cultural and linguistic factors;
— coordination of care transitions between and among health care practitioners and settings, including transitions involving referral to other clinicians, follow-up after an emergency department visit, or follow-up after discharges from hospitals, skilled nursing facilities, or other health care facilities;
— facilitating access to community-based social services (e.g., housing, utilities, transportation, likely to promote personalized and effective treatment of their condition;
— health care access/health system navigation;
— helping the patient access health care, including identifying appropriate practitioners or providers for clinical care, and helping secure appointments with them;
— providing the patient with information/resources to consider participation in clinical trials or clinical research as applicable;
— facilitating behavioral change as necessary for meeting diagnosis and treatment goals, including promoting patient motivation to participate in care and reach person-centered diagnosis or treatment goals; facilitating and providing social and emotional support to help the patient cope with the condition, SDOH need(s), and adjust daily routines to better meet diagnosis and treatment goals;
— leverage knowledge of the serious, high-risk condition, and/or lived experience when applicable to provide support, mentorship, or inspiration to meet treatment goals

● **G0024**　**Principal illness navigation services, additional 30 minutes per calendar month (list separately in addition to G0023)**

Semen Analysis

G0027　**Semen analysis; presence and/or motility of sperm excluding Huhner**　　　　　　　　　　　　　　　　　　♂ Ⓠ

Quality Measures

G0029　**Tobacco screening not performed or tobacco cessation intervention not provided during the measurement period or in the 6 months prior to the measurement period**

G0030　**Patient screened for tobacco use and received tobacco cessation intervention during the measurement period or in the 6 months prior to the measurement period (counseling, pharmacotherapy, or both), if identified as a tobacco user**

G0031　**Palliative care services given to patient any time during the measurement period**

G0032　**Two or more antipsychotic prescriptions ordered for patients who had a diagnosis of schizophrenia, schizoaffective disorder, or bipolar disorder on or between January 1 of the year prior to the measurement period and the index prescription start date (IPSD) for antipsychotics**

G0033　**Two or more benzodiazepine prescriptions ordered for patients who had a diagnosis of seizure disorders, rapid eye movement sleep behavior disorder, benzodiazepine withdrawal, ethanol withdrawal, or severe generalized anxiety disorder on or between January 1 of the year prior to the measurement period and the IPSD for benzodiazepines**

G0034　**Patients receiving palliative care during the measurement period**

G0035　**Patient has any emergency department encounter during the performance period with place of service indicator 23**

G0036　**Patient or care partner decline assessment**

G0037　**On date of encounter, patient is not able to participate in assessment or screening, including nonverbal patients, delirious, severely aphasic, severely developmentally delayed, severe visual or hearing impairment and for those patients, no knowledgeable informant available**

G0038　**Clinician determines patient does not require referral**

G0039　**Patient not referred, reason not otherwise specified**

G0040　**Patient already receiving physical/occupational/speech/recreational therapy during the measurement period**

G0041　**Patient and/or care partner decline referral**

G0042　**Referral to physical, occupational, speech, or recreational therapy**

G0043　**Patients with mechanical prosthetic heart valve**

G0044　**Patients with moderate or severe mitral stenosis**

G0045　**Clinical follow-up and MRS score assessed at 90 days following endovascular stroke intervention**

G0046　**Clinical follow-up and MRS score not assessed at 90 days following endovascular stroke intervention**

G0047　**Pediatric patient with minor blunt head trauma and PECARN prediction criteria are not assessed**

G0048　**Patients who receive palliative care services any time during the intake period through the end of the measurement year**

G0049　**With maintenance hemodialysis (in-center and home HD) for the complete reporting month**

G0050　**Patients with a catheter that have limited life expectancy**

G0051　**Patients under hospice care in the current reporting month**

G0052　**Patients on peritoneal dialysis for any portion of the reporting month**

G0053　**Advancing rheumatology patient care MIPS value pathways**

G0054　**Coordinating stroke care to promote prevention and cultivate positive outcomes MIPS value pathways**

G0055　**Advancing care for heart disease MIPS value pathways**

G0056　~~**Optimizing chronic disease management MIPS value pathways**~~

G0057　**Proposed adopting best practices and promoting patient safety within emergency medicine MIPS value pathways**

G0058　**Improving care for lower extremity joint repair MIPS value pathways**

G0059　**Patient safety and support of positive experiences with anesthesia MIPS value pathways**

G0060　**Allergy/Immunology MIPS specialty set**

Special Coverage Instructions　　Noncovered by Medicare　　Carrier Discretion　　☑ Quantity Alert　● New Code　○ Recycled/Reinstated　▲ Revised Code

50 — G Codes　　　Ⓐ Age Edit　　Ⓜ Maternity Edit　♀ Female Only　♂ Male Only　Ⓐ-Ⓨ OPPS Status Indicators　　© 2023 Optum360, LLC

G0061	Anesthesiology MIPS specialty set
G0062	Audiology MIPS specialty set
G0063	Cardiology MIPS specialty set
G0064	Certified Nurse Midwife MIPS specialty set
G0065	Chiropractic Medicine MIPS specialty set
G0066	Clinical Social Work MIPS specialty set
G0067	Dentistry MIPS specialty set

Professional Services

G0068 Professional services for the administration of anti-infective, pain management, chelation, pulmonary hypertension, inotropic, or other intravenous infusion drug or biological (excluding chemotherapy or other highly complex drug or biological) for each infusion drug administration calendar day in the individual's home, each 15 min
CMS: 100-04,20,180; 100-04,32,411.3; 100-04,32,411.4; 100-04,32,411.5; 100-04,32,411.6

G0069 Professional services for the administration of subcutaneous immunotherapy or other subcutaneous infusion drug or biological for each infusion drug administration calendar day in the individual's home, each 15 min
CMS: 100-04,20,180; 100-04,32,411.3; 100-04,32,411.4; 100-04,32,411.5; 100-04,32,411.6

G0070 Professional services for the administration of intravenous chemotherapy or other intravenous highly complex drug or biological infusion for each infusion drug administration calendar day in the individual's home, each 15 min
CMS: 100-04,20,180; 100-04,32,411.3; 100-04,32,411.4; 100-04,32,411.5; 100-04,32,411.6

G0071 Payment for communication technology-based services for 5 minutes or more of a virtual (nonface-to-face) communication between a rural health clinic (RHC) or federally qualified health center (FQHC) practitioner and RHC or FQHC patient, or 5 minutes or more of remote evaluation of recorded video and/or images by an RHC or FQHC practitioner, occurring in lieu of an office visit; RHC or FQHC only
CMS: 100-04,9,70.7

G0076 Brief (20 minutes) care management home visit for a new patient. For use only in a Medicare-approved CMMI model (services must be furnished within a beneficiary's home, domiciliary, rest home, assisted living and/or nursing facility)

G0077 Limited (30 minutes) care management home visit for a new patient. For use only in a Medicare-approved CMMI model (services must be furnished within a beneficiary's home, domiciliary, rest home, assisted living and/or nursing facility)

G0078 Moderate (45 minutes) care management home visit for a new patient. For use only in a Medicare-approved CMMI model (services must be furnished within a beneficiary's home, domiciliary, rest home, assisted living and/or nursing facility)

G0079 Comprehensive (60 minutes) care management home visit for a new patient. For use only in a Medicare-approved CMMI model (services must be furnished within a beneficiary's home, domiciliary, rest home, assisted living and/or nursing facility)

G0080 Extensive (75 minutes) care management home visit for a new patient. For use only in a Medicare-approved CMMI model (services must be furnished within a beneficiary's home, domiciliary, rest home, assisted living and/or nursing facility)

G0081 Brief (20 minutes) care management home visit for an existing patient. For use only in a Medicare-approved CMMI model (services must be furnished within a beneficiary's home, domiciliary, rest home, assisted living and/or nursing facility)

G0082 Limited (30 minutes) care management home visit for an existing patient. For use only in a Medicare-approved CMMI model (services must be furnished within a beneficiary's home, domiciliary, rest home, assisted living and/or nursing facility)

G0083 Moderate (45 minutes) care management home visit for an existing patient. For use only in a Medicare-approved CMMI model (services must be furnished within a beneficiary's home, domiciliary, rest home, assisted living and/or nursing facility)

G0084 Comprehensive (60 minutes) care management home visit for an existing patient. For use only in a Medicare-approved CMMI model (services must be furnished within a beneficiary's home, domiciliary, rest home, assisted living and/or nursing facility)

G0085 Extensive (75 minutes) care management home visit for an existing patient. For use only in a Medicare-approved CMMI model (services must be furnished within a beneficiary's home, domiciliary, rest home, assisted living and/or nursing facility)

G0086 Limited (30 minutes) care management home care plan oversight. For use only in a Medicare-approved CMMI model (services must be furnished within a beneficiary's home, domiciliary, rest home, assisted living and/or nursing facility)

G0087 Comprehensive (60 minutes) care management home care plan oversight. For use only in a Medicare-approved CMMI model (services must be furnished within a beneficiary's home, domiciliary, rest home, assisted living and/or nursing facility)

G0088 Professional services, initial visit, for the administration of anti-infective, pain management, chelation, pulmonary hypertension, inotropic, or other intravenous infusion drug or biological (excluding chemotherapy or other highly complex drug or biological) for each infusion drug administration calendar day in the individual's home, each 15 min
CMS: 100-04,32,411.3; 100-04,32,411.4; 100-04,32,411.5; 100-04,32,411.6

G0089 Professional services, initial visit, for the administration of subcutaneous immunotherapy or other subcutaneous infusion drug or biological for each infusion drug administration calendar day in the individual's home, each 15 min
CMS: 100-04,32,411.3; 100-04,32,411.4; 100-04,32,411.5; 100-04,32,411.6

G0090 Professional services, initial visit, for the administration of intravenous chemotherapy or other highly complex infusion drug or biological for each infusion drug administration calendar day in the individual's home, each 15 min
CMS: 100-04,32,411.3; 100-04,32,411.4; 100-04,32,411.5; 100-04,32,411.6

Screening Services

G0101 Cervical or vaginal cancer screening; pelvic and clinical breast examination   A ♀ S ⊘
G0101 can be reported with an E/M code when a separately identifiable E/M service was provided.
CMS: 100-02,13,220; 100-02,13,220.1; 100-03,210.2; 100-04,18,1.2; 1004-04,13,220.1

G0102 Prostate cancer screening; digital rectal examination   ♂ N ⊘
CMS: 100-02,13,220; 100-02,13,220.1; 100-02,13,220.3; 100-04,18,1.2; 100-04,18,50.3; 100-04,18,50.4

G0103 Prostate cancer screening; prostate specific antigen test (PSA)   ♂ A
CMS: 100-04,18,1.2; 100-04,18,50.3

G0104 Colorectal cancer screening; flexible sigmoidoscopy   T P3 ⊘
Medicare covers colorectal screening for cancer via flexible sigmoidoscopy once every four years for patients 50 years or older.
CMS: 100-02,15,280.2.2; 100-04,18,1.2; 100-04,18,60; 100-04,18,60.1; 100-04,18,60.1.1; 100-04,18,60.2; 100-04,18,60.2.1; 100-04,18,60.6; 100-04,18,60.7

Special Coverage Instructions   Noncovered by Medicare   Carrier Discretion   ☑ Quantity Alert   ● New Code   ○ Recycled/Reinstated   ▲ Revised Code

© 2023 Optum360, LLC   A2-Z3 ASC Pmt   **CMS:** IOM   **AHA:** Coding Clinic   ♿ DMEPOS Paid   ⊘ SNF Excluded   **G Codes — 51**

Procedures/Professional Services (Temporary)

G0105 — G0137

G0105 Colorectal cancer screening; colonoscopy on individual at high risk ⬚T ⬚A2 ⊘

An individual with ulcerative enteritis or a history of a malignant neoplasm of the lower gastrointestinal tract is considered at high-risk for colorectal cancer, as defined by CMS.

CMS: 100-02,15,280.2.2; 100-04,12,30.1; 100-04,18,1.2; 100-04,18,60; 100-04,18,60.1; 100-04,18,60.1.1; 100-04,18,60.2; 100-04,18,60.2.1; 100-04,18,60.2.2; 100-04,18,60.6; 100-04,18,60.7; 100-04,18,60.8; 100-04,23,30.2; 100-04,4,250.18

AHA: 3Q,23; 4Q,22; 2Q,18

G0106 Colorectal cancer screening; alternative to G0104, screening sigmoidoscopy, barium enema ⬚S

CMS: 100-02,15,280.2.2; 100-04,18,1.2; 100-04,18,60; 100-04,18,60.1; 100-04,18,60.1.1; 100-04,18,60.2; 100-04,18,60.2.1; 100-04,18,60.6; 100-04,18,60.7

G0108 Diabetes outpatient self-management training services, individual, per 30 minutes ⬚A ☑ ⊘

CMS: 100-02,13,220.3; 100-02,15,300; 100-02,15,300.2; 100-02,15,300.3; 100-02,15,300.4; 100-04,12,190.3; 100-04,12,190.3.6; 100-04,12,190.6; 100-04,12,190.6.1; 100-04,12,190.7; 100-04,18,1.2; 100-04,18,120.1; 100-04,4,300.6

AHA: 3Q,19

G0109 Diabetes outpatient self-management training services, group session (two or more), per 30 minutes ⬚A ☑ ⊘

CMS: 100-02,15,300.2; 100-02,15,300.3; 100-04,12,190.3; 100-04,12,190.3.6; 100-04,12,190.6; 100-04,12,190.6.1; 100-04,12,190.7; 100-04,18,1.2; 100-04,4,300.6

AHA: 3Q,19

G0117 Glaucoma screening for high risk patients furnished by an optometrist or ophthalmologist ⬚S ⊘

CMS: 100-02,13,220; 100-02,13,220.1; 100-02,13,220.3; 100-02,15,280.1; 100-04,18,1.2; 100-04,18,70.1.1; 1004-04,13,220.1

G0118 Glaucoma screening for high risk patient furnished under the direct supervision of an optometrist or ophthalmologist ⬚S ⊘

CMS: 100-02,13,220; 100-02,13,220.1; 100-02,13,220.3; 100-02,15,280.1; 100-04,18,1.2; 100-04,18,70.1.1; 1004-04,13,220.1

G0120 Colorectal cancer screening; alternative to G0105, screening colonoscopy, barium enema ⬚S

CMS: 100-02,15,280.2.2; 100-04,18,1.2; 100-04,18,60; 100-04,18,60.1; 100-04,18,60.1.1; 100-04,18,60.2; 100-04,18,60.2.1; 100-04,18,60.6; 100-04,18,60.7; 100-04,18,60.8

G0121 Colorectal cancer screening; colonoscopy on individual not meeting criteria for high risk ⬚T ⬚A2 ⊘

CMS: 100-02,15,280.2.2; 100-04,12,30.1; 100-04,18,1.2; 100-04,18,60; 100-04,18,60.1; 100-04,18,60.1.1; 100-04,18,60.2; 100-04,18,60.2.1; 100-04,18,60.2.2; 100-04,18,60.5; 100-04,18,60.6; 100-04,23,30.2; 100-04,4,250.18

AHA: 3Q,23; 4Q,22; 2Q,18

G0122 Colorectal cancer screening; barium enema ⬚E1

CMS: 100-02,15,280.2.2; 100-04,18,60; 100-04,18,60.2; 100-04,18,60.2.1; 100-04,18,60.5; 100-04,18,60.6; 100-04,18,60.7; 100-04,18,60.8

G0123 Screening cytopathology, cervical or vaginal (any reporting system), collected in preservative fluid, automated thin layer preparation, screening by cytotechnologist under physician supervision ⬚A ♀ ⬚A

See also P3000-P3001.

CMS: 100-03,210.2.1; 100-04,18,1.2; 100-04,18,30.2.1; 100-04,18,30.5; 100-04,18,30.6

G0124 Screening cytopathology, cervical or vaginal (any reporting system), collected in preservative fluid, automated thin layer preparation, requiring interpretation by physician ⬚A ♀ ⬚B ⊘

See also P3000-P3001.

CMS: 100-03,210.2.1; 100-04,18,1.2; 100-04,18,30.2.1; 100-04,18,30.5; 100-04,18,30.6

Miscellaneous Services

G0127 Trimming of dystrophic nails, any number ⬚01 ⊘

CMS: 100-02,15,290

G0128 Direct (face-to-face with patient) skilled nursing services of a registered nurse provided in a comprehensive outpatient rehabilitation facility, each 10 minutes beyond the first 5 minutes ⬚B ☑ ⊘

CMS: 100-02,12,30.1; 100-02,12,40.8; 100-02,17,40.1.2; 100-04,39,30.6; 100-04,39,30.8; 100-04,5,100.3; 100-04,5,20.4

▲ **G0129** Occupational therapy services requiring the skills of a qualified occupational therapist, furnished as a component of a partial hospitalization or intensive outpatient treatment program, per session (45 minutes or more) ⬚P ☑

CMS: 100-04,4,260.1; 100-04,4,260.1.1

G0130 Single energy x-ray absorptiometry (SEXA) bone density study, one or more sites; appendicular skeleton (peripheral) (e.g., radius, wrist, heel) ⬚S ⬚Z3

CMS: 100-04,18,1.2

● **G0136** Administration of a standardized, evidence-based social determinants of health risk assessment tool, 5 to 15 minutes

● **G0137** Intensive outpatient services, weekly bundle, minimum of 9 services over a 7 contiguous day period, which can include:

— individual and group therapy with physicians or psychologists (or other mental health professionals to the extent authorized under state law);

— occupational therapy requiring the skills of a qualified occupational therapist;

— services of social workers, trained psychiatric nurses, and other staff trained to work with psychiatric patients;

— individualized activity therapies that are not primarily recreational or diversionary; family counseling (the primary purpose of which is treatment of the individual's condition);

— patient training and education (to the extent that training and educational activities are closely and clearly related to individual's care and treatment);

— diagnostic services;

— such other items and services (excluding meals and transportation) that are reasonable and necessary for the diagnosis or active treatment of the individual's condition, reasonably expected to improve or maintain the individual's condition and functional level, and to prevent relapse or hospitalization, and furnished pursuant to such guidelines relating to frequency and duration of services in accordance with a physician certification and plan of treatment (provision of the services by a Medicare-enrolled opioid treatment program) (List separately in addition to code for primary procedure)

Special Coverage Instructions Noncovered by Medicare Carrier Discretion ☑ Quantity Alert ● New Code ○ Recycled/Reinstated ▲ Revised Code

52 — G Codes ⬚A Age Edit ⬚M Maternity Edit ♀ Female Only ♂ Male Only ⬚A-Y OPPS Status Indicators © 2023 Optum360, LLC

● **G0140**   **Principal illness navigation-peer support by certified or trained auxiliary personnel under the direction of a physician or other practitioner, including a certified peer specialist, 60 minutes per calendar month, in the following activities:**
— person-centered interview, performed to better understand the individual context of the serious, high-risk condition;
— conducting a person-centered interview to understand the patient's life story, strengths, needs, goals, preferences, and desired outcomes, including understanding cultural and linguistic factors, and including unmet SDOH needs (that are not billed separately);
— facilitating patient-driven goal setting and establishing an action plan;
— providing tailored support as needed to accomplish the person-centered goals in the practitioner's treatment plan;
— identifying or referring patient (and caregiver or family, if applicable) to appropriate supportive services;
— practitioner, home-, and community-based care communication;
— assist the patient in communicating with their practitioners, home-, and community-based service providers, hospitals, and skilled nursing facilities (or other health care facilities) regarding the patient's psychosocial strengths and needs, goals, preferences, and desired outcomes, including cultural and linguistic factors;
— facilitating access to community-based social services (e.g., housing, utilities, transportation, food assistance) as needed to address SDOH need(s);
— health education-helping the patient contextualize health education provided by the patient's treatment team with the patient's individual needs, goals, preferences, and SDOH need(s), and educating the patient (and caregiver if applicable) on how to best participate in medical decision-making;
— building patient self-advocacy skills, so that the patient can interact with members of the health care team and related community-based services (as needed), in ways that are more likely to promote personalized and effective treatment of their condition;
— developing and proposing strategies to help meet person-centered treatment goals and supporting the patient in using chosen strategies to reach person-centered treatment goals;
— facilitating and providing social and emotional support to help the patient cope with the condition, SDOH need(s), and adjust daily routines to better meet person-centered diagnosis and treatment goals;
— leverage knowledge of the serious, high risk condition and/or lived experience when applicable to provide support, mentorship, or inspiration to meet treatment goals

G0141   **Screening cytopathology smears, cervical or vaginal, performed by automated system, with manual rescreening, requiring interpretation by physician**   Ⓐ ♀Ⓑ ⊘
CMS: 100-03,210.2.1; 100-04,18,1.2; 100-04,18,30.2.1; 100-04,18,30.5; 100-04,18,30.6

G0143   **Screening cytopathology, cervical or vaginal (any reporting system), collected in preservative fluid, automated thin layer preparation, with manual screening and rescreening by cytotechnologist under physician supervision**   Ⓐ ♀Ⓐ
CMS: 100-03,210.2.1; 100-04,18,1.2; 100-04,18,30.2.1; 100-04,18,30.5; 100-04,18,30.6

G0144   **Screening cytopathology, cervical or vaginal (any reporting system), collected in preservative fluid, automated thin layer preparation, with screening by automated system, under physician supervision**   Ⓐ ♀Ⓐ
CMS: 100-03,210.2.1; 100-04,18,30.2.1; 100-04,18,30.5; 100-04,18,30.6

G0145   **Screening cytopathology, cervical or vaginal (any reporting system), collected in preservative fluid, automated thin layer preparation, with screening by automated system and manual rescreening under physician supervision**   Ⓐ ♀Ⓐ
CMS: 100-03,210.2.1; 100-04,18,1.2; 100-04,18,30.2.1; 100-04,18,30.5; 100-04,18,30.6

● **G0146**   **Principal illness navigation-peer support, additional 30 minutes per calendar month (list separately in addition to G0140)**
CMS: 100-03,210.2.1; 100-04,18,30.2.1; 100-04,18,30.5; 100-04,18,30.6

G0147   **Screening cytopathology smears, cervical or vaginal, performed by automated system under physician supervision**   Ⓐ ♀Ⓐ
CMS: 100-03,210.2.1; 100-04,18,1.2; 100-04,18,30.2.1; 100-04,18,30.5; 100-04,18,30.6

G0148   **Screening cytopathology smears, cervical or vaginal, performed by automated system with manual rescreening**   Ⓐ ♀Ⓐ
CMS: 100-03,210.2.1; 100-04,18,1.2; 100-04,18,30.2.1; 100-04,18,30.5; 100-04,18,30.6

G0151   **Services performed by a qualified physical therapist in the home health or hospice setting, each 15 minutes**   Ⓑ ☑
CMS: 100-01,3,30.3; 100-04,10,40.2; 100-04,11,10; 100-04,11,130.1; 100-04,11,30.3

G0152   **Services performed by a qualified occupational therapist in the home health or hospice setting, each 15 minutes**   Ⓑ ☑
CMS: 100-01,3,30.3; 100-04,10,40.2; 100-04,11,10; 100-04,11,130.1; 100-04,11,30.3

G0153   **Services performed by a qualified speech-language pathologist in the home health or hospice setting, each 15 minutes**   Ⓑ ☑
CMS: 100-01,3,30.3; 100-04,10,40.2; 100-04,11,10; 100-04,11,130.1; 100-04,11,30.3

G0155   **Services of clinical social worker in home health or hospice settings, each 15 minutes**   Ⓑ ☑
CMS: 100-01,3,30.3; 100-04,10,40.2; 100-04,11,10; 100-04,11,130.1; 100-04,11,30.3

G0156   **Services of home health/hospice aide in home health or hospice settings, each 15 minutes**   Ⓑ ☑
CMS: 100-01,3,30.3; 100-04,10,40.2; 100-04,11,10; 100-04,11,130.1; 100-04,11,30.3

G0157   **Services performed by a qualified physical therapist assistant in the home health or hospice setting, each 15 minutes**   Ⓑ ☑
CMS: 100-04,10,40.2; 100-04,11,10

G0158   **Services performed by a qualified occupational therapist assistant in the home health or hospice setting, each 15 minutes**   Ⓑ ☑
CMS: 100-04,10,40.2; 100-04,11,10

G0159   **Services performed by a qualified physical therapist, in the home health setting, in the establishment or delivery of a safe and effective physical therapy maintenance program, each 15 minutes**   Ⓑ ☑
CMS: 100-04,10,40.2

G0160   **Services performed by a qualified occupational therapist, in the home health setting, in the establishment or delivery of a safe and effective occupational therapy maintenance program, each 15 minutes**   Ⓑ ☑
CMS: 100-04,10,40.2

G0161   **Services performed by a qualified speech-language pathologist, in the home health setting, in the establishment or delivery of a safe and effective speech-language pathology maintenance program, each 15 minutes**   Ⓑ ☑
CMS: 100-04,10,40.2

G0162   **Skilled services by a registered nurse (RN) for management and evaluation of the plan of care; each 15 minutes (the patient's underlying condition or complication requires an RN to ensure that essential nonskilled care achieves its purpose in the home health or hospice setting)**   Ⓑ ☑
CMS: 100-04,10,40.2; 100-04,11,10

G0166   **External counterpulsation, per treatment session**   Ⓝ ☑ ⊘
CMS: 100-04,32,130; 100-04,32,130.1

G0168   **Wound closure utilizing tissue adhesive(s) only**   Ⓑ ⊘

G0175   **Scheduled interdisciplinary team conference (minimum of three exclusive of patient care nursing staff) with patient present**   Ⓥ
CMS: 100-04,4,160

G0176 Activity therapy, such as music, dance, art or play therapies not for recreation, related to the care and treatment of patient's disabling mental health problems, per session (45 minutes or more) P
CMS: 100-04,4,260.1; 100-04,4,260.1.1; 100-04,4,260.5

G0177 Training and educational services related to the care and treatment of patient's disabling mental health problems per session (45 minutes or more) N
CMS: 100-04,4,260.1; 100-04,4,260.1.1

G0179 Physician or allowed practitioner re-certification for Medicare-covered home health services under a home health plan of care (patient not present), including contacts with home health agency and review of reports of patient status required by physicians and allowed practitioners to affirm the initial implementation of the plan of care M ⊘
CMS: 100-02,7,30.5.4; 100-04,10,20.1.2; 100-04,12,180; 100-04,12,180.1

G0180 Physician or allowed practitioner certification for Medicare-covered home health services under a home health plan of care (patient not present), including contacts with home health agency and review of reports of patient status required by physicians or allowed practitioners to affirm the initial implementation of the plan of care M ⊘
CMS: 100-02,7,30.5.4; 100-04,10,20.1.2; 100-04,12,180; 100-04,12,180.1

G0181 Physician or allowed practitioner supervision of a patient receiving Medicare-covered services provided by a participating home health agency (patient not present) requiring complex and multidisciplinary care modalities involving regular physician or allowed practitioner development and/or revision of care plans M ⊘
CMS: 100-04,12,100.1.4; 100-04,12,180; 100-04,12,180.1

G0182 Physician supervision of a patient under a Medicare-approved hospice (patient not present) requiring complex and multidisciplinary care modalities involving regular physician development and/or revision of care plans, review of subsequent reports of patient status, review of laboratory and other studies, communication (including telephone calls) with other health care professionals involved in the patient's care, integration of new information into the medical treatment plan and/or adjustment of medical therapy, within a calendar month, 30 minutes or more M ⊘
CMS: 100-04,11,40.1.3.1; 100-04,12,100.1.4; 100-04,12,180; 100-04,12,180.1

G0186 Destruction of localized lesion of choroid (for example, choroidal neovascularization); photocoagulation, feeder vessel technique (one or more sessions) T R2 ⊘

G0219 PET imaging whole body; melanoma for noncovered indications E1
CMS: 100-03,220.6.10; 100-03,220.6.12; 100-03,220.6.17; 100-03,220.6.3; 100-03,220.6.4; 100-03,220.6.6; 100-03,220.6.7; 100-04,13,60; 100-04,13,60.16

G0235 PET imaging, any site, not otherwise specified E1 Z2
CMS: 100-03,220.6.10; 100-03,220.6.12; 100-03,220.6.13; 100-03,220.6.17; 100-03,220.6.2; 100-03,220.6.3; 100-03,220.6.4; 100-03,220.6.5; 100-03,220.6.6; 100-03,220.6.7; 100-03,220.6.9; 100-04,13,60; 100-04,13,60.13; 100-04,13,60.14; 100-04,13,60.16; 100-04,13,60.17

G0237 Therapeutic procedures to increase strength or endurance of respiratory muscles, face-to-face, one-on-one, each 15 minutes (includes monitoring) S ☑ ⊘
CMS: 100-02,12,30.1; 100-02,12,40.5

G0238 Therapeutic procedures to improve respiratory function, other than described by G0237, one-on-one, face-to-face, per 15 minutes (includes monitoring) S ☑
CMS: 100-02,12,30.1; 100-02,12,40.5

G0239 Therapeutic procedures to improve respiratory function or increase strength or endurance of respiratory muscles, two or more individuals (includes monitoring) S
CMS: 100-02,12,30.1; 100-02,12,40.5

G0245 Initial physician evaluation and management of a diabetic patient with diabetic sensory neuropathy resulting in a loss of protective sensation (LOPS) which must include: (1) the diagnosis of LOPS, (2) a patient history, (3) a physical examination that consists of at least the following elements: (a) visual inspection of the forefoot, hindfoot, and toe web spaces, (b) evaluation of a protective sensation, (c) evaluation of foot structure and biomechanics, (d) evaluation of vascular status and skin integrity, and (e) evaluation and recommendation of footwear, and (4) patient education V ⊘
CMS: 100-04,32,80.2; 100-04,32,80.3; 100-04,32,80.6; 100-04,32,80.8

G0246 Follow-up physician evaluation and management of a diabetic patient with diabetic sensory neuropathy resulting in a loss of protective sensation (LOPS) to include at least the following: (1) a patient history, (2) a physical examination that includes: (a) visual inspection of the forefoot, hindfoot, and toe web spaces, (b) evaluation of protective sensation, (c) evaluation of foot structure and biomechanics, (d) evaluation of vascular status and skin integrity, and (e) evaluation and recommendation of footwear, and (3) patient education V ⊘
CMS: 100-03,70.2.1; 100-04,32,80; 100-04,32,80.2; 100-04,32,80.3; 100-04,32,80.6; 100-04,32,80.8

G0247 Routine foot care by a physician of a diabetic patient with diabetic sensory neuropathy resulting in a loss of protective sensation (LOPS) to include the local care of superficial wounds (i.e., superficial to muscle and fascia) and at least the following, if present: (1) local care of superficial wounds, (2) debridement of corns and calluses, and (3) trimming and debridement of nails 01 ⊘
CMS: 100-03,70.2.1; 100-04,32,80; 100-04,32,80.2; 100-04,32,80.3; 100-04,32,80.6; 100-04,32,80.8

G0248 Demonstration, prior to initiation of home INR monitoring, for patient with either mechanical heart valve(s), chronic atrial fibrillation, or venous thromboembolism who meets Medicare coverage criteria, under the direction of a physician; includes: face-to-face demonstration of use and care of the INR monitor, obtaining at least one blood sample, provision of instructions for reporting home INR test results, and documentation of patient's ability to perform testing and report results V
CMS: 100-03,190.11; 100-04,32,80

G0249 Provision of test materials and equipment for home INR monitoring of patient with either mechanical heart valve(s), chronic atrial fibrillation, or venous thromboembolism who meets Medicare coverage criteria; includes: provision of materials for use in the home and reporting of test results to physician; testing not occurring more frequently than once a week; testing materials, billing units of service include four tests V ☑
CMS: 100-03,190.11

G0250 Physician review, interpretation, and patient management of home INR testing for patient with either mechanical heart valve(s), chronic atrial fibrillation, or venous thromboembolism who meets Medicare coverage criteria; testing not occurring more frequently than once a week; billing units of service include four tests M ☑ ⊘
CMS: 100-03,190.11

G0252 PET imaging, full and partial-ring PET scanners only, for initial diagnosis of breast cancer and/or surgical planning for breast cancer (e.g., initial staging of axillary lymph nodes) E1
CMS: 100-03,220.6.10; 100-03,220.6.3; 100-04,13,60; 100-04,13,60.16

G0255 Current perception threshold/sensory nerve conduction test, (SNCT) per limb, any nerve E1

Special Coverage Instructions   Noncovered by Medicare   Carrier Discretion   ☑ Quantity Alert   ● New Code   ○ Recycled/Reinstated   ▲ Revised Code

54 — G Codes   A Age Edit   M Maternity Edit   ♀ Female Only   ♂ Male Only   A-Y OPPS Status Indicators   © 2023 Optum360, LLC

G0257 Unscheduled or emergency dialysis treatment for an ESRD patient in a hospital outpatient department that is not certified as an ESRD facility ⑤
CMS: 100-04,4,200.2; 100-04,8,60.4.7

G0259 Injection procedure for sacroiliac joint; arthrography Ⓝ

G0260 Injection procedure for sacroiliac joint; provision of anesthetic, steroid and/or other therapeutic agent, with or without arthrography Ⓣ A2
AHA: 4Q,21

G0268 Removal of impacted cerumen (one or both ears) by physician on same date of service as audiologic function testing Ⓝ ⊘

G0269 Placement of occlusive device into either a venous or arterial access site, postsurgical or interventional procedure (e.g., angioseal plug, vascular plug) Ⓝ ⊘
AHA: 3Q,22

G0270 Medical nutrition therapy; reassessment and subsequent intervention(s) following second referral in same year for change in diagnosis, medical condition or treatment regimen (including additional hours needed for renal disease), individual, face-to-face with the patient, each 15 minutes Ⓐ ☑ ⊘
CMS: 100-04,12,190.3; 100-04,12,190.6; 100-04,12,190.6.1; 100-04,12,190.7; 100-04,18,1.2
AHA: 3Q,19

G0271 Medical nutrition therapy, reassessment and subsequent intervention(s) following second referral in same year for change in diagnosis, medical condition, or treatment regimen (including additional hours needed for renal disease), group (two or more individuals), each 30 minutes Ⓐ ☑ ⊘
CMS: 100-04,18,1.2

G0276 Blinded procedure for lumbar stenosis, percutaneous image-guided lumbar decompression (PILD) or placebo-control, performed in an approved coverage with evidence development (CED) clinical trial Ⓙ B2
CMS: 100-03,150.13; 100-04,32,330.1; 100-04,32,330.2

G0277 Hyperbaric oxygen under pressure, full body chamber, per 30 minute interval ⑤
CMS: 100 04,32,30.1

G0278 Iliac and/or femoral artery angiography, nonselective, bilateral or ipsilateral to catheter insertion, performed at the same time as cardiac catheterization and/or coronary angiography, includes positioning or placement of the catheter in the distal aorta or ipsilateral femoral or iliac artery, injection of dye, production of permanent images, and radiologic supervision and interpretation (List separately in addition to primary procedure) Ⓝ N1 ⊘
AHA: 3Q,22

G0279 Diagnostic digital breast tomosynthesis, unilateral or bilateral (list separately in addition to 77065 or 77066) Ⓐ
CMS: 100-04,18,20.2; 100-04,18,20.2.1; 100-04,18,20.2.2; 100-04,18,20.6

G0281 Electrical stimulation, (unattended), to one or more areas, for chronic Stage III and Stage IV pressure ulcers, arterial ulcers, diabetic ulcers, and venous stasis ulcers not demonstrating measurable signs of healing after 30 days of conventional care, as part of a therapy plan of care Ⓐ
CMS: 100-02,15,220.4; 100-04,32,11.1; 100 04,5,10.3.2; 100-04,5,10.3.3

G0282 Electrical stimulation, (unattended), to one or more areas, for wound care other than described in G0281 EI
CMS: 100-04,32,11.1

G0283 Electrical stimulation (unattended), to one or more areas for indication(s) other than wound care, as part of a therapy plan of care Ⓐ
CMS: 100-02,15,220.4; 100-04,5,10.3.2; 100-04,5,10.3.3

G0288 Reconstruction, computed tomographic angiography of aorta for surgical planning for vascular surgery Ⓝ

G0289 Arthroscopy, knee, surgical, for removal of loose body, foreign body, debridement/shaving of articular cartilage (chondroplasty) at the time of other surgical knee arthroscopy in a different compartment of the same knee Ⓝ ⊘
AHA: 4Q,20

G0293 Noncovered surgical procedure(s) using conscious sedation, regional, general, or spinal anesthesia in a Medicare qualifying clinical trial, per day 01 ☑

G0294 Noncovered procedure(s) using either no anesthesia or local anesthesia only, in a Medicare qualifying clinical trial, per day 01 ☑

G0295 Electromagnetic therapy, to one or more areas, for wound care other than described in G0329 or for other uses EI

G0296 Counseling visit to discuss need for lung cancer screening using low dose CT scan (LDCT) (service is for eligibility determination and shared decision making) ⑤
CMS: 100-02,13,220; 100-02,13,220.1; 100-02,13,220.3; 100-04,18,1.2; 100-04,18,220; 100-04,18,220.1; 100-04,18,220.2; 100-04,18,220.3; 100-04,18,220.4; 100-04,18,220.5; 1004-04,13,220.1
AHA: 3Q,19

G0299 Direct skilled nursing services of a registered nurse (RN) in the home health or hospice setting, each 15 minutes Ⓡ
CMS: 100-01,3,30.3; 100-04,10,40.2; 100-04,11,130.1; 100-04,11,30.3

G0300 Direct skilled nursing services of a licensed practical nurse (LPN) in the home health or hospice setting, each 15 minutes Ⓑ
CMS: 100-01,3,30.3; 100-04,10,40.2; 100-04,11,130.1; 100-04,11,30.3

G0302 Preoperative pulmonary surgery services for preparation for LVRS, complete course of services, to include a minimum of 16 days of services ⑤ ☑

G0303 Preoperative pulmonary surgery services for preparation for LVRS, 10 to 15 days of services ⑤ ☑

G0304 Preoperative pulmonary surgery services for preparation for LVRS, 1 to 9 days of services ⑤ ☑

G0305 Postdischarge pulmonary surgery services after LVRS, minimum of 6 days of services ⑤ ☑

G0306 Complete CBC, automated (HgB, HCT, RBC, WBC, without platelet count) and automated WBC differential count Ⓠ
CMS: 100-02,11,20.2

G0307 Complete CBC, automated (HgB, HCT, RBC, WBC; without platelet count) Ⓠ
CMS: 100-02,11,20.2

G0310 Immunization counseling by a physician or other qualified health care professional when the vaccine(s) is not administered on the same date of service, 5-15 minutes time (This code is used for Medicaid billing purposes)
AHA: 4Q,22

G0311 Immunization counseling by a physician or other qualified health care professional when the vaccine(s) is not administered on the same date of service, 16-30 minutes time (This code is used for Medicaid billing purposes)
AHA: 4Q,22

G0312 Immunization counseling by a physician or other qualified health care professional when the vaccine(s) is not administered on the same date of service for ages under 21, 5-15 minutes time (This code is used for Medicaid billing purposes)
AHA: 4Q,22

Special Coverage Instructions   Noncovered by Medicare   Carrier Discretion   ☑ Quantity Alert   ● New Code   ○ Recycled/Reinstated   ▲ Revised Code

G0313 Immunization counseling by a physician or other qualified health care professional when the vaccine(s) is not administered on the same date of service for ages under 21, 16-30 minutes time (This code is used for Medicaid billing purposes)
AHA: 4Q,22

G0314 Immunization counseling by a physician or other qualified health care professional for COVID-19, ages under 21, 16-30 minutes time (This code is used for the Medicaid Early and Periodic Screening, Diagnostic, and Treatment Benefit [EPSDT])
AHA: 4Q,22

G0315 Immunization counseling by a physician or other qualified health care professional for COVID-19, ages under 21, 5-15 minutes time (This code is used for the Medicaid Early and Periodic Screening, Diagnostic, and Treatment Benefit [EPSDT])
AHA: 4Q,22

G0316 Prolonged hospital inpatient or observation care evaluation and management service(s) beyond the total time for the primary service (when the primary service has been selected using time on the date of the primary service); each additional 15 minutes by the physician or qualified healthcare professional, with or without direct patient contact (list separately in addition to CPT codes 99223, 99233, and 99236 for hospital inpatient or observation care evaluation and management services). (Do not report G0316 on the same date of service as other prolonged services for evaluation and management codes 99358, 99359, 99418, 99415, 99416). (Do not report G0316 for any time unit less than 15 minutes)
CMS: 100-04,12,30.6.15.3
AHA: 1Q,23

G0317 Prolonged nursing facility evaluation and management service(s) beyond the total time for the primary service (when the primary service has been selected using time on the date of the primary service); each additional 15 minutes by the physician or qualified healthcare professional, with or without direct patient contact (list separately in addition to CPT codes 99306, 99310 for nursing facility evaluation and management services). (Do not report G0317 on the same date of service as other prolonged services for evaluation and management codes 99358, 99359, 99418). (Do not report G0317 for any time unit less than 15 minutes)
CMS: 100-04,12,30.6.13; 100-04,12,30.6.15.3

G0318 Prolonged home or residence evaluation and management service(s) beyond the total time for the primary service (when the primary service has been selected using time on the date of the primary service); each additional 15 minutes by the physician or qualified healthcare professional, with or without direct patient contact (list separately in addition to CPT codes 99345, 99350 for home or residence evaluation and management services). (Do not report G0318 on the same date of service as other prolonged services for evaluation and management codes 99358, 99359, 99417). (Do not report G0318 for any time unit less than 15 minutes)
CMS: 100-04,12,30.6.15.3

G0320 Home health services furnished using synchronous telemedicine rendered via a real-time two-way audio and video telecommunications system
CMS: 100-04,10,40.2
AHA: 1Q,23

G0321 Home health services furnished using synchronous telemedicine rendered via telephone or other real-time interactive audio-only telecommunications system
CMS: 100-04,10,40.2
AHA: 1Q,23

G0322 The collection of physiologic data digitally stored and/or transmitted by the patient to the home health agency (i.e., remote patient monitoring)
CMS: 100-04,10,40.2
AHA: 1Q,23

G0323 Care management services for behavioral health conditions, at least 20 minutes of clinical psychologist or clinical social worker time, per calendar month. (These services include the following required elements: initial assessment or follow-up monitoring, including the use of applicable validated rating scales; behavioral health care planning in relation to behavioral/psychiatric health problems, including revision for patients who are not progressing or whose status changes; facilitating and coordinating treatment such as psychotherapy, coordination with and/or referral to physicians and practitioners who are authorized by Medicare to prescribe medications and furnish E/M services, counseling and/or psychiatric consultation; and continuity of care with a designated member of the care team)

G0327 Colorectal cancer screening; blood-based biomarker
CMS: 100-02,15,280.2.2; 100-04,18,1.2; 100-04,18,60; 100-04,18,60.1; 100-04,18,60.1.1; 100-04,18,60.2; 100-04,18,60.2.1; 100-04,18,60.6; 100-04,18,60.7; 100-04,18,60.8
AHA: 3Q,21

G0328 Colorectal cancer screening; fecal occult blood test, immunoassay, one to three simultaneous determinations Ⓐ
CMS: 100-02,15,280.2.2; 100-04,16,70.8; 100-04,18,1.2; 100-04,18,60; 100-04,18,60.1; 100-04,18,60.1.1; 100-04,18,60.2; 100-04,18,60.2.1; 100-04,18,60.6; 100-04,18,60.7
AHA: 3Q,23

G0329 Electromagnetic therapy, to one or more areas for chronic Stage III and Stage IV pressure ulcers, arterial ulcers, diabetic ulcers and venous stasis ulcers not demonstrating measurable signs of healing after 30 days of conventional care as part of a therapy plan of care Ⓐ
CMS: 100-02,15,220.4; 100-04,32,11.2; 100-04,5,10.3.2; 100-04,5,10.3.3

G0330 Facility services for dental rehabilitation procedure(s) performed on a patient who requires monitored anesthesia (e.g., general, intravenous sedation (monitored anesthesia care) and use of an operating room

G0333 Pharmacy dispensing fee for inhalation drug(s); initial 30-day supply as a beneficiary Ⓜ

G0337 Hospice evaluation and counseling services, preelection Ⓑ
CMS: 100-04,11,10

G0339 Image guided robotic linear accelerator-based stereotactic radiosurgery, complete course of therapy in one session or first session of fractionated treatment Ⓑ ⊘

G0340 Image guided robotic linear accelerator-based stereotactic radiosurgery, delivery including collimator changes and custom plugging, fractionated treatment, all lesions, per session, second through fifth sessions, maximum five sessions per course of treatment Ⓑ ⊘

G0341 Percutaneous islet cell transplant, includes portal vein catheterization and infusion Ⓒ ⊘
CMS: 100-04,32,70

G0342 Laparoscopy for islet cell transplant, includes portal vein catheterization and infusion Ⓒ ⊘
CMS: 100-04,32,70

G0343 Laparotomy for islet cell transplant, includes portal vein catheterization and infusion Ⓒ ⊘
CMS: 100-04,32,70

G0372 Physician service required to establish and document the need for a power mobility device Ⓜ ⊘
CMS: 100-04,12,30.6.15.4

Special Coverage Instructions   Noncovered by Medicare   Carrier Discretion   ☑ Quantity Alert   ● New Code   ○ Recycled/Reinstated   ▲ Revised Code

56 — G Codes   Ⓐ Age Edit   Ⓜ Maternity Edit   ♀ Female Only   ♂ Male Only   Ⓐ-Ⓨ OPPS Status Indicators   © 2023 Optum360, LLC

Observation/Emergency Department Services

G0378 Hospital observation service, per hour ☒N
CMS: 100-02,6,20.6; 100-04,01,50.3.2; 100-04,4,290.1; 100-04,4,290.2.2; 100-04,4,290.4.1; 100-04,4,290.4.2; 100-04,4,290.4.3; 100-04,4,290.5.1; 100-04,4,290.5.2; 100-04,4,290.5.3

G0379 Direct admission of patient for hospital observation care ☒J
CMS: 100-02,6,20.6; 100-04,4,290.4.1; 100-04,4,290.4.2; 100-04,4,290.4.3; 100-04,4,290.5.1; 100-04,4,290.5.2; 100-04,4,290.5.3

G0380 Level 1 hospital emergency department visit provided in a type B emergency department; (the ED must meet at least one of the following requirements: (1) it is licensed by the state in which it is located under applicable state law as an emergency room or emergency department; (2) it is held out to the public (by name, posted signs, advertising, or other means) as a place that provides care for emergency medical conditions on an urgent basis without requiring a previously scheduled appointment; or (3) during the calendar year immediately preceding the calendar year in which a determination under 42 CFR 489.24 is being made, based on a representative sample of patient visits that occurred during that calendar year, it provides at least one-third of all of its outpatient visits for the treatment of emergency medical conditions on an urgent basis without requiring a previously scheduled appointment) ☒J
CMS: 100-04,4,160

G0381 Level 2 hospital emergency department visit provided in a type B emergency department; (the ED must meet at least one of the following requirements: (1) it is licensed by the state in which it is located under applicable state law as an emergency room or emergency department; (2) it is held out to the public (by name, posted signs, advertising, or other means) as a place that provides care for emergency medical conditions on an urgent basis without requiring a previously scheduled appointment; or (3) during the calendar year immediately preceding the calendar year in which a determination under 42 CFR 489.24 is being made, based on a representative sample of patient visits that occurred during that calendar year, it provides at least one-third of all of its outpatient visits for the treatment of emergency medical conditions on an urgent basis without requiring a previously scheduled appointment) ☒J
CMS: 100-04,4,160

G0382 Level 3 hospital emergency department visit provided in a type B emergency department; (the ED must meet at least one of the following requirements: (1) it is licensed by the state in which it is located under applicable state law as an emergency room or emergency department; (2) it is held out to the public (by name, posted signs, advertising, or other means) as a place that provides care for emergency medical conditions on an urgent basis without requiring a previously scheduled appointment; or (3) during the calendar year immediately preceding the calendar year in which a determination under 42 CFR 489.24 is being made, based on a representative sample of patient visits that occurred during that calendar year, it provides at least one-third of all of its outpatient visits for the treatment of emergency medical conditions on an urgent basis without requiring a previously scheduled appointment) ☒J
CMS: 100-04,4,160

G0383 Level 4 hospital emergency department visit provided in a type B emergency department; (the ED must meet at least one of the following requirements: (1) it is licensed by the state in which it is located under applicable state law as an emergency room or emergency department; (2) it is held out to the public (by name, posted signs, advertising, or other means) as a place that provides care for emergency medical conditions on an urgent basis without requiring a previously scheduled appointment; or (3) during the calendar year immediately preceding the calendar year in which a determination under 42 CFR 489.24 is being made, based on a representative sample of patient visits that occurred during that calendar year, it provides at least one-third of all of its outpatient visits for the treatment of emergency medical conditions on an urgent basis without requiring a previously scheduled appointment) ☒J
CMS: 100-04,4,160

G0384 Level 5 hospital emergency department visit provided in a type B emergency department; (the ED must meet at least one of the following requirements: (1) it is licensed by the state in which it is located under applicable state law as an emergency room or emergency department; (2) it is held out to the public (by name, posted signs, advertising, or other means) as a place that provides care for emergency medical conditions on an urgent basis without requiring a previously scheduled appointment; or (3) during the calendar year immediately preceding the calendar year in which a determination under 42 CFR 489.24 is being made, based on a representative sample of patient visits that occurred during that calendar year, it provides at least one-third of all of its outpatient visits for the treatment of emergency medical conditions on an urgent basis without requiring a previously scheduled appointment) ☒J
CMS: 100-04,4,160; 100-04,4,290.5.1

Other Services

G0390 Trauma response team associated with hospital critical care service ☒6
CMS: 100-04,4,160.1

Alcohol or Substance Abuse

G0396 Alcohol and/or substance (other than tobacco) misuse structured assessment (e.g., audit, dast), and brief intervention 15 to 30 minutes ☒S ☑ ⊘
CMS: 100-04,12,190.3; 100-04,12,190.6; 100-04,12,190.6.1; 100-04,12,190.7; 100-04,4,200.6
AHA: 3Q,19

G0397 Alcohol and/or substance (other than tobacco) misuse structured assessment (e.g., audit, dast), and intervention, greater than 30 minutes ☒S ☑ ⊘
CMS: 100-04,12,190.3; 100-04,12,190.6; 100-04,12,190.6.1; 100-04,12,190.7; 100-04,4,200.6
AHA: 3Q,19

Home Sleep Study

G0398 Home sleep study test (HST) with type II portable monitor, unattended; minimum of 7 channels: EEG, EOG, EMG, ECG/heart rate, airflow, respiratory effort and oxygen saturation ☒S
CMS: 100-03,240.4

G0399 Home sleep test (HST) with type III portable monitor, unattended; minimum of 4 channels: 2 respiratory movement/airflow, 1 ECG/heart rate and 1 oxygen saturation ☒S
CMS: 100-03,240.4

G0400 Home sleep test (HST) with type IV portable monitor, unattended; minimum of 3 channels ☒S
CMS: 100-03,240.4

Procedures/Professional Services (Temporary)

G0402 — G0429

Initial Physical Exam

G0402 Initial preventive physical examination; face-to-face visit, services limited to new beneficiary during the first 12 months of Medicare enrollment   V ⊘
CMS: 100-02,13,220; 100-02,13,220.1; 100-02,13,220.3; 100-04,12,100.1.1; 100-04,18,1.2; 100-04,18,140.6; 100-04,18,80; 100-04,18,80.1; 100-04,18,80.2; 100-04,18,80.3.3; 100-04,18,80.4; 1004-04,13,220.1

G0403 Electrocardiogram, routine ECG with 12 leads; performed as a screening for the initial preventive physical examination with interpretation and report   M
CMS: 100-04,18,1.2; 100-04,18,80; 100-04,18,80.1; 100-04,18,80.2

G0404 Electrocardiogram, routine ECG with 12 leads; tracing only, without interpretation and report, performed as a screening for the initial preventive physical examination   S
CMS: 100-04,18,1.2; 100-04,18,80; 100-04,18,80.1; 100-04,18,80.2; 100-04,18,80.3.3

G0405 Electrocardiogram, routine ECG with 12 leads; interpretation and report only, performed as a screening for the initial preventive physical examination   B ⊘
CMS: 100-04,18,1.2; 100-04,18,80; 100-04,18,80.1; 100-04,18,80.2

Follow-up Telehealth

G0406 Follow-up inpatient consultation, limited, physicians typically spend 15 minutes communicating with the patient via telehealth   B ⊘
CMS: 100-04,12,190.3; 100-04,12,190.3.1; 100-04,12,190.3.3; 100-04,12,190.3.5; 100-04,12,190.6; 100-04,12,190.6.1; 100-04,12,190.7
AHA: 3Q,19

G0407 Follow-up inpatient consultation, intermediate, physicians typically spend 25 minutes communicating with the patient via telehealth   B ⊘
CMS: 100-04,12,190.3; 100-04,12,190.3.1; 100-04,12,190.3.3; 100-04,12,190.3.5; 100-04,12,190.6; 100-04,12,190.6.1; 100-04,12,190.7
AHA: 3Q,19

G0408 Follow-up inpatient consultation, complex, physicians typically spend 35 minutes communicating with the patient via telehealth   B ⊘
CMS: 100-04,12,190.3; 100-04,12,190.3.1; 100-04,12,190.3.3; 100-04,12,190.3.5; 100-04,12,190.6; 100-04,12,190.6.1; 100-04,12,190.7
AHA: 3Q,19

Psychological Services

G0409 Social work and psychological services, directly relating to and/or furthering the patient's rehabilitation goals, each 15 minutes, face-to-face; individual (services provided by a CORF qualified social worker or psychologist in a CORF)   B ☑
CMS: 100-02,12,30.1; 100-04,5,100.11; 100-04,5,100.4

▲ **G0410** Group psychotherapy other than of a multiple-family group, in a partial hospitalization or intensive outpatient setting, approximately 45 to 50 minutes   P
CMS: 100-04,4,260.1; 100-04,4,260.1.1

▲ **G0411** Interactive group psychotherapy, in a partial hospitalization or intensive outpatient setting, approximately 45 to 50 minutes   P
CMS: 100-04,4,260.1; 100-04,4,260.1.1

Fracture Care

G0412 Open treatment of iliac spine(s), tuberosity avulsion, or iliac wing fracture(s), unilateral or bilateral for pelvic bone fracture patterns which do not disrupt the pelvic ring, includes internal fixation, when performed   C ⊘

G0413 Percutaneous skeletal fixation of posterior pelvic bone fracture and/or dislocation, for fracture patterns which disrupt the pelvic ring, unilateral or bilateral, (includes ilium, sacroiliac joint and/or sacrum)   J ⊘

G0414 Open treatment of anterior pelvic bone fracture and/or dislocation for fracture patterns which disrupt the pelvic ring, unilateral or bilateral, includes internal fixation when performed (includes pubic symphysis and/or superior/inferior rami)   C ⊘

G0415 Open treatment of posterior pelvic bone fracture and/or dislocation, for fracture patterns which disrupt the pelvic ring, unilateral or bilateral, includes internal fixation, when performed (includes ilium, sacroiliac joint and/or sacrum)   C ⊘

Surgical Pathology

G0416 Surgical pathology, gross and microscopic examinations, for prostate needle biopsy, any method   ♂ Q2
AHA: 2Q,22

Educational Services

G0420 Face-to-face educational services related to the care of chronic kidney disease; individual, per session, per 1 hour   A ☑ ⊘
CMS: 100-02,15,200; 100-02,15,310; 100-02,15,310.1; 100-02,15,310.2; 100-02,15,310.4; 100-02,15,310.5; 100-04,12,190.3; 100-04,12,190.6; 100-04,12,190.6.1; 100-04,12,190.7
AHA: 3Q,19

G0421 Face-to-face educational services related to the care of chronic kidney disease; group, per session, per 1 hour   A ☑ ⊘
CMS: 100-02,15,200; 100-02,15,310; 100-02,15,310.1; 100-02,15,310.2; 100-02,15,310.4; 100-02,15,310.5; 100-04,12,190.3; 100-04,12,190.6; 100-04,12,190.6.1; 100-04,12,190.7
AHA: 3Q,19

Cardiac and Pulmonary Rehabilitation

G0422 Intensive cardiac rehabilitation; with or without continuous ECG monitoring with exercise, per session   S ☑ ⊘
CMS: 100-02,15,232; 100-04,32,140.2.2.1; 100-04,32,140.2.2.2; 100-04,32,140.3; 100-04,32,140.3.1; 100-08,15,4.2.8

G0423 Intensive cardiac rehabilitation; with or without continuous ECG monitoring; without exercise, per session   S ☑ ⊘
CMS: 100-02,15,232; 100-04,32,140.2.2.1; 100-04,32,140.2.2.2; 100-04,32,140.3; 100-04,32,140.3.1; 100-08,15,4.2.8

Inpatient Telehealth

G0425 Telehealth consultation, emergency department or initial inpatient, typically 30 minutes communicating with the patient via telehealth   B ☑ ⊘
CMS: 100-04,12,190.3; 100-04,12,190.3.1; 100-04,12,190.3.2; 100-04,12,190.6; 100-04,12,190.6.1; 100-04,12,190.7
AHA: 3Q,19

G0426 Telehealth consultation, emergency department or initial inpatient, typically 50 minutes communicating with the patient via telehealth   B ☑ ⊘
CMS: 100-04,12,190.3; 100-04,12,190.3.1; 100-04,12,190.3.2; 100-04,12,190.6; 100-04,12,190.6.1; 100-04,12,190.7
AHA: 3Q,19

G0427 Telehealth consultation, emergency department or initial inpatient, typically 70 minutes or more communicating with the patient via telehealth   B ☑ ⊘
CMS: 100-04,12,190.3; 100-04,12,190.3.1; 100-04,12,190.3.2; 100-04,12,190.6; 100-04,12,190.6.1; 100-04,12,190.7
AHA: 3Q,19

Defect Fillers

G0428 Collagen meniscus implant procedure for filling meniscal defects (e.g., CMI, collagen scaffold, Menaflex)   E1
CMS: 100-03,150.12

G0429 Dermal filler injection(s) for the treatment of facial lipodystrophy syndrome (LDS) (e.g., as a result of highly active antiretroviral therapy)   T P3
CMS: 100-03,250.5; 100-04,32,260.1; 100-04,32,260.2.1; 100-04,32,260.2.2

Special Coverage Instructions   Noncovered by Medicare   Carrier Discretion   ☑ Quantity Alert   ● New Code   ○ Recycled/Reinstated   ▲ Revised Code

58 — G Codes   A Age Edit   M Maternity Edit   ♀ Female Only   ♂ Male Only   A-Y OPPS Status Indicators   © 2023 Optum360, LLC

Laboratory Services

G0432 Infectious agent antibody detection by enzyme immunoassay (EIA) technique, HIV-1 and/or HIV-2, screening [A]
CMS: 100-03,190.14; 100-03,190.9; 100-03,210.7; 100-04,18,1.2; 100-04,18,130.1; 100-04,18,130.2; 100-04,18,130.3; 100-04,18,130.4; 100-04,18,130.5

G0433 Infectious agent antibody detection by enzyme-linked immunosorbent assay (ELISA) technique, HIV-1 and/or HIV-2, screening [A]
CMS: 100-03,190.14; 100-03,190.9; 100-03,210.7; 100-04,16,70.8; 100-04,18,1.2; 100-04,18,130.1; 100-04,18,130.2; 100-04,18,130.3; 100-04,18,130.4; 100-04,18,130.5

G0435 Infectious agent antibody detection by rapid antibody test, HIV-1 and/or HIV-2, screening [A]
CMS: 100-03,190.14; 100-03,190.9; 100-03,210.7; 100-04,18,1.2; 100-04,18,130.1; 100-04,18,130.2; 100-04,18,130.3; 100-04,18,130.4; 100-04,18,130.5

Counseling and Wellness Visit

G0438 Annual wellness visit; includes a personalized prevention plan of service (PPS), initial visit [A]
CMS: 100-02,13,220; 100-02,13,220.1; 100-02,13,220.3; 100-02,15,280.5; 100-02,15,280.5.1; 100-04,12,100.1.1; 100-04,18,1.2; 100-04,18,140; 100-04,18,140.1; 100-04,18,140.5; 100-04,18,140.6; 100-04,18,140.8; 100-04.4.200.11; 1004-04,13,220.1
AHA: 3Q,19

G0439 Annual wellness visit, includes a personalized prevention plan of service (PPS), subsequent visit [A]
CMS: 100-02,13,220; 100-02,13,220.1; 100-02,13,220.3; 100-02,15,280.5; 100-02,15,280.5.1; 100-04,12,100.1.1; 100-04,18,1.2; 100-04,18,140; 100-04,18,140.1; 100-04,18,140.5; 100-04,18,140.6; 100-04,18,140.8; 100-04,4,200.11; 1004-04,13,220.1
AHA: 3Q,19

Other Services

G0442 Annual alcohol misuse screening, 5 to 15 minutes [S] [✓]
CMS: 100-03,210.8; 100-04,12,190.3; 100-04,12,190.6; 100-04,12,190.6.1; 100-04,12,190.7; 100-04,18,180; 100-04,18,180.1; 100-04,18,180.2; 100-04,18,180.3; 100-04,18,180.4; 100-04,18,180.5; 100-04,32,180.4; 100-04,32,180.5
AHA: 3Q,19

G0443 Brief face-to-face behavioral counseling for alcohol misuse, 15 minutes [S] [✓]
CMS: 100-03,210.8; 100-04,12,190.3; 100-04,12,190.6; 100-04,12,190.6.1; 100-04,12,190.7; 100-04,18,180; 100-04,18,180.1; 100-04,18,180.2; 100-04,18,180.3; 100-04,18,180.4; 100-04,18,180.5; 100-04,32,180.4; 100-04,32,180.5
AHA: 3Q,19

G0444 Annual depression screening, 5 to 15 minutes [S] [✓]
CMS: 100-04,12,190.3; 100-04,12,190.6; 100-04,12,190.6.1; 100-04,12,190.7; 100-04,18,190; 100-04,18,190.1; 100-04,18,190.2; 100-04,18,190.3
AHA: 3Q,19

G0445 Semiannual high intensity behavioral counseling to prevent STIs, individual, face-to-face, includes education skills training & guidance on how to change sexual behavior [S] [✓]
CMS: 100-03,210.10; 100-04,12,190.3; 100-04,12,190.6; 100-04,12,190.6.1; 100-04,12,190.7; 100 04,18,170.1; 100-04,18,170.2; 100-04,18,170.3; 100-04,18,170.4; 100-04,18,170.4.1; 100-04,18,170.5
AHA: 3Q,19

G0446 Annual, face-to-face intensive behavioral therapy for cardiovascular disease, individual, 15 minutes [S] [✓]
CMS: 100-03,210.11; 100-04,12,190.3; 100-04,12,190.6; 100-04,12,190.6.1; 100-04,12,190.7; 100-04,18,160; 100-04,18,160.1; 100-04,18,160.2.1; 100-04,18,160.2.2; 100-04,18,160.3; 100-04,18,160.4; 100-04,18,160.5
AHA: 3Q,19

G0447 Face-to-face behavioral counseling for obesity, 15 minutes [S] [✓]
CMS: 100-03,210.12; 100-04,12,190.3; 100-04,12,190.6; 100-04,12,190.6.1; 100-04,12,190.7; 100-04,18,1.2; 100-04,18,200; 100-04,18,200.1; 100-04,18,200.2; 100-04,18,200.3; 100-04,18,200.4; 100-04,18,200.5
AHA: 3Q,19

G0448 Insertion or replacement of a permanent pacing cardioverter-defibrillator system with transvenous lead(s), single or dual chamber with insertion of pacing electrode, cardiac venous system, for left ventricular pacing [B]
CMS: 100-04,32,270; 100-04,32,270.1; 100-04,32,270.2; 100-04,32,270.3

G0451 Development testing, with interpretation and report, per standardized instrument form [Q3]
CMS: 100-02,15,220.4; 100-04,5,10.3.2; 100-04,5,10.3.3

Molecular Pathology

G0452 Molecular pathology procedure; physician interpretation and report [B]

Neurophysiology Monitoring

G0453 Continuous intraoperative neurophysiology monitoring, from outside the operating room (remote or nearby), per patient, (attention directed exclusively to one patient) each 15 minutes (list in addition to primary procedure) [N]

Documentation and Preparation

G0454 Physician documentation of face-to-face visit for durable medical equipment determination performed by nurse practitioner, physician assistant or clinical nurse specialist [B]

G0455 Preparation with instillation of fecal microbiota by any method, including assessment of donor specimen [QI]

Prostate Brachytherapy

G0458 Low dose rate (LDR) prostate brachytherapy services, composite rate [♂] [B]

Inpatient Telehealth Pharmacologic Management

G0459 Inpatient telehealth pharmacologic management, including prescription, use, and review of medication with no more than minimal medical psychotherapy [B]
CMS: 100-04,12,190.3; 100-04,12,190.6; 100-04,12,190.6.1; 100-04,12,190.7
AHA: 3Q,19

Other Wound/Ulcer Care

▲ G0460 Autologous platelet rich plasma (PRP) or other blood-derived product for nondiabetic chronic wounds/ulcers (includes, as applicable: administration, dressings, phlebotomy, centrifugation or mixing, and all other preparatory procedures, per treatment) [T]
CMS: 100-03,270.3; 100-04,32,11.3.1; 100-04,32,11.3.2; 100-04,32,11.3.3; 100-04,32,11.3.4; 100-04,32,11.3.5; 100-04,32,11.3.6
AHA: 3Q,23; 3Q,22

Hospital Outpatient Visit

G0463 Hospital outpatient clinic visit for assessment and management of a patient [J]
CMS: 100-04,32,130.1; 100-04,4,160.2; 100-04,4,260.1; 100-04,4,260.1.1; 100-04,4,290.5.1; 100-04,4,290.5.3; 100-04,6,20.1.1.2; 100-04,6,30.4.1
AHA: 4Q,20; 2Q,20

Platelet Rich Plasma

▲ G0465 Autologous platelet rich plasma (PRP) or other blood-derived product for diabetic chronic wounds/ulcers, using an FDA-cleared device for this indication, (includes, as applicable: administration, dressings, phlebotomy, centrifugation or mixing, and all other preparatory procedures, per treatment)
CMS: 100-04,32,11.3.1; 100-04,32,11.3.2; 100-04,32,11.3.3; 100-04,32,11.3.4; 100-04,32,11.3.5; 100-04,32,11.3.6
AHA: 3Q,23; 3Q,22

Special Coverage Instructions   Noncovered by Medicare   Carrier Discretion   ☑ Quantity Alert   ● New Code   ○ Recycled/Reinstated   ▲ Revised Code

© 2023 Optum360, LLC   [A2-Z3] ASC Pmt   **CMS:** IOM   **AHA:** Coding Clinic   ⅋ DMEPOS Paid   ⊘ SNF Excluded   G Codes — 59

Federally Qualified Health Center Visits

G0466 Federally qualified health center (FQHC) visit, new patient Ⓐ
CMS: 100-04,9,60.6

G0467 Federally qualified health center (FQHC) visit, established patient Ⓐ
CMS: 100-04,9,60.6

G0468 Federally qualified health center (FQHC) visit, initial preventive physical exam (IPPE) or annual wellness visit (AWV) Ⓐ
CMS: 100-04,9,60.6

G0469 Federally qualified health center (FQHC) visit, mental health, new patient Ⓐ
CMS: 100-04,9,60.6

G0470 Federally qualified health center (FQHC) visit, mental health, established patient Ⓐ
CMS: 100-04,9,60.6

HHA and SNF Specimen Collection

G0471 Collection of venous blood by venipuncture or urine sample by catheterization from an individual in a skilled nursing facility (SNF) or by a laboratory on behalf of a home health agency (HHA) Ⓐ
CMS: 100-04,16,60.1.2; 100-04,16,60.1.4

Hepatitis C Screening

G0472 Hepatitis C antibody screening for individual at high risk and other covered indication(s) Ⓐ
CMS: 100-02,13,220; 100-02,13,220.1; 100-02,13,220.3; 100-03,210.13; 100-04,18,1.2; 100-04,18,210; 100-04,18,210.2; 100-04,18,210.3; 100-04,18,210.4; 1004-04,13,220.1

Behavioral Counseling

G0473 Face-to-face behavioral counseling for obesity, group (2-10), 30 minutes Ⓢ
CMS: 100-04,18,1.2; 100-04,18,200.1; 100-04,18,200.2; 100-04,18,200.3; 100-04,18,200.4; 100-04,18,200.5

Screening Measures

G0475 HIV antigen/antibody, combination assay, screening Ⓐ
CMS: 100-03,210.7; 100-04,18,130.1; 100-04,18,130.2; 100-04,18,130.3; 100-04,18,130.5

G0476 Infectious agent detection by nucleic acid (DNA or RNA); human papillomavirus HPV), high-risk types (e.g., 16, 18, 31, 33, 35, 39, 45, 51, 52, 56, 58, 59, 68) for cervical cancer screening, must be performed in addition to pap test ♀Ⓐ
CMS: 100-03,210.2.1; 100-04,18,30.2.1; 100-04,18,30.5; 100-04,18,30.6; 100-04,18,30.8; 100-04,18,30.9

Drug Testing

G0480 Drug test(s), definitive, utilizing (1) drug identification methods able to identify individual drugs and distinguish between structural isomers (but not necessarily stereoisomers), including, but not limited to, GC/MS (any type, single or tandem) and LC/MS (any type, single or tandem and excluding immunoassays (e.g., IA, EIA, ELISA, EMIT, FPIA) and enzymatic methods (e.g., alcohol dehydrogenase)), (2) stable isotope or other universally recognized internal standards in all samples (e.g., to control for matrix effects, interferences and variations in signal strength), and (3) method or drug-specific calibration and matrix-matched quality control material (e.g., to control for instrument variations and mass spectral drift); qualitative or quantitative, all sources, includes specimen validity testing, per day; 1-7 drug class(es), including metabolite(s) if performed Ⓠ
AHA: 2Q,22; 1Q,18

G0481 Drug test(s), definitive, utilizing (1) drug identification methods able to identify individual drugs and distinguish between structural isomers (but not necessarily stereoisomers), including, but not limited to, GC/MS (any type, single or tandem) and LC/MS (any type, single or tandem and excluding immunoassays (e.g., IA, EIA, ELISA, EMIT, FPIA) and enzymatic methods (e.g., alcohol dehydrogenase)), (2) stable isotope or other universally recognized internal standards in all samples (e.g., to control for matrix effects, interferences and variations in signal strength), and (3) method or drug-specific calibration and matrix-matched quality control material (e.g., to control for instrument variations and mass spectral drift); qualitative or quantitative, all sources, includes specimen validity testing, per day; 8-14 drug class(es), including metabolite(s) if performed Ⓠ
AHA: 2Q,22; 1Q,18

G0482 Drug test(s), definitive, utilizing (1) drug identification methods able to identify individual drugs and distinguish between structural isomers (but not necessarily stereoisomers), including, but not limited to, GC/MS (any type, single or tandem) and LC/MS (any type, single or tandem and excluding immunoassays (e.g., IA, EIA, ELISA, EMIT, FPIA) and enzymatic methods (e.g., alcohol dehydrogenase)), (2) stable isotope or other universally recognized internal standards in all samples (e.g., to control for matrix effects, interferences and variations in signal strength), and (3) method or drug-specific calibration and matrix-matched quality control material (e.g., to control for instrument variations and mass spectral drift); qualitative or quantitative, all sources, includes specimen validity testing, per day; 15-21 drug class(es), including metabolite(s) if performed Ⓠ
AHA: 2Q,22; 1Q,18

G0483 Drug test(s), definitive, utilizing (1) drug identification methods able to identify individual drugs and distinguish between structural isomers (but not necessarily stereoisomers), including, but not limited to, GC/MS (any type, single or tandem) and LC/MS (any type, single or tandem and excluding immunoassays (e.g., IA, EIA, ELISA, EMIT, FPIA) and enzymatic methods (e.g., alcohol dehydrogenase)), (2) stable isotope or other universally recognized internal standards in all samples (e.g., to control for matrix effects, interferences and variations in signal strength), and (3) method or drug-specific calibration and matrix-matched quality control material (e.g., to control for instrument variations and mass spectral drift); qualitative or quantitative, all sources, includes specimen validity testing, per day; 22 or more drug class(es), including metabolite(s) if performed Ⓠ
AHA: 2Q,22; 1Q,18

Home Health Nursing Visit

G0490 Face-to-face home health nursing visit by a rural health clinic (RHC) or federally qualified health center (FQHC) in an area with a shortage of home health agencies; (services limited to RN or LPN only) Ⓐ

Dialysis Procedures

G0491 Dialysis procedure at a Medicare certified ESRD facility for acute kidney injury without ESRD Ⓑ
CMS: 100-04,8,40; 100-04,8,50.2

G0492 Dialysis procedure with single evaluation by a physician or other qualified health care professional for acute kidney injury without ESRD Ⓑ

Skilled Nursing Services

G0493 Skilled services of a registered nurse (RN) for the observation and assessment of the patient's condition, each 15 minutes (the change in the patient's condition requires skilled nursing personnel to identify and evaluate the patient's need for possible modification of treatment in the home health or hospice setting) Ⓑ
CMS: 100-04,10,40.2

Special Coverage Instructions   Noncovered by Medicare   Carrier Discretion   ☑ Quantity Alert ● New Code   ○ Recycled/Reinstated ▲ Revised Code

G0494 Skilled services of a licensed practical nurse (LPN) for the observation and assessment of the patient's condition, each 15 minutes (the change in the patient's condition requires skilled nursing personnel to identify and evaluate the patient's need for possible modification of treatment in the home health or hospice setting)   B
CMS: 100-04,10,40.2

G0495 Skilled services of a registered nurse (RN), in the training and/or education of a patient or family member, in the home health or hospice setting, each 15 minutes   B
CMS: 100-04,10,40.2

G0496 Skilled services of a licensed practical nurse (LPN), in the training and/or education of a patient or family member, in the home health or hospice setting, each 15 minutes   B
CMS: 100-04,10,40.2

Chemotherapy Infusion

G0498 Chemotherapy administration, intravenous infusion technique; initiation of infusion in the office/clinic setting using office/clinic pump/supplies, with continuation of the infusion in the community setting (e.g., home, domiciliary, rest home or assisted living) using a portable pump provided by the office/clinic, includes follow up office/clinic visit at the conclusion of the infusion   S

Hepatitis B Screening

G0499 Hepatitis B screening in nonpregnant, high-risk individual includes hepatitis B surface antigen (HBSAG), antibodies to HBSAG (anti-HBS) and antibodies to hepatitis B core antigen (anti-HBC), and is followed by a neutralizing confirmatory test, when performed, only for an initially reactive HBSAG result   A
CMS: 100-03,1,210.6; 100-04,18,230; 100-04,18,230.1; 100-04,18,230.2; 100-04,18,230.3; 100 04,18,230.4

Moderate Sedation

G0500 Moderate sedation services provided by the same physician or other qualified health care professional performing a gastrointestinal endoscopic service that sedation supports, requiring the presence of an independent trained observer to assist in the monitoring of the patient's level of consciousness and physiological status; initial 15 minutes of intra-service time; patient age 5 years or older (additional time may be reported with 99153, as appropriate)   N
CMS: 100-04,18,60.1.1

Mobility-Assistive Technology

G0501 Resource-intensive services for patients for whom the use of specialized mobility-assistive technology (such as adjustable height chairs or tables, patient lift, and adjustable padded leg supports) is medically necessary and used during the provision of an office/outpatient, evaluation and management visit (list separately in addition to primary service)   N

Care Management Services

G0506 Comprehensive assessment of and care planning for patients requiring chronic care management services (list separately in addition to primary monthly care management service)   N
AHA: 3Q,19

Telehealth Consultation

G0508 Telehealth consultation, critical care, initial, physicians typically spend 60 minutes communicating with the patient and providers via telehealth   B
AHA: 3Q,19

G0509 Telehealth consultation, critical care, subsequent, physicians typically spend 50 minutes communicating with the patient and providers via telehealth   B
AHA: 3Q,19

RHC or FQHC General Care Management

G0511 Rural health clinic or federally qualified health center (RHC or FQHC) only, general care management, 20 minutes or more of clinical staff time for chronic care management services or behavioral health integration services directed by an RHC or FQHC practitioner (physician, NP, PA, or CNM), per calendar month   A
CMS: 100-02,13,230.2; 100-04,9,70.8

G0512 Rural health clinic or federally qualified health center (RHC/FQHC) only, psychiatric collaborative care model (psychiatric COCM), 60 minutes or more of clinical staff time for psychiatric COCM services directed by an RHC or FQHC practitioner (physician, NP, PA, or CNM) and including services furnished by a behavioral health care manager and consultation with a psychiatric consultant, per calendar month   A
CMS: 100-02,13,230.2; 100-02,13,230.3; 100-04,9,70.8

Prolonged Services

G0513 Prolonged preventive service(s) (beyond the typical service time of the primary procedure), in the office or other outpatient setting requiring direct patient contact beyond the usual service; first 30 minutes (list separately in addition to code for preventive service)   N
AHA: 3Q,19

G0514 Prolonged preventive service(s) (beyond the typical service time of the primary procedure), in the office or other outpatient setting requiring direct patient contact beyond the usual service; each additional 30 minutes (list separately in addition to code G0513 for additional 30 minutes of preventive service)   N
AHA: 3Q,19

Drug Delivery Implants

G0516 Insertion of nonbiodegradable drug delivery implants, four or more (services for subdermal rod implant)   01 N1

G0517 Removal of nonbiodegradable drug delivery implants, four or more (services for subdermal implants)   01 N1

G0518 Removal with reinsertion, nonbiodegradable drug delivery implants, four or more (services for subdermal implants)   01 N1

Drug Test(s)

G0659 Drug test(s), definitive, utilizing drug identification methods able to identify individual drugs and distinguish between structural isomers (but not necessarily stereoisomers), including but not limited to GC/MS (any type, single or tandem) and LC/MS (any type, single or tandem), excluding immunoassays (e.g., IA, EIA, ELISA, EMIT, FPIA) and enzymatic methods (e.g., alcohol dehydrogenase), performed without method or drug-specific calibration, without matrix-matched quality control material, or without use of stable isotope or other universally recognized internal standard(s) for each drug, drug metabolite or drug class per specimen; qualitative or quantitative, all sources, includes specimen validity testing, per day, any number of drug classes   Q
AHA: 2Q,22

Quality Measures

G0913 Improvement in visual function achieved within 90 days following cataract surgery   M

G0914 Patient care survey was not completed by patient   M

G0915 Improvement in visual function not achieved within 90 days following cataract surgery   M

G0916 Satisfaction with care achieved within 90 days following cataract surgery   M

G0917 Patient care survey was not completed by patient   M

Special Coverage Instructions   Noncovered by Medicare   Carrier Discretion   ☑ Quantity Alert ● New Code   ○ Recycled/Reinstated ▲ Revised Code

Procedures/Professional Services (Temporary)

G0918 — G2007

G0918   Satisfaction with care not achieved within 90 days following cataract surgery   M

Clinical Decision Support Mechanism

G1001   Clinical Decision Support Mechanism eviCore, as defined by the Medicare Appropriate Use Criteria Program

G1002   Clinical Decision Support Mechanism MedCurrent, as defined by the Medicare Appropriate Use Criteria Program

G1003   Clinical Decision Support Mechanism Medicalis, as defined by the Medicare Appropriate Use Criteria Program

G1004   Clinical Decision Support Mechanism National Decision Support Company, as defined by the Medicare Appropriate Use Criteria Program

G1007   Clinical Decision Support Mechanism AIM Specialty Health, as defined by the Medicare Appropriate Use Criteria Program

G1008   Clinical Decision Support Mechanism Cranberry Peak, as defined by the Medicare Appropriate Use Criteria Program

G1010   Clinical Decision Support Mechanism Stanson, as defined by the Medicare Appropriate Use Criteria Program

G1011   Clinical Decision Support Mechanism, qualified tool not otherwise specified, as defined by the Medicare Appropriate Use Criteria Program

G1012   Clinical Decision Support Mechanism AgileMD, as defined by the Medicare Appropriate Use Criteria Program

G1013   Clinical Decision Support Mechanism EvidenceCare ImagingCare, as defined by the Medicare Appropriate Use Criteria Program

G1014   Clinical Decision Support Mechanism InveniQA Semantic Answers in Medicine, as defined by the Medicare Appropriate Use Criteria Program

G1015   Clinical Decision Support Mechanism Reliant Medical Group, as defined by the Medicare Appropriate Use Criteria Program

G1016   Clinical Decision Support Mechanism Speed of Care, as defined by the Medicare Appropriate Use Criteria Program

G1017   Clinical Decision Support Mechanism HealthHelp, as defined by the Medicare Appropriate Use Criteria Program

G1018   Clinical Decision Support Mechanism INFINX, as defined by the Medicare Appropriate Use Criteria Program

G1019   Clinical Decision Support Mechanism LogicNets, as defined by the Medicare Appropriate Use Criteria Program

G1020   Clinical Decision Support Mechanism Curbside Clinical Augmented Workflow, as defined by the Medicare Appropriate Use Criteria Program

G1021   Clinical Decision Support Mechanism EHealthLine Clinical Decision Support Mechanism, as defined by the Medicare Appropriate Use Criteria Program

G1022   Clinical Decision Support Mechanism Intermountain Clinical Decision Support Mechanism, as defined by the Medicare Appropriate Use Criteria Program

G1023   Clinical Decision Support Mechanism Persivia Clinical Decision Support, as defined by the Medicare Appropriate Use Criteria Program

G1024   Clinical decision support mechanism Radrite, as defined by the Medicare Appropriate Use Criteria Program

Patient-Month Quality Measures

G1025   Patient-months where there are more than one Medicare capitated payment (MCP) provider listed for the month

G1026   The number of adult patient-months in the denominator who were on maintenance hemodialysis using a catheter continuously for 3 months or longer under the care of the same practitioner or group partner as of the last hemodialysis session of the reporting month

G1027   The number of adult patient-months in the denominator who were on maintenance hemodialysis under the care of the same practitioner or group partner as of the last hemodialysis session of the reporting month using a catheter continuously for less than 3 months

Nasal Naloxone

G1028   Take-home supply of nasal naloxone; 2-pack of 8 mg per 0.1 ml nasal spray (provision of the services by a Medicare-enrolled Opioid Treatment Program); list separately in addition to code for primary procedure
     CMS: 100-02,17,20; 100-02,17,40.1.1; 100-04,39,30.6.1

Convulsive Therapy Procedure

G2000   Blinded administration of convulsive therapy procedure, either electroconvulsive therapy (ECT, current covered gold standard) or magnetic seizure therapy (MST, noncovered experimental therapy), performed in an approved IDE-based clinical trial, per treatment session

Assessments, Evaluations, and CMMI Home Visits

G2001   Brief (20 minutes) in-home visit for a new patient postdischarge. For use only in a Medicare-approved CMMI model. (Services must be furnished within a beneficiary's home, domiciliary, rest home, assisted living and/or nursing facility within 90 days following discharge from an inpatient facility and no more than nine times.)

G2002   Limited (30 minutes) in-home visit for a new patient postdischarge. For use only in a Medicare-approved CMMI model. (Services must be furnished within a beneficiary's home, domiciliary, rest home, assisted living and/or nursing facility within 90 days following discharge from an inpatient facility and no more than nine times.)

G2003   Moderate (45 minutes) in-home visit for a new patient postdischarge. For use only in a Medicare-approved CMMI model. (Services must be furnished within a beneficiary's home, domiciliary, rest home, assisted living and/or nursing facility within 90 days following discharge from an inpatient facility and no more than nine times.)

G2004   Comprehensive (60 minutes) in-home visit for a new patient postdischarge. For use only in a Medicare-approved CMMI model. (Services must be furnished within a beneficiary's home, domiciliary, rest home, assisted living and/or nursing facility within 90 days following discharge from an inpatient facility and no more than nine times.)

G2005   Extensive (75 minutes) in-home visit for a new patient postdischarge. For use only in a Medicare-approved CMMI model. (Services must be furnished within a beneficiary's home, domiciliary, rest home, assisted living and/or nursing facility within 90 days following discharge from an inpatient facility and no more than nine times.)

G2006   Brief (20 minutes) in-home visit for an existing patient postdischarge. For use only in a Medicare-approved CMMI model. (Services must be furnished within a beneficiary's home, domiciliary, rest home, assisted living and/or nursing facility within 90 days following discharge from an inpatient facility and no more than nine times.)

G2007   Limited (30 minutes) in-home visit for an existing patient postdischarge. For use only in a Medicare-approved CMMI model. (Services must be furnished within a beneficiary's home, domiciliary, rest home, assisted living and/or nursing facility within 90 days following discharge from an inpatient facility and no more than nine times.)

Special Coverage Instructions   Noncovered by Medicare   Carrier Discretion   ☑ Quantity Alert   ● New Code   ○ Recycled/Reinstated   ▲ Revised Code

62 — G Codes   A Age Edit   M Maternity Edit   ♀ Female Only   ♂ Male Only   A-Y OPPS Status Indicators   © 2023 Optum360, LLC

G2008   Moderate (45 minutes) in-home visit for an existing patient postdischarge. For use only in a Medicare-approved CMMI model. (Services must be furnished within a beneficiary's home, domiciliary, rest home, assisted living and/or nursing facility within 90 days following discharge from an inpatient facility and no more than nine times.)

G2009   Comprehensive (60 minutes) in-home visit for an existing patient postdischarge. For use only in a Medicare-approved CMMI model. (Services must be furnished within a beneficiary's home, domiciliary, rest home, assisted living and/or nursing facility within 90 days following discharge from an inpatient facility and no more than nine times.)

G2010   Remote evaluation of recorded video and/or images submitted by an established patient (e.g., store and forward), including interpretation with follow-up with the patient within 24 business hours, not originating from a related E/M service provided within the previous 7 days nor leading to an E/M service or procedure within the next 24 hours or soonest available appointment

G2011   Alcohol and/or substance (other than tobacco) misuse structured assessment (e.g., audit, dast), and brief intervention, 5-14 minutes

G2012   Brief communication technology-based service, e.g., virtual check-in, by a physician or other qualified health care professional who can report evaluation and management services, provided to an established patient, not originating from a related E/M service provided within the previous 7 days nor leading to an E/M service or procedure within the next 24 hours or soonest available appointment; 5-10 minutes of medical discussion

G2013   Extensive (75 minutes) in-home visit for an existing patient postdischarge. For use only in a Medicare-approved CMMI model. (Services must be furnished within a beneficiary's home, domiciliary, rest home, assisted living and/or nursing facility within 90 days following discharge from an inpatient facility and no more than nine times.)

G2014   Limited (30 minutes) care plan oversight. For use only in a Medicare-approved CMMI model. (Services must be furnished within a beneficiary's home, domiciliary, rest home, assisted living and/or nursing facility within 90 days following discharge from an inpatient facility and no more than nine times.)

G2015   Comprehensive (60 minutes) home care plan oversight. For use only in a Medicare-approved CMMI model. (Services must be furnished within a beneficiary's home, domiciliary, rest home, assisted living and/or nursing facility within 90 days following discharge from an inpatient facility.)

Treatment in Place

G2020   Services for high intensity clinical services associated with the initial engagement and outreach of beneficiaries assigned to the SIP component of the PCF model (do not bill with chronic care management codes)
         AHA: 2Q,21

G2021   Health care practitioners rendering treatment in place (TIP)

G2022   A model participant (ambulance supplier/provider), the beneficiary refuses services covered under the model (transport to an alternate destination/treatment in place)

COVID-19 Specimen Collection

May be reported by clinical diagnostic laboratories.

G2023   Specimen collection for Severe Acute Respiratory Syndrome Coronavirus 2 (SARS-CoV-2) (Coronavirus disease [COVID-19]), any specimen source

G2024   Specimen collection for severe acute respiratory syndrome coronavirus 2 (SARS-CoV-2) (coronavirus disease [COVID-19]) from an individual in a SNF or by a laboratory on behalf of a HHA, any specimen source

G2025   Payment for a telehealth distant site service furnished by a Rural Health Clinic (RHC) or Federally Qualified Health Center (FQHC) only
         AHA: 2Q,20

Device Evaluation/Interrogation

G2066   Interrogation device evaluation(s), (remote) up to 30 days; implantable cardiovascular physiologic monitor system, implantable loop recorder system, or subcutaneous cardiac rhythm monitor system, remote data acquisition(s), receipt of transmissions and technician review, technical support and distribution of results

Medication Assisted Treatment and Other Services

G2067   Medication assisted treatment, methadone; weekly bundle including dispensing and/or administration, substance use counseling, individual and group therapy, and toxicology testing, if performed (provision of the services by a Medicare-enrolled opioid treatment program)
         CMS: 100-02,17,20; 100-02,17,40.1.1; 100-02,17,40.1.2; 100-04,26,10.5; 100-04,39,30.6; 100-04,39,30.6.1; 100-04,39,30.7; 100-04,39,30.8; 100-04,39,30.9; 100-04,39,40; 100-04,39,40.2; 100-04,39,50; 100-04,39,50.1

G2068   Medication assisted treatment, buprenorphine (oral); weekly bundle including dispensing and/or administration, substance use counseling, individual and group therapy, and toxicology testing if performed (provision of the services by a Medicare-enrolled opioid treatment program)
         CMS: 100-02,17,20; 100-02,17,40.1.1; 100-02,17,40.1.2; 100-04,26,10.5; 100-04,39,30.6; 100-04,39,30.6.1; 100-04,39,30.7; 100-04,39,30.8; 100-04,39,30.9; 100-04,39,40; 100-04,39,40.2; 100-04,39,50; 100-04,39,50.1

G2069   Medication assisted treatment, buprenorphine (injectable); weekly bundle including dispensing and/or administration, substance use counseling, individual and group therapy, and toxicology testing if performed (provision of the services by a Medicare-enrolled opioid treatment program)
         CMS: 100-02,17,20; 100-02,17,40.1.1; 100-02,17,40.1.2; 100-04,26,10.5; 100-04,39,30.6; 100-04,39,30.6.1; 100-04,39,30.7; 100-04,39,30.8; 100-04,39,30.9; 100-04,39,40; 100-04,39,40.2; 100-04,39,50; 100-04,39,50.1

G2070   Medication assisted treatment, buprenorphine (implant insertion); weekly bundle including dispensing and/or administration, substance use counseling, individual and group therapy, and toxicology testing if performed (provision of the services by a Medicare-enrolled opioid treatment program)
         CMS: 100-02,17,20; 100-02,17,40.1.1; 100-02,17,40.1.2; 100-04,26,10.5; 100-04,39,30.6; 100-04,39,30.6.1; 100-04,39,30.7; 100-04,39,30.8; 100-04,39,30.9; 100-04,39,40; 100-04,39,40.2; 100-04,39,50; 100-04,39,50.1

G2071   Medication assisted treatment, buprenorphine (implant removal); weekly bundle including dispensing and/or administration, substance use counseling, individual and group therapy, and toxicology testing if performed (provision of the services by a Medicare-enrolled opioid treatment program)
         CMS: 100-02,17,20; 100-02,17,40.1.1; 100-02,17,40.1.2; 100-04,26,10.5; 100-04,39,30.6; 100-04,39,30.6.1; 100-04,39,30.7; 100-04,39,30.8; 100-04,39,30.9; 100-04,39,40; 100-04,39,40.2; 100-04,39,50; 100-04,39,50.1

G2072   Medication assisted treatment, buprenorphine (implant insertion and removal); weekly bundle including dispensing and/or administration, substance use counseling, individual and group therapy, and toxicology testing if performed (provision of the services by a Medicare-enrolled opioid treatment program)
         CMS: 100-02,17,20; 100-02,17,40.1.1; 100-02,17,40.1.2; 100-04,26,10.5; 100-04,39,30.6; 100-04,39,30.6.1; 100-04,39,30.7; 100-04,39,30.8; 100-04,39,30.9; 100-04,39,40; 100-04,39,40.2; 100-04,39,50; 100-04,39,50.1

Special Coverage Instructions   Noncovered by Medicare   Carrier Discretion   ☑ Quantity Alert ● New Code   ○ Recycled/Reinstated ▲ Revised Code

© 2023 Optum360, LLC   A2-Z3 ASC Pmt   CMS: IOM   AHA: Coding Clinic   ⅋ DMEPOS Paid   ⊘ SNF Excluded   G Codes — 63

G2073 Medication assisted treatment, naltrexone; weekly bundle including dispensing and/or administration, substance use counseling, individual and group therapy, and toxicology testing if performed (provision of the services by a Medicare-enrolled opioid treatment program)
CMS: 100-02,17,20; 100-02,17,40.1.1; 100-02,17,40.1.2; 100-04,26,10.5; 100-04,39,30.6; 100-04,39,30.6.1; 100-04,39,30.7; 100-04,39,30.8; 100-04,39,30.9; 100-04,39,40; 100-04,39,40.2; 100-04,39,50; 100-04,39,50.1

G2074 Medication assisted treatment, weekly bundle not including the drug, including substance use counseling, individual and group therapy, and toxicology testing if performed (provision of the services by a Medicare-enrolled opioid treatment program)
CMS: 100-02,17,20; 100-02,17,40.1.1; 100-02,17,40.1.2; 100-04,26,10.5; 100-04,39,30.2; 100-04,39,30.3; 100-04,39,30.6; 100-04,39,30.6.1; 100-04,39,30.7; 100-04,39,30.8; 100-04,39,30.9; 100-04,39,40; 100-04,39,40.2; 100-04,39,50; 100-04,39,50.1

G2075 Medication assisted treatment, medication not otherwise specified; weekly bundle including dispensing and/or administration, substance use counseling, individual and group therapy, and toxicology testing, if performed (provision of the services by a Medicare-enrolled opioid treatment program)
CMS: 100-02,17,20; 100-02,17,40.1.1; 100-02,17,40.1.2; 100-04,26,10.5; 100-04,39,30.4; 100-04,39,30.6; 100-04,39,30.6.1; 100-04,39,30.7; 100-04,39,30.8; 100-04,39,30.9; 100-04,39,40; 100-04,39,40.2; 100-04,39,50; 100-04,39,50.1

G2076 Intake activities, including initial medical examination that is a complete, fully documented physical evaluation and initial assessment by a program physician or a primary care physician, or an authorized health care professional under the supervision of a program physician qualified personnel that includes preparation of a treatment plan that includes the patient's short-term goals and the tasks the patient must perform to complete the short-term goals; the patient's requirements for education, vocational rehabilitation, and employment; and the medical, psycho-social, economic, legal, or other supportive services that a patient needs, conducted by qualified personnel (provision of the services by a Medicare-enrolled opioid treatment program); list separately in addition to code for primary procedure
CMS: 100-02,17,20; 100-02,17,40.1.1; 100-02,17,40.1.2; 100-04,26,10.5; 100-04,39,30.6; 100-04,39,30.6.1; 100-04,39,30.7; 100-04,39,30.8; 100-04,39,30.9; 100-04,39,40; 100-04,39,40.2; 100-04,39,50; 100-04,39,50.1

G2077 Periodic assessment; assessing periodically by qualified personnel to determine the most appropriate combination of services and treatment (provision of the services by a Medicare-enrolled opioid treatment program); list separately in addition to code for primary procedure
CMS: 100-02,17,20; 100-02,17,40.1.1; 100-02,17,40.1.2; 100-04,26,10.5; 100-04,39,30.6; 100-04,39,30.6.1; 100-04,39,30.7; 100-04,39,30.8; 100-04,39,30.9; 100-04,39,40; 100-04,39,40.2; 100-04,39,50; 100-04,39,50.1

G2078 Take home supply of methadone; up to 7 additional day supply (provision of the services by a Medicare-enrolled opioid treatment program); list separately in addition to code for primary procedure
CMS: 100-02,17,20; 100-02,17,40.1.1; 100-02,17,40.1.2; 100-04,26,10.5; 100-04,39,30.6; 100-04,39,30.6.1; 100-04,39,30.7; 100-04,39,30.8; 100-04,39,30.9; 100-04,39,40; 100-04,39,40.2; 100-04,39,50; 100-04,39,50.1

G2079 Take home supply of buprenorphine (oral); up to 7 additional day supply (provision of the services by a Medicare-enrolled opioid treatment program); list separately in addition to code for primary procedure
CMS: 100-02,17,20; 100-02,17,40.1.1; 100-02,17,40.1.2; 100-04,26,10.5; 100-04,39,30.6; 100-04,39,30.6.1; 100-04,39,30.7; 100-04,39,30.8; 100-04,39,30.9; 100-04,39,40; 100-04,39,40.2; 100-04,39,50; 100-04,39,50.1

G2080 Each additional 30 minutes of counseling in a week of medication assisted treatment, (provision of the services by a Medicare-enrolled opioid treatment program); list separately in addition to code for primary procedure
CMS: 100-02,17,20; 100-02,17,40.1.1; 100-02,17,40.1.2; 100-04,26,10.5; 100-04,39,30.5; 100-04,39,30.6; 100-04,39,30.6.1; 100-04,39,30.7; 100-04,39,30.8; 100-04,39,30.9; 100-04,39,40; 100-04,39,40.2; 100-04,39,50; 100-04,39,50.1

G2081 Patients age 66 and older in institutional special needs plans (SNP) or residing in long-term care with a POS code 32, 33, 34, 54 or 56 for more than 90 consecutive days during the measurement period Ⓐ

G2082 Office or other outpatient visit for the evaluation and management of an established patient that requires the supervision of a physician or other qualified health care professional and provision of up to 56 mg of esketamine nasal self administration, includes 2 hours post administration observation

G2083 Office or other outpatient visit for the evaluation and management of an established patient that requires the supervision of a physician or other qualified health care professional and provision of greater than 56 mg esketamine nasal self administration, includes 2 hours post administration observation

G2086 Office-based treatment for opioid use disorder, including development of the treatment plan, care coordination, individual therapy and group therapy and counseling; at least 70 minutes in the first calendar month
AHA: 1Q,20

G2087 Office-based treatment for opioid use disorder, including care coordination, individual therapy and group therapy and counseling; at least 60 minutes in a subsequent calendar month
AHA: 1Q,20

G2088 Office-based treatment for opioid use disorder, including care coordination, individual therapy and group therapy and counseling; each additional 30 minutes beyond the first 120 minutes (list separately in addition to code for primary procedure)
AHA: 1Q,20

G2090 Patients 66 years of age and older with at least one claim/encounter for frailty during the measurement period and a dispensed medication for dementia during the measurement period or the year prior to the measurement period Ⓐ

G2091 Patients 66 years of age and older with at least one claim/encounter for frailty during the measurement period and either one acute inpatient encounter with a diagnosis of advanced illness or two outpatient, observation, ED or nonacute inpatient encounters on different dates of service with an advanced illness diagnosis during the measurement period or the year prior to the measurement period Ⓐ

G2092 Angiotensin converting enzyme (ACE) inhibitor or angiotensin receptor blocker (ARB) or angiotensin receptor-neprilysin inhibitor (ARNI) therapy prescribed or currently being taken

G2093 Documentation of medical reason(s) for not prescribing ACE inhibitor or ARB or ARNI therapy (e.g., hypotensive patients who are at immediate risk of cardiogenic shock, hospitalized patients who have experienced marked azotemia, allergy, intolerance, other medical reasons)

G2094 Documentation of patient reason(s) for not prescribing ACE inhibitor or ARB or ARNI therapy (e.g., patient declined, other patient reasons)

G2096 Angiotensin converting enzyme (ACE) inhibitor or angiotensin receptor blocker (ARB) or angiotensin receptor-neprilysin inhibitor (ARNI) therapy was not prescribed, reason not given

---

G2097 Episodes where the patient had a competing diagnosis on or within 3 days after the episode date (e.g., intestinal infection, pertussis, bacterial infection, Lyme disease, otitis media, acute sinusitis, chronic sinusitis, infection of the adenoids, prostatitis, cellulitis, mastoiditis, or bone infections, acute lymphadenitis, impetigo, skin staph infections, pneumonia/gonococcal infections, venereal disease (syphilis, chlamydia, inflammatory diseases [female reproductive organs]), infections of the kidney, cystitis or UTI)

G2098 Patients 66 years of age and older with at least one claim/encounter for frailty during the measurement period and a dispensed medication for dementia during the measurement period or the year prior to the measurement period ⬛A

G2099 Patients 66 years of age and older with at least one claim/encounter for frailty during the measurement period and either one acute inpatient encounter with a diagnosis of advanced illness or two outpatient, observation, ED or nonacute inpatient encounters on different dates of service with an advanced illness diagnosis during the measurement period or the year prior to the measurement period ⬛A

G2100 Patients 66 years of age and older with at least one claim/encounter for frailty during the measurement period and a dispensed medication for dementia during the measurement period or the year prior to the measurement period ⬛A

G2101 Patients 66 years of age and older with at least one claim/encounter for frailty during the measurement period and either one acute inpatient encounter with a diagnosis of advanced illness or two outpatient, observation, ED or nonacute inpatient encounters on different dates of service with an advanced illness diagnosis during the measurement period or the year prior to the measurement period ⬛A

G2105 Patient age 66 or older in institutional special needs plans (SNP) or residing in long-term care with POS code 32, 33, 34, 54 or 56 for more than 90 consecutive days during the measurement period ⬛A

G2106 Patients 66 years of age and older with at least one claim/encounter for frailty during the measurement period and a dispensed medication for dementia during the measurement period or the year prior to the measurement period ⬛A

G2107 Patients 66 years of age and older with at least one claim/encounter for frailty during the measurement period and either one acute inpatient encounter with a diagnosis of advanced illness or two outpatient, observation, ED or nonacute inpatient encounters on different dates of service with an advanced illness diagnosis during the measurement period or the year prior to the measurement period ⬛A

G2108 ~~Patient age 66 or older in institutional special needs plans (SNP) or residing in long-term care with POS code 32, 33, 34, 54 or 56 for more than 90 consecutive days during the measurement period~~

G2109 ~~Patients 66 years of age and older with at least one claim/encounter for frailty during the measurement period and a dispensed medication for dementia during the measurement period or the year prior to the measurement period~~

G2110 ~~Patients 66 years of age and older with at least one claim/encounter for frailty during the measurement period and either one acute inpatient encounter with a diagnosis of advanced illness or two outpatient, observation, ED or nonacute inpatient encounters on different dates of service with an advanced illness diagnosis during the measurement period or the year prior to the measurement period~~

G2112 Patient receiving <=5 mg daily prednisone (or equivalent), or RA activity is worsening, or glucocorticoid use is for less than 6 months

G2113 Patient receiving >5 mg daily prednisone (or equivalent) for longer than 6 months, and improvement or no change in disease activity

G2115 Patients 66 - 80 years of age with at least one claim/encounter for frailty during the measurement period and a dispensed medication for dementia during the measurement period or the year prior to the measurement period ⬛A

G2116 Patients 66 - 80 years of age with at least one claim/encounter for frailty during the measurement period and either one acute inpatient encounter with a diagnosis of advanced illness or two outpatient, observation, ED or nonacute inpatient encounters on different dates of service with an advanced illness diagnosis during the measurement period or the year prior to the measurement period ⬛A

G2118 Patients 81 years of age and older with at least one claim/encounter for frailty during the measurement period ⬛A

G2121 Depression, anxiety, apathy, and psychosis assessed

G2122 Depression, anxiety, apathy, and psychosis not assessed

G2125 Patients 81 years of age and older with at least one claim/encounter for frailty during the six months prior to the measurement period through December 31 of the measurement period ⬛A

G2126 Patients 66 - 80 years of age with at least one claim/encounter for frailty during the measurement period and either one acute inpatient encounter with a diagnosis of advanced illness or two outpatient, observation, ED or nonacute inpatient encounters on different dates of service with an advanced illness diagnosis during the measurement period or the year prior to the measurement period ⬛A

G2127 Patients 66 - 80 years of age with at least one claim/encounter for frailty during the measurement period and a dispensed medication for dementia during the measurement period or the year prior to the measurement period ⬛A

G2128 Documentation of medical reason(s) for not on a daily aspirin or other antiplatelet (e.g., history of gastrointestinal bleed, intracranial bleed, blood disorders, idiopathic thrombocytopenic purpura (ITP), gastric bypass or documentation of active anticoagulant use during the measurement period)

G2129 Procedure related BP's not taken during an outpatient visit. Examples include same day surgery, ambulatory service center, GI, lab, dialysis, infusion center, chemotherapy

G2136 Back pain measured by the visual analog scale (VAS) or numeric pain scale at 3 months (6 to 20 weeks) postoperatively was less than or equal to 3.0 or back pain measured by the visual analog scale (VAS) or numeric pain scale within 3 months preoperatively and at 3 months (6 to 20 weeks) postoperatively demonstrated an improvement of 5.0 points or greater

▲ **G2137** Back pain measured by the visual analog scale (VAS) or numeric pain scale at 3 months (6 to 20 weeks) postoperatively was greater than 3.0 and back pain measured by the visual analog scale (VAS) or numeric pain scale within 3 months preoperatively and at 3 months (6 to 20 weeks) postoperatively demonstrated improvement of less than 5.0 points

G2138 Back pain as measured by the visual analog scale (VAS) or numeric pain scale at 1 year (9 to 15 months) postoperatively was less than or equal to 3.0 or back pain measured by the visual analog scale (VAS) or numeric pain scale within 3 months preoperatively and at 1 year (9 to 15 months) postoperatively demonstrated an improvement of 5.0 points or greater

---

Special Coverage Instructions   Noncovered by Medicare   Carrier Discretion   ☑ Quantity Alert   ● New Code   ○ Recycled/Reinstated   ▲ Revised Code

© 2023 Optum360, LLC   N2-Z3 ASC Pmt   **CMS:** IOM   **AHA:** Coding Clinic   ⅃ DMEPOS Paid   ⊘ SNF Excluded   **G Codes — 65**

Procedures/Professional Services (Temporary)

G2139 — G2188

▲ **G2139** Back pain measured by the visual analog scale (VAS) or numeric pain scale at 1 year (9 to 15 months) postoperatively was greater than 3.0 and back pain measured by the visual analog scale (VAS) or numeric pain scale within 3 months preoperatively and at 1 year (9 to 15 months) postoperatively demonstrated improvement of less than 5.0 points

G2140 Leg pain measured by the visual analog scale (VAS) or numeric pain scale at 3 months (6 to 20 weeks) postoperatively was less than or equal to 3.0 or leg pain measured by the visual analog scale (VAS) or numeric pain scale within 3 months preoperatively and at 3 months (6 to 20 weeks) postoperatively demonstrated an improvement of 5.0 points or greater
AHA: 2Q,21

▲ **G2141** Leg pain measured by the visual analog scale (VAS) or numeric pain scale at 3 months (6 to 20 weeks) postoperatively was greater than 3.0 and leg pain measured by the visual analog scale (VAS) or numeric pain scale within 3 months preoperatively and at 3 months (6 to 20 weeks) postoperatively demonstrated improvement of less than 5.0 points

G2142 Functional status measured by the Oswestry Disability Index (ODI version 2.1a) at 1 year (9 to 15 months) postoperatively was less than or equal to 22 or functional status measured by the ODI version 2.1a within 3 months preoperatively and at 1 year (9 to 15 months) postoperatively demonstrated an improvement of 30 points or greater

G2143 Functional status measured by the Oswestry Disability Index (ODI version 2.1a) at 1 year (9 to 15 months) postoperatively was greater than 22 and functional status measured by the ODI version 2.1a within 3 months preoperatively and at 1 year (9 to 15 months) postoperatively demonstrated an improvement of less than 30 points

G2144 Functional status measured by the Oswestry Disability Index (ODI version 2.1a) at 3 months (6 to 20 weeks) postoperatively was less than or equal to 22 or functional status measured by the ODI version 2.1a within 3 months preoperatively and at 3 months (6 to 20 weeks) postoperatively demonstrated an improvement of 30 points or greater

G2145 Functional status measured by the Oswestry Disability Index (ODI version 2.1a) at 3 months (6 to 20 weeks) postoperatively was greater than 22 and functional status measured by the ODI version 2.1a within 3 months preoperatively and at 3 months (6 to 20 weeks) postoperatively demonstrated an improvement of less than 30 points

G2146 Leg pain as measured by the visual analog scale (VAS) or numeric pain scale at 1 year (9 to 15 months) postoperatively was less than or equal to 3.0 or leg pain measured by the visual analog scale (VAS) or numeric pain scale within 3 months preoperatively and at 1 year (9 to 15 months) postoperatively demonstrated an improvement of 5.0 points or greater

▲ **G2147** Leg pain measured by the visual analog scale (VAS) or numeric pain scale at 1 year (9 to 15 months) postoperatively was greater than 3.0 and leg pain measured by the visual analog scale (VAS) or numeric pain scale within 3 months preoperatively and at 1 year (9 to 15 months) postoperatively demonstrated improvement of less than 5.0 points

G2148 Multimodal pain management was used

G2149 Documentation of medical reason(s) for not using multimodal pain management (e.g., allergy to multiple classes of analgesics, intubated patient, hepatic failure, patient reports no pain during PACU stay, other medical reason(s))

G2150 Multimodal pain management was not used

G2151 Documentation stating patient has a diagnosis of a degenerative neurological condition such as ALS, MS, or Parkinson's diagnosed at any time before or during the episode of care

G2152 Residual score for the neck impairment successfully calculated and the score was equal to zero (0) or greater than zero (> 0)

G2167 Residual score for the neck impairment successfully calculated and the score was less than zero (< 0)

Home Health

G2168 Services performed by a physical therapist assistant in the home health setting in the delivery of a safe and effective physical therapy maintenance program, each 15 minutes
CMS: 100-04,10,40.2

G2169 Services performed by an occupational therapist assistant in the home health setting in the delivery of a safe and effective occupational therapy maintenance program, each 15 minutes
CMS: 100-04,10,40.2

Quality Measures

G2172 All inclusive payment for services related to highly coordinated and integrated opioid use disorder (OUD) treatment services furnished for the demonstration project
AHA: 2Q,21

G2173 URI episodes where the patient had a comorbid condition during the 12 months prior to or on the episode date (e.g., tuberculosis, neutropenia, cystic fibrosis, chronic bronchitis, pulmonary edema, respiratory failure, rheumatoid lung disease)

▲ **G2174** URI episodes where the patient is taking antibiotics (Table 1) in the 30 days prior to the episode date

G2175 Episodes where the patient had a comorbid condition during the 12 months prior to or on the episode date (e.g., tuberculosis, neutropenia, cystic fibrosis, chronic bronchitis, pulmonary edema, respiratory failure, rheumatoid lung disease)

G2176 Outpatient, ED, or observation visits that result in an inpatient admission

G2177 Acute bronchitis/bronchiolitis episodes when the patient had a new or refill prescription of antibiotics (table 1) in the 30 days prior to the episode date

G2178 Clinician documented that patient was not an eligible candidate for lower extremity neurological exam measure, for example patient bilateral amputee; patient has condition that would not allow them to accurately respond to a neurological exam (dementia, Alzheimer's, etc.); patient has previously documented diabetic peripheral neuropathy with loss of protective sensation

G2179 Clinician documented that patient had medical reason for not performing lower extremity neurological exam

G2180 Clinician documented that patient was not an eligible candidate for evaluation of footwear as patient is bilateral lower extremity amputee

G2181 BMI not documented due to medical reason or patient refusal of height or weight measurement

G2182 Patient receiving first-time biologic and/or immune response modifier therapy

G2183 Documentation patient unable to communicate and informant not available

G2184 Patient does not have a caregiver

G2185 Documentation caregiver is trained and certified in dementia care

G2186 Patient /caregiver dyad has been referred to appropriate resources and connection to those resources is confirmed

G2187 Patients with clinical indications for imaging of the head: head trauma

G2188 Patients with clinical indications for imaging of the head: new or change in headache above 50 years of age

---

Special Coverage Instructions   Noncovered by Medicare   Carrier Discretion   ☑ Quantity Alert   ● New Code   ○ Recycled/Reinstated   ▲ Revised Code

G2189 Patients with clinical indications for imaging of the head: abnormal neurologic exam

G2190 Patients with clinical indications for imaging of the head: headache radiating to the neck

G2191 Patients with clinical indications for imaging of the head: positional headaches

G2192 Patients with clinical indications for imaging of the head: temporal headaches in patients over 55 years of age

G2193 Patients with clinical indications for imaging of the head: new onset headache in preschool children or younger (<6 years of age)

G2194 Patients with clinical indications for imaging of the head: new onset headache in pediatric patients with disabilities for which headache is a concern as inferred from behavior

G2195 Patients with clinical indications for imaging of the head: occipital headache in children

G2196 Patient identified as an unhealthy alcohol user when screened for unhealthy alcohol use using a systematic screening method

G2197 Patient screened for unhealthy alcohol use using a systematic screening method and not identified as an unhealthy alcohol user

G2199 Patient not screened for unhealthy alcohol use using a systematic screening method

G2200 Patient identified as an unhealthy alcohol user received brief counseling

G2202 Patient did not receive brief counseling if identified as an unhealthy alcohol user

G2204 Patients between 45 and 85 years of age who received a screening colonoscopy during the performance period

G2205 Patients with pregnancy during adjuvant treatment course

G2206 Patient received adjuvant treatment course including both chemotherapy and HER2-targeted therapy

G2207 Reason for not administering adjuvant treatment course including both chemotherapy and HER2-targeted therapy (e.g., poor performance status (ECOG 3-4; Karnofsky <=50), cardiac contraindications, insufficient renal function, insufficient hepatic function, other active or secondary cancer diagnoses, other medical contraindications, patients who died during initial treatment course or transferred during or after initial treatment course)

G2208 Patient did not receive adjuvant treatment course including both chemotherapy and HER2-targeted therapy

G2209 Patient refused to participate

G2210 Residual score for the neck impairment not measured because the patient did not complete the neck FS PROM at initial evaluation and/or near discharge, reason not given

G2211 Visit complexity inherent to evaluation and management associated with medical care services that serve as the continuing focal point for all needed health care services and/or with medical care services that are part of ongoing care related to a patient's single, serious condition or a complex condition. (add-on code, list separately in addition to office/outpatient evaluation and management visit, new or established)

G2212 Prolonged office or other outpatient evaluation and management service(s) beyond the maximum required time of the primary procedure which has been selected using total time on the date of the primary service; each additional 15 minutes by the physician or qualified healthcare professional, with or without direct patient contact (list separately in addition to CPT codes 99205, 99215, 99483 for office or other outpatient evaluation and management services.) (Do not report G2212 on the same date of service as codes 99358, 99359, 99415, 99416). (Do not report G2212 for any time unit less than 15 minutes)
CMS: 100-04,12,30.6.15.1; 100-04,12,30.6.15.2; 100-04,12,30.6.15.3; 100-04,12,30.6.18

G2213 Initiation of medication for the treatment of opioid use disorder in the emergency department setting, including assessment, referral to ongoing care, and arranging access to supportive services (list separately in addition to code for primary procedure)

G2214 Initial or subsequent psychiatric collaborative care management, first 30 minutes in a month of behavioral health care manager activities, in consultation with a psychiatric consultant, and directed by the treating physician or other qualified health care professional

G2215 Take home supply of nasal naloxone; 2-pack of 4 mg per 0.1 ml nasal spray (provision of the services by a Medicare-enrolled Opioid Treatment Program); list separately in addition to code for primary procedure
CMS: 100-02,17,20; 100-02,17,40.1.1; 100-02,17,40.1.2; 100-04,39,30.6; 100-04,39,30.6.1; 100-04,39,30.7; 100-04,39,30.8; 100-04,39,40

G2216 Take home supply of injectable naloxone (provision of the services by a Medicare-enrolled opioid treatment program); list separately in addition to code for primary procedure
CMS: 100-02,17,20; 100-02,17,40.1.1; 100-02,17,40.1.2; 100-04,39,30.6; 100-04,39,30.6.1; 100-04,39,30.7; 100-04,39,30.8; 100-04,39,40

G2250 Remote assessment of recorded video and/or images submitted by an established patient (e.g., store and forward), including interpretation with follow-up with the patient within 24 business hours, not originating from a related service provided within the previous 7 days nor leading to a service or procedure within the next 24 hours or soonest available appointment

G2251 Brief communication technology-based service, e.g. virtual check-in, by a qualified health care professional who cannot report evaluation and management services, provided to an established patient, not originating from a related service provided within the previous 7 days nor leading to a service or procedure within the next 24 hours or soonest available appointment; 5-10 minutes of clinical discussion

G2252 Brief communication technology-based service, e.g. virtual check-in, by a physician or other qualified health care professional who can report evaluation and management services, provided to an established patient, not originating from a related EM service provided within the previous 7 days nor leading to an EM service or procedure within the next 24 hours or soonest available appointment; 11-20 minutes of medical discussion

Special Coverage Instructions · Noncovered by Medicare · Carrier Discretion · ☑ Quantity Alert · ● New Code · ○ Recycled/Reinstated · ▲ Revised Code

© 2023 Optum360, LLC · A2-Z3 ASC Pmt · CMS: IOM · AHA: Coding Clinic · ⅛ DMEPOS Paid · ⊘ SNF Excluded · G Codes — 67

Chronic Pain Management

G3002 Chronic pain management and treatment, monthly bundle including, diagnosis; assessment and monitoring; administration of a validated pain rating scale or tool; the development, implementation, revision, and/or maintenance of a person-centered care plan that includes strengths, goals, clinical needs, and desired outcomes; overall treatment management; facilitation and coordination of any necessary behavioral health treatment; medication management; pain and health literacy counseling; any necessary chronic pain related crisis care; and ongoing communication and care coordination between relevant practitioners furnishing care e.g., physical therapy and occupational therapy, complementary and integrative approaches, and community-based care, as appropriate. Requires initial face-to-face visit at least 30 minutes provided by a physician or other qualified health professional; first 30 minutes personally provided by physician or other qualified health care professional, per calendar month. (When using G3002, 30 minutes must be met or exceeded)

G3003 Each additional 15 minutes of chronic pain management and treatment by a physician or other qualified health care professional, per calendar month. (List separately in addition to code for G3002. When using G3003, 15 minutes must be met or exceeded)

MIPS Specialty Sets

G4000 Dermatology MIPS specialty set

G4001 Diagnostic Radiology MIPS specialty set

G4002 Electrophysiology Cardiac Specialist MIPS specialty set

G4003 Emergency Medicine MIPS specialty set

G4004 Endocrinology MIPS specialty set

G4005 Family Medicine MIPS specialty set

G4006 Gastroenterology MIPS specialty set

G4007 General Surgery MIPS specialty set

G4008 Geriatrics MIPS specialty set

G4009 Hospitalists MIPS specialty set

G4010 Infectious Disease MIPS specialty set

G4011 Internal Medicine MIPS specialty set

G4012 Interventional Radiology MIPS specialty set

G4013 Mental/behavioral and Psychiatry MIPS specialty set

G4014 Nephrology MIPS specialty set

G4015 Neurology MIPS specialty set

G4016 Neurosurgical MIPS specialty set

G4017 Nutrition/Dietician MIPS specialty set

G4018 Obstetrics/Gynecology MIPS specialty set

G4019 Oncology/Hematology MIPS specialty set

G4020 Ophthalmology/Optometry MIPS specialty set

G4021 Orthopedic surgery MIPS specialty set

G4022 Otolaryngology MIPS specialty set

G4023 Pathology MIPS specialty set

G4024 Pediatrics MIPS specialty set

G4025 Physical Medicine MIPS specialty set

G4026 Physical Therapy/Occupational Therapy MIPS specialty set

G4027 Plastic Surgery MIPS specialty set

G4028 Podiatry MIPS specialty set

G4029 Preventive Medicine MIPS specialty set

G4030 Pulmonology MIPS specialty set

G4031 Radiation Oncology MIPS specialty set

G4032 Rheumatology MIPS specialty set

G4033 Skilled Nursing Facility MIPS specialty set

G4034 Speech Language Pathology MIPS specialty set

G4035 Thoracic Surgery MIPS specialty set

G4036 Urgent Care MIPS specialty set

G4037 Urology MIPS specialty set

G4038 Vascular Surgery MIPS specialty set

Radiation Therapy

G6001 Ultrasonic guidance for placement of radiation therapy fields ☐B

G6002 Stereoscopic x-ray guidance for localization of target volume for the delivery of radiation therapy ☐B

G6003 Radiation treatment delivery, single treatment area, single port or parallel opposed ports, simple blocks or no blocks: up to 5 mev ☐B

G6004 Radiation treatment delivery, single treatment area, single port or parallel opposed ports, simple blocks or no blocks: 6-10 mev ☐B

G6005 Radiation treatment delivery, single treatment area, single port or parallel opposed ports, simple blocks or no blocks: 11-19 mev ☐B

G6006 Radiation treatment delivery, single treatment area, single port or parallel opposed ports, simple blocks or no blocks: 20 mev or greater ☐B

G6007 Radiation treatment delivery, two separate treatment areas, three or more ports on a single treatment area, use of multiple blocks: up to 5 mev ☐B

G6008 Radiation treatment delivery, two separate treatment areas, three or more ports on a single treatment area, use of multiple blocks: 6-10 mev ☐B

G6009 Radiation treatment delivery, two separate treatment areas, three or more ports on a single treatment area, use of multiple blocks: 11-19 mev ☐B

G6010 Radiation treatment delivery, two separate treatment areas, three or more ports on a single treatment area, use of multiple blocks: 20 mev or greater ☐B

G6011 Radiation treatment delivery, three or more separate treatment areas, custom blocking, tangential ports, wedges, rotational beam, compensators, electron beam; up to 5 mev ☐B

G6012 Radiation treatment delivery, three or more separate treatment areas, custom blocking, tangential ports, wedges, rotational beam, compensators, electron beam; 6-10 mev ☐B

G6013 Radiation treatment delivery, three or more separate treatment areas, custom blocking, tangential ports, wedges, rotational beam, compensators, electron beam; 11-19 mev ☐B

G6014 Radiation treatment delivery, three or more separate treatment areas, custom blocking, tangential ports, wedges, rotational beam, compensators, electron beam; 20 mev or greater ☐B

G6015 Intensity modulated treatment delivery, single or multiple fields/arcs, via narrow spatially and temporally modulated beams, binary, dynamic MLC, per treatment session ☐B

G6016 Compensator-based beam modulation treatment delivery of inverse planned treatment using three or more high resolution (milled or cast) compensator, convergent beam modulated fields, per treatment session ☐B

Special Coverage Instructions   Noncovered by Medicare   Carrier Discretion   ☑ Quantity Alert ● New Code   ○ Recycled/Reinstated ▲ Revised Code

68 — G Codes   Ⓐ Age Edit   Ⓜ Maternity Edit   ♀ Female Only   ♂ Male Only   Ⓐ-Ⓨ OPPS Status Indicators   © 2023 Optum360, LLC

G6017 Intra-fraction localization and tracking of target or patient motion during delivery of radiation therapy (e.g., 3D positional tracking, gating, 3D surface tracking), each fraction of treatment ⓑ

Quality Measures

G8395 Left ventricular ejection fraction (LVEF) ≥ 40% or documentation as normal or mildly depressed left ventricular systolic function Ⓜ

G8396 Left ventricular ejection fraction (LVEF) not performed or documented Ⓜ

G8397 Dilated macular or fundus exam performed, including documentation of the presence or absence of macular edema and level of severity of retinopathy Ⓜ

G8399 Patient with documented results of a central dual-energy x-ray absorptiometry (DXA) ever being performed Ⓜ

G8400 Patient with central dual-energy x-ray absorptiometry (DXA) results not documented, reason not given Ⓜ

G8404 Lower extremity neurological exam performed and documented Ⓜ

G8405 Lower extremity neurological exam not performed Ⓜ

G8410 Footwear evaluation performed and documented Ⓜ

G8415 Footwear evaluation was not performed Ⓜ

G8416 Clinician documented that patient was not an eligible candidate for footwear evaluation measure Ⓜ

G8417 BMI is documented above normal parameters and a follow-up plan is documented Ⓜ

G8418 BMI is documented below normal parameters and a follow-up plan is documented Ⓜ

G8419 BMI documented outside normal parameters, no follow-up plan documented, no reason given Ⓜ

G8420 BMI is documented within normal parameters and no follow-up plan is required Ⓜ

G8421 BMI not documented and no reason is given Ⓜ

G8427 Eligible clinician attests to documenting in the medical record they obtained, updated, or reviewed the patient's current medications Ⓜ

G8428 Current list of medications not documented as obtained, updated, or reviewed by the eligible clinician, reason not given Ⓜ

G8430 Documentation of a medical reason(s) for not documenting, updating, or reviewing the patient's current medications list (e.g., patient is in an urgent or emergent medical situation) Ⓜ

G8431 Screening for depression is documented as being positive and a follow-up plan is documented Ⓜ

G8432 Depression screening not documented, reason not given Ⓜ

G8433 Screening for depression not completed, documented patient or medical reason Ⓜ

G8450 Beta-blocker therapy prescribed Ⓜ

G8451 Beta-blocker therapy for LVEF <=40% not prescribed for reasons documented by the clinician (e.g., low blood pressure, fluid overload, asthma, patients recently treated with an intravenous positive inotropic agent, allergy, intolerance, other medical reasons, patient declined, other patient reasons) Ⓜ

G8452 Beta-blocker therapy not prescribed Ⓜ

G8465 High or very high risk of recurrence of prostate cancer Ⓜ

G8473 Angiotensin converting enzyme (ACE) inhibitor or angiotensin receptor blocker (ARB) therapy prescribed Ⓜ

▲ **G8474** Angiotensin converting enzyme (ACE) inhibitor or angiotensin receptor blocker (ARB) therapy not prescribed for reasons documented by the clinician (e.g., allergy, intolerance, pregnancy, renal failure due to ACE inhibitor, diseases of the aortic or mitral valve, other medical reasons) or (e.g., patient declined, other patient reasons) Ⓜ

G8475 Angiotensin converting enzyme (ACE) inhibitor or angiotensin receptor blocker (ARB) therapy not prescribed, reason not given Ⓜ

G8476 Most recent blood pressure has a systolic measurement of < 140 mm Hg and a diastolic measurement of < 90 mm Hg Ⓜ

G8477 Most recent blood pressure has a systolic measurement of >=140 mm Hg and/or a diastolic measurement of >=90 mm Hg Ⓜ

G8478 Blood pressure measurement not performed or documented, reason not given Ⓜ

G8482 Influenza immunization administered or previously received Ⓜ

G8483 Influenza immunization was not administered for reasons documented by clinician (e.g., patient allergy or other medical reasons, patient declined or other patient reasons, vaccine not available or other system reasons) Ⓜ

G8484 Influenza immunization was not administered, reason not given Ⓜ

G8506 Patient receiving angiotensin converting enzyme (ACE) inhibitor or angiotensin receptor blocker (ARB) therapy

G8510 Screening for depression is documented as negative, a follow-up plan is not required Ⓜ

G8511 Screening for depression documented as positive, follow-up plan not documented, reason not given Ⓜ

▲ **G8535** Elder maltreatment screen not documented; documentation that patient is not eligible for the elder maltreatment screen at the time of the encounter related to one of the following reasons: (1) patient refuses to participate in the screening and has reasonable decisional capacity for self-protection, or (2) patient is in an urgent or emergent situation where time is of the essence and to delay treatment to perform the screening would jeopardize the patient's health status Ⓜ

G8536 No documentation of an elder maltreatment screen, reason not given Ⓜ

G8539 Functional outcome assessment documented as positive using a standardized tool and a care plan based on identified deficiencies is documented within 2 days of the functional outcome assessment Ⓜ

G8540 Functional outcome assessment not documented as being performed, documentation the patient is not eligible for a functional outcome assessment using a standardized tool at the time of the encounter Ⓜ

G8541 Functional outcome assessment using a standardized tool, not documented, reason not given Ⓜ

G8542 Functional outcome assessment using a standardized tool is documented; no functional deficiencies identified, care plan not required Ⓜ

G8543 Documentation of a positive functional outcome assessment using a standardized tool; care plan not documented within 2 days of assessment, reason not given Ⓜ

G8559 Patient referred to a physician (preferably a physician with training in disorders of the ear) for an otologic evaluation Ⓜ

Special Coverage Instructions | Noncovered by Medicare | Carrier Discretion | ☑ Quantity Alert | ● New Code | ○ Recycled/Reinstated | ▲ Revised Code

© 2023 Optum360, LLC | Ⓐ-Ⓩ ASC Pmt | **CMS:** IOM | **AHA:** Coding Clinic | ♿ DMEPOS Paid | ⊘ SNF Excluded | G Codes — 69

G8560 Patient has a history of active drainage from the ear within the previous 90 days Ⓜ

G8561 Patient is not eligible for the referral for otologic evaluation for patients with a history of active drainage measure Ⓜ

G8562 Patient does not have a history of active drainage from the ear within the previous 90 days Ⓜ

G8563 Patient not referred to a physician (preferably a physician with training in disorders of the ear) for an otologic evaluation, reason not given Ⓜ

G8564 Patient was referred to a physician (preferably a physician with training in disorders of the ear) for an otologic evaluation, reason not specified) Ⓜ

G8565 Verification and documentation of sudden or rapidly progressive hearing loss Ⓜ

G8566 Patient is not eligible for the "referral for otologic evaluation for sudden or rapidly progressive hearing loss" measure Ⓜ

G8567 Patient does not have verification and documentation of sudden or rapidly progressive hearing loss Ⓜ

G8568 Patient was not referred to a physician (preferably a physician with training in disorders of the ear) for an otologic evaluation, reason not given Ⓜ

G8569 Prolonged postoperative intubation (> 24 hrs) required Ⓜ

G8570 Prolonged postoperative intubation (> 24 hrs) not required Ⓜ

G8575 Developed postoperative renal failure or required dialysis Ⓜ

G8576 No postoperative renal failure/dialysis not required Ⓜ

G8577 Re-exploration required due to mediastinal bleeding with or without tamponade, graft occlusion, valve dysfunction or other cardiac reason Ⓜ

G8578 Re-exploration not required due to mediastinal bleeding with or without tamponade, graft occlusion, valve dysfunction or other cardiac reason Ⓜ

G8598 Aspirin or another antiplatelet therapy used Ⓜ

G8599 Aspirin or another antiplatelet therapy not used, reason not given Ⓜ

G8600 IV tPA initiated within 3 hours (≤ 180 minutes) of time last known well Ⓜ

▲ **G8601** IV thrombolytic therapy not initiated within 4.5 hours (<= 270 minutes) of time last known well for reasons documented by clinician (e.g., patient enrolled in clinical trial for stroke, patient admitted for elective carotid intervention) Ⓜ

G8602 IV tPA not initiated within 3 hours (≤ 180 minutes) of time last known well, reason not given Ⓜ

G8633 Pharmacologic therapy (other than minerals/vitamins) for osteoporosis prescribed Ⓜ

G8635 Pharmacologic therapy for osteoporosis was not prescribed, reason not given Ⓜ

G8647 Residual score for the knee impairment successfully calculated and the score was equal to zero (0) or greater than zero (> 0) Ⓜ ☑

G8648 Residual score for the knee impairment successfully calculated and the score was less than zero (< 0) Ⓜ ☑

G8650 Residual score for the knee impairment not measured because the patient did not complete the LEPF PROM at initial evaluation and/or near discharge, reason not given Ⓜ

G8651 Residual score for the hip impairment successfully calculated and the score was equal to zero (0) or greater than zero (> 0) Ⓜ ☑

G8652 Residual score for the hip impairment successfully calculated and the score was less than zero (< 0) Ⓜ ☑

G8654 Residual score for the hip impairment not measured because the patient did not complete the LEPF PROM at initial evaluation and/or near discharge, reason not given Ⓜ

G8655 Risk-adjusted functional status change residual score for the foot or ankle successfully calculated and the score was equal to zero (0) or greater than zero (> 0) Ⓜ ☑

G8656 Residual score for the lower leg, foot or ankle impairment successfully calculated and the score was less than zero (< 0) Ⓜ ☑

G8658 Residual score for the lower leg, foot or ankle impairment not measured because the patient did not complete the LEPF PROM at initial evaluation and/or near discharge, reason not given Ⓜ

G8659 Residual score for the low back impairment successfully calculated and the score was equal to zero (0) or greater than zero (> 0) Ⓜ

G8660 Residual score for the low back impairment successfully calculated and the score was less than zero (< 0) Ⓜ ☑

G8661 Risk-adjusted functional status change residual score for the low back impairment not measured because the patient did not complete the FS status survey near discharge, patient not appropriate Ⓜ

G8662 Residual score for the low back impairment not measured because the patient did not complete the low back FS PROM at initial evaluation and/or near discharge, reason not given Ⓜ

G8663 Residual score for the shoulder impairment successfully calculated and the score was equal to zero (0) or greater than zero (> 0) Ⓜ ☑

G8664 Residual score for the shoulder impairment successfully calculated and the score was less than zero (< 0) Ⓜ ☑

G8666 Residual score for the shoulder impairment not measured because the patient did not complete the shoulder FS PROM at initial evaluation and/or near discharge, reason not given Ⓜ

G8667 Residual score for the elbow, wrist or hand impairment successfully calculated and the score was equal to zero (0) or greater than zero (> 0) Ⓜ ☑

G8668 Residual score for the elbow, wrist or hand impairment successfully calculated and the score was less than zero (< 0) Ⓜ ☑

G8670 Residual score for the elbow, wrist or hand impairment not measured because the patient did not complete the elbow/wrist/hand FS PROM at initial evaluation and/or near discharge, reason not given Ⓜ

G8694 Left ventricular ejection fraction (LVEF) < = 40% or documentation of moderate or severe LVSD Ⓜ ☑

G8708 Patient not prescribed antibiotic Ⓜ

G8709 URI episodes when the patient had competing diagnoses on or three days after the episode date (e.g., intestinal infection, pertussis, bacterial infection, Lyme disease, otitis media, acute sinusitis, acute pharyngitis, acute tonsillitis, chronic sinusitis, infection of the pharynx/larynx/tonsils/adenoids, prostatitis, cellulitis, mastoiditis, or bone infections, acute lymphadenitis, impetigo, skin staph infections, pneumonia/gonococcal infections, venereal disease (syphilis, chlamydia, inflammatory diseases [female reproductive organs]), infections of the kidney, cystitis or UTI, and acne) Ⓜ

G8710 Patient prescribed antibiotic Ⓜ

| Special Coverage Instructions | Noncovered by Medicare | Carrier Discretion | ☑ Quantity Alert ● New Code ○ Recycled/Reinstated ▲ Revised Code |

70 — G Codes   Ⓐ Age Edit   Ⓜ Maternity Edit   ♀ Female Only   ♂ Male Only   Ⓐ-Ⓨ OPPS Status Indicators   © 2023 Optum360, LLC

G8711	Prescribed antibiotic on or within 3 days after the episode date [M]
G8712	Antibiotic not prescribed or dispensed [M]
G8721	PT category (primary tumor), PN category (regional lymph nodes), and histologic grade were documented in pathology report [M]
G8722	Documentation of medical reason(s) for not including the PT category, the PN category or the histologic grade in the pathology report (e.g., re-excision without residual tumor; noncarcinomasanal canal) [M]
G8723	Specimen site is other than anatomic location of primary tumor [M]
G8724	PT category, PN category and histologic grade were not documented in the pathology report, reason not given [M]
G8733	Elder maltreatment screen documented as positive and a follow-up plan is documented [M]
G8734	Elder maltreatment screen documented as negative, follow-up is not required [M]
G8735	Elder maltreatment screen documented as positive, follow-up plan not documented, reason not given [M]
G8749	Absence of signs of melanoma (tenderness, jaundice, localized neurologic signs such as weakness, or any other sign suggesting systemic spread) or absence of symptoms of melanoma (cough, dyspnea, pain, paresthesia, or any other symptom suggesting the possibility of systemic spread of melanoma) [M]
G8752	Most recent systolic blood pressure < 140 mm Hg [M] ☑
G8753	Most recent systolic blood pressure ≥ 140 mm Hg [M] ☑
G8754	Most recent diastolic blood pressure < 90 mm Hg [M] ☑
G8755	Most recent diastolic blood pressure ≥ 90 mm Hg [M] ☑
G8756	No documentation of blood pressure measurement, reason not given [M]
G8783	Normal blood pressure reading documented, follow-up not required [M]
G8785	Blood pressure reading not documented, reason not given [M]
G8797	Specimen site other than anatomic location of esophagus [M]
G8798	Specimen site other than anatomic location of prostate [M]
G8806	Performance of trans-abdominal or trans-vaginal ultrasound and pregnancy location documented [A] [♀] [M]
▲ **G8807**	Transabdominal or transvaginal ultrasound not performed for reasons documented by clinician (e.g., patient has a documented intrauterine pregnancy [IUP]) [A] [♀] [M]
G8808	Transabdominal or transvaginal ultrasound not performed, reason not given [A] [♀] [M]
G8815	Documented reason in the medical records for why the statin therapy was not prescribed (i.e., lower extremity bypass was for a patient with nonartherosclerotic disease) [M]
G8816	Statin medication prescribed at discharge [M]
G8817	Statin therapy not prescribed at discharge, reason not given [M]
G8818	~~Patient discharge to home no later than postoperative day #7~~
G8825	~~Patient not discharged to home by postoperative day #7~~
G8826	Patient discharged to home no later than postoperative day #2 following EVAR [M]
G8833	Patient not discharged to home by postoperative day #2 following EVAR [M]
G8834	Patient discharged to home no later than postoperative day #2 following CEA [M]
G8838	Patient not discharged to home by postoperative day #2 following CEA [M]
G8839	Sleep apnea symptoms assessed, including presence or absence of snoring and daytime sleepiness [M]
G8840	Documentation of reason(s) for not documenting an assessment of sleep symptoms (e.g., patient didn't have initial daytime sleepiness, patient visited between initial testing and initiation of therapy) [M]
G8841	Sleep apnea symptoms not assessed, reason not given [M]
G8842	Apnea hypopnea index (AHI), respiratory disturbance index (RDI) or respiratory event index (REI) documented or measured within 2 months of initial evaluation for suspected obstructive sleep apnea [M]
G8843	Documentation of reason(s) for not measuring an apnea hypopnea index (AHI), a respiratory disturbance index (RDI), or a respiratory event index (REI) within 2 months of initial evaluation for suspected obstructive sleep apnea (e.g., medical, neurological, or psychiatric disease that prohibits successful completion of a sleep study, patients for whom a sleep study would present a bigger risk than benefit or would pose an undue burden, dementia, patients who decline AHI/RDI/REI measurement, patients who had a financial reason for not completing testing, test was ordered but not completed, patients decline because their insurance (payer) does not cover the expense)) [M]
G8844	Apnea hypopnea index (AHI), respiratory disturbance index (RDI), or respiratory event index (REI) not documented or measured within 2 months of initial evaluation for suspected obstructive sleep apnea, reason not given [M]
G8845	Positive airway pressure therapy prescribed [M]
G8846	Moderate or severe obstructive sleep apnea (apnea hypopnea index (AHI) or respiratory disturbance index (RDI) of 15 or greater) [M] ☑
G8849	Documentation of reason(s) for not prescribing positive airway pressure therapy (e.g., patient unable to tolerate, alternative therapies use, patient declined, financial, insurance coverage) [M]
G8850	Positive airway pressure therapy not prescribed, reason not given [M]
▲ **G8851**	Adherence to therapy was assessed at least annually through an objective informatics system or through self-reporting (if objective reporting is not available, documented) [M]
G8852	~~Positive airway pressure therapy was prescribed~~
▲ **G8854**	Documentation of reason(s) for not objectively reporting adherence to evidence-based therapy (e.g., patients who have been diagnosed with a terminal or advanced disease with an expected life span of less than 6 months, patients who decline therapy, patients who do not return for follow-up at least annually, patients unable to access/afford therapy, patient's insurance will not cover therapy) [M]
▲ **G8855**	Adherence to therapy was not assessed at least annually through an objective informatics system or through self-reporting (if objective reporting is not available), reason not given [M]
G8856	Referral to a physician for an otologic evaluation performed [M]
G8857	Patient is not eligible for the referral for otologic evaluation measure (e.g., patients who are already under the care of a physician for acute or chronic dizziness) [M]

Special Coverage Instructions   Noncovered by Medicare   Carrier Discretion   ☑ Quantity Alert   ● New Code   ○ Recycled/Reinstated   ▲ Revised Code

© 2023 Optum360, LLC   A2-Z3 ASC Pmt   **CMS:** IOM   **AHA:** Coding Clinic   ⅙ DMEPOS Paid   ⊘ SNF Excluded   **G Codes — 71**

G8858 Referral to a physician for an otologic evaluation not performed, reason not given Ⓜ

G8863 Patients not assessed for risk of bone loss, reason not given Ⓜ

G8864 Pneumococcal vaccine administered or previously received Ⓜ

G8865 Documentation of medical reason(s) for not administering or previously receiving pneumococcal vaccine (e.g., patient allergic reaction, potential adverse drug reaction) Ⓜ

G8866 Documentation of patient reason(s) for not administering or previously receiving pneumococcal vaccine (e.g., patient refusal) Ⓜ

G8867 Pneumococcal vaccine not administered or previously received, reason not given Ⓜ

G8869 Patient has documented immunity to hepatitis B and initiating anti-TNF therapy Ⓜ

G8875 Clinician diagnosed breast cancer preoperatively by a minimally invasive biopsy method Ⓜ

G8876 Documentation of reason(s) for not performing minimally invasive biopsy to diagnose breast cancer preoperatively (e.g., lesion too close to skin, implant, chest wall, etc., lesion could not be adequately visualized for needle biopsy, patient condition prevents needle biopsy [weight, breast thickness, etc.], duct excision without imaging abnormality, prophylactic mastectomy, reduction mammoplasty, excisional biopsy performed by another physician) Ⓜ

G8877 Clinician did not attempt to achieve the diagnosis of breast cancer preoperatively by a minimally invasive biopsy method, reason not given Ⓜ

G8878 Sentinel lymph node biopsy procedure performed Ⓜ

G8880 Documentation of reason(s) sentinel lymph node biopsy not performed (e.g., reasons could include but not limited to: noninvasive cancer, incidental discovery of breast cancer on prophylactic mastectomy, incidental discovery of breast cancer on reduction mammoplasty, preoperative biopsy proven lymph node (LN) metastases, inflammatory carcinoma, Stage III locally advanced cancer, recurrent invasive breast cancer, clinically node positive after neoadjuvant systemic therapy, patient refusal after informed consent, patient with significant age, comorbidities, or limited life expectancy and favorable tumor; adjuvant systemic therapy unlikely to change) Ⓜ

G8881 Stage of breast cancer is greater than T1N0M0 or T2N0M0 Ⓜ

G8882 Sentinel lymph node biopsy procedure not performed, reason not given Ⓜ

G8883 ~~Biopsy results reviewed, communicated, tracked and documented~~

G8884 ~~Clinician documented reason that patient's biopsy results were not reviewed~~

G8885 ~~Biopsy results not reviewed, communicated, tracked or documented~~

G8907 Patient documented not to have experienced any of the following events: a burn prior to discharge; a fall within the facility; wrong site/side/patient/procedure/implant event; or a hospital transfer or hospital admission upon discharge from the facility Ⓜ

G8908 Patient documented to have received a burn prior to discharge Ⓜ

G8909 Patient documented not to have received a burn prior to discharge Ⓜ

G8910 Patient documented to have experienced a fall within ASC Ⓜ

G8911 Patient documented not to have experienced a fall within ASC Ⓜ

G8912 Patient documented to have experienced a wrong site, wrong side, wrong patient, wrong procedure or wrong implant event Ⓜ

G8913 Patient documented not to have experienced a wrong site, wrong side, wrong patient, wrong procedure or wrong implant event Ⓜ

G8914 Patient documented to have experienced a hospital transfer or hospital admission upon discharge from ASC Ⓜ

G8915 Patient documented not to have experienced a hospital transfer or hospital admission upon discharge from ASC Ⓜ

G8916 Patient with preoperative order for IV antibiotic surgical site infection (SSI) prophylaxis, antibiotic initiated on time Ⓜ

G8917 Patient with preoperative order for IV antibiotic surgical site infection (SSI) prophylaxis, antibiotic not initiated on time Ⓜ

G8918 Patient without preoperative order for IV antibiotic surgical site infection (SSI) prophylaxis Ⓜ

G8923 Left ventricular ejection fraction (LVEF) <= 40% or documentation of moderately or severely depressed left ventricular systolic function Ⓜ

▲ **G8924** Spirometry results documented (FEV1/FVC < 70%) Ⓜ

G8934 Left ventricular ejection fraction (LVEF) <=40% or documentation of moderately or severely depressed left ventricular systolic function Ⓜ

G8935 Clinician prescribed angiotensin converting enzyme (ACE) inhibitor or angiotensin receptor blocker (ARB) therapy Ⓜ

▲ **G8936** Clinician documented that patient was not an eligible candidate for angiotensin converting enzyme (ACE) inhibitor or angiotensin receptor blocker (ARB) therapy (e.g., allergy, intolerance, pregnancy, renal failure due to ACE inhibitor, diseases of the aortic or mitral valve, other medical reasons) or (e.g., patient declined, other patient reasons) Ⓜ

G8937 Clinician did not prescribe angiotensin converting enzyme (ACE) inhibitor or angiotensin receptor blocker (ARB) therapy, reason not given Ⓜ

G8941 ~~Elder maltreatment screen documented as positive, follow-up plan not documented, documentation the patient is not eligible for follow-up plan at the time of the encounter~~

▲ **G8942** Functional outcome assessment using a standardized tool is documented within the previous 30 days and a care plan, based on identified deficiencies is documented within 2 days of the functional outcome assessment Ⓜ

G8944 AJCC melanoma cancer stage 0 through IIC melanoma Ⓜ

G8946 Minimally invasive biopsy method attempted but not diagnostic of breast cancer (e.g., high risk lesion of breast such as atypical ductal hyperplasia, lobular neoplasia, atypical lobular hyperplasia, lobular carcinoma in situ, atypical columnar hyperplasia, flat epithelial atypia, radial scar, complex sclerosing lesion, papillary lesion, or any lesion with spindle cells) Ⓜ

G8950 Elevated or hypertensive blood pressure reading documented, and the indicated follow-up is documented Ⓜ

G8952 Elevated or hypertensive blood pressure reading documented, indicated follow-up not documented, reason not given Ⓜ

G8955 Most recent assessment of adequacy of volume management documented Ⓜ

G8956 Patient receiving maintenance hemodialysis in an outpatient dialysis facility Ⓜ

Special Coverage Instructions   Noncovered by Medicare   Carrier Discretion   ☑ Quantity Alert ● New Code   ○ Recycled/Reinstated ▲ Revised Code

72 — G Codes   Ⓐ Age Edit   Ⓜ Maternity Edit   ♀ Female Only   ♂ Male Only   Ⓐ-Ⓨ OPPS Status Indicators   © 2023 Optum360, LLC

G8958	Assessment of adequacy of volume management not documented, reason not given [M]
G8961	Cardiac stress imaging test primarily performed on low-risk surgery patient for preoperative evaluation within 30 days preceding this surgery [M]
G8962	Cardiac stress imaging test performed on patient for any reason including those who did not have low risk surgery or test that was performed more than 30 days preceding low risk surgery [M]
G8963	~~Cardiac stress imaging performed primarily for monitoring of asymptomatic patient who had PCI wihin 2 years~~
G8964	~~Cardiac stress imaging test performed primarily for any other reason than monitoring of asymptomatic patient who had PCI wthin 2 years (e.g., symptomatic patient, patient greater than 2 years since PCI, initial evaluation, etc.)~~
G8965	Cardiac stress imaging test primarily performed on low CHD risk patient for initial detection and risk assessment [M]
G8966	Cardiac stress imaging test performed on symptomatic or higher than low CHD risk patient or for any reason other than initial detection and risk assessment [M]
G8967	FDA-approved oral anticoagulant is prescribed [M]
▲ **G8968**	Documentation of medical reason(s) for not prescribing an FDA-approved anticoagulant (e.g., present or planned atrial appendage occlusion or ligation or patient being currently enrolled in a clinical trial related to AF/atrial flutter treatment) [M]
G8969	Documentation of patient reason(s) for not prescribing an oral anticoagulant that is FDA-approved for the prevention of thromboembolism (e.g., patient preference for not receiving anticoagulation) [M]
G8970	No risk factors or one moderate risk factor for thromboembolism [M]

Coordinated Care

G9001	Coordinated care fee, initial rate [B]
G9002	Coordinated care fee [B]
G9003	Coordinated care fee, risk adjusted high, initial [B]
G9004	Coordinated care fee, risk adjusted low, initial [B]
G9005	Coordinated care fee risk adjusted maintenance [B]
G9006	Coordinated care fee, home monitoring [B]
G9007	Coordinated care fee, scheduled team conference [B]
G9008	Coordinated care fee, physician coordinated care oversight services [B]
G9009	Coordinated care fee, risk adjusted maintenance, Level 3 [B]
G9010	Coordinated care fee, risk adjusted maintenance, Level 4 [B]
G9011	Coordinated care fee, risk adjusted maintenance, Level 5 [B]
G9012	Other specified case management service not elsewhere classified [B]

Demonstration Project

G9013	ESRD demo basic bundle Level I [EI]
G9014	ESRD demo expanded bundle including venous access and related services [EI]
G9016	Smoking cessation counseling, individual, in the absence of or in addition to any other evaluation and management service, per session (6-10 minutes) [demo project code only] [EI] [☑] **CMS:** 100-03,210.4.1

G9050	Oncology; primary focus of visit; work-up, evaluation, or staging at the time of cancer diagnosis or recurrence (for use in a Medicare-approved demonstration project) [EI]
G9051	Oncology; primary focus of visit; treatment decision-making after disease is staged or restaged, discussion of treatment options, supervising/coordinating active cancer-directed therapy or managing consequences of cancer-directed therapy (for use in a Medicare-approved demonstration project) [EI]
G9052	Oncology; primary focus of visit; surveillance for disease recurrence for patient who has completed definitive cancer-directed therapy and currently lacks evidence of recurrent disease; cancer-directed therapy might be considered in the future (for use in a Medicare-approved demonstration project) [EI]
G9053	Oncology; primary focus of visit; expectant management of patient with evidence of cancer for whom no cancer-directed therapy is being administered or arranged at present; cancer-directed therapy might be considered in the future (for use in a Medicare-approved demonstration project) [EI]
G9054	Oncology; primary focus of visit; supervising, coordinating or managing care of patient with terminal cancer or for whom other medical illness prevents further cancer treatment; includes symptom management, end-of-life care planning, management of palliative therapies (for use in a Medicare-approved demonstration project) [EI]
G9055	Oncology; primary focus of visit; other, unspecified service not otherwise listed (for use in a Medicare-approved demonstration project) [EI]
G9056	Oncology; practice guidelines; management adheres to guidelines (for use in a Medicare-approved demonstration project) [EI]
G9057	Oncology; practice guidelines; management differs from guidelines as a result of patient enrollment in an institutional review board-approved clinical trial (for use in a Medicare-approved demonstration project) [EI]
G9058	Oncology; practice guidelines; management differs from guidelines because the treating physician disagrees with guideline recommendations (for use in a Medicare-approved demonstration project) [EI]
G9059	Oncology; practice guidelines; management differs from guidelines because the patient, after being offered treatment consistent with guidelines, has opted for alternative treatment or management, including no treatment (for use in a Medicare-approved demonstration project) [EI]
G9060	Oncology; practice guidelines; management differs from guidelines for reason(s) associated with patient comorbid illness or performance status not factored into guidelines (for use in a Medicare-approved demonstration project) [EI]
G9061	Oncology; practice guidelines; patient's condition not addressed by available guidelines (for use in a Medicare-approved demonstration project) [EI]
G9062	Oncology; practice guidelines; management differs from guidelines for other reason(s) not listed (for use in a Medicare-approved demonstration project) [EI]
G9063	Oncology; disease status; limited to nonsmall cell lung cancer; extent of disease initially established as Stage I (prior to neoadjuvant therapy, if any) with no evidence of disease progression, recurrence, or metastases (for use in a Medicare-approved demonstration project) [M]

Special Coverage Instructions — Noncovered by Medicare — Carrier Discretion — ☑ Quantity Alert — ● New Code — ○ Recycled/Reinstated — ▲ Revised Code

© 2023 Optum360, LLC — A2–Z3 ASC Pmt — **CMS:** IOM — **AHA:** Coding Clinic — ⅙ DMEPOS Paid — ⊘ SNF Excluded — G Codes — 73

Procedures/Professional Services (Temporary)

G9064 — G9091

G9064 Oncology; disease status; limited to nonsmall cell lung cancer; extent of disease initially established as Stage II (prior to neoadjuvant therapy, if any) with no evidence of disease progression, recurrence, or metastases (for use in a Medicare-approved demonstration project) Ⓜ

G9065 Oncology; disease status; limited to nonsmall cell lung cancer; extent of disease initially established as Stage III a (prior to neoadjuvant therapy, if any) with no evidence of disease progression, recurrence, or metastases (for use in a Medicare-approved demonstration project) Ⓜ

G9066 Oncology; disease status; limited to nonsmall cell lung cancer; Stage III B-IV at diagnosis, metastatic, locally recurrent, or progressive (for use in a Medicare-approved demonstration project) Ⓜ

G9067 Oncology; disease status; limited to nonsmall cell lung cancer; extent of disease unknown, staging in progress, or not listed (for use in a Medicare-approved demonstration project) Ⓜ

G9068 Oncology; disease status; limited to small cell and combined small cell/nonsmall cell; extent of disease initially established as limited with no evidence of disease progression, recurrence, or metastases (for use in a Medicare-approved demonstration project) Ⓜ

G9069 Oncology; disease status; small cell lung cancer, limited to small cell and combined small cell/nonsmall cell; extensive Stage at diagnosis, metastatic, locally recurrent, or progressive (for use in a Medicare-approved demonstration project) Ⓜ

G9070 Oncology; disease status; small cell lung cancer, limited to small cell and combined small cell/nonsmall; extent of disease unknown, staging in progress, or not listed (for use in a Medicare-approved demonstration project) Ⓜ

G9071 Oncology; disease status; invasive female breast cancer (does not include ductal carcinoma in situ); adenocarcinoma as predominant cell type; Stage I or Stage IIA-IIB; or T3, N1, M0; and ER and/or PR positive; with no evidence of disease progression, recurrence, or metastases (for use in a Medicare-approved demonstration project) ♀ Ⓜ

G9072 Oncology; disease status; invasive female breast cancer (does not include ductal carcinoma in situ); adenocarcinoma as predominant cell type; Stage I, or Stage IIA-IIB; or T3, N1, M0; and ER and PR negative; with no evidence of disease progression, recurrence, or metastases (for use in a Medicare-approved demonstration project) ♀ Ⓜ

G9073 Oncology; disease status; invasive female breast cancer (does not include ductal carcinoma in situ); adenocarcinoma as predominant cell type; Stage IIIA-IIIB; and not T3, N1, M0; and ER and/or PR positive; with no evidence of disease progression, recurrence, or metastases (for use in a Medicare-approved demonstration project) ♀ Ⓜ

G9074 Oncology; disease status; invasive female breast cancer (does not include ductal carcinoma in situ); adenocarcinoma as predominant cell type; Stage IIIA-IIIB; and not T3, N1, M0; and ER and PR negative; with no evidence of disease progression, recurrence, or metastases (for use in a Medicare-approved demonstration project) ♀ Ⓜ

G9075 Oncology; disease status; invasive female breast cancer (does not include ductal carcinoma in situ); adenocarcinoma as predominant cell type; M1 at diagnosis, metastatic, locally recurrent, or progressive (for use in a Medicare-approved demonstration project) ♀ Ⓜ

G9077 Oncology; disease status; prostate cancer, limited to adenocarcinoma as predominant cell type; T1-T2c and Gleason 2-7 and PSA < or equal to 20 at diagnosis with no evidence of disease progression, recurrence, or metastases (for use in a Medicare-approved demonstration project) ♂ Ⓜ

G9078 Oncology; disease status; prostate cancer, limited to adenocarcinoma as predominant cell type; T2 or T3a Gleason 8-10 or PSA > 20 at diagnosis with no evidence of disease progression, recurrence, or metastases (for use in a Medicare-approved demonstration project) ♂ Ⓜ

G9079 Oncology; disease status; prostate cancer, limited to adenocarcinoma as predominant cell type; T3b-T4, any N; any T, N1 at diagnosis with no evidence of disease progression, recurrence, or metastases (for use in a Medicare-approved demonstration project) ♂ Ⓜ

G9080 Oncology; disease status; prostate cancer, limited to adenocarcinoma; after initial treatment with rising PSA or failure of PSA decline (for use in a Medicare-approved demonstration project) ♂ Ⓜ

G9083 Oncology; disease status; prostate cancer, limited to adenocarcinoma; extent of disease unknown, staging in progress, or not listed (for use in a Medicare-approved demonstration project) ♂ Ⓜ

G9084 Oncology; disease status; colon cancer, limited to invasive cancer, adenocarcinoma as predominant cell type; extent of disease initially established as T1-3, N0, M0 with no evidence of disease progression, recurrence or metastases (for use in a Medicare-approved demonstration project) Ⓜ

G9085 Oncology; disease status; colon cancer, limited to invasive cancer, adenocarcinoma as predominant cell type; extent of disease initially established as T4, N0, M0 with no evidence of disease progression, recurrence, or metastases (for use in a Medicare-approved demonstration project) Ⓜ

G9086 Oncology; disease status; colon cancer, limited to invasive cancer, adenocarcinoma as predominant cell type; extent of disease initially established as T1-4, N1-2, M0 with no evidence of disease progression, recurrence, or metastases (for use in a Medicare-approved demonstration project) Ⓜ

G9087 Oncology; disease status; colon cancer, limited to invasive cancer, adenocarcinoma as predominant cell type; M1 at diagnosis, metastatic, locally recurrent, or progressive with current clinical, radiologic, or biochemical evidence of disease (for use in a Medicare-approved demonstration project) Ⓜ

G9088 Oncology; disease status; colon cancer, limited to invasive cancer, adenocarcinoma as predominant cell type; M1 at diagnosis, metastatic, locally recurrent, or progressive without current clinical, radiologic, or biochemical evidence of disease (for use in a Medicare-approved demonstration project) Ⓜ

G9089 Oncology; disease status; colon cancer, limited to invasive cancer, adenocarcinoma as predominant cell type; extent of disease unknown, staging in progress or not listed (for use in a Medicare-approved demonstration project) Ⓜ

G9090 Oncology; disease status; rectal cancer, limited to invasive cancer, adenocarcinoma as predominant cell type; extent of disease initially established as T1-2, N0, M0 (prior to neoadjuvant therapy, if any) with no evidence of disease progression, recurrence, or metastases (for use in a Medicare-approved demonstration project) Ⓜ

G9091 Oncology; disease status; rectal cancer, limited to invasive cancer, adenocarcinoma as predominant cell type; extent of disease initially established as T3, N0, M0 (prior to neoadjuvant therapy, if any) with no evidence of disease progression, recurrence, or metastases (for use in a Medicare-approved demonstration project) Ⓜ

Special Coverage Instructions   Noncovered by Medicare   Carrier Discretion   ☑ Quantity Alert   ● New Code   ○ Recycled/Reinstated   ▲ Revised Code

74 — G Codes   Ⓐ Age Edit   Ⓜ Maternity Edit   ♀ Female Only   ♂ Male Only   Ⓐ-Ⓨ OPPS Status Indicators   © 2023 Optum360, LLC

G9092 Oncology; disease status; rectal cancer, limited to invasive cancer, adenocarcinoma as predominant cell type; extent of disease initially established as T1-3, N1-2, M0 (prior to neoadjuvant therapy, if any) with no evidence of disease progression, recurrence or metastases (for use in a Medicare-approved demonstration project) Ⓜ

G9093 Oncology; disease status; rectal cancer, limited to invasive cancer, adenocarcinoma as predominant cell type; extent of disease initially established as T4, any N, M0 (prior to neoadjuvant therapy, if any) with no evidence of disease progression, recurrence, or metastases (for use in a Medicare-approved demonstration project) Ⓜ

G9094 Oncology; disease status; rectal cancer, limited to invasive cancer, adenocarcinoma as predominant cell type; M1 at diagnosis, metastatic, locally recurrent, or progressive (for use in a Medicare-approved demonstration project) Ⓜ

G9095 Oncology; disease status; rectal cancer, limited to invasive cancer, adenocarcinoma as predominant cell type; extent of disease unknown, staging in progress or not listed (for use in a Medicare-approved demonstration project) Ⓜ

G9096 Oncology; disease status; esophageal cancer, limited to adenocarcinoma or squamous cell carcinoma as predominant cell type; extent of disease initially established as T1-T3, N0-N1 or NX (prior to neoadjuvant therapy, if any) with no evidence of disease progression, recurrence, or metastases (for use In a Medicare-approved demonstration project) Ⓜ

G9097 Oncology; disease status; esophageal cancer, limited to adenocarcinoma or squamous cell carcinoma as predominant cell type; extent of disease initially established as T4, any N, M0 (prior to neoadjuvant therapy, if any) with no evidence of disease progression, recurrence, or metastases (for use in a Medicare-approved demonstration project) Ⓜ

G9098 Oncology; disease status; esophageal cancer, limited to adenocarcinoma or squamous cell carcinoma as predominant cell type; M1 at diagnosis, metastatic, locally recurrent, or progressive (for use in a Medicare-approved demonstration project) Ⓜ

G9099 Oncology; disease status; esophageal cancer, limited to adenocarcinoma or squamous cell carcinoma as predominant cell type; extent of disease unknown, staging in progress, or not listed (for use in a Medicare-approved demonstration project) Ⓜ

G9100 Oncology; disease status; gastric cancer, limited to adenocarcinoma as predominant cell type; post R0 resection (with or without neoadjuvant therapy) with no evidence of disease recurrence, progression, or metastases (for use in a Medicare-approved demonstration project) Ⓜ

G9101 Oncology; disease status; gastric cancer, limited to adenocarcinoma as predominant cell type; post R1 or R2 resection (with or without neoadjuvant therapy) with no evidence of disease progression, or metastases (for use in a Medicare-approved demonstration project) Ⓜ

G9102 Oncology; disease status; gastric cancer, limited to adenocarcinoma as predominant cell type; clinical or pathologic M0, unresectable with no evidence of disease progression, or metastases (for use In a Medicare-approved demonstration project) Ⓜ

G9103 Oncology; disease status; gastric cancer, limited to adenocarcinoma as predominant cell type; clinical or pathologic M1 at diagnosis, metastatic, locally recurrent, or progressive (for use in a Medicare-approved demonstration project) Ⓜ

G9104 Oncology; disease status; gastric cancer, limited to adenocarcinoma as predominant cell type; extent of disease unknown, staging in progress, or not listed (for use in a Medicare-approved demonstration project) Ⓜ

G9105 Oncology; disease status; pancreatic cancer, limited to adenocarcinoma as predominant cell type; post R0 resection without evidence of disease progression, recurrence, or metastases (for use in a Medicare-approved demonstration project) Ⓜ

G9106 Oncology; disease status; pancreatic cancer, limited to adenocarcinoma; post R1 or R2 resection with no evidence of disease progression, or metastases (for use in a Medicare-approved demonstration project) Ⓜ

G9107 Oncology; disease status; pancreatic cancer, limited to adenocarcinoma; unresectable at diagnosis, M1 at diagnosis, metastatic, locally recurrent, or progressive (for use in a Medicare-approved demonstration project) Ⓜ

G9108 Oncology; disease status; pancreatic cancer, limited to adenocarcinoma; extent of disease unknown, staging in progress, or not listed (for use in a Medicare-approved demonstration project) Ⓜ

G9109 Oncology; disease status; head and neck cancer, limited to cancers of oral cavity, pharynx and larynx with squamous cell as predominant cell type; extent of disease initially established as T1-T2 and N0, M0 (prior to neoadjuvant therapy, if any) with no evidence of disease progression, recurrence, or metastases (for use in a Medicare-approved demonstration project) Ⓜ

G9110 Oncology; disease status; head and neck cancer, limited to cancers of oral cavity, pharynx and larynx with squamous cell as predominant cell type; extent of disease Initially established as T3-4 and/or N1-3, M0 (prior to neoadjuvant therapy, if any) with no evidence of disease progression, recurrence, or metastases (for use in a Medicare-approved demonstration project) Ⓜ

G9111 Oncology; disease status; head and neck cancer, limited to cancers of oral cavity, pharynx and larynx with squamous cell as predominant cell type; M1 at diagnosis, metastatic, locally recurrent, or progressive (for use in a Medicare-approved demonstration project) Ⓜ

G9112 Oncology; disease status; head and neck cancer, limited to cancers of oral cavity, pharynx and larynx with squamous cell as predominant cell type; extent of disease unknown, staging in progress, or not listed (for use in a Medicare-approved demonstration project) Ⓜ

G9113 Oncology; disease status; ovarian cancer, limited to epithelial cancer; pathologic Stage IA-B (Grade 1) without evidence of disease progression, recurrence, or metastases (for use in a Medicare-approved demonstration project) ♀ Ⓜ

G9114 Oncology; disease status; ovarian cancer, limited to epithelial cancer; pathologic Stage IA-B (Grade 2-3); or Stage IC (all grades); or Stage II; without evidence of disease progression, recurrence, or metastases (for use in a Medicare-approved demonstration project) ♀ Ⓜ

G9115 Oncology; disease status; ovarian cancer, limited to epithelial cancer; pathologic Stage III-IV; without evidence of progression, recurrence, or metastases (for use in a Medicare-approved demonstration project) ♀ Ⓜ

G9116 Oncology; disease status; ovarian cancer, limited to epithelial cancer; evidence of disease progression, or recurrence, and/or platinum resistance (for use in a Medicare-approved demonstration project) ♀ Ⓜ

Special Coverage Instructions   Noncovered by Medicare   Carrier Discretion   ☑ Quantity Alert   ● New Code   ○ Recycled/Reinstated   ▲ Revised Code

© 2023 Optum360, LLC   A2-Z3 ASC Pmt   **CMS:** IOM   **AHA:** Coding Clinic   ♿ DMEPOS Paid   ○ SNF Excluded   **G Codes — 75**

G9117 Oncology; disease status; ovarian cancer, limited to epithelial cancer; extent of disease unknown, staging in progress, or not listed (for use in a Medicare-approved demonstration project) ♀ Ⓜ

G9123 Oncology; disease status; chronic myelogenous leukemia, limited to Philadelphia chromosome positive and/or BCR-ABL positive; chronic phase not in hematologic, cytogenetic, or molecular remission (for use in a Medicare-approved demonstration project) Ⓜ

G9124 Oncology; disease status; chronic myelogenous leukemia, limited to Philadelphia chromosome positive and /or BCR-ABL positive; accelerated phase not in hematologic cytogenetic, or molecular remission (for use in a Medicare-approved demonstration project) Ⓜ

G9125 Oncology; disease status; chronic myelogenous leukemia, limited to Philadelphia chromosome positive and/or BCR-ABL positive; blast phase not in hematologic, cytogenetic, or molecular remission (for use in a Medicare-approved demonstration project) Ⓜ

G9126 Oncology; disease status; chronic myelogenous leukemia, limited to Philadelphia chromosome positive and/or BCR-ABL positive; in hematologic, cytogenetic, or molecular remission (for use in a Medicare-approved demonstration project) Ⓜ

G9128 Oncology; disease status; limited to multiple myeloma, systemic disease; smoldering, Stage I (for use in a Medicare-approved demonstration project) Ⓜ

G9129 Oncology; disease status; limited to multiple myeloma, systemic disease; Stage II or higher (for use in a Medicare-approved demonstration project) Ⓜ

G9130 Oncology; disease status; limited to multiple myeloma, systemic disease; extent of disease unknown, staging in progress, or not listed (for use in a Medicare-approved demonstration project) Ⓜ

G9131 Oncology; disease status; invasive female breast cancer (does not include ductal carcinoma in situ); adenocarcinoma as predominant cell type; extent of disease unknown, staging in progress, or not listed (for use in a Medicare-approved demonstration project) ♀ Ⓜ

G9132 Oncology; disease status; prostate cancer, limited to adenocarcinoma; hormone-refractory/androgen-independent (e.g., rising PSA on antiandrogen therapy or postorchiectomy); clinical metastases (for use in a Medicare-approved demonstration project) ♂ Ⓜ

G9133 Oncology; disease status; prostate cancer, limited to adenocarcinoma; hormone-responsive; clinical metastases or M1 at diagnosis (for use in a Medicare-approved demonstration project) ♂ Ⓜ

G9134 Oncology; disease status; non-Hodgkin's lymphoma, any cellular classification; Stage I, II at diagnosis, not relapsed, not refractory (for use in a Medicare-approved demonstration project) Ⓜ

G9135 Oncology; disease status; non-Hodgkin's lymphoma, any cellular classification; Stage III, IV, not relapsed, not refractory (for use in a Medicare-approved demonstration project) Ⓜ

G9136 Oncology; disease status; non-Hodgkin's lymphoma, transformed from original cellular diagnosis to a second cellular classification (for use in a Medicare-approved demonstration project) Ⓜ

G9137 Oncology; disease status; non-Hodgkin's lymphoma, any cellular classification; relapsed/refractory (for use in a Medicare-approved demonstration project) Ⓜ

G9138 Oncology; disease status; non-Hodgkin's lymphoma, any cellular classification; diagnostic evaluation, stage not determined, evaluation of possible relapse or nonresponse to therapy, or not listed (for use in a Medicare-approved demonstration project) Ⓜ

G9139 Oncology; disease status; chronic myelogenous leukemia, limited to Philadelphia chromosome positive and/or BCR-ABL positive; extent of disease unknown, staging in progress, not listed (for use in a Medicare-approved demonstration project) Ⓜ

G9140 Frontier Extended Stay Clinic demonstration; for a patient stay in a clinic approved for the CMS demonstration project; the following measures should be present: the stay must be equal to or greater than 4 hours; weather or other conditions must prevent transfer or the case falls into a category of monitoring and observation cases that are permitted by the rules of the demonstration; there is a maximum Frontier Extended Stay Clinic (FESC) visit of 48 hours, except in the case when weather or other conditions prevent transfer; payment is made on each period up to 4 hours, after the first 4 hours Ⓐ ☑

Warfarin Testing

G9143 Warfarin responsiveness testing by genetic technique using any method, any number of specimen(s) Ⓝ
CMS: 100-03,90.1; 100-04,32,250.1; 100-04,32,250.2; 100-04,32,250.3

Outpatient IV Insulin TX

G9147 Outpatient Intravenous Insulin Treatment (OIVIT) either pulsatile or continuous, by any means, guided by the results of measurements for: respiratory quotient; and/or, urine urea nitrogen (UUN); and/or, arterial, venous or capillary glucose; and/or potassium concentration Ⓔ
CMS: 100-03,40.7; 100-04,4,320.1; 100-04,4,320.2

Quality Assurance

G9148 National Committee for Quality Assurance-Level 1 Medical Home Ⓜ

G9149 National Committee for Quality Assurance-Level 2 Medical Home Ⓜ

G9150 National Committee for Quality Assurance-Level 3 Medical Home Ⓜ

G9151 MAPCP Demonstration-state provided services Ⓜ

G9152 MAPCP Demonstration-Community Health Teams Ⓜ

G9153 MAPCP Demonstration-Physician Incentive Pool Ⓜ

Wheelchair Evaluation

G9156 Evaluation for wheelchair requiring face-to-face visit with physician Ⓜ

Monitor

G9157 Transesophageal Doppler used for cardiac monitoring Ⓑ
CMS: 100-04,32,310; 100-04,32,310.2; 100-04,32,310.3

BPCI Services

G9187 Bundled payments for care improvement initiative home visit for patient assessment performed by a qualified health care professional for individuals not considered homebound including, but not limited to, assessment of safety, falls, clinical status, fluid status, medication reconciliation/management, patient compliance with orders/plan of care, performance of activities of daily living, appropriateness of care setting; (for use only in the Medicare-approved bundled payments for care improvement initiative); may not be billed for a 30-day period covered by a transitional care management code Ⓔ

Miscellaneous Quality Measures

G9188 Beta-blocker therapy not prescribed, reason not given Ⓜ

Special Coverage Instructions   Noncovered by Medicare   Carrier Discretion   ☑ Quantity Alert ● New Code   ○ Recycled/Reinstated   ▲ Revised Code

76 — G Codes   Ⓐ Age Edit   Ⓜ Maternity Edit   ♀ Female Only   ♂ Male Only   Ⓐ-Ⓨ OPPS Status Indicators   © 2023 Optum360, LLC

G9189 Beta-blocker therapy prescribed or currently being taken ☒

G9190 Documentation of medical reason(s) for not prescribing beta-blocker therapy (e.g., allergy, intolerance, other medical reasons) ☒

G9191 Documentation of patient reason(s) for not prescribing beta-blocker therapy (e.g., patient declined, other patient reasons) ☒

G9192 ~~Documentation of system reason(s) for not prescribing beta-blocker therapy (e.g., other reasons attributable to the health care system)~~

G9212 DSM-IVTM criteria for major depressive disorder documented at the initial evaluation ☒

G9213 DSM-IV-TR criteria for major depressive disorder not documented at the initial evaluation, reason not otherwise specified ☒

G9223 Pneumocystis jiroveci pneumonia prophylaxis prescribed within 3 months of low CD4+ cell count below 500 cells/mm3 or a CD4 percentage below 15% ☒

G9225 Foot exam was not performed, reason not given ☒

G9226 Foot examination performed (includes examination through visual inspection, sensory exam with 10-g monofilament plus testing any one of the following: vibration using 128-Hz tuning fork, pinprick sensation, ankle reflexes, or vibration perception threshold, and pulse exam; report when all of the three components are completed) ☒

G9227 Functional outcome assessment documented, care plan not documented, documentation the patient is not eligible for a care plan at the time of the encounter ☒

G9228 Chlamydia, gonorrhea and syphilis screening results documented (report when results are present for all of the three screenings) ☒

G9229 ~~Chlamydia, gonorrhea, and syphilis screening results not documented (patient refusal is the only allowed exception)~~

G9230 Chlamydia, gonorrhea, and syphilis not screened, reason not given ☒

G9231 Documentation of end stage renal disease (ESRD), dialysis, renal transplant before or during the measurement period or pregnancy during the measurement period ☒

G9242 Documentation of viral load equal to or greater than 200 copies/ml or viral load not performed ☒

G9243 Documentation of viral load less than 200 copies/ml ☒

G9246 Patient did not have at least one medical visit in each 6 month period of the 24 month measurement period, with a minimum of 60 days between medical visits ☒

G9247 Patient had at least one medical visit in each 6 month period of the 24 month measurement period, with a minimum of 60 days between medical visits ☒

G9254 Documentation of patient discharged to home later than post-operative day 2 following CAS ☒

G9255 Documentation of patient discharged to home no later than post operative day 2 following CAS ☒

G9273 Blood pressure has a systolic value of < 140 and a diastolic value of < 90 ☒

G9274 Blood pressure has a systolic value of = 140 and a diastolic value of = 90 or systolic value < 140 and diastolic value = 90 or systolic value = 140 and diastolic value < 90 ☒

G9275 Documentation that patient is a current nontobacco user ☒

G9276 Documentation that patient is a current tobacco user ☒

G9277 Documentation that the patient is on daily aspirin or antiplatelet or has documentation of a valid contraindication or exception to aspirin/antiplatelet; contraindications/exceptions include anticoagulant use, allergy to aspirin or antiplatelets, history of gastrointestinal bleed and bleeding disorder. Additionally, the following exceptions documented by the physician as a reason for not taking daily aspirin or antiplatelet are acceptable (use of nonsteroidal anti-inflammatory agents, documented risk for drug interaction, uncontrolled hypertension defined as > 180 systolic or > 110 diastolic or gastroesophageal reflux) ☒

G9278 Documentation that the patient is not on daily aspirin or antiplatelet regimen ☒

G9279 Pneumococcal screening performed and documentation of vaccination received prior to discharge ☒

G9280 Pneumococcal vaccination not administered prior to discharge, reason not specified ☒

G9281 Screening performed and documentation that vaccination not indicated/patient refusal ☒

G9282 Documentation of medical reason(s) for not reporting the histological type or NSCLC-NOS classification with an explanation (e.g., biopsy taken for other purposes in a patient with a history of nonsmall cell lung cancer or other documented medical reasons) ☒

G9283 Nonsmall cell lung cancer biopsy and cytology specimen report documents classification into specific histologic type or classified as NSCLC-NOS with an explanation ☒

G9284 Nonsmall cell lung cancer biopsy and cytology specimen report does not document classification into specific histologic type or classified as NSCLC-NOS with an explanation ☒

G9285 Specimen site other than anatomic location of lung or is not classified as nonsmall cell lung cancer ☒

G9286 Antibiotic regimen prescribed within 10 days after onset of symptoms ☒

G9287 Antibiotic regimen not prescribed within 10 days after onset of symptoms ☒

G9288 Documentation of medical reason(s) for not reporting the histological type or NSCLC-NOS classification with an explanation (e.g., a solitary fibrous tumor in a person with a history of nonsmall cell carcinoma or other documented medical reasons) ☒

G9289 Nonsmall cell lung cancer biopsy and cytology specimen report documents classification into specific histologic type or classified as NSCLC-NOS with an explanation ☒

G9290 Nonsmall cell lung cancer biopsy and cytology specimen report does not document classification into specific histologic type or classified as NSCLC-NOS with an explanation ☒

G9291 Specimen site other than anatomic location of lung, is not classified as nonsmall cell lung cancer or classified as NSCLC-NOS ☒

G9292 Documentation of medical reason(s) for not reporting PT category and a statement on thickness and ulceration and for PT1, mitotic rate (e.g., negative skin biopsies in a patient with a history of melanoma or other documented medical reasons) ☒

G9293 Pathology report does not include the PT category and a statement on thickness and ulceration and for PT1, mitotic rate ☒

G9294 Pathology report includes the PT category and a statement on thickness and ulceration and for PT1, mitotic rate ☒

G9295 Specimen site other than anatomic cutaneous location ☒

Special Coverage Instructions   Noncovered by Medicare   Carrier Discretion   ☑ Quantity Alert ● New Code   ○ Recycled/Reinstated   ▲ Revised Code

© 2023 Optum360, LLC   A2–Z3 ASC Pmt   **CMS:** IOM   **AHA:** Coding Clinic   ⚕ DMEPOS Paid   ⊘ SNF Excluded   **G Codes — 77**

Procedures/Professional Services (Temporary)

G9296 — G9368

G9296 Patients with documented shared decision-making including discussion of conservative (nonsurgical) therapy (e.g., NSAIDs, analgesics, weight loss, exercise, injections) prior to the procedure M

G9297 Shared decision-making including discussion of conservative (nonsurgical) therapy (e.g., NSAIDs, analgesics, weight loss, exercise, injections) prior to the procedure, not documented, reason not given M

G9298 Patients who are evaluated for venous thromboembolic and cardiovascular risk factors within 30 days prior to the procedure (e.g., history of DVT, PE, MI, arrhythmia and stroke) M

G9299 Patients who are not evaluated for venous thromboembolic and cardiovascular risk factors within 30 days prior to the procedure (e.g., history of DVT, PE, MI, arrhythmia and stroke, reason not given) M

G9305 Intervention for presence of leak of endoluminal contents through an anastomosis not required M

G9306 Intervention for presence of leak of endoluminal contents through an anastomosis required M

G9307 No return to the operating room for a surgical procedure, for complications of the principal operative procedure, within 30 days of the principal operative procedure M

G9308 Unplanned return to the operating room for a surgical procedure, for complications of the principal operative procedure, within 30 days of the principal operative procedure M

G9309 No unplanned hospital readmission within 30 days of principal procedure M

G9310 Unplanned hospital readmission within 30 days of principal procedure M

G9311 No surgical site infection M

G9312 Surgical site infection M

G9313 Amoxicillin, with or without clavulanate, not prescribed as first line antibiotic at the time of diagnosis for documented reason M

G9314 Amoxicillin, with or without clavulanate, not prescribed as first line antibiotic at the time of diagnosis, reason not given M

G9315 Amoxicillin, with or without clavulanate, prescribed as a first line antibiotic at the time of diagnosis M

G9316 Documentation of patient-specific risk assessment with a risk calculator based on multi-institutional clinical data, the specific risk calculator used, and communication of risk assessment from risk calculator with the patient or family M

G9317 Documentation of patient-specific risk assessment with a risk calculator based on multi-institutional clinical data, the specific risk calculator used, and communication of risk assessment from risk calculator with the patient or family not completed M

G9318 Imaging study named according to standardized nomenclature M

G9319 Imaging study not named according to standardized nomenclature, reason not given M

G9321 Count of previous CT (any type of CT) and cardiac nuclear medicine (myocardial perfusion) studies documented in the 12-month period prior to the current study M

G9322 Count of previous CT and cardiac nuclear medicine (myocardial perfusion) studies not documented in the 12-month period prior to the current study, reason not given M

G9341 Search conducted for prior patient CT studies completed at nonaffiliated external health care facilities or entities within the past 12-months and are available through a secure, authorized, media-free, shared archive prior to an imaging study being performed M

G9342 Search not conducted prior to an imaging study being performed for prior patient CT studies completed at nonaffiliated external health care facilities or entities within the past 12 months and are available through a secure, authorized, media-free, shared archive, reason not given M

G9344 Due to system reasons search not conducted for DICOM format images for prior patient CT imaging studies completed at nonaffiliated external health care facilities or entities within the past 12 months that are available through a secure, authorized, media-free, shared archive (e.g., nonaffiliated external health care facilities or entities does not have archival abilities through a shared archival system) M

G9345 Follow-up recommendations documented according to recommended guidelines for incidentally detected pulmonary nodules (e.g., follow-up CT imaging studies needed or that no follow-up is needed) based at a minimum on nodule size and patient risk factors M

G9347 Follow-up recommendations not documented according to recommended guidelines for incidentally detected pulmonary nodules, reason not given M

G9351 More than one CT scan of the paranasal sinuses ordered or received within 90 days after diagnosis M

G9352 More than one CT scan of the paranasal sinuses ordered or received within 90 days after the date of diagnosis, reason not given M

G9353 More than one CT scan of the paranasal sinuses ordered or received within 90 days after the date of diagnosis for documented reasons (e.g., patients with complications, second CT obtained prior to surgery, other medical reasons) M

G9354 One CT scan or no CT scan of the paranasal sinuses ordered within 90 days after the date of diagnosis M

G9355 Elective delivery (without medical indication) by Cesarean birth or induction of labor not performed (<39 weeks of gestation) M

G9356 Elective delivery (without medical indication) by Cesarean birth or induction of labor performed (<39 weeks of gestation) M

G9357 Post-partum screenings, evaluations and education performed M

G9358 Post-partum screenings, evaluations and education not performed M

G9361 Medical indication for delivery by Cesarean birth or induction of labor (<39 weeks of gestation) [documentation of reason(s) for elective delivery (e.g., hemorrhage and placental complications, hypertension, preeclampsia and eclampsia, rupture of membranes (premature or prolonged), maternal conditions complicating pregnancy/delivery, fetal conditions complicating pregnancy/delivery, late pregnancy, prior uterine surgery, or participation in clinical trial)] M

G9364 Sinusitis caused by, or presumed to be caused by, bacterial infection M

G9367 At least two orders for high risk medications from the same drug class M

G9368 At least two orders for high risk medications from the same drug class not ordered M

Special Coverage Instructions   Noncovered by Medicare   Carrier Discretion   ☑ Quantity Alert ● New Code ○ Recycled/Reinstated ▲ Revised Code

78 — G Codes   A Age Edit   M Maternity Edit   ♀ Female Only   ♂ Male Only   A-Y OPPS Status Indicators   © 2023 Optum360, LLC

▲ **G9380** Patient offered assistance with end of life issues or existing end of life plan was reviewed or updated during the measurement period ⓜ

▲ **G9382** Patient not offered assistance with end of life issues or existing end of life plan was not reviewed or updated during the measurement period ⓜ

G9383 Patient received screening for HCV infection within the 12 month reporting period ⓜ

G9384 Documentation of medical reason(s) for not receiving annual screening for HCV infection (e.g., decompensated cirrhosis indicating advanced disease [i.e., ascites, esophageal variceal bleeding, hepatic encephalopathy], hepatocellular carcinoma, waitlist for organ transplant, limited life expectancy, other medical reasons) ⓜ

G9385 Documentation of patient reason(s) for not receiving annual screening for HCV infection (e.g., patient declined, other patient reasons) ⓜ

G9386 Screening for HCV infection not received within the twelve-month reporting period, reason not given ⓜ

G9393 Patient with an initial PHQ-9 score greater than nine who achieves remission at twelve months as demonstrated by a twelve-month (+/- 30 days) PHQ-9 score of less than five ⓜ

G9394 Patient who had a diagnosis of bipolar disorder or personality disorder, death, permanent nursing home resident or receiving hospice or palliative care any time during the measurement or assessment period ⓜ

G9395 Patient with an initial PHQ-9 score greater than nine who did not achieve remission at twelve months as demonstrated by a twelve-month (+/- 30 days) PHQ-9 score greater than or equal to five ⓜ

G9396 Patient with an initial PHQ-9 score greater than nine who was not assessed for remission at twelve months (+/- 30 days) ⓜ

G9402 Patient received follow-up within 30 days after discharge ⓜ

G9403 Clinician documented reason patient was not able to complete 30-day follow-up from acute inpatient setting discharge (e.g., patient death prior to follow-up visit, patient noncompliant for visit follow-up) ⓜ

G9404 Patient did not receive follow-up within 30 days after discharge ⓜ

G9405 Patient received follow up within 7 days after discharge ⓜ

G9406 Clinician documented reason patient was not able to complete 7-day follow-up from acute inpatient setting discharge (i.e., patient death prior to follow-up visit, patient noncompliance for visit follow-up) ⓜ

G9407 Patient did not receive follow-up within 7 days after discharge ⓜ

G9408 Patients with cardiac tamponade and/or pericardiocentesis occurring within 30 days ⓜ

G9409 Patients without cardiac tamponade and/or pericardiocentesis occurring within 30 days ⓜ

G9410 Patient admitted within 180 days, status post CIED implantation, replacement, or revision with an infection requiring device removal or surgical revision ⓜ

G9411 Patient not admitted within 180 days, status post CIED implantation, replacement, or revision with an infection requiring device removal or surgical revision ⓜ

G9412 Patient admitted within 180 days, status post CIED implantation, replacement, or revision with an infection requiring device removal or surgical revision ⓜ

G9413 Patient not admitted within 180 days, status post CIED implantation, replacement, or revision with an infection requiring device removal or surgical revision ⓜ

G9414 Patient had one dose of meningococcal vaccine (serogroups A, C, W, Y) on or between the patient's 11th and 13th birthdays ⓜ

G9415 Patient did not have one dose of meningococcal vaccine (serogroups A, C, W, Y) on or between the patient's 11th and 13th birthdays ⓜ

G9416 Patient had one tetanus, diphtheria toxoids and acellular pertussis vaccine (TDaP) on or between the patient's 10th and 13th birthdays ⓜ

G9417 Patient did not have one tetanus, diphtheria toxoids and acellular pertussis vaccine (TDaP) on or between the patient's 10th and 13th birthdays ⓜ

G9418 Primary nonsmall cell lung cancer lung biopsy and cytology specimen report documents classification into specific histologic type following IASLC guidance or classified as NSCLC-NOS with an explanation ⓜ

G9419 Documentation of medical reason(s) for not including the histological type or NSCLC-NOS classification with an explanation (e.g. specimen insufficient or non-diagnostic, specimen does not contain cancer, or other documented medical reasons) ⓜ

G9420 Specimen site other than anatomic location of lung or is not classified as primary nonsmall cell lung cancer ⓜ

G9421 Primary nonsmall cell lung cancer lung biopsy and cytology specimen report does not document classification into specific histologic type or histologic type does not follow IASLC guidance or is classified as NSCLC-NOS but without an explanation ⓜ

G9422 Primary lung carcinoma resection report documents PT category, PN category and for nonsmall cell lung cancer, histologic type (e.g., squamous cell carcinoma, adenocarcinoma and not NSCLC-NOS) ⓜ

G9423 Documentation of medical reason for not including PT category, PN category and histologic type (for patient with appropriate exclusion criteria [e.g., metastatic disease, benign tumors, malignant tumors other than carcinomas, inadequate surgical specimens]) ⓜ

G9424 Specimen site other than anatomic location of lung, or classified as NSCLC-NOS ⓜ

G9425 Primary lung carcinoma resection report does not document PT category, PN category and for nonsmall cell lung cancer, histologic type (e.g., squamous cell carcinoma, adenocarcinoma) ⓜ

G9426 Improvement in median time from ED arrival to initial ED oral or parenteral pain medication administration performed for ED admitted patients ⓜ

G9427 Improvement in median time from ED arrival to initial ED oral or parenteral pain medication administration not performed for ED admitted patients ⓜ

G9428 Pathology report includes the PT category, thickness, ulceration and mitotic rate, peripheral and deep margin status and presence or absence of microsatellitosis for invasive tumors ⓜ

G9429 Documentation of medical reason(s) for not including PT category, thickness, ulceration and mitotic rate, peripheral and deep margin status and presence or absence of microsatellitosis for invasive tumors (e.g., negative skin biopsies, insufficient tissue, or other documented medical reasons) ⓜ

G9430 Specimen site other than anatomic cutaneous location ⓜ

Special Coverage Instructions   Noncovered by Medicare   Carrier Discretion   ☑ Quantity Alert   ● New Code   ○ Recycled/Reinstated   ▲ Revised Code

G9431 Pathology report does not include the PT category, thickness, ulceration and mitotic rate, peripheral and deep margin status and presence or absence of microsatellitosis for invasive tumors [M]

G9432 Asthma well-controlled based on the ACT, C-ACT, ACQ, or ATAQ score and results documented [M]

G9434 Asthma not well-controlled based on the ACT, C-ACT, ACQ, or ATAQ score, or specified asthma control tool not used, reason not given [M]

G9451 ~~Patient received one-time screening for HCV infection~~

▲ **G9452** Documentation of medical reason(s) for not receiving HCV antibody test due to limited life expectancy [M]

G9453 ~~Documentation of patient reason(s) for not receiving one-time screening for HCV infection (e.g., patient declined, other patient reasons)~~

G9454 ~~One-time screening for HCV infection not received within 12-month reporting period and no documentation of prior screening for HCV infection, reason not given~~

G9455 Patient underwent abdominal imaging with ultrasound, contrast enhanced CT or contrast MRI for HCC [M]

G9456 Documentation of medical or patient reason(s) for not ordering or performing screening for HCC. Medical reason: comorbid medical conditions with expected survival < 5 years, hepatic decompensation and not a candidate for liver transplantation, or other medical reasons; patient reasons: patient declined or other patient reasons (e.g., cost of tests, time related to accessing testing equipment) [M]

G9457 Patient did not undergo abdominal imaging and did not have a documented reason for not undergoing abdominal imaging in the submission period [M]

G9458 Patient documented as tobacco user and received tobacco cessation intervention (must include at least one of the following: advice given to quit smoking or tobacco use, counseling on the benefits of quitting smoking or tobacco use, assistance with or referral to external smoking or tobacco cessation support programs, or current enrollment in smoking or tobacco use cessation program) if identified as a tobacco user [M]

G9459 Currently a tobacco nonuser [M]

G9460 Tobacco assessment or tobacco cessation intervention not performed, reason not given [M]

G9468 Patient not receiving corticosteroids greater than or equal to 10 mg/day of prednisone equivalents for 60 or greater consecutive days or a single prescription equating to 600 mg prednisone or greater for all fills [M]

G9470 Patients not receiving corticosteroids greater than or equal to 10 mg/day of prednisone equivalents for 60 or greater consecutive days or a single prescription equating to 600 mg prednisone or greater for all fills [M]

G9471 Within the past 2 years, central dual-energy x-ray absorptiometry (DXA) not ordered or documented [M]

Hospice Services

G9473 Services performed by chaplain in the hospice setting, each 15 minutes [B]

G9474 Services performed by dietary counselor in the hospice setting, each 15 minutes [B]

G9475 Services performed by other counselor in the hospice setting, each 15 minutes [B]

G9476 Services performed by volunteer in the hospice setting, each 15 minutes [B]

G9477 Services performed by care coordinator in the hospice setting, each 15 minutes [B]

G9478 Services performed by other qualified therapist in the hospice setting, each 15 minutes [B]

G9479 Services performed by qualified pharmacist in the hospice setting, each 15 minutes [B]

Medicare Care Choice Model Program

G9480 Admission to Medicare Care Choice Model Program (MCCM) [B]

CMS Innovation Center Demonstration Project

G9481 Remote in-home visit for the evaluation and management of a new patient for use only in a Medicare-approved CMS Innovation Center Demonstration Project, which requires these three key components: a problem focused history; a problem focused examination; straightforward medical decision making, furnished in real time using interactive audio and video technology. Counseling and coordination of care with other physicians, other qualified health care professionals or agencies are provided consistent with the nature of the problem(s) and the needs of the patient or the family or both. Usually, the presenting problem(s) are self limited or minor. Typically, 10 minutes are spent with the patient or family or both via real time, audio and video intercommunications technology [B]

G9482 Remote in-home visit for the evaluation and management of a new patient for use only in a Medicare-approved CMS Innovation Center Demonstration Project, which requires these three key components: an expanded problem focused history; an expanded problem focused examination; straightforward medical decision making, furnished in real time using interactive audio and video technology. Counseling and coordination of care with other physicians, other qualified health care professionals or agencies are provided consistent with the nature of the problem(s) and the needs of the patient or the family or both. Usually, the presenting problem(s) are of low to moderate severity. Typically, 20 minutes are spent with the patient or family or both via real time, audio and video intercommunications technology [B]

G9483 Remote in-home visit for the evaluation and management of a new patient for use only in a Medicare-approved CMS Innovation Center Demonstration Project, which requires these three key components: a detailed history; a detailed examination; medical decision making of low complexity, furnished in real time using interactive audio and video technology. Counseling and coordination of care with other physicians, other qualified health care professionals or agencies are provided consistent with the nature of the problem(s) and the needs of the patient or the family or both. Usually, the presenting problem(s) are of moderate severity. Typically, 30 minutes are spent with the patient or family or both via real time, audio and video intercommunications technology [B]

G9484 Remote in-home visit for the evaluation and management of a new patient for use only in a Medicare-approved CMS Innovation Center Demonstration Project, which requires these three key components: a comprehensive history; a comprehensive examination; medical decision making of moderate complexity, furnished in real time using interactive audio and video technology. Counseling and coordination of care with other physicians, other qualified health care professionals or agencies are provided consistent with the nature of the problem(s) and the needs of the patient or the family or both. Usually, the presenting problem(s) are of moderate to high severity. Typically, 45 minutes are spent with the patient or family or both via real time, audio and video intercommunications technology [B]

Special Coverage Instructions   Noncovered by Medicare   Carrier Discretion   ☑ Quantity Alert ● New Code   ○ Recycled/Reinstated ▲ Revised Code

80 — G Codes   [A] Age Edit   [M] Maternity Edit   ♀ Female Only   ♂ Male Only   [A]-[Y] OPPS Status Indicators   © 2023 Optum360, LLC

G9485 Remote in-home visit for the evaluation and management of a new patient for use only in a Medicare-approved CMS Innovation Center Demonstration Project, which requires these three key components: a comprehensive history; a comprehensive examination; medical decision making of high complexity, furnished in real time using interactive audio and video technology. Counseling and coordination of care with other physicians, other qualified health care professionals or agencies are provided consistent with the nature of the problem(s) and the needs of the patient or the family or both. Usually, the presenting problem(s) are of moderate to high severity. Typically, 60 minutes are spent with the patient or family or both via real time, audio and video intercommunications technology   Ⓑ

G9486 Remote in-home visit for the evaluation and management of an established patient for use only in a Medicare-approved CMS Innovation Center Demonstration Project, which requires at least two of the following three key components: a problem focused history; a problem focused examination; straightforward medical decision making, furnished in real time using interactive audio and video technology. Counseling and coordination of care with other physicians, other qualified health care professionals or agencies are provided consistent with the nature of the problem(s) and the needs of the patient or the family or both. Usually, the presenting problem(s) are self limited or minor. Typically, 10 minutes are spent with the patient or family or both via real time, audio and video intercommunications technology   Ⓑ

G9487 Remote in-home visit for the evaluation and management of an established patient for use only in a Medicare-approved CMS Innovation Center Demonstration Project, which requires at least two of the following three key components: an expanded problem focused history; an expanded problem focused examination; medical decision making of low complexity, furnished in real time using interactive audio and video technology. Counseling and coordination of care with other physicians, other qualified health care professionals or agencies are provided consistent with the nature of the problem(s) and the needs of the patient or the family or both. Usually, the presenting problem(s) are of low to moderate severity. Typically, 15 minutes are spent with the patient or family or both via real time, audio and video intercommunications technology   Ⓑ

G9488 Remote in-home visit for the evaluation and management of an established patient for use only in a Medicare-approved CMS Innovation Center Demonstration Project, which requires at least two of the following three key components: a detailed history; a detailed examination; medical decision making of moderate complexity, furnished in real time using interactive audio and video technology. Counseling and coordination of care with other physicians, other qualified health care professionals or agencies are provided consistent with the nature of the problem(s) and the needs of the patient or the family or both. Usually, the presenting problem(s) are of moderate to high severity. Typically, 25 minutes are spent with the patient or family or both via real time, audio and video intercommunications technology   Ⓑ

G9489 Remote in-home visit for the evaluation and management of an established patient for use only in a Medicare-approved CMS Innovation Center Demonstration Project, which requires at least two of the following three key components: a comprehensive history; a comprehensive examination; medical decision making of high complexity, furnished in real time using interactive audio and video technology. Counseling and coordination of care with other physicians, other qualified health care professionals or agencies are provided consistent with the nature of the problem(s) and the needs of the patient or the family or both. Usually, the presenting problem(s) are of moderate to high severity. Typically, 40 minutes are spent with the patient or family or both via real time, audio and video intercommunications technology   Ⓑ

G9490 CMS Innovation Center Models, home visit for patient assessment performed by clinical staff for an individual not considered homebound, including, but not necessarily limited to patient assessment of clinical status, safety/fall prevention, functional status/ambulation, medication reconciliation/management, compliance with orders/plan of care, performance of activities of daily living, and ensuring beneficiary connections to community and other services. (For use only in Medicare-approved CMS Innovation Center Models); may not be billed for a 30 day period covered by a transitional care management code   Ⓑ

Quality Measures

G9497 Received instruction from the anesthesiologist or proxy prior to the day of surgery to abstain from smoking on the day of surgery   Ⓜ

G9498 Antibiotic regimen prescribed   Ⓜ

G9500 Radiation exposure indices documented in final report for procedure using fluoroscopy   Ⓜ

G9501 Radiation exposure indices not documented in final report for procedure using fluoroscopy, reason not given   Ⓜ

G9502 Documentation of medical reason for not performing foot exam (i.e., patients who have had either a bilateral amputation above or below the knee, or both a left and right amputation above or below the knee before or during the measurement period)   Ⓜ

G9504 Documented reason for not assessing hepatitis B virus (HBV) status (e.g., patient not initiating anti-TNF therapy, patient declined) prior to initiating anti-TNF therapy   Ⓜ

G9505 Antibiotic regimen prescribed within 10 days after onset of symptoms for documented medical reason   Ⓜ

G9507 Documentation that the patient is on a statin medication or has documentation of a valid contraindication or exception to statin medications; contraindications/exceptions that can be defined by diagnosis codes include pregnancy during the measurement period, active liver disease, rhabdomyolysis, end stage renal disease on dialysis and heart failure; provider documented contraindications/exceptions include breastfeeding during the measurement period, woman of child-bearing age not actively taking birth control, allergy to statin, drug interaction (HIV protease inhibitors, nefazodone, cyclosporine, gemfibrozil, and danazol) and intolerance (with supporting documentation of trying a statin at least once within the last 5 years or diagnosis codes for myostitis or toxic myopathy related to drugs)   Ⓜ

G9508 Documentation that the patient is not on a statin medication   Ⓜ

G9509 Adult patients 18 years of age or older with major depression or dysthymia who reached remission at twelve months as demonstrated by a twelve-month (+/-60 days) PHQ-9 or PHQ-9M score of less than 5   Ⓜ

Special Coverage Instructions   Noncovered by Medicare   Carrier Discretion   ☑ Quantity Alert   ● New Code   ○ Recycled/Reinstated   ▲ Revised Code

© 2023 Optum360, LLC   A2-Z3 ASC Pmt   **CMS:** IOM   **AHA:** Coding Clinic   ⅊ DMEPOS Paid   ⊘ SNF Excluded   **G Codes — 81**

G9510 Adult patients 18 years of age or older with major depression or dysthymia who did not reach remission at 12 months as demonstrated by a 12 month (+/-60 days) PHQ-9 or PHQ-9M score of less than 5. Either PHQ-9 or PHQ-9M score was not assessed or is greater than or equal to 5 Ⓜ

G9511 Index PHQ-9 or PHQ-9M score greater than 9 documented during the twelve-month denominator identification period Ⓜ

G9512 Individual had a PDC of 0.8 or greater Ⓜ

G9513 Individual did not have a PDC of 0.8 or greater Ⓜ

G9514 Patient required a return to the operating room within 90 days of surgery Ⓜ

G9515 Patient did not require a return to the operating room within 90 days of surgery Ⓜ

G9516 Patient achieved an improvement in visual acuity, from their preoperative level, within 90 days of surgery Ⓜ

G9517 Patient did not achieve an improvement in visual acuity, from their preoperative level, within 90 days of surgery, reason not given Ⓜ

G9518 Documentation of active injection drug use Ⓜ

G9519 Patient achieves final refraction (spherical equivalent) +/- 1.0 diopters of their planned refraction within 90 days of surgery Ⓜ

G9520 Patient does not achieve final refraction (spherical equivalent) +/- 1.0 diopters of their planned refraction within 90 days of surgery Ⓜ

G9521 Total number of emergency department visits and inpatient hospitalizations less than two in the past 12 months Ⓜ

G9522 Total number of emergency department visits and inpatient hospitalizations equal to or greater than two in the past 12 months or patient not screened, reason not given Ⓜ

Blunt Head Trauma

G9529 Patient with minor blunt head trauma had an appropriate indication(s) for a head CT Ⓜ

G9530 Patient presented with a minor blunt head trauma and had a head CT ordered for trauma by an emergency care provider Ⓜ

G9531 Patient has documentation of ventricular shunt, brain tumor, multisystem trauma, or is currently taking an antiplatelet medication including: abciximab, anagrelide, cangrelor, cilostazol, clopidogrel, dipyridamole, eptifibatide, prasugrel, ticlopidine, ticagrelor, tirofiban, or vorapaxar Ⓜ

G9533 Patient with minor blunt head trauma did not have an appropriate indication(s) for a head CT Ⓜ

Miscellaneous Quality Measures

G9537 Imaging needed as part of a clinical trial; or other clinician ordered the study Ⓜ

G9539 Intent for potential removal at time of placement Ⓜ

G9540 Patient alive 3 months post procedure Ⓜ

G9541 Filter removed within 3 months of placement Ⓜ

G9542 Documented reassessment for the appropriateness of filter removal within 3 months of placement Ⓜ

G9543 Documentation of at least two attempts to reach the patient to arrange a clinical reassessment for the appropriateness of filter removal within 3 months of placement Ⓜ

G9544 Patients that do not have the filter removed, documented reassessment for the appropriateness of filter removal, or documentation of at least two attempts to reach the patient to arrange a clinical reassessment for the appropriateness of filter removal within 3 months of placement Ⓜ

G9547 Cystic renal lesion that is simple appearing (Bosniak I or II), or adrenal lesion less than or equal to 1.0 cm or adrenal lesion greater than 1.0 cm but less than or equal to 4.0 cm classified as likely benign by unenhanced CT or washout protocol CT, or MRI with in- and opposed-phase sequences or other equivalent institutional imaging protocols Ⓜ

G9548 Final reports for imaging studies stating no follow up imaging is recommended Ⓜ

G9549 Documentation of medical reason(s) that follow up imaging is indicated (e.g., patient has lymphadenopathy, signs of metastasis or an active diagnosis or history of cancer, and other medical reason(s)) Ⓜ

G9550 Final reports for imaging studies with follow-up imaging recommended, or final reports that do not include a specific recommendation of no follow-up Ⓜ

G9551 Final reports for imaging studies without an incidentally found lesion noted Ⓜ

G9552 Incidental thyroid nodule < 1.0 cm noted in report Ⓜ

G9553 Prior thyroid disease diagnosis Ⓜ

G9554 Final reports for CT, CTA, MRI or MRA of the chest or neck with follow-up imaging recommended Ⓜ

G9555 Documentation of medical reason(s) for recommending follow up imaging (e.g., patient has multiple endocrine neoplasia, patient has cervical lymphadenopathy, other medical reason(s)) Ⓜ

G9556 Final reports for CT, CTA, MRI or MRA of the chest or neck with follow-up imaging not recommended Ⓜ

G9557 Final reports for CT, CTA, MRI or MRA studies of the chest or neck without an incidentally found thyroid nodule < 1.0 cm noted or no nodule found Ⓜ

Stroke Therapy

G9580 Door to puncture time of 90 minutes or less Ⓜ

G9582 Door to puncture time of greater than 90 minutes, no reason given Ⓜ

Blunt Head Trauma

G9593 Pediatric patient with minor blunt head trauma classified as low risk according to the PECARN prediction rules Ⓜ

G9594 Patient presented with a minor blunt head trauma and had a head CT ordered for trauma by an emergency care provider Ⓜ

G9595 Patient has documentation of ventricular shunt, brain tumor, or coagulopathy Ⓜ

G9596 ~~Pediatric patient had a head CT for trauma ordered by someone other than an emergency care provider or was ordered for a reason other than trauma~~

G9597 Pediatric patient with minor blunt head trauma not classified as low risk according to the PECARN prediction rules Ⓜ

Aortic Aneurysm

G9598 Aortic aneurysm 5.5-5.9 cm maximum diameter on centerline formatted CT or minor diameter on axial formatted CT Ⓜ

G9599 Aortic aneurysm 6.0 cm or greater maximum diameter on centerline formatted CT or minor diameter on axial formatted CT Ⓜ

Special Coverage Instructions   Noncovered by Medicare   Carrier Discretion   ☑ Quantity Alert ● New Code   ○ Recycled/Reinstated ▲ Revised Code

82 — G Codes   Ⓐ Age Edit   Ⓜ Maternity Edit   ♀ Female Only   ♂ Male Only   Ⓐ-Ⓨ OPPS Status Indicators   © 2023 Optum360, LLC

Patient Survey

G9603   Patient survey score improved from baseline following treatment Ⓜ

G9604   Patient survey results not available Ⓜ

G9605   Patient survey score did not improve from baseline following treatment Ⓜ

Intraoperative Cystoscopy

G9606   Intraoperative cystoscopy performed to evaluate for lower tract injury Ⓜ

G9607   Documented medical reasons for not performing intraoperative cystoscopy (e.g., urethral pathology precluding cystoscopy, any patient who has a congenital or acquired absence of the urethra) or in the case of patient death Ⓜ

G9608   Intraoperative cystoscopy not performed to evaluate for lower tract injury Ⓜ

Aspirin/Antiplatelet Therapy

G9609   Documentation of an order for antiplatelet agents Ⓜ

G9610   Documentation of medical reason(s) in the patient's record for not ordering antiplatelet agents Ⓜ

G9611   Order for antiplatelet agents was not documented in the patient's record, reason not given Ⓜ

Colonoscopy Documentation

G9612   ~~Photodocumentation of two or more cecal landmarks to establish a complete examination~~

G9613   ~~Documentation of postsurgical anatomy (e.g., right hemicolectomy, ileocecal resection, etc.)~~

G9614   ~~Photodocumentation of less than two cecal landmarks (i.e., no cecal landmarks or only one cecal landmark) to establish a complete examination~~

Uterine Malignancy Screening

Alcohol Use

G9621   Patient identified as an unhealthy alcohol user when screened for unhealthy alcohol use using a systematic screening method and received brief counseling Ⓜ

G9622   Patient not identified as an unhealthy alcohol user when screened for unhealthy alcohol use using a systematic screening method Ⓜ

G9624   Patient not screened for unhealthy alcohol use using a systematic screening method or patient did not receive brief counseling if identified as an unhealthy alcohol user Ⓜ

Bladder/Ureter Injury

G9625   Patient sustained bladder injury at the time of surgery or discovered subsequently up to 30 days post-surgery Ⓜ

G9626   Documented medical reason for not reporting bladder injury (e.g., gynecologic or other pelvic malignancy documented, concurrent surgery involving bladder pathology, injury that occurs during urinary incontinence procedure, patient death from nonmedical causes not related to surgery, patient died during procedure without evidence of bladder injury) Ⓜ

G9627   Patient did not sustain bladder injury at the time of surgery nor discovered subsequently up to 30 days post-surgery Ⓜ

G9628   Patient sustained bowel injury at the time of surgery or discovered subsequently up to 30 days post-surgery Ⓜ

G9629   Documented medical reasons for not reporting bowel injury (e.g., gynecologic or other pelvic malignancy documented, planned (e.g., not due to an unexpected bowel injury) resection and/or re-anastomosis of bowel, or patient death from nonmedical causes not related to surgery, patient died during procedure without evidence of bowel injury) Ⓜ

G9630   Patient did not sustain a bowel injury at the time of surgery nor discovered subsequently up to 30 days post-surgery Ⓜ

Quality Measures

G9637   Final reports with documentation of one or more dose reduction techniques (e.g., automated exposure control, adjustment of the mA and/or kV according to patient size, use of iterative reconstruction technique) Ⓜ

G9638   Final reports without documentation of one or more dose reduction techniques (e.g., automated exposure control, adjustment of the mA and/or kV according to patient size, use of iterative reconstruction technique) Ⓜ

G9642   Current smoker (e.g., cigarette, cigar, pipe, e-cigarette or marijuana) Ⓜ

G9643   Elective surgery Ⓜ

G9644   Patients who abstained from smoking prior to anesthesia on the day of surgery or procedure Ⓜ

G9645   Patients who did not abstain from smoking prior to anesthesia on the day of surgery or procedure Ⓜ

G9646   Patients with 90 day MRS score of 0 to 2 Ⓜ

G9648   Patients with 90 day MRS score greater than 2 Ⓜ

Psoriasis Therapy

G9649   Psoriasis assessment tool documented meeting any one of the specified benchmarks (e.g., (PGA; 5-point or 6-point scale), body surface area (BSA), psoriasis area and severity index (PASI) and/or dermatology life quality index (DLQI)) Ⓜ

G9651   Psoriasis assessment tool documented not meeting any one of the specified benchmarks (e.g., (PGA; 5-point or 6-point scale), body surface area (BSA), psoriasis area and severity index (PASI) and/or dermatology life quality index (DLQI)) or psoriasis assessment tool not documented Ⓜ

Anesthesia Services

G9654   Monitored anesthesia care (MAC) Ⓜ

G9655   A transfer of care protocol or handoff tool/checklist that includes the required key handoff elements is used Ⓜ

G9656   Patient transferred directly from anesthetizing location to PACU or other non-ICU location Ⓜ

G9658   A transfer of care protocol or handoff tool/checklist that includes the required key handoff elements is not used Ⓜ

Reason for Colonoscopy

G9659   Patients greater than or equal to 86 years of age who underwent a screening colonoscopy and did not have a history of colorectal cancer or other valid medical reason for the colonoscopy, including: iron deficiency anemia, lower gastrointestinal bleeding, Crohn's disease (i.e., regional enteritis), familial adenomatous polyposis, Lynch syndrome (i.e., hereditary nonpolyposis colorectal cancer), inflammatory bowel disease, ulcerative colitis, abnormal finding of gastrointestinal tract, or changes in bowel habits Ⓜ

Special Coverage Instructions   Noncovered by Medicare   Carrier Discretion   ☑ Quantity Alert   ● New Code   ○ Recycled/Reinstated   ▲ Revised Code

© 2023 Optum360, LLC   A2-Z3 ASC Pmt   **CMS:** IOM   **AHA:** Coding Clinic   ⅏ DMEPOS Paid   ⊘ SNF Excluded   **G Codes — 83**

Procedures/Professional Services (Temporary)

G9660 — G9711

G9660 Documentation of medical reason(s) for a colonoscopy performed on a patient greater than or equal to 86 years of age (e.g., iron deficiency anemia, lower gastrointestinal bleeding, Crohn's disease (i.e., regional enteritis), familial history of adenomatous polyposis, Lynch syndrome (i.e., hereditary nonpolyposis colorectal cancer), inflammatory bowel disease, ulcerative colitis, abnormal finding of gastrointestinal tract, or changes in bowel habits) Ⓜ

G9661 Patients greater than or equal to 86 years of age who received a colonoscopy for an assessment of signs/symptoms of GI tract illness, and/or because the patient meets high risk criteria, and/or to follow-up on previously diagnosed advanced lesions Ⓜ

Statin Therapy

G9662 Previously diagnosed or have a diagnosis of clinical ASCVD, including ASCVD procedure Ⓜ

G9663 Any LDL-C laboratory result >= 190 mg/dl Ⓜ

G9664 Patients who are currently statin therapy users or received an order (prescription) for statin therapy Ⓜ

G9665 Patients who are not currently statin therapy users or did not receive an order (prescription) for statin therapy Ⓜ

Cardiovascular Measures

G9674 Patients with clinical ASCVD diagnosis Ⓜ

G9675 Patients who have ever had a fasting or direct laboratory result of LDL-C = 190 mg/dl Ⓜ

G9676 Patients aged 40 to 75 years at the beginning of the measurement period with type 1 or type 2 diabetes and with an ldl-c result of 70-189 mg/dl recorded as the highest fasting or direct laboratory test result in the measurement year or during the two years prior to the beginning of the measurement period Ⓜ

Nursing Facility Care

G9679 Onsite acute care treatment of a nursing facility resident with pneumonia. May only be billed once per day per beneficiary Ⓑ

G9680 Onsite acute care treatment of a nursing facility resident with CHF. May only be billed once per day per beneficiary Ⓑ

G9681 Onsite acute care treatment of a nursing facility resident with COPD or asthma. May only be billed once per day per beneficiary Ⓑ

G9682 Onsite acute care treatment of a nursing facility resident with a skin infection. May only be billed once per day per beneficiary Ⓑ

G9683 Facility service(s) for the onsite acute care treatment of a nursing facility resident with fluid or electrolyte disorder. (May only be billed once per day per beneficiary.) This service is for a demonstration project Ⓑ

G9684 Onsite acute care treatment of a nursing facility resident for a UTI. May only be billed once per day per beneficiary Ⓑ

G9685 Physician service or other qualified health care professional for the evaluation and management of a beneficiary's acute change in condition in a nursing facility. This service is for a demonstration project Ⓜ

Other Quality Measures

G9687 Hospice services provided to patient any time during the measurement period Ⓜ

G9688 Patients using hospice services any time during the measurement period Ⓜ

G9689 Patient admitted for performance of elective carotid intervention Ⓜ

G9690 Patient receiving hospice services any time during the measurement period Ⓜ

G9691 Patient had hospice services any time during the measurement period Ⓜ

G9692 Hospice services received by patient any time during the measurement period Ⓜ

G9693 Patient use of hospice services any time during the measurement period Ⓜ

G9694 Hospice services utilized by patient any time during the measurement period Ⓜ

G9695 Long-acting inhaled bronchodilator prescribed Ⓜ

▲ **G9696** Documentation of medical reason(s) for not prescribing a long-acting inhaled bronchodilator (e.g., patient intolerance or history of side effects) Ⓜ

G9697 ~~Documentation of patient reason(s) for not prescribing a long-acting inhaled bronchodilator~~

▲ **G9698** Documentation of system reason(s) for not prescribing a long-acting inhaled bronchodilator (e.g., cost of treatment or lack of insurance) Ⓜ

G9699 Long-acting inhaled bronchodilator not prescribed, reason not otherwise specified Ⓜ

G9700 Patients who use hospice services any time during the measurement period Ⓜ

G9702 Patients who use hospice services any time during the measurement period Ⓜ

▲ **G9703** Episodes where the patient is taking antibiotics (Table 1) in the 30 days prior to the episode date Ⓜ

G9704 AJCC breast cancer Stage I: T1 mic or T1a documented Ⓜ

G9705 AJCC breast cancer Stage I: T1b (tumor > 0.5 cm but <= 1 cm in greatest dimension) documented Ⓜ

G9706 Low (or very low) risk of recurrence, prostate cancer Ⓜ

G9707 Patient received hospice services any time during the measurement period Ⓜ

G9708 Women who had a bilateral mastectomy or who have a history of a bilateral mastectomy or for whom there is evidence of a right and a left unilateral mastectomy Ⓜ

G9709 Hospice services used by patient any time during the measurement period Ⓜ

G9710 Patient was provided hospice services any time during the measurement period Ⓜ

G9711 Patients with a diagnosis or past history of total colectomy or colorectal cancer Ⓜ

Special Coverage Instructions   Noncovered by Medicare   Carrier Discretion   ☑ Quantity Alert   ● New Code   ○ Recycled/Reinstated   ▲ Revised Code

84 — G Codes   Ⓐ Age Edit   Ⓜ Maternity Edit   ♀ Female Only   ♂ Male Only   Ⓐ-Ⓨ OPPS Status Indicators   © 2023 Optum360, LLC

G9712 Documentation of medical reason(s) for prescribing or dispensing antibiotic (e.g., intestinal infection, pertussis, bacterial infection, lyme disease, otitis media, acute sinusitis, acute pharyngitis, acute tonsillitis, chronic sinusitis, infection of the pharynx/larynx/tonsils/adenoids, prostatitis, cellulitis/mastoiditis/bone infections, acute lymphadenitis, impetigo, skin staph infections, pneumonia, gonococcal infections/venereal disease (syphilis, chlamydia, inflammatory diseases [female reproductive organs]), infections of the kidney, cystitis/UTI, acne, HIV disease/asymptomatic HIV, cystic fibrosis, disorders of the immune system, malignancy neoplasms, chronic bronchitis, emphysema, bronchiectasis, extrinsic allergic alveolitis, chronic airway obstruction, chronic obstructive asthma, pneumoconiosis and other lung disease due to external agents, other diseases of the respiratory system, and tuberculosis [M]

G9713 Patients who use hospice services any time during the measurement period [M]

G9714 Patient is using hospice services any time during the measurement period [M]

G9715 ~~Patients who use hospice services any time during the measurement period~~

G9716 BMI is documented as being outside of normal parameters, follow-up plan is not completed for documented medical reason [M]

▲ **G9717** Documentation stating the patient has had a diagnosis of bipolar disorder [M]

G9719 Patient is not ambulatory, bed ridden, immobile, confined to chair, wheelchair bound, dependent on helper pushing wheelchair, independent in wheelchair or minimal help in wheelchair [M]

G9720 Hospice services for patient occurred any time during the measurement period [M]

G9721 Patient not ambulatory, bed ridden, immobile, confined to chair, wheelchair bound, dependent on helper pushing wheelchair, independent in wheelchair or minimal help in wheelchair [M]

G9722 Documented history of renal failure or baseline serum creatinine >= 4.0 mg/dl; renal transplant recipients are not considered to have preoperative renal failure, unless, since transplantation the CR has been or is 4.0 or higher [M]

G9723 Hospice services for patient received any time during the measurement period [M]

G9724 Patients who had documentation of use of anticoagulant medications overlapping the measurement year [M]

G9725 ~~Patients who use hospice services any time during the measurement period~~

G9726 Patient refused to participate [M]

G9727 Patient unable to complete the LEPF PROM at initial evaluation and/or discharge due to blindness, illiteracy, severe mental incapacity or language incompatibility and an adequate proxy is not available [M]

G9728 Patient refused to participate [M]

G9729 Patient unable to complete the LEPF PROM at initial evaluation and/or discharge due to blindness, illiteracy, severe mental incapacity or language incompatibility and an adequate proxy is not available [M]

G9730 Patient refused to participate [M]

G9731 Patient unable to complete the LEPF PROM at initial evaluation and/or discharge due to blindness, illiteracy, severe mental incapacity or language incompatibility and an adequate proxy is not available [M]

G9732 Patient refused to participate [M]

G9733 Patient unable to complete the low back FS PROM at initial evaluation and/or discharge due to blindness, illiteracy, severe mental incapacity or language incompatibility and an adequate proxy is not available [M]

G9734 Patient refused to participate [M]

G9735 Patient unable to complete the shoulder FS PROM at initial evaluation and/or discharge due to blindness, illiteracy, severe mental incapacity or language incompatibility and an adequate proxy is not available [M]

G9736 Patient refused to participate [M]

G9737 Patient unable to complete the elbow/wrist/hand FS PROM at initial evaluation and/or discharge due to blindness, illiteracy, severe mental incapacity or language incompatibility and an adequate proxy is not available [M]

G9740 Hospice services given to patient any time during the measurement period [M]

G9741 Patients who use hospice services any time during the measurement period [M]

G9744 Patient not eligible due to active diagnosis of hypertension [M]

G9745 Documented reason for not screening or recommending a follow-up for high blood pressure [M]

G9746 Patient has mitral stenosis or prosthetic heart valves or patient has transient or reversible cause of AF (e.g., pneumonia, hyperthyroidism, pregnancy, cardiac surgery) [M]

G9751 Patient died at any time during the 24-month measurement period [M]

G9752 Emergency surgery [M]

G9753 Documentation of medical reason for not conducting a search for DICOM format images for prior patient CT imaging studies completed at nonaffiliated external healthcare facilities or entities within the past 12 months that are available through a secure, authorized, media-free, shared archive (e.g., trauma, acute myocardial infarction, stroke, aortic aneurysm where time is of the essence) [M]

G9754 A finding of an incidental pulmonary nodule [M]

G9755 Documentation of medical reason(s) for not including a recommended interval and modality for follow-up or for no follow-up, and source of recommendations (e.g., patients with unexplained fever, immunocompromised patients who are at risk for infection) [M]

G9756 Surgical procedures that included the use of silicone oil [M]

G9757 Surgical procedures that included the use of silicone oil [M]

G9758 Patient in hospice at any time during the measurement period [M]

G9760 Patients who use hospice services any time during the measurement period [M]

G9761 Patients who use hospice services any time during the measurement period [M]

G9762 Patient had at least two HPV vaccines (with at least 146 days between the two) or three HPV vaccines on or between the patient's 9th and 13th birthdays [M]

G9763 Patient did not have at least two HPV vaccines (with at least 146 days between the two) or three HPV vaccines on or between the patient's 9th and 13th birthdays [M]

G9764 Patient has been treated with a systemic medication for psoriasis vulgaris [M]

Special Coverage Instructions   Noncovered by Medicare   Carrier Discretion   ☑ Quantity Alert   ● New Code   ○ Recycled/Reinstated   ▲ Revised Code

G9765 Documentation that the patient declined change in medication or alternative therapies were unavailable, has documented contraindications, or has not been treated with a systemic medication for at least six consecutive months (e.g., experienced adverse effects or lack of efficacy with all other therapy options) in order to achieve better disease control as measured by PGA, BSA, PASI, or DLQI ⓜ

G9766 Patients who are transferred from one institution to another with a known diagnosis of CVA for endovascular stroke treatment ⓜ

G9767 Hospitalized patients with newly diagnosed CVA considered for endovascular stroke treatment ⓜ

G9768 Patients who utilize hospice services any time during the measurement period ⓜ

G9769 Patient had a bone mineral density test in the past two years or received osteoporosis medication or therapy in the past 12 months ⓜ

G9770 Peripheral nerve block (PNB) ⓜ

▲ **G9771** At least one body temperature measurement equal to or greater than 35.5 degrees Celsius (or 95.9 degrees Fahrenheit) achieved within the 30 minutes immediately before or 15 minutes immediately after anesthesia end time ⓜ

▲ **G9772** Documentation of medical reason(s) for not achieving at least one body temperature measurement equal to or greater than 35.5 degrees Celsius (or 95.9 degrees Fahrenheit) within the 30 minutes immediately before or 15 minutes immediately after anesthesia end time (e.g., emergency cases, intentional hypothermia, etc.) ⓜ

▲ **G9773** At least one body temperature measurement equal to or greater than 35.5 degrees Celsius (or 95.9 degrees Fahrenheit) not achieved within the 30 minutes immediately before or 15 minutes immediately after anesthesia end time, reason not given ⓜ

G9775 Patient received at least two prophylactic pharmacologic antiemetic agents of different classes preoperatively and/or intraoperatively ⓜ

G9776 Documentation of medical reason for not receiving at least two prophylactic pharmacologic antiemetic agents of different classes preoperatively and/or intraoperatively (e.g., intolerance or other medical reason) ⓜ

G9777 Patient did not receive at least two prophylactic pharmacologic antiemetic agents of different classes preoperatively and/or intraoperatively ⓜ

▲ **G9779** Patients who are breastfeeding at any time during the performance period ⓜ

▲ **G9780** Patients who have a diagnosis of rhabdomyolysis at any time during the performance period ⓜ

G9781 Documentation of medical reason(s) for not currently being a statin therapy user or receiving an order (prescription) for statin therapy (e.g., patients with statin-associated muscle symptoms or an allergy to statin medication therapy, patients who are receiving palliative or hospice care, patients with active liver disease or hepatic disease or insufficiency, patients with end stage renal disease [ESRD], or other medical reasons) ⓜ

G9782 History of or active diagnosis of familial hypercholesterolemia ⓜ

G9784 Pathologists/dermatopathologists providing a second opinion on a biopsy ⓜ

G9785 Pathology report diagnosing cutaneous basal cell carcinoma, squamous cell carcinoma, or melanoma (to include in situ disease) sent from the pathologist/dermatopathologist to the biopsying clinician for review within 7 days from the time when the tissue specimen was received by the pathologist ⓜ

G9786 Pathology report diagnosing cutaneous basal cell carcinoma, squamous cell carcinoma, or melanoma (to include in situ disease) was not sent from the pathologist/dermatopathologist to the biopsying clinician for review within 7 days from the time when the tissue specimen was received by the pathologist ⓜ

G9787 Patient alive as of the last day of the measurement year ⓜ

G9788 Most recent BP is less than or equal to 140/90 mm Hg ⓜ

G9789 Blood pressure recorded during inpatient stays, emergency room visits, or urgent care visits ⓜ

G9790 Most recent BP is greater than 140/90 mm Hg, or blood pressure not documented ⓜ

G9791 Most recent tobacco status is tobacco free ⓜ

G9792 Most recent tobacco status is not tobacco free ⓜ

G9793 Patient is currently on a daily aspirin or other antiplatelet ⓜ

G9794 Documentation of medical reason(s) for not on a daily aspirin or other antiplatelet (e.g., history of gastrointestinal bleed, intracranial bleed, idiopathic thrombocytopenic purpura (ITP), gastric bypass or documentation of active anticoagulant use during the measurement period) ⓜ

G9795 Patient is not currently on a daily aspirin or other antiplatelet ⓜ

G9796 Patient is currently on a statin therapy ⓜ

G9797 Patient is not on a statin therapy ⓜ

G9805 Patients who use hospice services any time during the measurement period ⓜ

G9806 Patients who received cervical cytology or an HPV test ⓜ

G9807 Patients who did not receive cervical cytology or an HPV test ⓜ

G9812 Patient died including all deaths occurring during the hospitalization in which the operation was performed, even if after 30 days, and those deaths occurring after discharge from the hospital, but within 30 days of the procedure ⓜ

G9813 Patient did not die within 30 days of the procedure or during the index hospitalization ⓜ

G9818 Documentation of sexual activity ⓜ

G9819 Patients who use hospice services any time during the measurement period ⓜ

G9820 Documentation of a chlamydia screening test with proper follow-up ⓜ

G9821 No documentation of a chlamydia screening test with proper follow-up ⓜ

G9822 Patients who had an endometrial ablation procedure during the 12 months prior to the index date (exclusive of the index date) ⓜ

G9823 Endometrial sampling or hysteroscopy with biopsy and results documented during the 12 months prior to the index date (exclusive of the index date) of the endometrial ablation ⓜ

G9824 Endometrial sampling or hysteroscopy with biopsy and results not documented during the 12 months prior to the index date (exclusive of the index date) of the endometrial ablation ⓜ

G9830 HER2/neu positive ⓜ

Special Coverage Instructions ▪ Noncovered by Medicare ▪ Carrier Discretion ☑ Quantity Alert ● New Code ○ Recycled/Reinstated ▲ Revised Code

86 — G Codes · Ⓐ Age Edit · ⓜ Maternity Edit · ♀ Female Only · ♂ Male Only · Ⓐ-Ⓨ OPPS Status Indicators · © 2023 Optum360, LLC

G9831 AJCC Stage at breast cancer diagnosis = II or III ☐M

G9832 AJCC Stage at breast cancer diagnosis = I (Ia or Ib) and T-Stage at breast cancer diagnosis does not equal = T1, T1a, T1b ☐M

G9838 Patient has metastatic disease at diagnosis ☐M

G9839 Anti-EGFR monoclonal antibody therapy ☐M

G9840 RAS (KRAS and NRAS) gene mutation testing performed before initiation of anti-EGFR MoAb ☐M

G9841 RAS (KRAS and NRAS) gene mutation testing not performed before initiation of anti-EGFR MoAb ☐M

G9842 Patient has metastatic disease at diagnosis ☐M

G9843 RAS (KRAS or NRAS) gene mutation ☐M

G9844 Patient did not receive anti-EGFR monoclonal antibody therapy ☐M

G9845 Patient received anti-EGFR monoclonal antibody therapy ☐M

G9846 Patients who died from cancer ☐M

G9847 Patient received systemic cancer-directed therapy in the last 14 days of life ☐M

G9848 Patient did not receive systemic cancer-directed therapy in the last 14 days of life ☐M

G9852 ~~Patients who died from cancer~~

G9853 ~~Patient admitted to the ICU in the last 30 days of life~~

G9854 ~~Patient was not admitted to the ICU in the last 30 days of life~~

G9858 Patient enrolled in hospice ☐M

G9859 Patients who died from cancer ☐M

G9860 Patient spent less than three days in hospice care ☐M

G9861 Patient spent greater than or equal to three days in hospice care ☐M

G9862 Documentation of medical reason(s) for not recommending at least a 10 year follow-up interval (e.g., inadequate prep, familial or personal history of colonic polyps, patient had no adenoma and age is = 66 years old, or life expectancy < 10 years old, other medical reasons) ☐M

G9868 Receipt and analysis of remote, asynchronous images for dermatologic and/or ophthalmologic evaluation, for use only in a Medicare-approved CMMI model, less than 10 minutes ☐B
AHA: 2Q,21

G9869 Receipt and analysis of remote, asynchronous images for dermatologic and/or ophthalmologic evaluation, for use only in a Medicare-approved CMMI model, 10 to 20 minutes ☐B
AHA: 2Q,21

G9870 Receipt and analysis of remote, asynchronous images for dermatologic and/or ophthalmologic evaluation, for use only in a Medicare-approved CMMI model, more than 20 minutes ☐B
AHA: 2Q,21

G9873 First Medicare Diabetes Prevention Program (MDPP) core session was attended by an MDPP beneficiary under the MDPP Expanded Model (EM). A core session is an MDPP service that: (1) is furnished by an MDPP supplier during months 1 through 6 of the MDPP services period; (2) is approximately 1 hour in length; and (3) adheres to a CDC-approved DPP curriculum for core sessions ☐M

G9874 Four total Medicare Diabetes Prevention Program (MDPP) core sessions were attended by an MDPP beneficiary under the MDPP Expanded Model (EM). A core session is an MDPP service that: (1) is furnished by an MDPP supplier during months 1 through 6 of the MDPP services period; (2) is approximately 1 hour in length; and (3) adheres to a CDC-approved DPP curriculum for core sessions ☐M

G9875 Nine total Medicare Diabetes Prevention Program (MDPP) core sessions were attended by an MDPP beneficiary under the MDPP Expanded Model (EM). A core session is an MDPP service that: (1) is furnished by an MDPP supplier during months 1 through 6 of the MDPP services period; (2) is approximately 1 hour in length; and (3) adheres to a CDC-approved DPP curriculum for core sessions ☐M

G9876 Two Medicare Diabetes Prevention Program (MDPP) core maintenance sessions (MS) were attended by an MDPP beneficiary in months (mo) 7-9 under the MDPP Expanded Model (EM). A core maintenance session is an MDPP service that: (1) is furnished by an MDPP supplier during months 7 through 12 of the MDPP services period; (2) is approximately 1 hour in length; and (3) adheres to a CDC-approved DPP curriculum for maintenance sessions. The beneficiary did not achieve at least 5% weight loss (WL) from his/her baseline weight, as measured by at least one in-person weight measurement at a core maintenance session in months 7-9 ☐M

G9877 Two Medicare Diabetes Prevention Program (MDPP) core maintenance sessions (MS) were attended by an MDPP beneficiary in months (mo) 10-12 under the MDPP Expanded Model (EM). A core maintenance session is an MDPP service that: (1) is furnished by an MDPP supplier during months 7 through 12 of the MDPP services period; (2) is approximately 1 hour in length; and (3) adheres to a CDC-approved DPP curriculum for maintenance sessions. The beneficiary did not achieve at least 5% weight loss (WL) from his/her baseline weight, as measured by at least one in-person weight measurement at a core maintenance session in months 10-12 ☐M

G9878 Two Medicare Diabetes Prevention Program (MDPP) core maintenance sessions (MS) were attended by an MDPP beneficiary in months (mo) 7-9 under the MDPP Expanded Model (EM). A core maintenance session is an MDPP service that: (1) is furnished by an MDPP supplier during months 7 through 12 of the MDPP services period; (2) is approximately 1 hour in length; and (3) adheres to a CDC-approved DPP curriculum for maintenance sessions. The beneficiary achieved at least 5% weight loss (WL) from his/her baseline weight, as measured by at least one in-person weight measurement at a core maintenance session in months 7-9 ☐M

G9879 Two Medicare Diabetes Prevention Program (MDPP) core maintenance sessions (MS) were attended by an MDPP beneficiary in months (mo) 10-12 under the MDPP Expanded Model (EM). A core maintenance session is an MDPP service that: (1) is furnished by an MDPP supplier during months 7 through 12 of the MDPP services period; (2) is approximately 1 hour in length; and (3) adheres to a CDC-approved DPP curriculum for maintenance sessions. The beneficiary achieved at least 5% weight loss (WL) from his/her baseline weight, as measured by at least one in-person weight measurement at a core maintenance session in months 10-12 ☐M

G9880 The MDPP beneficiary achieved at least 5% weight loss (WL) from his/her baseline weight in months 1-12 of the MDPP services period under the MDPP Expanded Model (EM). This is a one-time payment available when a beneficiary first achieves at least 5% weight loss from baseline as measured by an in-person weight measurement at a core session or core maintenance session ☐M

Special Coverage Instructions   Noncovered by Medicare   Carrier Discretion   ☑ Quantity Alert   ● New Code   ○ Recycled/Reinstated   ▲ Revised Code

© 2023 Optum360, LLC   A2-Z3 ASC Pmt   CMS: IOM   AHA: Coding Clinic   ⅊ DMEPOS Paid   ⊘ SNF Excluded   G Codes — 87

G9881 The MDPP beneficiary achieved at least 9% weight loss (WL) from his/her baseline weight in months 1-24 under the MDPP Expanded Model (EM). This is a one-time payment available when a beneficiary first achieves at least 9% weight loss from baseline as measured by an in-person weight measurement at a core session, core maintenance session, or ongoing maintenance session ☒

G9882 Two Medicare Diabetes Prevention Program (MDPP) ongoing maintenance sessions (MS) were attended by an MDPP beneficiary in months (mo) 13-15 under the MDPP Expanded Model (EM). An ongoing maintenance session is an MDPP service that: (1) is furnished by an MDPP supplier during months 13 through 24 of the MDPP services period; (2) is approximately 1 hour in length; and (3) adheres to a CDC-approved DPP curriculum for maintenance sessions. The beneficiary maintained at least 5% weight loss (WL) from his/her baseline weight, as measured by at least one in-person weight measurement at an ongoing maintenance session in months 13-15 ☒

G9883 Two Medicare Diabetes Prevention Program (MDPP) ongoing maintenance sessions (MS) were attended by an MDPP beneficiary in months (mo) 16-18 under the MDPP Expanded Model (EM). An ongoing maintenance session is an MDPP service that: (1) is furnished by an MDPP supplier during months 13 through 24 of the MDPP services period; (2) is approximately 1 hour in length; and (3) adheres to a CDC-approved DPP curriculum for maintenance sessions. The beneficiary maintained at least 5% weight loss (WL) from his/her baseline weight, as measured by at least one in-person weight measurement at an ongoing maintenance session in months 16-18 ☒

G9884 Two Medicare Diabetes Prevention Program (MDPP) ongoing maintenance sessions (MS) were attended by an MDPP beneficiary in months (mo) 19-21 under the MDPP Expanded Model (EM). An ongoing maintenance session is an MDPP service that: (1) is furnished by an MDPP supplier during months 13 through 24 of the MDPP services period; (2) is approximately 1 hour in length; and (3) adheres to a CDC-approved DPP curriculum for maintenance sessions. The beneficiary maintained at least 5% weight loss (WL) from his/her baseline weight, as measured by at least one in-person weight measurement at an ongoing maintenance session in months 19-21 ☒

G9885 Two Medicare Diabetes Prevention Program (MDPP) ongoing maintenance sessions (MS) were attended by an MDPP beneficiary in months (mo) 22-24 under the MDPP Expanded Model (EM). An ongoing maintenance session is an MDPP service that: (1) is furnished by an MDPP supplier during months 13 through 24 of the MDPP services period; (2) is approximately 1 hour in length; and (3) adheres to a CDC-approved DPP curriculum for maintenance sessions. The beneficiary maintained at least 5% weight loss (WL) from his/her baseline weight, as measured by at least one in-person weight measurement at an ongoing maintenance session in months 22-24 ☒

G9890 Bridge Payment: A one-time payment for the first Medicare Diabetes Prevention Program (MDPP) core session, core maintenance session, or ongoing maintenance session furnished by an MDPP supplier to an MDPP beneficiary during months 1-24 of the MDPP Expanded Model (EM) who has previously received MDPP services from a different MDPP supplier under the MDPP Expanded Model. A supplier may only receive one bridge payment per MDPP beneficiary ☒

G9891 MDPP session reported as a line-item on a claim for a payable MDPP Expanded Model (EM) HCPCS code for a session furnished by the billing supplier under the MDPP Expanded Model and counting toward achievement of the attendance performance goal for the payable MDPP Expanded Model HCPCS code. (This code is for reporting purposes only) ☒

G9892 Documentation of patient reason(s) for not performing a dilated macular examination ☒

G9893 Dilated macular exam was not performed, reason not otherwise specified ☒

G9894 Androgen deprivation therapy prescribed/administered in combination with external beam radiotherapy to the prostate ☒

G9895 Documentation of medical reason(s) for not prescribing/administering androgen deprivation therapy in combination with external beam radiotherapy to the prostate (e.g., salvage therapy) ☒

G9896 Documentation of patient reason(s) for not prescribing/administering androgen deprivation therapy in combination with external beam radiotherapy to the prostate ☒

G9897 Patients who were not prescribed/administered androgen deprivation therapy in combination with external beam radiotherapy to the prostate, reason not given ☒

G9898 Patients age 66 or older in institutional special needs plans (SNP) or residing in long-term care with POS code 32, 33, 34, 54, or 56 for more than 90 consecutive days during the measurement period ☒

G9899 Screening, diagnostic, film, digital or digital breast tomosynthesis (3D) mammography results documented and reviewed ☒

G9900 Screening, diagnostic, film, digital or digital breast tomosynthesis (3D) mammography results were not documented and reviewed, reason not otherwise specified ☒

G9901 Patient age 66 or older in institutional special needs plans (SNP) or residing in long-term care with POS code 32, 33, 34, 54, or 56 for more than 90 consecutive days during the measurement period ☒

G9902 Patient screened for tobacco use and identified as a tobacco user ☒

G9903 Patient screened for tobacco use and identified as a tobacco nonuser ☒

G9905 Patient not screened for tobacco use ☒

G9906 Patient identified as a tobacco user received tobacco cessation intervention during the measurement period or in the 6 months prior to the measurement period (counseling and/or pharmacotherapy) ☒

G9908 Patient identified as tobacco user did not receive tobacco cessation intervention during the measurement period or in the 6 months prior to the measurement period (counseling and/or pharmacotherapy) ☒

G9910 Patients age 66 or older in institutional special needs plans (SNP) or residing in long-term care with POS code 32, 33, 34, 54 or 56 for more than 90 consecutive days during the measurement period ☒

G9911 Clinically node negative (T1N0M0 or T2N0M0) invasive breast cancer before or after neoadjuvant systemic therapy ☒

G9912 Hepatitis B virus (HBV) status assessed and results interpreted prior to initiating anti-TNF (tumor necrosis factor) therapy ☒

G9913 Hepatitis B virus (HBV) status not assessed and results interpreted prior to initiating anti-TNF (tumor necrosis factor) therapy, reason not otherwise specified ☒

▲ **G9914** Patient initiated an anti-TNF agent ☒

G9915 No record of HBV results documented ☒

G9916 Functional status performed once in the last 12 months ☒

Special Coverage Instructions   Noncovered by Medicare   Carrier Discretion   ☑ Quantity Alert ● New Code   ○ Recycled/Reinstated ▲ Revised Code

88 — G Codes   Ⓐ Age Edit   Ⓜ Maternity Edit   ♀ Female Only   ♂ Male Only   Ⓐ-Ⓨ OPPS Status Indicators   © 2023 Optum360, LLC

G9917 Documentation of advanced stage dementia and caregiver knowledge is limited ⓜ

G9918 Functional status not performed, reason not otherwise specified ⓜ

G9919 Screening performed and positive and provision of recommendations ⓜ

G9920 Screening performed and negative ⓜ

G9921 No screening performed, partial screening performed or positive screen without recommendations and reason is not given or otherwise specified ⓜ

G9922 Safety concerns screen provided and if positive then documented mitigation recommendations ⓜ

G9923 Safety concerns screen provided and negative ⓜ

G9925 Safety concerns screening not provided, reason not otherwise specified ⓜ

G9926 Safety concerns screening positive screen is without provision of mitigation recommendations, including but not limited to referral to other resources ⓜ

G9927 ~~Documentation of system reason(s) for not prescribing an FDA-approved anticoagulation due to patient being currently enrolled in a clinical trial related to AF/atrial flutter treatment~~

G9928 FDA-approved anticoagulant not prescribed, reason not given ⓜ

G9929 Patient with transient or reversible cause of AF (e.g., pneumonia, hyperthyroidism, pregnancy, cardiac surgery) ⓜ

G9930 Patients who are receiving comfort care only ⓜ

G9931 Documentation of CHA2DS2-VASc risk score of 0 or 1 for men; or 0, 1, or 2 for women ⓜ

▲ **G9938** Patients aged 66 or older in institutional special needs plans (SNP) or residing in long-term care with POS code 32, 33, 34, 54, or 56 for more than 90 consecutive days during the 6 months prior to the measurement period through December 31 of the measurement period ⓜ

G9939 Pathologist(s)/dermatopathologist(s) is the same clinician who performed the biopsy ⓜ

G9940 Documentation of medical reason(s) for not on a statin (e.g., pregnancy, in vitro fertilization, clomiphene Rx, ESRD, cirrhosis, muscular pain and disease during the measurement period or prior year) ⓜ

G9943 Back pain was not measured by the visual analog scale (VAS) or numeric pain scale at three months (6 to 20 weeks) postoperatively ⓜ

G9945 Patient had cancer, acute fracture or infection related to the lumbar spine or patient had neuromuscular, idiopathic or congenital lumbar scoliosis ⓜ

G9946 Back pain was not measured by the visual analog scale (VAS) or numeric pain scale at one year (9 to 15 months) postoperatively ⓜ

G9949 Leg pain was not measured by the visual analog scale (VAS) or numeric pain scale at three months (6 to 20 weeks) postoperatively ⓜ

G9954 Patient exhibits 2 or more risk factors for postoperative vomiting ⓜ

G9955 Cases in which an inhalational anesthetic is used only for induction ⓜ

G9956 Patient received combination therapy consisting of at least two prophylactic pharmacologic antiemetic agents of different classes preoperatively and/or intraoperatively ⓜ

G9957 Documentation of medical reason for not receiving combination therapy consisting of at least two prophylactic pharmacologic antiemetic agents of different classes preoperatively and/or intraoperatively (e.g., intolerance or other medical reason) ⓜ

G9958 Patient did not receive combination therapy consisting of at least two prophylactic pharmacologic antiemetic agents of different classes preoperatively and/or intraoperatively ⓜ

G9959 Systemic antimicrobials not prescribed ⓜ

G9960 Documentation of medical reason(s) for prescribing systemic antimicrobials ⓜ

G9961 Systemic antimicrobials prescribed ⓜ

G9962 Embolization endpoints are documented separately for each embolized vessel and ovarian artery angiography or embolization performed in the presence of variant uterine artery anatomy ⓜ

G9963 Embolization endpoints are not documented separately for each embolized vessel or ovarian artery angiography or embolization not performed in the presence of variant uterine artery anatomy ⓜ

G9964 Patient received at least one well-child visit with a PCP during the performance period ⓜ

G9965 Patient did not receive at least one well-child visit with PCP during the performance period ⓜ

G9968 Patient was referred to another clinician or specialist during the measurement period ⓜ

G9969 Clinician who referred the patient to another clinician received a report from the clinician to whom the patient was referred ⓜ

G9970 Clinician who referred the patient to another clinician did not receive a report from the clinician to whom the patient was referred ⓜ

G9974 Dilated macular exam performed, including documentation of the presence or absence of macular thickening or geographic atrophy or hemorrhage and the level of macular degeneration severity ⓜ

G9975 Documentation of medical reason(s) for not performing a dilated macular examination ⓜ

G9976 Documentation of patient reason(s) for not performing a dilated macular examination ⓜ

G9977 Dilated macular exam was not performed, reason not otherwise specified ⓜ

G9978 Remote in-home visit for the evaluation and management of a new patient for use only in a Medicare-approved Bundled Payments for Care Improvement Advanced (BPCI Advanced) model episode of care, which requires these three key components: a problem focused history; a problem focused examination; straightforward medical decision making, furnished in real time using interactive audio and video technology. Counseling and coordination of care with other physicians, other qualified health care professionals or agencies are provided consistent with the nature of the problem(s) and the needs of the patient or the family or both. Usually, the presenting problem(s) are self limited or minor. Typically, 10 minutes are spent with the patient or family or both via real time, audio and video intercommunications technology

Special Coverage Instructions   Noncovered by Medicare   Carrier Discretion   ☑ Quantity Alert   ● New Code   ○ Recycled/Reinstated   ▲ Revised Code

© 2023 Optum360, LLC   A2-Z3 ASC Pmt   **CMS:** IOM   **AHA:** Coding Clinic   ⅃ DMEPOS Paid   ⊘ SNF Excluded   **G Codes — 89**

Procedures/Professional Services (Temporary)

G9979 — G9986

G9979 Remote in-home visit for the evaluation and management of a new patient for use only in a Medicare-approved Bundled Payments for Care Improvement Advanced (BPCI Advanced) model episode of care, which requires these three key components: an expanded problem focused history; an expanded problem focused examination; straightforward medical decision making, furnished in real time using interactive audio and video technology. Counseling and coordination of care with other physicians, other qualified health care professionals or agencies are provided consistent with the nature of the problem(s) and the needs of the patient or the family or both. Usually, the presenting problem(s) are of low to moderate severity. Typically, 20 minutes are spent with the patient or family or both via real time, audio and video intercommunications technology

G9980 Remote in-home visit for the evaluation and management of a new patient for use only in a Medicare-approved Bundled Payments for Care Improvement Advanced (BPCI Advanced) model episode of care, which requires these three key components: a detailed history; a detailed examination; medical decision making of low complexity, furnished in real time using interactive audio and video technology. Counseling and coordination of care with other physicians, other qualified health care professionals or agencies are provided consistent with the nature of the problem(s) and the needs of the patient or the family or both. Usually, the presenting problem(s) are of moderate severity. Typically, 30 minutes are spent with the patient or family or both via real time, audio and video intercommunications technology

G9981 Remote in-home visit for the evaluation and management of a new patient for use only in a Medicare-approved Bundled Payments for Care Improvement Advanced (BPCI Advanced) model episode of care, which requires these three key components: a comprehensive history; a comprehensive examination; medical decision making of moderate complexity, furnished in real time using interactive audio and video technology. Counseling and coordination of care with other physicians, other qualified health care professionals or agencies are provided consistent with the nature of the problem(s) and the needs of the patient or the family or both. Usually, the presenting problem(s) are of moderate to high severity. Typically, 45 minutes are spent with the patient or family or both via real time, audio and video intercommunications technology

G9982 Remote in-home visit for the evaluation and management of a new patient for use only in a Medicare-approved Bundled Payments for Care Improvement Advanced (BPCI Advanced) model episode of care, which requires these three key components: a comprehensive history; a comprehensive examination; medical decision making of high complexity, furnished in real time using interactive audio and video technology. Counseling and coordination of care with other physicians, other qualified health care professionals or agencies are provided consistent with the nature of the problem(s) and the needs of the patient or the family or both. Usually, the presenting problem(s) are of moderate to high severity. Typically, 60 minutes are spent with the patient or family or both via real time, audio and video intercommunications technology

G9983 Remote in-home visit for the evaluation and management of an established patient for use only in a Medicare-approved Bundled Payments for Care Improvement Advanced (BPCI Advanced) model episode of care, which requires at least two of the following three key components: a problem focused history; a problem focused examination; straightforward medical decision making, furnished in real time using interactive audio and video technology. Counseling and coordination of care with other physicians, other qualified health care professionals or agencies are provided consistent with the nature of the problem(s) and the needs of the patient or the family or both. Usually, the presenting problem(s) are self limited or minor. Typically, 10 minutes are spent with the patient or family or both via real time, audio and video intercommunications technology

G9984 Remote in-home visit for the evaluation and management of an established patient for use only in a Medicare-approved Bundled Payments for Care Improvement Advanced (BPCI Advanced) model episode of care, which requires at least two of the following three key components: an expanded problem focused history; an expanded problem focused examination; medical decision making of low complexity, furnished in real time using interactive audio and video technology. Counseling and coordination of care with other physicians, other qualified health care professionals or agencies are provided consistent with the nature of the problem(s) and the needs of the patient or the family or both. Usually, the presenting problem(s) are of low to moderate severity. Typically, 15 minutes are spent with the patient or family or both via real time, audio and video intercommunications technology

G9985 Remote in-home visit for the evaluation and management of an established patient for use only in a Medicare-approved Bundled Payments for Care Improvement Advanced (BPCI Advanced) model episode of care, which requires at least two of the following three key components: a detailed history; a detailed examination; medical decision making of moderate complexity, furnished in real time using interactive audio and video technology. Counseling and coordination of care with other physicians, other qualified health care professionals or agencies are provided consistent with the nature of the problem(s) and the needs of the patient or the family or both. Usually, the presenting problem(s) are of moderate to high severity. Typically, 25 minutes are spent with the patient or family or both via real time, audio and video intercommunications technology

G9986 Remote in-home visit for the evaluation and management of an established patient for use only in a Medicare-approved Bundled Payments for Care Improvement Advanced (BPCI Advanced) model episode of care, which requires at least two of the following three key components: a comprehensive history; a comprehensive examination; medical decision making of high complexity, furnished in real time using interactive audio and video technology. Counseling and coordination of care with other physicians, other qualified health care professionals or agencies are provided consistent with the nature of the problem(s) and the needs of the patient or the family or both. Usually, the presenting problem(s) are of moderate to high severity. Typically, 40 minutes are spent with the patient or family or both via real time, audio and video intercommunications technology

Special Coverage Instructions   Noncovered by Medicare   Carrier Discretion   ☑ Quantity Alert ● New Code   ○ Recycled/Reinstated ▲ Revised Code

90 — G Codes   🅰 Age Edit   Ⓜ Maternity Edit   ♀ Female Only   ♂ Male Only   🅰-🆈 OPPS Status Indicators   © 2023 Optum360, LLC

G9987   Bundled Payments for Care Improvement Advanced (BPCI Advanced) model home visit for patient assessment performed by clinical staff for an individual not considered homebound, including, but not necessarily limited to patient assessment of clinical status, safety/fall prevention, functional status/ambulation, medication reconciliation/management, compliance with orders/plan of care, performance of activities of daily living, and ensuring beneficiary connections to community and other services; for use only for a BPCI Advanced model episode of care; may not be billed for a 30-day period covered by a transitional care management code

G9988   Palliative care services provided to patient any time during the measurement period

▲ **G9990**   Patient did not receive any pneumococcal conjugate or polysaccharide vaccine on or after their 19th birthday and before the end of the measurement period

▲ **G9991**   Patient received any pneumococcal conjugate or polysaccharide vaccine on or after their 19th birthday and before the end of the measurement period

G9992   Palliative care services used by patient any time during the measurement period

G9993   Patient was provided palliative care services any time during the measurement period

G9994   Patient is using palliative care services any time during the measurement period

G9995   ~~Patients who use palliative care services any time during the measurement period~~

G9996   Documentation stating the patient has received or is currently receiving palliative or hospice care

G9997   Documentation of patient pregnancy anytime during the measurement period prior to and including the current encounter

▲ **G9998**   Documentation of medical reason(s) for an interval of less than 3 years since the last colonoscopy (e.g., last colonoscopy incomplete, last colonoscopy had inadequate prep, piecemeal removal of adenomas, or sessile serrated polyps >= 20 mm in size, last colonoscopy found greater than 10 adenomas, lower gastrointestinal bleeding, or patient at high risk for colon cancer due to underlying medical history [i.e., Crohn's disease, ulcerative colitis, personal or family history of colon cancer, hereditary colorectal cancer syndromes])

G9999   Documentation of system reason(s) for an interval of less than 3 years since the last colonoscopy (e.g., unable to locate previous colonoscopy report, previous colonoscopy report was incomplete)

Special Coverage Instructions   Noncovered by Medicare   Carrier Discretion   ☑ Quantity Alert   ● New Code   ○ Recycled/Reinstated   ▲ Revised Code

© 2023 Optum360, LLC   A2-Z3 ASC Pmt   **CMS:** IOM   **AHA:** Coding Clinic   ⅄ DMEPOS Paid   ⊘ SNF Excluded   **G Codes — 91**

Alcohol and Drug Abuse Treatment Services H0001-H2041

The H codes are used by those state Medicaid agencies that are mandated by state law to establish separate codes for identifying mental health services that include alcohol and drug treatment services.

H0001	Alcohol and/or drug assessment	
H0002	Behavioral health screening to determine eligibility for admission to treatment program	
H0003	Alcohol and/or drug screening; laboratory analysis of specimens for presence of alcohol and/or drugs	
H0004	Behavioral health counseling and therapy, per 15 minutes	☑
H0005	Alcohol and/or drug services; group counseling by a clinician	
H0006	Alcohol and/or drug services; case management	
H0007	Alcohol and/or drug services; crisis intervention (outpatient)	
H0008	Alcohol and/or drug services; subacute detoxification (hospital inpatient)	
H0009	Alcohol and/or drug services; acute detoxification (hospital inpatient)	
H0010	Alcohol and/or drug services; subacute detoxification (residential addiction program inpatient)	
H0011	Alcohol and/or drug services; acute detoxification (residential addiction program inpatient)	
H0012	Alcohol and/or drug services; subacute detoxification (residential addiction program outpatient)	
H0013	Alcohol and/or drug services; acute detoxification (residential addiction program outpatient)	
H0014	Alcohol and/or drug services; ambulatory detoxification	
H0015	Alcohol and/or drug services; intensive outpatient (treatment program that operates at least 3 hours/day and at least 3 days/week and is based on an individualized treatment plan), including assessment, counseling; crisis intervention, and activity therapies or education	
H0016	Alcohol and/or drug services; medical/somatic (medical intervention in ambulatory setting)	
H0017	Behavioral health; residential (hospital residential treatment program), without room and board, per diem	☑
H0018	Behavioral health; short-term residential (nonhospital residential treatment program), without room and board, per diem	☑
H0019	Behavioral health; long-term residential (nonmedical, nonacute care in a residential treatment program where stay is typically longer than 30 days), without room and board, per diem	☑
H0020	Alcohol and/or drug services; methadone administration and/or service (provision of the drug by a licensed program)	
H0021	Alcohol and/or drug training service (for staff and personnel not employed by providers)	
H0022	Alcohol and/or drug intervention service (planned facilitation)	
H0023	Behavioral health outreach service (planned approach to reach a targeted population)	
H0024	Behavioral health prevention information dissemination service (one-way direct or nondirect contact with service audiences to affect knowledge and attitude)	
H0025	Behavioral health prevention education service (delivery of services with target population to affect knowledge, attitude and/or behavior)	
H0026	Alcohol and/or drug prevention process service, community-based (delivery of services to develop skills of impactors)	

H0027	Alcohol and/or drug prevention environmental service (broad range of external activities geared toward modifying systems in order to mainstream prevention through policy and law)	
H0028	Alcohol and/or drug prevention problem identification and referral service (e.g., student assistance and employee assistance programs), does not include assessment	
H0029	Alcohol and/or drug prevention alternatives service (services for populations that exclude alcohol and other drug use e.g., alcohol free social events)	
H0030	Behavioral health hotline service	
H0031	Mental health assessment, by nonphysician	
H0032	Mental health service plan development by nonphysician	
H0033	Oral medication administration, direct observation	
H0034	Medication training and support, per 15 minutes	☑
H0035	Mental health partial hospitalization, treatment, less than 24 hours	☑
H0036	Community psychiatric supportive treatment, face-to-face, per 15 minutes	☑
H0037	Community psychiatric supportive treatment program, per diem	☑
H0038	Self-help/peer services, per 15 minutes	☑
H0039	Assertive community treatment, face-to-face, per 15 minutes	☑
H0040	Assertive community treatment program, per diem	☑
H0041	Foster care, child, nontherapeutic, per diem	A ☑
H0042	Foster care, child, nontherapeutic, per month	A ☑
H0043	Supported housing, per diem	☑
H0044	Supported housing, per month	☑
H0045	Respite care services, not in the home, per diem	☑
H0046	Mental health services, not otherwise specified	
H0047	Alcohol and/or other drug abuse services, not otherwise specified	
H0048	Alcohol and/or other drug testing: collection and handling only, specimens other than blood	
H0049	Alcohol and/or drug screening	
H0050	Alcohol and/or drug services, brief intervention, per 15 minutes	☑
H1000	Prenatal care, at-risk assessment	M ♀
H1001	Prenatal care, at-risk enhanced service; antepartum management	M ♀
H1002	Prenatal care, at risk enhanced service; care coordination	M ♀
H1003	Prenatal care, at-risk enhanced service; education	M ♀
H1004	Prenatal care, at-risk enhanced service; follow-up home visit	M ♀
H1005	Prenatal care, at-risk enhanced service package (includes H1001-H1004)	M ♀
H1010	Nonmedical family planning education, per session	☑
H1011	Family assessment by licensed behavioral health professional for state defined purposes	
H2000	Comprehensive multidisciplinary evaluation	
H2001	Rehabilitation program, per 1/2 day	☑
H2010	Comprehensive medication services, per 15 minutes	☑

Special Coverage Instructions   Noncovered by Medicare   Carrier Discretion   ☑ Quantity Alert ● New Code   ○ Recycled/Reinstated ▲ Revised Code

92 — H Codes   A Age Edit   M Maternity Edit   ♀ Female Only   ♂ Male Only   A-Y OPPS Status Indicators   © 2023 Optum360, LLC

Code	Description	
H2011	Crisis intervention service, per 15 minutes	☑
H2012	Behavioral health day treatment, per hour	☑
H2013	Psychiatric health facility service, per diem	☑
H2014	Skills training and development, per 15 minutes	☑
H2015	Comprehensive community support services, per 15 minutes	☑
H2016	Comprehensive community support services, per diem	☑
H2017	Psychosocial rehabilitation services, per 15 minutes	☑
H2018	Psychosocial rehabilitation services, per diem	☑
H2019	Therapeutic behavioral services, per 15 minutes	☑
H2020	Therapeutic behavioral services, per diem	☑
H2021	Community-based wrap-around services, per 15 minutes	☑
H2022	Community-based wrap-around services, per diem	☑
H2023	Supported employment, per 15 minutes	☑
H2024	Supported employment, per diem	☑
H2025	Ongoing support to maintain employment, per 15 minutes	☑
H2026	Ongoing support to maintain employment, per diem	☑
H2027	Psychoeducational service, per 15 minutes	☑
H2028	Sexual offender treatment service, per 15 minutes	☑
H2029	Sexual offender treatment service, per diem	☑
H2030	Mental health clubhouse services, per 15 minutes	☑
H2031	Mental health clubhouse services, per diem	☑
H2032	Activity therapy, per 15 minutes	☑
H2033	Multisystemic therapy for juveniles, per 15 minutes	☑
H2034	Alcohol and/or drug abuse halfway house services, per diem	☑
H2035	Alcohol and/or other drug treatment program, per hour	☑
H2036	Alcohol and/or other drug treatment program, per diem	☑
H2037	Developmental delay prevention activities, dependent child of client, per 15 minutes	Ⓐ ☑
H2038	Skills training and development, per diem	
● H2040	Coordinated specialty care, team-based, for first episode psychosis, per month	
● H2041	Coordinated specialty care, team-based, for first episode psychosis, per encounter	

Special Coverage Instructions   Noncovered by Medicare   Carrier Discretion   ☑ Quantity Alert   ● New Code   ○ Recycled/Reinstated   ▲ Revised Code

© 2023 Optum360, LLC   A2-Z3 ASC Pmt   CMS: IOM   AHA: Coding Clinic   ♿ DMEPOS Paid   ⊘ SNF Excluded   H Codes — 93

J Codes Drugs J0120-J8499

J codes include drugs that ordinarily cannot be self-administered, chemotherapy drugs, immunosuppressive drugs, inhalation solutions, and other miscellaneous drugs and solutions.

Miscellaneous Drugs

J0120 Injection, tetracycline, up to 250 mg ☒ ☒ ☑
AHA: 4Q,18

J0121 Injection, omadacycline, 1 mg K2
Use this code for Nuzyra.
AHA: 4Q,19

J0122 Injection, eravacycline, 1 mg N1
Use this code for Xerava.
AHA: 4Q,19

J0129 Injection, abatacept, 10 mg (code may be used for Medicare when drug administered under the direct supervision of a physician, not for use when drug is self-administered) K K2 ☑
Use this code for Orencia.
CMS: 100-02,15,50.5
AHA: 4Q,18

J0130 Injection abciximab, 10 mg N N1 ☑
Use this code for ReoPro.
AHA: 4Q,18

J0131 Injection, acetaminophen, not otherwise specified, 10 mg N N1 ☑
AHA: 1Q,23; 4Q,18

J0132 Injection, acetylcysteine, 100 mg N N1 ☑
Use this code for Acetadote.
AHA: 4Q,18

J0133 Injection, acyclovir, 5 mg N N1 ☑
Use this code for Zovirax.
CMS: 100-04,20,180; 100-04,32,411.3
AHA: 4Q,18

J0134 Injection, acetaminophen (Fresenius Kabi) not therapeutically equivalent to J0131, 10 mg
Use this code for acetaminophen manufactured by Fresenius Kabi.
AHA: 1Q,23

J0135 Injection, adalimumab, 20 mg K K2 ☑
Use this code for Humira.
CMS: 100-02,15,50.5
AHA: 4Q,18

J0136 Injection, acetaminophen (B. Braun) not therapeutically equivalent to J0131, 10 mg
Use this code for acetaminophen manufactured by B. Braun.
AHA: 1Q,23

● **J0137** Injection, acetaminophen (Hikma) not therapeutically equivalent to J0131, 10 mg
Use this code for acetaminophen manufactured by Hikma.
AHA: 3Q,23

J0153 Injection, adenosine, 1 mg (not to be used to report any adenosine phosphate compounds) N N1 ☑
Use this code for Adenocard, Adenoscan.
AHA: 4Q,18

J0171 Injection, adrenalin, epinephrine, 0.1 mg N N1 ☑
AHA: 4Q,18

J0172 Injection, aducanumab-avwa, 2 mg K2
Use this code for Aduhelm.
AHA: 1Q,22

J0173 Injection, epinephrine (Belcher) not therapeutically equivalent to J0171, 0.1 mg
Use this code for epinephrine manufactured by Belcher.
AHA: 1Q,23

● **J0174** Injection, lecanemab-irmb, 1 mg K2
Use this code for Leqembi.
AHA: 3Q,23

J0178 Injection, aflibercept, 1 mg K K2 ☑
Use this code for Eylea.
AHA: 4Q,18

J0179 Injection, brolucizumab-dbll, 1 mg K2
Use this code for Beovu.
AHA: 1Q,20

J0180 Injection, agalsidase beta, 1 mg K K2 ☑
Use this code for Fabrazyme.
AHA: 4Q,18

● **J0184** Injection, amisulpride, 1 mg
Use this code for Barhemsys.

J0185 Injection, aprepitant, 1 mg K2
Use this code for Cinvanti.
AHA: 1Q,19; 4Q,18

J0190 Injection, biperiden lactate, per 5 mg E1 ☑
AHA: 4Q,18

J0200 Injection, alatrofloxacin mesylate, 100 mg E1 ☑
AHA: 4Q,18

J0202 Injection, alemtuzumab, 1 mg K K2 ☑
Use this code for Lemtrada.
AHA: 4Q,18

J0205 Injection, alglucerase, per 10 units E1 ☑
Use this code for Ceredase.
AHA: 4Q,18

● **J0206** Injection, allopurinol sodium, 1 mg
AHA: 3Q,23

J0207 Injection, amifostine, 500 mg K N1 ☑
Use this code for Ethyol.
AHA: 4Q,18

● **J0208** Injection, sodium thiosulfate, 100 mg K2
Use this code for Pedmark.
AHA: 2Q,23

J0210 Injection, methyldopate HCl, up to 250 mg N ☑
Use this code for Aldomet.
AHA: 4Q,18

J0215 Injection, alefacept, 0.5 mg E1 ☑
Use this for Amevive.
AHA: 4Q,18

● **J0216** Injection, alfentanil HCl, 500 mcg
AHA: 3Q,23

● **J0217** Injection, velmanase alfa-tycv, 1 mg
Use this code for Lamzede.

● **J0218** Injection, olipudase alfa-rpcp, 1 mg K2
Use this code for Xenpozyme.
AHA: 2Q,23

J0219 Injection, avalglucosidase alfa-ngpt, 4 mg K2
Use this code for Nexviazyme.
AHA: 2Q,22

Special Coverage Instructions   Noncovered by Medicare   Carrier Discretion   ☑ Quantity Alert ● New Code ○ Recycled/Reinstated ▲ Revised Code

Drugs Administered Other Than Oral Method

J0220 — J0457

Code	Description	Indicators
J0220	**Injection, alglucosidase alfa, 10 mg, not otherwise specified** Use this code for Myozyme. **AHA:** 4Q,18	K K2 ☑
J0221	**Injection, alglucosidase alfa, (Lumizyme), 10 mg** **AHA:** 4Q,18	K K2 ☑
J0222	**Injection, patisiran, 0.1 mg** Use this code for Onpattro. **AHA:** 4Q,19	K2
J0223	**Injection, givosiran, 0.5 mg** Use this code for Givlaari. **AHA:** 2Q,20	K2
J0224	**Injection, lumasiran, 0.5 mg** **AHA:** 3Q,21	K2
J0225	**Injection, vutrisiran, 1 mg** **AHA:** 1Q,23	K2
J0248	**Injection, remdesivir, 1 mg** **AHA:** 1Q,22	
J0256	**Injection, alpha 1-proteinase inhibitor (human), not otherwise specified, 10 mg** Use this code for Aralast, Aralast NP, Prolastin C, Zemaira. **AHA:** 4Q,18	K K2 ☑
J0257	**Injection, alpha 1 proteinase inhibitor (human), (GLASSIA), 10 mg** **AHA:** 4Q,18	K K2 ☑
J0270	**Injection, alprostadil, 1.25 mcg (code may be used for Medicare when drug administered under the direct supervision of a physician, not for use when drug is self-administered)** Use this code for Alprostadil, Caverject, Edex, Prostin VR Pediatric. **AHA:** 4Q,18	B ☑
J0275	**Alprostadil urethral suppository (code may be used for Medicare when drug administered under the direct supervision of a physician, not for use when drug is self-administered)** Use this code for Muse. **AHA:** 4Q,18	B ☑
J0278	**Injection, amikacin sulfate, 100 mg** Use this code for Amikin. **AHA:** 4Q,18	N N1 ☑
J0280	**Injection, aminophylline, up to 250 mg** **AHA:** 4Q,18	N N1 ☑
J0282	**Injection, amiodarone HCl, 30 mg** Use this code for Cordarone IV. **AHA:** 4Q,18	N N1 ☑
J0283	**Injection, amiodarone HCl (Nexterone), 30 mg** **AHA:** 1Q,23	
J0285	**Injection, amphotericin B, 50 mg** Use this for Amphocin, Fungizone. **CMS:** 100-04,20,180; 100-04,32,411.3 **AHA:** 4Q,18	N N1 ☑
J0287	**Injection, amphotericin B lipid complex, 10 mg** Use this code for Abelcet. **CMS:** 100-04,20,180; 100-04,32,411.3 **AHA:** 4Q,18	K K2 ☑
J0288	**Injection, amphotericin B cholesteryl sulfate complex, 10 mg** Use this code for Amphotec. **CMS:** 100-04,20,180; 100-04,32,411.3 **AHA:** 4Q,18	EI ☑
J0289	**Injection, amphotericin B liposome, 10 mg** Use this code for Ambisome. **CMS:** 100-04,20,180; 100-04,32,411.3 **AHA:** 4Q,18	K K2 ☑
J0290	**Injection, ampicillin sodium, 500 mg** **AHA:** 4Q,18	N N1 ☑
J0291	**Injection, plazomicin, 5 mg** Use this code for Zemdri. **AHA:** 4Q,19	K2
J0295	**Injection, ampicillin sodium/sulbactam sodium, per 1.5 g** Use this code for Unasyn. **AHA:** 4Q,18	N N1 ☑
J0300	**Injection, amobarbital, up to 125 mg** Use this code for Amytal. **AHA:** 4Q,18	K K2 ☑
J0330	**Injection, succinylcholine chloride, up to 20 mg** Use this code for Anectine, Quelicin. **AHA:** 4Q,18	N N1 ☑
J0348	**Injection, anidulafungin, 1 mg** Use this code for Eraxis. **AHA:** 4Q,18	N N1 ☑
● **J0349**	**Injection, rezafungin, 1 mg** Use this code for Rezzayo.	K2
J0350	**Injection, anistreplase, per 30 units** Use this code for Eminase. **AHA:** 4Q,18	EI ☑
J0360	**Injection, hydralazine HCl, up to 20 mg** **AHA:** 4Q,18	N N1 ☑
J0364	**Injection, apomorphine HCl, 1 mg** Use this code for Apokyn. **CMS:** 100-02,15,50.5 **AHA:** 4Q,18	EI ☑
J0365	**Injection, aprotinin, 10,000 kiu** Use this code for Trasylol. **AHA:** 4Q,18	EI ☑
J0380	**Injection, metaraminol bitartrate, per 10 mg** Use this code for Aramine. **AHA:** 4Q,18	N ☑
J0390	**Injection, chloroquine HCl, up to 250 mg** Use this code for Aralen. **AHA:** 4Q,18	N K2 ☑
● **J0391**	**Injection, artesunate, 1 mg**	
J0395	**Injection, arbutamine HCl, 1 mg** **AHA:** 4Q,18	EI ☑
J0400	**Injection, aripiprazole, intramuscular, 0.25 mg** Use this code for Abilify. **AHA:** 4Q,18	K K2 ☑
J0401	**Injection, aripiprazole, extended release, 1 mg** Use this code for the Abilify Maintena kit. **AHA:** 4Q,18	K K2 ☑
● **J0402**	**Injection, aripiprazole (Abilify Asimtufii), 1 mg**	
J0456	**Injection, azithromycin, 500 mg** Use this code for Zithromax. **AHA:** 4Q,18	N N1 ☑
● **J0457**	**Injection, aztreonam, 100 mg** Use this code for Azactam. **AHA:** 3Q,23	

Special Coverage Instructions   Noncovered by Medicare   Carrier Discretion   ☑ Quantity Alert   ● New Code   ○ Recycled/Reinstated   ▲ Revised Code

   A Age Edit   M Maternity Edit   ♀ Female Only   ♂ Male Only   A-Y OPPS Status Indicators   © 2023 Optum360, LLC

J0461	**Injection, atropine sulfate, 0.01 mg**	N N1 ☑
	Use this code for AtroPen.	
	AHA: 4Q,18	
J0470	**Injection, dimercaprol, per 100 mg**	K K2 ☑
	Use this code for BAL.	
	AHA: 4Q,18	
J0475	**Injection, baclofen, 10 mg**	K K2 ☑
	Use this code for Lioresal, Gablofen.	
	AHA: 4Q,18	
J0476	**Injection, baclofen, 50 mcg for intrathecal trial**	K N1 ☑
	Use this code for Lioresal, Gablofen.	
	AHA: 4Q,18	
J0480	**Injection, basiliximab, 20 mg**	K K2 ☑
	Use this code for Simulect.	
	AHA: 4Q,18	
J0485	**Injection, belatacept, 1 mg**	K K2 ☑
	Use this code for Nulojix.	
	AHA: 4Q,18	
J0490	**Injection, belimumab, 10 mg**	K K2 ☑
	Use this code for BENLYSTA.	
	AHA: 4Q,18	
J0491	**Injection, anifrolumab-fnia, 1 mg**	K2
	Use this code for Saphnelo.	
	AHA: 2Q,22	
J0500	**Injection, dicyclomine HCl, up to 20 mg**	N N1 ☑
	Use this code for Bentyl.	
	AHA: 4Q,18	
J0515	**Injection, benztropine mesylate, per 1 mg**	N N1 ☑
	Use this code for Cogentin.	
	AHA: 4Q,18	
J0517	**Injection, benralizumab, 1 mg**	K2
	Use this code for Fasenra.	
	AHA: 1Q,19; 4Q,18	
J0520	**Injection, bethanechol chloride, Myotonachol or Urecholine, up to 5 mg**	EI ☑
	AHA: 4Q,18	
J0558	**Injection, penicillin G benzathine and penicillin G procaine, 100,000 units**	N K2 ☑
	Use this code for Bicillin CR, Bicillin CR 900/300, Bicillin CR Tubex.	
	AHA: 4Q,18	
J0561	**Injection, penicillin G benzathine, 100,000 units**	K K2 ☑
	AHA: 4Q,18	
J0565	**Injection, bezlotoxumab, 10 mg**	G K2
	Use this code for Zinplava.	
	AHA: 4Q,18; 1Q,18	
J0567	**Injection, cerliponase alfa, 1 mg**	
	Use this code for Brineura.	
	AHA: 1Q,19; 4Q,18	
J0570	**Buprenorphine implant, 74.2 mg**	G K2 ☑
	Use this code for Probuphine.	
J0571	**Buprenorphine, oral, 1 mg**	EI ☑
	Use this code for Subutex.	
J0572	**Buprenorphine/naloxone, oral, less than or equal to 3 mg buprenorphine**	EI ☑
	Use this code for Bunavail, Suboxone, Zubsolv.	
J0573	**Buprenorphine/naloxone, oral, greater than 3 mg, but less than or equal to 6 mg buprenorphine**	EI ☑
	Use this code for Bunavail, Suboxone, Zubsolv.	

J0574	**Buprenorphine/naloxone, oral, greater than 6 mg, but less than or equal to 10 mg buprenorphine**	EI ☑
	Use this code for Bunavail, Suboxone.	
J0575	**Buprenorphine/naloxone, oral, greater than 10 mg buprenorphine**	EI ☑
	Use this code for Suboxone.	
● **J0576**	**Injection, buprenorphine extended-release (Brixadi), 1 mg**	
J0583	**Injection, bivalirudin, 1 mg**	N N1 ☑
	Use this code for Angiomax.	
	AHA: 4Q,18	
J0584	**Injection, burosumab-twza, 1 mg**	K2
	Use this code for Crysvita.	
	CMS: 100-04,4,260.1; 100-04,4,260.1.1	
	AHA: 1Q,19; 4Q,18	
J0585	**Injection, onabotulinumtoxinA, 1 unit**	K K2 ☑
	Use this code for Botox, Botox Cosmetic.	
	AHA: 2Q,21; 4Q,18	
J0586	**Injection, abobotulinumtoxinA, 5 units**	K K2 ☑
	Use this code for Dysport.	
	AHA: 4Q,18	
J0587	**Injection, rimabotulinumtoxinB, 100 units**	K K2 ☑
	Use this code for Myobloc.	
	AHA: 4Q,18	
J0588	**Injection, incobotulinumtoxinA, 1 unit**	K K2 ☑
	Use this code for XEOMIN.	
	AHA: 4Q,18	
J0591	**Injection, deoxycholic acid, 1 mg**	
	Use this code for Kybella.	
	AHA: 2Q,20	
J0592	**Injection, buprenorphine HCl, 0.1 mg**	N N1 ☑
	Use this code for Buprenex.	
	AHA: 4Q,18	
J0593	**Injection, lanadelumab-flyo, 1 mg (code may be used for Medicare when drug administered under direct supervision of a physician, not for use when drug is self-administered)**	
	Use this code for Takhzyro.	
	AHA: 4Q,19	
J0594	**Injection, busulfan, 1 mg**	K K2 ☑
	Use this code for Busulfex.	
	AHA: 4Q,18	
J0595	**Injection, butorphanol tartrate, 1 mg**	N N1 ☑
	Use this code for Stadol.	
	AHA: 4Q,18	
J0596	**Injection, C1 esterase inhibitor (recombinant), Ruconest, 10 units**	K K2 ☑
	CMS: 100-02,15,50.5	
	AHA: 4Q,18	
J0597	**Injection, C1 esterase inhibitor (human), Berinert, 10 units**	K K2 ☑
	AHA: 4Q,18	
J0598	**Injection, C1 esterase inhibitor (human), Cinryze, 10 units**	K K2 ☑
	AHA: 4Q,18	
J0599	**Injection, C1 esterase inhibitor (human), (Haegarda), 10 units**	
	AHA: 1Q,19; 4Q,18	
J0600	**Injection, edetate calcium disodium, up to 1,000 mg**	K K2 ☑
	Use this code for Calcium Disodium Versenate, Calcium EDTA.	
	AHA: 4Q,18	

Special Coverage Instructions   Noncovered by Medicare   Carrier Discretion   ☑ Quantity Alert   ● New Code   ○ Recycled/Reinstated   ▲ Revised Code

J0604 Cinacalcet, oral, 1 mg, (for ESRD on dialysis) 🅱
Use this code for Sensipar.
AHA: 4Q,18; 1Q,18

J0606 Injection, etelcalcetide, 0.1 mg 🅚 N1
Use this code for Parsabiv.
AHA: 4Q,18; 2Q,18; 1Q,18

J0610 ~~Injection, calcium gluconate (Fresenius Kabi), per 10 ml~~
To report, see ~J0612

J0611 ~~Injection, calcium gluconate (WG Critical Care), per 10 ml~~
To report, see ~J0613

● **J0612** Injection, calcium gluconate (Fresenius Kabi), per 10 mg N1
Use this code for calcium gluconate manufactured by Fresenius Kabi.
AHA: 2Q,23

● **J0613** Injection, calcium gluconate (WG Critical Care), per 10 mg N1
Use this code for calcium gluconate manufactured by WG Critical Care.
AHA: 2Q,23

J0620 Injection, calcium glycerophosphate and calcium lactate, per 10 ml N N1 ☑
AHA: 4Q,18

J0630 Injection, calcitonin salmon, up to 400 units 🅚 K2 ☑
Use this code for Calcimar, Miacalcin.
CMS: 100-04,10,90.1
AHA: 4Q,18

J0636 Injection, calcitriol, 0.1 mcg N N1 ☑
Use this code for Calcijex.
AHA: 4Q,18

J0637 Injection, caspofungin acetate, 5 mg 🅚 N1 ☑
Use this code for Cancidas.
AHA: 4Q,18

J0638 Injection, canakinumab, 1 mg 🅚 K2 ☑
Use this code for ILARIS.
AHA: 4Q,18

J0640 Injection, leucovorin calcium, per 50 mg N N1 ☑
AHA: 4Q,18

J0641 Injection, levoleucovorin, not otherwise specified, 0.5 mg 🅚 K2 ☑
AHA: 4Q,19; 4Q,18

J0642 Injection, levoleucovorin (Khapzory), 0.5 mg N1
AHA: 1Q,20; 4Q,19

● **J0665** Injection, bupivicaine, not otherwise specified, 0.5 mg
AHA: 3Q,23

J0670 Injection, mepivacaine HCl, per 10 ml N N1 ☑
Use this code for Carbocaine, Polocaine, Isocaine HCl, Scandonest
AHA: 4Q,18

● **J0688** Injection, cefazolin sodium (Hikma), not therapeutically equivalent to J0690, 500 mg

J0689 Injection, cefazolin sodium (Baxter), not therapeutically equivalent to J0690, 500 mg
Use this code for cefazolin sodium manufactured by Baxter.
AHA: 1Q,23

J0690 Injection, cefazolin sodium, 500 mg N N1 ☑
AHA: 4Q,18

J0691 Injection, lefamulin, 1 mg N1
Use this code for Xenleta.
AHA: 2Q,20

J0692 Injection, cefepime HCl, 500 mg N N1 ☑
AHA: 4Q,18

J0694 Injection, cefoxitin sodium, 1 g N N1 ☑
AHA: 4Q,18

J0695 Injection, ceftolozane 50 mg and tazobactam 25 mg 🅚 K2 ☑
Use this code for Zerbaxa.
AHA: 4Q,18

J0696 Injection, ceftriaxone sodium, per 250 mg N N1 ☑
AHA: 4Q,18

J0697 Injection, sterile cefuroxime sodium, per 750 mg N N1 ☑
AHA: 4Q,18

J0698 Injection, cefotaxime sodium, per g N N1 ☑
AHA: 4Q,18

J0699 Injection, cefiderocol, 10 mg K2
Use this code for Fetroja.
AHA: 4Q,21

J0701 Injection, cefepime HCl (Baxter), not therapeutically equivalent to Maxipime, 500 mg
Use this code for cefepime HCl manufactured by Baxter.
AHA: 1Q,23

J0702 Injection, betamethasone acetate 3 mg and betamethasone sodium phosphate 3 mg N N1 ☑
AHA: 4Q,18

J0703 Injection, cefepime HCl (B. Braun), not therapeutically equivalent to Maxipime, 500 mg
Use this code for cefepime HCl manufactured by B. Braun.

J0706 Injection, caffeine citrate, 5 mg N N1 ☑
AHA: 4Q,18

J0710 Injection, cephapirin sodium, up to 1 g 🇪🇮 ☑
AHA: 4Q,18

J0712 Injection, ceftaroline fosamil, 10 mg 🅚 K2 ☑
AHA: 4Q,18

J0713 Injection, ceftazidime, per 500 mg N N1 ☑
AHA: 4Q,18

J0714 Injection, ceftazidime and avibactam, 0.5 g/0.125 g 🅚 K2 ☑
Use this code for Avycaz.
AHA: 4Q,18

J0715 Injection, ceftizoxime sodium, per 500 mg N N1 ☑
AHA: 4Q,18

J0716 Injection, Centruroides immune f(ab)2, up to 120 mg 🅚 K2 ☑
Use this code for Anascorp.
AHA: 4Q,18

J0717 Injection, certolizumab pegol, 1 mg (code may be used for Medicare when drug administered under the direct supervision of a physician, not for use when drug is self-administered) 🅚 K2 ☑
CMS: 100-02,15,50.5
AHA: 4Q,18

J0720 Injection, chloramphenicol sodium succinate, up to 1 g N N1 ☑
AHA: 4Q,18

J0725 Injection, chorionic gonadotropin, per 1,000 USP units N N1 ☑
CMS: 100-02,15,50.5
AHA: 4Q,18

J0735 Injection, clonidine HCl, 1 mg N N1 ☑
AHA: 4Q,18

● **J0736** Injection, clindamycin phosphate, 300 mg
AHA: 3Q,23

Special Coverage Instructions   Noncovered by Medicare   Carrier Discretion   ☑ Quantity Alert   ● New Code   ○ Recycled/Reinstated   ▲ Revised Code

98 — J Codes   🅐 Age Edit   🅜 Maternity Edit   ♀ Female Only   ♂ Male Only   🅐-🆈 OPPS Status Indicators   © 2023 Optum360, LLC

● **J0737** **Injection, clindamycin phosphate (Baxter), not therapeutically equivalent to J0736, 300 mg**
Use this code for clindamycin phosphate manufactured by Baxter.
AHA: 3Q,23

▲ **J0739** **Injection, cabotegravir, 1 mg, FDA-approved prescription, only for use as HIV pre-exposure prophylaxis (not for use as treatment for HIV)**
Use this code for Apretude, Vocabria.
AHA: 3Q,22

J0740 **Injection, cidofovir, 375 mg** ⓚ ⓚ² ☑
AHA: 4Q,18

J0741 **Injection, cabotegravir and rilpivirine, 2 mg/3 mg** ⓚ²
Use this code for Cabenuva.
AHA: 4Q,21

J0742 **Injection, imipenem 4 mg, cilastatin 4 mg and relebactam 2 mg** ⓚ²
Use this code for Recarbrio.
AHA: 2Q,20

J0743 **Injection, cilastatin sodium; imipenem, per 250 mg** Ⓝ Ⓝ¹ ☑
AHA: 4Q,18

J0744 **Injection, ciprofloxacin for intravenous infusion, 200 mg** Ⓝ Ⓝ¹ ☑
AHA: 4Q,18

J0745 **Injection, codeine phosphate, per 30 mg** Ⓝ ⓚ² ☑
AHA: 4Q,18

● **J0750** **Emtricitabine 200 mg and tenofovir disoproxil fumarate 300 mg, oral, FDA-approved prescription, only for use as HIV pre-exposure prophylaxis (not for use as treatment of HIV)**
Use this code for Truvada for PReP.

● **J0751** **Emtricitabine 200 mg and tenofovir alafenamide 25 mg, oral, FDA-approved prescription, only for use as HIV pre-exposure prophylaxis (not for use as treatment of HIV)**
Use this code for Descovy for PReP.

J0770 **Injection, colistimethate sodium, up to 150 mg** Ⓝ Ⓝ¹ ☑
AHA: 4Q,18

J0775 **Injection, collagenase, clostridium histolyticum, 0.01 mg** ⓚ ⓚ² ☑
AHA: 4Q,18

J0780 **Injection, prochlorperazine, up to 10 mg** Ⓝ Ⓝ¹ ☑
AHA: 4Q,18

J0791 **Injection, crizanlizumab-tmca, 5 mg** ⓚ²
Use this code for ADAKVEO.
AHA: 2Q,20

J0795 **Injection, corticorelin ovine triflutate, 1 mcg** ⓚ Ⓝ¹ ☑
AHA: 4Q,18

● **J0799** **FDA-approved prescription drug, only for use as HIV pre-exposure prophylaxis (not for use as treatment of HIV), not otherwise classified**

~~J0800~~ ~~Injection, corticotropin, up to 40 units~~

● **J0801** **Injection, corticotropin (Acthar Gel), up to 40 units** ⓚ²

● **J0802** **Injection, corticotropin (ANI), up to 40 units** ⓚ²
Use this code for corticotropin manufactured by ANI.

J0834 **Injection, cosyntropin, 0.25 mg** Ⓝ Ⓝ¹ ☑
Use this code for Cortrosyn.
AHA: 4Q,18

J0840 **Injection, crotalidae polyvalent immune fab (ovine), up to 1 g** ⓚ ⓚ² ☑
AHA: 4Q,18

J0841 **Injection, crotalidae immune F(ab')2 (equine), 120 mg** ⓚ²
Use this code for Anavip.
CMS: 100-04,4,260.1; 100-04,4,260.1.1
AHA: 1Q,19; 4Q,18

J0850 **Injection, cytomegalovirus immune globulin intravenous (human), per vial** ⓚ ⓚ² ☑
AHA: 4Q,18

● **J0873** **Injection, daptomycin (Xellia), not therapeutically equivalent to J0878, 1 mg**

● **J0874** **Injection, daptomycin (Baxter), not therapeutically equivalent to J0878, 1 mg**

J0875 **Injection, dalbavancin, 5 mg** ⓚ ⓚ² ☑
Use this code for Dalvance.
AHA: 4Q,18

J0877 **Injection, daptomycin (Hospira), not therapeutically equivalent to J0878, 1 mg**
Use this code for daptomycin manufactured by Hospira.
AHA: 1Q,23

J0878 **Injection, daptomycin, 1 mg** ⓚ Ⓝ¹ ☑
Use this code for Cubicin.
AHA: 4Q,18

J0879 **Injection, difelikefalin, 0.1 mcg, (for ESRD on dialysis)** ⓚ²
Use this code for Korsuva.
AHA: 2Q,22

J0881 **Injection, darbepoetin alfa, 1 mcg (non-ESRD use)** ⓚ ⓚ² ☑
Use this code for Aranesp.
CMS: 100-03,110.21; 100-04,17,80.12
AHA: 4Q,18

J0882 **Injection, darbepoetin alfa, 1 mcg (for ESRD on dialysis)** ⓚ ⓚ² ☑ ⊘
Use this code for Aranesp.
CMS: 100-04,8,60.4; 100-04,8,60.4.1; 100-04,8,60.4.2; 100-04,8,60.4.5.1; 100-04,8,60.4.6.3; 100-04,8,60.4.6.4; 100-04,8,60.4.6.5
AHA: 4Q,18

J0883 **Injection, argatroban, 1 mg (for non-ESRD use)** ⓚ ⓚ² ☑
AHA: 4Q,18

J0884 **Injection, argatroban, 1 mg (for ESRD on dialysis)** ⓚ ⓚ² ☑
AHA: 4Q,18

J0885 **Injection, epoetin alfa, (for non-ESRD use), 1000 units** ⓚ ⓚ² ☑
Use this code for Epogen/Procrit.
CMS: 100-03,110.21; 100-04,17,80.12
AHA: 4Q,18

J0887 **Injection, epoetin beta, 1 mcg, (for ESRD on dialysis)** Ⓝ ⓚ² ☑
Use this code for Mircera.
AHA: 4Q,18

J0888 **Injection, epoetin beta, 1 mcg, (for non-ESRD use)** ⓚ Ⓝ¹ ☑
Use this code for Mircera.
AHA: 4Q,18

● **J0889** **Daprodustat, oral, 1 mg, (for ESRD on dialysis)**
Use this code for Jesduvroq.

J0890 **Injection, peginesatide, 0.1 mg (for ESRD on dialysis)** Ⓔ ☑
Use this code for Omontys.
CMS: 100-04,8,60.4; 100-04,8,60.4.1; 100-04,8,60.4.2; 100-04,8,60.4.5.1; 100-04,8,60.4.7
AHA: 4Q,18

J0891 **Injection, argatroban (Accord), not therapeutically equivalent to J0883, 1 mg (for non-ESRD use)** ⓚ²
Use this code for argatroban manufactured by Accord; for non-ESRD use.
AHA: 1Q,23

Special Coverage Instructions   Noncovered by Medicare   Carrier Discretion   ☑ Quantity Alert   ● New Code   ○ Recycled/Reinstated   ▲ Revised Code

Drugs Administered Other Than Oral Method

J0892 — J1230

J0892 Injection, argatroban (Accord), not therapeutically equivalent to J0884, 1 mg (for ESRD on dialysis) K2
Use this code for argatroban manufactured by Accord; for patients on ESRD dialysis.
AHA: 1Q,23

J0893 Injection, decitabine (Sun Pharma) not therapeutically equivalent to J0894, 1 mg
Use this code for decitabine manufactured by Sun Pharma.
AHA: 1Q,23

J0894 Injection, decitabine, 1 mg K N1 ✓ ⊘
Use this code for Dacogen.
AHA: 4Q,18

J0895 Injection, deferoxamine mesylate, 500 mg N N1 ✓
Use this code for Desferal.
CMS: 100-04,20,180; 100-04,32,411.3
AHA: 4Q,18

J0896 Injection, luspatercept-aamt, 0.25 mg K2
Use this code for REBLOZYL.
AHA: 2Q,20

J0897 Injection, denosumab, 1 mg K K2 ✓
Use this code for XGEVA, Prolia.
CMS: 100-04,10,90.1
AHA: 4Q,18

J0898 Injection, argatroban (AuroMedics), not therapeutically equivalent to J0883, 1 mg (for non-ESRD use) K2
Use this code for argatroban manufactured by AuroMedics; for non-ESRD use.
AHA: 1Q,23

J0899 Injection, argatroban (AuroMedics), not therapeutically equivalent to J0884, 1 mg (for ESRD on dialysis) K2
Use this code for argatroban manufactured by AuroMedics; for patients on ESRD dialysis.
AHA: 1Q,23

J0945 Injection, brompheniramine maleate, per 10 mg N ✓
AHA: 4Q,18

J1000 Injection, depo-estradiol cypionate, up to 5 mg N N1 ✓
Use this code for depGynogen, Depogen, Estradiol Cypionate.
AHA: 4Q,18

J1020 Injection, methylprednisolone acetate, 20 mg N N1 ✓
Use this code for Depo-Medrol.
AHA: 3Q,19; 4Q,18

J1030 Injection, methylprednisolone acetate, 40 mg N N1 ✓
Use this code for DepoMedalone40, Depo-Medrol, Sano-Drol.
AHA: 4Q,22; 3Q,19; 4Q,18

J1040 Injection, methylprednisolone acetate, 80 mg N N1 ✓
Use this code for Cortimed, DepMedalone 40, DepMedalone 80, Depo-Medrol, Duro Cort, Methylcotolone, Pri-Methylate, Sano-Drol.
AHA: 4Q,18

J1050 Injection, medroxyprogesterone acetate, 1 mg N N1 ✓
AHA: 4Q,18

J1071 Injection, testosterone cypionate, 1 mg N N1 ✓
Use this code for Depo-testosterone.
AHA: 4Q,18

J1094 Injection, dexamethasone acetate, 1 mg N N1 ✓
Use this code for Cortastat LA, Dalalone L.A., Dexamethasone Acetate Anhydrous, Dexone LA.
AHA: 4Q,18

J1095 Injection, dexamethasone 9%, intraocular, 1 mcg N1
AHA: 1Q,19; 4Q,18

J1096 Dexamethasone, lacrimal ophthalmic insert, 0.1 mg K2
Use this code for Dextenza.
AHA: 4Q,19

J1097 Phenylephrine 10.16 mg/ml and ketorolac 2.88 mg/ml ophthalmic irrigation solution, 1 ml K2
Use this code for Omidria.
AHA: 4Q,19

J1100 Injection, dexamethasone sodium phosphate, 1 mg N N1 ✓
Use this code for Cortastat, Dalalone, Decaject, Dexone, Solurex, Adrenocort, Primethasone, Dexasone, Dexim, Medidex, Spectro-Dex.
AHA: 4Q,18

● **J1105** Dexmedetomidine, oral, 1 mcg
Use this code for Igalmi.

J1110 Injection, dihydroergotamine mesylate, per 1 mg K N1 ✓
Use this code for D.H.E. 45.
AHA: 4Q,18

J1120 Injection, acetazolamide sodium, up to 500 mg N N1 ✓
Use this code for Diamox.
AHA: 4Q,18

J1130 Injection, diclofenac sodium, 0.5 mg K N1 ✓
Use this code for Dyloject.
AHA: 4Q,18; 1Q,17

J1160 Injection, digoxin, up to 0.5 mg N N1 ✓
Use this code for Lanoxin.
AHA: 4Q,18

J1162 Injection, digoxin immune fab (ovine), per vial K K2 ✓
Use this code for Digibind, Digifab.
AHA: 4Q,18

J1165 Injection, phenytoin sodium, per 50 mg N N1 ✓
Use this code for Dilantin.
AHA: 4Q,18

J1170 Injection, hydromorphone, up to 4 mg N N1 ✓
Use this code for Dilaudid, Dilaudid-HP.
CMS: 100-04,20,180; 100-04,32,411.3
AHA: 4Q,18

J1180 Injection, dyphylline, up to 500 mg E ✓
AHA: 4Q,18

J1190 Injection, dexrazoxane HCl, per 250 mg K K2 ✓
Use this code for Zinecard.
AHA: 4Q,18

J1200 Injection, diphenhydramine HCl, up to 50 mg N N1 ✓
Use this code for Benadryl, Benahist 10, Benahist 50, Benoject-10, Benoject-50, Bena-D 10, Bena-D 50, Nordryl, Dihydrex, Diphenacen-50, Hyrexin-50, Truxadryl, Wehdryl.
AHA: 4Q,18

J1201 Injection, cetirizine HCl, 0.5 mg K2
Use this code for Quzyttir.
AHA: 2Q,20

J1205 Injection, chlorothiazide sodium, per 500 mg N N1 ✓
Use this code for Diuril Sodium.
AHA: 4Q,18

J1212 Injection, DMSO, dimethyl sulfoxide, 50%, 50 ml K K2 ✓
Use this code for Rimso 50. DMSO is covered only as a treatment of interstitial cystitis.
AHA: 4Q,18

J1230 Injection, methadone HCl, up to 10 mg N N1 ✓
Use this code for Dolophine HCl.
AHA: 4Q,18

Special Coverage Instructions   Noncovered by Medicare   Carrier Discretion   ☑ Quantity Alert ● New Code   ○ Recycled/Reinstated   ▲ Revised Code

100 — J Codes   A Age Edit   M Maternity Edit   ♀ Female Only   ♂ Male Only   A-Y OPPS Status Indicators   © 2023 Optum360, LLC

J1240 **Injection, dimenhydrinate, up to 50 mg** ☒ N1 ☑
Use this code for Dramamine, Dinate, Dommanate, Dramanate, Dramilin, Dramocen, Dramoject, Dymenate, Hydrate, Marmine, Wehamine.
AHA: 4Q,18

J1245 **Injection, dipyridamole, per 10 mg** ☒ N1 ☑
Use this code for Persantine IV.
AHA: 4Q,18

● **J1246** **Injection, dinutuximab, 0.1 mg**
Use this code for Unituxin.

J1250 **Injection, dobutamine HCl, per 250 mg** ☒ N1 ☑
CMS: 100-04,20,180; 100-04,32,411.3
AHA: 4Q,18

J1260 **Injection, dolasetron mesylate, 10 mg** ☒ N1 ☑
Use this code for Anzemet.
AHA: 4Q,18

J1265 **Injection, dopamine HCl, 40 mg** ☒ N1 ☑
CMS: 100-04,20,180; 100-04,32,411.3
AHA: 4Q,18

J1267 **Injection, doripenem, 10 mg** ☒ ☑
Use this code for Doribax.
AHA: 4Q,18

J1270 **Injection, doxercalciferol, 1 mcg** ☒ N1 ☑
Use this code for Hectorol.
AHA: 4Q,18

J1290 **Injection, ecallantide, 1 mg** ☒ K2 ☑
Use this code for KALBITOR.
AHA: 4Q,18

J1300 **Injection, eculizumab, 10 mg** ☒ K2 ☑
Use this code for Soliris.
AHA: 4Q,18

J1301 **Injection, edaravone, 1 mg** K2
Use this code for Radicava.
AHA: 1Q,19; 4Q,18

J1302 **Injection, sutimlimab-jome, 10 mg** K2
Use this code for Enjaymo.
AHA: 4Q,22

J1303 **Injection, ravulizumab-cwvz, 10 mg** K2
Use this code for Ultomiris.
AHA: 4Q,19

● **J1304** **Injection, tofersen, 1 mg**
Use this code for Qalsody.

J1305 **Injection, evinacumab-dgnb, 5 mg** K2
Use this code for Evkeeza.
AHA: 4Q,21

J1306 **Injection, inclisiran, 1 mg** K2
Use this code for Leqvio.
AHA: 3Q,22

J1320 **Injection, amitriptyline HCl, up to 20 mg** ☒ N1 ☑
Use this code for Elavil.
AHA: 4Q,18

J1322 **Injection, elosulfase alfa, 1 mg** ☒ K2 ☑
Use this code for Vimizim.
AHA: 4Q,18

J1324 **Injection, enfuvirtide, 1 mg** EI ☑
Use this code for Fuzeon.
CMS: 100-02,15,50.5
AHA: 4Q,18

J1325 **Injection, epoprostenol, 0.5 mg** ☒ N1 ☑
Use this code for Flolan and Veletri.
CMS: 100-04,20,180; 100-04,32,411.3
AHA: 4Q,18

J1327 **Injection, eptifibatide, 5 mg** ☒ N1 ☑
Use this code for Integrilin.
AHA: 4Q,18

J1330 **Injection, ergonovine maleate, up to 0.2 mg** ☒ ☑
Medicare jurisdiction: local contractor. Use this code for Ergotrate Maleate.
AHA: 4Q,18

J1335 **Injection, ertapenem sodium, 500 mg** ☒ N1 ☑
Use this code for Invanz.
AHA: 4Q,18

J1364 **Injection, erythromycin lactobionate, per 500 mg** ☒ K2 ☑
AHA: 4Q,18

J1380 **Injection, estradiol valerate, up to 10 mg** ☒ N1 ☑
Use this code for Delestrogen, Dioval, Dioval XX, Dioval 40, Duragen-10, Duragen-20, Duragen-40, Estradiol L.A., Estradiol L.A. 20, Estradiol L.A. 40, Gynogen L.A. 10, Gynogen L.A. 20, Gynogen L.A. 40, Valergen 10, Valergen 20, Valergen 40, Estra-L 20, Estra-L 40, L.A.E. 20.
AHA: 4Q,18

J1410 **Injection, estrogen conjugated, per 25 mg** ☒ K2 ☑
Use this code for Natural Estrogenic Substance, Premarin Intravenous, Primestrin Aqueous.
AHA: 4Q,18

● **J1411** **Injection, etranacogene dezaparvovec-drlb, per therapeutic dose**
Use this code for Hemgenix.
AHA: 2Q,23

● **J1412** **Injection, valoctocogene roxaparvovec-rvox, per ml, containing nominal 2×10^{13} vector genomes**
Use this code for Roctavian.

● **J1413** **Injection, delandistrogene moxeparvovec-rokl, per therapeutic dose**
Use this code for Elevidys.

J1426 **Injection, casimersen, 10 mg** K2
Use this code for Amondys 45.
AHA: 4Q,21

J1427 **Injection, viltolarsen, 10 mg** K2
Use this code for Viltepso.
AHA: 1Q,21

J1428 **Injection, eteplirsen, 10 mg** G
Use this code for Exondys 51.
AHA: 4Q,18; 1Q,18

J1429 **Injection, golodirsen, 10 mg** K2
Use this code for Vyondys 53.
AHA: 2Q,20

J1430 **Injection, ethanolamine oleate, 100 mg** ☒ K2 ☑
Use this code for Ethamolin.
AHA: 4Q,18

J1435 **Injection, estrone, per 1 mg** EI ☑
Use this code for Estrone Aqueous, Estragyn, Estro-A, Estrone, Estronol, Theelin Aqueous, Estrone 5, Kestrone 5.
AHA: 4Q,18

J1436 **Injection, etidronate disodium, per 300 mg** EI ☑
Use this code for Didronel.
AHA: 4Q,18

J1437 **Injection, ferric derisomaltose, 10 mg** K2
Use this code for Monoferric.
AHA: 4Q,20

Special Coverage Instructions   Noncovered by Medicare   Carrier Discretion   ☑ Quantity Alert ● New Code   ○ Recycled/Reinstated ▲ Revised Code

Drugs Administered Other Than Oral Method

J1240 — J1437

Drugs Administered Other Than Oral Method

J1438 — J1566

J1438 Injection, etanercept, 25 mg (code may be used for Medicare when drug administered under the direct supervision of a physician, not for use when drug is self-administered) K K2 ☑
Use this code for Enbrel.
CMS: 100-02,15,50.5
AHA: 4Q,18

J1439 Injection, ferric carboxymaltose, 1 mg K K2 ☑
Use this code for Injectafer.
AHA: 4Q,18

○ **J1440** Fecal microbiota, live - jslm, 1 ml K2
Use this code for Rebyota.
AHA: 3Q,23

J1442 Injection, filgrastim (G-CSF), excludes biosimilars, 1 mcg K K2 ☑
Use this code for Neupogen.
AHA: 4Q,18

J1443 Injection, ferric pyrophosphate citrate solution (Triferic), 0.1 mg of iron N ☑
Use this code for Triferic solution.
AHA: 4Q,18

J1444 Injection, ferric pyrophosphate citrate powder, 0.1 mg of iron
Use this code for Triferic powder.
AHA: 3Q,19

J1445 Injection, ferric pyrophosphate citrate solution (Triferic AVNU), 0.1 mg of iron
AHA: 4Q,21

J1447 Injection, tbo-filgrastim, 1 mcg K K2 ☑
Use this code for Granix.
AHA: 4Q,18

J1448 Injection, trilaciclib, 1 mg K2
Use this code for Cosela.
AHA: 4Q,21

● **J1449** Injection, eflapegrastim-xnst, 0.1 mg K2
Use this code for Rolvedon.
AHA: 2Q,23

J1450 Injection, fluconazole, 200 mg N N1 ☑
Use this code for Diflucan.
CMS: 100-02,15,50.6
AHA: 4Q,18

J1451 Injection, fomepizole, 15 mg K K2 ☑
Use this code for Antizol.
CMS: 100-02,15,50.6
AHA: 4Q,18

J1452 Injection, fomivirsen sodium, intraocular, 1.65 mg EI ☑
Use this code for Vitravene.
CMS: 100-02,15,50.4.2; 100-02,15,50.6
AHA: 4Q,18

J1453 Injection, fosaprepitant, 1 mg K N1 ☑
Use this code for Emend.
CMS: 100-02,15,50.6
AHA: 4Q,18

J1454 Injection, fosnetupitant 235 mg and palonosetron 0.25 mg K2
Use this code for Akynzeo.
CMS: 100-02,15,50.6
AHA: 1Q,19; 4Q,18

J1455 Injection, foscarnet sodium, per 1,000 mg K K2 ☑
Use this code for Foscavir.
CMS: 100-02,15,50.6; 100-04,20,180; 100-04,32,411.3
AHA: 4Q,18

J1456 Injection, fosaprepitant (Teva), not therapeutically equivalent to J1453, 1 mg
Use this code for fosaprepitant manufactured by Teva.
CMS: 100-02,15,50.6
AHA: 1Q,23

J1457 Injection, gallium nitrate, 1 mg EI ☑
Use this code for Ganite.
CMS: 100-02,15,50.6; 100-04,20,180; 100-04,32,411.3
AHA: 4Q,18

J1458 Injection, galsulfase, 1 mg K N1 ☑
Use this code for Naglazyme.
CMS: 100-02,15,50.6
AHA: 4Q,18

J1459 Injection, immune globulin (Privigen), intravenous, nonlyophilized (e.g., liquid), 500 mg K K2 ☑
CMS: 100-02,15,50.6
AHA: 4Q,18

J1460 Injection, gamma globulin, intramuscular, 1 cc K K2 ☑
Use this code for GamaSTAN SD.
CMS: 100-02,15,50.6; 100-04,17,80.6
AHA: 4Q,18

J1551 Injection, immune globulin (Cutaquig), 100 mg K2
CMS: 100-02,15,50.6; 100-04,32,411.3
AHA: 3Q,22

J1554 Injection, immune globulin (Asceniv), 500 mg K2
CMS: 100-02,15,50.6
AHA: 1Q,21

J1555 Injection, immune globulin (Cuvitru), 100 mg K K2
CMS: 100-02,15,50.6; 100-04,20,180; 100-04,32,411.3
AHA: 4Q,18; 1Q,18

J1556 Injection, immune globulin (Bivigam), 500 mg K K2 ☑
CMS: 100-02,15,50.6
AHA: 4Q,18

J1557 Injection, immune globulin, (Gammaplex), intravenous, nonlyophilized (e.g., liquid), 500 mg K K2 ☑
CMS: 100-02,15,50.6
AHA: 4Q,18

J1558 Injection, immune globulin (xembify), 100 mg K2
CMS: 100-02,15,50.6; 100-04,32,411.3
AHA: 2Q,20

J1559 Injection, immune globulin (Hizentra), 100 mg K K2 ☑
CMS: 100-02,15,50.6; 100-04,20,180; 100-04,32,411.3
AHA: 4Q,18

J1560 Injection, gamma globulin, intramuscular, over 10 cc K K2 ☑
Use this code for GamaSTAN SD.
CMS: 100-02,15,50.6; 100-04,17,80.6
AHA: 4Q,18

J1561 Injection, immune globulin, (Gamunex/Gamunex-C/Gammaked), nonlyophilized (e.g., liquid), 500 mg K K2 ☑
CMS: 100-02,15,50.6; 100-04,20,180; 100-04,32,411.3
AHA: 4Q,18

J1562 Injection, immune globulin (Vivaglobin), 100 mg EI ☑
CMS: 100-02,15,50.6; 100-04,20,180; 100-04,32,411.3
AHA: 4Q,18

J1566 Injection, immune globulin, intravenous, lyophilized (e.g., powder), not otherwise specified, 500 mg K K2 ☑
Use this code for Carimune, Gammagard S/D, Iveegam, Polygam, Polygam S/D.
CMS: 100-02,15,50.6
AHA: 4Q,18

Special Coverage Instructions   Noncovered by Medicare   Carrier Discretion   ☑ Quantity Alert ● New Code   ○ Recycled/Reinstated ▲ Revised Code

102 — J Codes   A Age Edit   M Maternity Edit   ♀ Female Only   ♂ Male Only   A-Y OPPS Status Indicators   © 2023 Optum360, LLC

J1568   **Injection, immune globulin, (Octagam), intravenous, nonlyophilized (e.g., liquid), 500 mg**   K K2 ☑
CMS: 100-02,15,50.6
AHA: 4Q,18

J1569   **Injection, immune globulin, (Gammagard liquid), nonlyophilized, (e.g., liquid), 500 mg**   K K2 ☑
CMS: 100-02,15,50.6; 100-04,20,180; 100-04,32,411.3
AHA: 4Q,18

J1570   **Injection, ganciclovir sodium, 500 mg**   N N1 ☑
Use this code for Cytovene.
CMS: 100-04,20,180; 100-04,32,411.3
AHA: 4Q,18

J1571   **Injection, hepatitis B immune globulin (Hepagam B), intramuscular, 0.5 ml**   K K2 ☑
AHA: 4Q,18

J1572   **Injection, immune globulin, (Flebogamma/Flebogamma Dif), intravenous, nonlyophilized (e.g., liquid), 500 mg**   K K2 ☑
AHA: 4Q,18

J1573   **Injection, hepatitis B immune globulin (Hepagam B), intravenous, 0.5 ml**   K K2 ☑
AHA: 4Q,18

J1574   **Injection, ganciclovir sodium (Exela) not therapeutically equivalent to J1570, 500 mg**
Use this code for ganciclovir manufactured by Exela.
AHA: 1Q,23

J1575   **Injection, immune globulin/hyaluronidase, 100 mg immuneglobulin**   K K2 ☑
Use this code for HyOvia.
CMS: 100-04,20,180; 100-04,32,411.3
AHA: 4Q,18

● **J1576**   **Injection, immune globulin (Panzyga), intravenous, non-lyophilized (e.g., liquid), 500 mg**   K2
AHA: 3Q,23

J1580   **Injection, garamycin, gentamicin, up to 80 mg**   N N1 ☑
Use this code for Gentamicin Sulfate, Jenamicin.
AHA: 4Q,18

J1595   **Injection, glatiramer acetate, 20 mg**   K K2 ☑
Use this code for Copaxone.
CMS: 100-02,15,50.5
AHA: 4Q,18

● **J1596**   **Injection, glycopyrrolate, 0.1 mg**

J1599   **Injection, immune globulin, intravenous, nonlyophilized (e.g., liquid), not otherwise specified, 500 mg**   N N1 ☑
AHA: 4Q,18

J1600   **Injection, gold sodium thiomalate, up to 50 mg**   EI ☑
Use this code for Myochrysine.
CMS: 100-04,4,20.6.4
AHA: 4Q,18

J1602   **Injection, golimumab, 1 mg, for intravenous use**   K K2 ☑
Use this code for Simponi.
AHA: 4Q,18

J1610   **Injection, glucagon HCl, per 1 mg**   K K2 ☑
Use this code for Glucagon.
AHA: 4Q,18

J1611   **Injection, glucagon HCl (Fresenius Kabi), not therapeutically equivalent to J1610, per 1 mg**   K2
Use this code for glucagon HCl manufactured by Fresenius Kabi.
AHA: 1Q,23

J1620   **Injection, gonadorelin HCl, per 100 mcg**   EI ☑
Use this code for Factrel, Lutrepulse.
AHA: 4Q,18

J1626   **Injection, granisetron HCl, 100 mcg**   N N1 ☑
Use this code for Kytril.
CMS: 100-04,4,20.6.4
AHA: 4Q,18

J1627   **Injection, granisetron, extended-release, 0.1 mg**   G K2
Use this code for Sustol.
AHA: 4Q,18; 1Q,18

J1628   **Injection, guselkumab, 1 mg**   K2
Use this code for Tremfya.
AHA: 1Q,19; 4Q,18

J1630   **Injection, haloperidol, up to 5 mg**   N N1 ☑
Use this code for Haldol.
CMS: 100-04,4,20.6.4
AHA: 4Q,18

J1631   **Injection, haloperidol decanoate, per 50 mg**   N N1 ☑
Use this code for Haldol Decanoate-50.
CMS: 100-04,4,20.6.4
AHA: 4Q,18

J1632   **Injection, brexanolone, 1 mg**   N1
Use this code for Zulresso.
AHA: 4Q,20

J1640   **Injection, hemin, 1 mg**   K K2 ☑
Use this code for Panhematin.
AHA: 4Q,18

J1642   **Injection, heparin sodium, (heparin lock flush), per 10 units**   N N1 ☑
Use this code for Hep-Lock, Hep-Lock U/P, Hep-Pak, Lok-Pak.
CMS: 100-04,4,20.6.4
AHA: 4Q,18

J1643   **Injection, heparin sodium (Pfizer), not therapeutically equivalent to J1644, per 1000 units**
Use this code for heparin sodium manufactured by Pfizer.
AHA: 1Q,23

J1644   **Injection, Heparin sodium, per 1000 units**   N N1 ☑
Use this code for Heparin Sodium, Liquaemin Sodium.
CMS: 100-04,4,20.6.4
AHA: 4Q,18

J1645   **Injection, dalteparin sodium, per 2500 IU**   N N1 ☑
Use this code for Fragmin.
CMS: 100-02,15,50.5; 100-04,4,20.6.4
AHA: 4Q,18

J1650   **Injection, enoxaparin sodium, 10 mg**   N N1 ☑
Use this code for Lovenox.
CMS: 100-02,15,50.5; 100-04,4,20.6.4
AHA: 4Q,18

J1652   **Injection, fondaparinux sodium, 0.5 mg**   N N1 ☑
Use this code for Atrixtra.
CMS: 100-02,15,50.5
AHA: 4Q,18

J1655   **Injection, tinzaparin sodium, 1000 IU**   N ☑
Use this code for Innohep.
CMS: 100-02,15,50.5; 100-04,4,20.6.4
AHA: 4Q,18

J1670   **Injection, tetanus immune globulin, human, up to 250 units**   K K2 ☑
Use this code for HyperTET SD.
AHA: 4Q,18

Drugs Administered Other Than Oral Method

J1568 — J1670

J1675 Injection, histrelin acetate, 10 mcg ☐B ☑
Use this code for Supprelin LA.
AHA: 4Q,18

J1700 Injection, hydrocortisone acetate, up to 25 mg ☐N ☐N1 ☑
Use this code for Hydrocortone Acetate.
CMS: 100-04,4,20.6.4
AHA: 4Q,18

J1710 Injection, hydrocortisone sodium phosphate, up to 50 mg ☐N ☐N1 ☑
Use this code for Hydrocortone Phosphate.
CMS: 100-04,4,20.6.4
AHA: 4Q,18

J1720 Injection, hydrocortisone sodium succinate, up to 100 mg ☐N ☐N1 ☑
Use this code for Solu-Cortef, A-Hydrocort.
CMS: 100-04,4,20.6.4
AHA: 4Q,18

J1726 Injection, hydroxyprogesterone caproate, (Makena), 10 mg ☐K ☐K2
AHA: 4Q,18; 1Q,18

J1729 Injection, hydroxyprogesterone caproate, not otherwise specified, 10 mg ☐N ☐K2
AHA: 4Q,18; 1Q,18

J1730 Injection, diazoxide, up to 300 mg ☐EI ☑
AHA: 4Q,18

J1738 Injection, meloxicam, 1 mg ☐N1
Use this code for Anjeso.
AHA: 4Q,20

J1740 Injection, ibandronate sodium, 1 mg ☐K ☐K2 ☑
Use this code for Boniva.
AHA: 4Q,18

J1741 Injection, ibuprofen, 100 mg ☐N ☐N1 ☑
Use this code for Caldolor.
AHA: 4Q,18

J1742 Injection, ibutilide fumarate, 1 mg ☐K ☐K2 ☑
Use this code for Corvert.
AHA: 4Q,18

J1743 Injection, idursulfase, 1 mg ☐K ☐K2 ☑
Use this code for Elaprase.
AHA: 4Q,18

J1744 Injection, icatibant, 1 mg ☐K ☐K2 ☑
Use this code for Firazyr.
CMS: 100-02,15,50.5
AHA: 4Q,18

J1745 Injection, infliximab, excludes biosimilar, 10 mg ☐K ☐K2 ☑
Use this code for Remicade.
AHA: 4Q,18

J1746 Injection, ibalizumab-uiyk, 10 mg ☐K2
Use this code for Trogarzo.
CMS: 100-04,4,260.1; 100-04,4,260.1.1
AHA: 1Q,19; 4Q,18

● **J1747** Injection, spesolimab-sbzo, 1 mg ☐K2
Use this code for Spevigo.
AHA: 2Q,23

J1750 Injection, iron dextran, 50 mg ☐K ☐K2 ☑
Use this code for INFeD.
AHA: 4Q,18

J1756 Injection, iron sucrose, 1 mg ☐N ☐N1 ☑
Use this code for Venofer.
CMS: 100-04,8,60.2.4; 100-04,8,60.2.4.2
AHA: 4Q,18

J1786 Injection, imiglucerase, 10 units ☐K ☐K2 ☑
Use this code for Cerezyme.
AHA: 4Q,18

J1790 Injection, droperidol, up to 5 mg ☐N ☐N1 ☑
Use this code for Inapsine.
CMS: 100-04,4,20.6.4
AHA: 4Q,18

J1800 Injection, propranolol HCl, up to 1 mg ☐N ☐N1 ☑
Use this code for Inderal.
CMS: 100-04,4,20.6.4
AHA: 4Q,18

● **J1805** Injection, esmolol HCl, 10 mg
AHA: 3Q,23

● **J1806** Injection, esmolol HCl (WG Critical Care) not therapeutically equivalent to J1805, 10 mg
Use this code for esmolol HCl manufactured by WG Critical Care.
AHA: 3Q,23

J1810 Injection, droperidol and fentanyl citrate, up to 2 ml ampule ☐EI ☑
AHA: 4Q,18

● **J1811** Insulin (Fiasp) for administration through DME (i.e., insulin pump) per 50 units
AHA: 3Q,23

● **J1812** Insulin (Fiasp), per 5 units
AHA: 3Q,23

● **J1813** Insulin (Lyumjev) for administration through DME (i.e., insulin pump) per 50 units
AHA: 3Q,23

● **J1814** Insulin (Lyumjev), per 5 units
AHA: 3Q,23

J1815 Injection, insulin, per 5 units ☐N ☐N1 ☑
Use this code for Humalog, Humulin, Iletin, Insulin Lispro, Lantus, Levemir, NPH, Pork insulin, Regular insulin, Ultralente, Velosulin, Humulin R, Iletin II Regular Pork, Insulin Purified Pork, Relion, Lente Iletin I, Novolin R, Humulin R U-500.
CMS: 100-04,4,20.6.4
AHA: 4Q,18

J1817 Insulin for administration through DME (i.e., insulin pump) per 50 units ☐N ☐N1 ☑
Use this code for Humalog, Humulin, Iletin II NPH Pork, Lispro-PFC, Novolin, Novolog, Novolog Flexpen, Novolog Mix, Relion Novolin.
AHA: 4Q,18

J1823 Injection, inebilizumab-cdon, 1 mg ☐K2
Use this code for Uplinza.
AHA: 1Q,21

J1826 Injection, interferon beta-1a, 30 mcg ☐K ☐K2 ☑
Use this code for AVONEX, Rebif.
AHA: 4Q,18

J1830 Injection interferon beta-1b, 0.25 mg (code may be used for Medicare when drug administered under the direct supervision of a physician, not for use when drug is self-administered) ☐K ☐N1 ☑
Use this code for Betaseron.
CMS: 100-02,15,50.5
AHA: 4Q,18

Special Coverage Instructions   Noncovered by Medicare   Carrier Discretion   ☑ Quantity Alert ● New Code   ○ Recycled/Reinstated   ▲ Revised Code

104 — J Codes   ☐A Age Edit   ☐M Maternity Edit   ♀ Female Only   ♂ Male Only   ☐A-Y OPPS Status Indicators   © 2023 Optum360, LLC

J1833 Injection, isavuconazonium, 1 mg K K2 ☑
Use this code for Cresemba.
AHA: 4Q,18

J1835 Injection, itraconazole, 50 mg EI ☑
Use this code for Sporonox IV.
CMS: 100-04,4,20.6.4
AHA: 4Q,18

● **J1836** Injection, metronidazole, 10 mg
AHA: 3Q,23

J1840 Injection, kanamycin sulfate, up to 500 mg N N1 ☑
Use this code for Kantrex.
CMS: 100-04,4,20.6.4
AHA: 4Q,18

J1850 Injection, kanamycin sulfate, up to 75 mg N ☑
Use this code for Kantrex.
CMS: 100-04,4,20.6.4
AHA: 4Q,18

J1885 Injection, ketorolac tromethamine, per 15 mg N N1 ☑
Use this code for Toradol.
CMS: 100-04,4,20.6.4
AHA: 4Q,18

J1890 Injection, cephalothin sodium, up to 1 g N ☑
CMS: 100-04,4,20.6.4
AHA: 4Q,18

● **J1920** Injection, labetalol HCl, 5 mg
AHA: 3Q,23

▲ **J1921** Injection, labetalol HCl (Hikma) not therapeutically equivalent to J1920, 5 mg N1
Use this code for labetalol HCl manufactured by Hikma.
AHA: 3Q,23

J1930 Injection, lanreotide, 1 mg K K2 ☑
Use this code for Somatuline.
AHA: 4Q,18

J1931 Injection, laronidase, 0.1 mg K K2 ☑
Use this code for Aldurazyme.
AHA: 4Q,18

J1932 Injection, lanreotide, (Cipla), 1 mg K2
AHA: 1Q,22

● **J1939** Injection, bumetanide, 0.5 mg
Use this code for Bumex.

J1940 Injection, furosemide, up to 20 mg N N1 ☑
Use this code for Lasix.
CMS: 100-04,4,20.6.4
AHA: 4Q,18

● **J1941** Injection, furosemide (Furoscix), 20 mg
Use this code for Furoscix.
AHA: 3Q,23

J1943 Injection, aripiprazole lauroxil, (Aristada Initio), 1 mg K2
AHA: 4Q,19

J1944 Injection, aripiprazole lauroxil, (Aristada), 1 mg K2
AHA: 4Q,19

J1945 Injection, lepirudin, 50 mg EI ☑
Use this code for Refludan.
This drug is used for patients with heparin-induced thrombocytopenia.
AHA: 4Q,18

J1950 Injection, leuprolide acetate (for depot suspension), per 3.75 mg K K2 ☑
Use this code for Lupron Depot-Pedi.
AHA: 2Q,19; 4Q,18

J1951 Injection, leuprolide acetate for depot suspension (Fensolvi), 0.25 mg K2
AHA: 3Q,21

J1952 Leuprolide injectable, camcevi, 1 mg K2
Use this code for Camcevi.
AHA: 1Q,22

J1953 Injection, levetiracetam, 10 mg N N1 ☑
Use this code for Keppra.
AHA: 4Q,18

▲ **J1954** Injection, leuprolide acetate for depot suspension (Cipla), 7.5 mg K2
AHA: 2Q,23; 1Q,23

J1955 Injection, levocarnitine, per 1 g B ☑
Use this code for Carnitor.
AHA: 4Q,18

J1956 Injection, levofloxacin, 250 mg N N1 ☑
Use this code for Levaquin.
CMS: 100-04,4,20.6.4
AHA: 4Q,18

J1960 Injection, levorphanol tartrate, up to 2 mg N N1 ☑
Use this code for Levo-Dromoran.
CMS: 100-04,4,20.6.4
AHA: 4Q,18

● **J1961** Injection, lenacapavir, 1 mg K2
Use this code for Sunlenca.
AHA: 3Q,23

J1980 Injection, hyoscyamine sulfate, up to 0.25 mg N N1 ☑
Use this code for Levsin.
CMS: 100-04,4,20.6.4
AHA: 4Q,18

J1990 Injection, chlordiazepoxide HCl, up to 100 mg N ☑
Use this code for Librium.
CMS: 100-04,4,20.6.4
AHA: 4Q,18

J2001 Injection, lidocaine HCl for intravenous infusion, 10 mg N N1 ☑
Use this code for Xylocaine.
CMS: 100-04,4,20.6.4
AHA: 3Q,23; 4Q,18

J2010 Injection, lincomycin HCl, up to 300 mg N N1 ☑
Use this code for Lincocin.
CMS: 100-04,4,20.6.4
AHA: 4Q,18

J2020 Injection, linezolid, 200 mg N N1 ☑
Use this code for Zyvok.
AHA: 4Q,18

J2021 Injection, linezolid (Hospira) not therapeutically equivalent to J2020, 200 mg
Use this code for linezolid manufactured by Hospira.
AHA: 1Q,23

J2060 Injection, lorazepam, 2 mg N N1 ☑
Use this code for Ativan.
CMS: 100 04,4,20.6.4
AHA: 4Q,18

J2062 Loxapine for inhalation, 1 mg
Use this code for Adasuve.
AHA: 1Q,19

J2150 Injection, mannitol, 25% in 50 ml N N1 ☑
Use this code for Osmitrol.
CMS: 100-04,4,20.6.4
AHA: 4Q,18

Special Coverage Instructions   Noncovered by Medicare   Carrier Discretion   ☑ Quantity Alert   ● New Code   ○ Recycled/Reinstated   ▲ Revised Code

J2170 Injection, mecasermin, 1 mg ☒ ☒ ☑
Use this code for Iplex, Increlex.
CMS: 100-02,15,50.5; 100-04,4,20.6.4
AHA: 4Q,18

J2175 Injection, meperidine HCl, per 100 mg ☒ ☒ ☑
Use this code for Demerol.
CMS: 100-04,20,180; 100-04,32,411.3; 100-04,4,20.6.4
AHA: 4Q,18

J2180 Injection, meperidine and promethazine HCl, up to 50 mg ☒ ☒ ☑
Use this code for Mepergan Injection.
CMS: 100-04,4,20.6.4
AHA: 4Q,18

J2182 Injection, mepolizumab, 1 mg ☒ ☒ ☑
Use this code for Nucala.
AHA: 4Q,18

J2184 Injection, meropenem (B. Braun) not therapeutically equivalent to J2185, 100 mg
Use this code for meropenem manufactured by B. Braun.
AHA: 1Q,23

J2185 Injection, meropenem, 100 mg ☒ ☒ ☑
Use this code for Merrem.
CMS: 100-04,4,20.6.4
AHA: 4Q,18

J2186 Injection, meropenem, vaborbactam, 10 mg/10 mg, (20 mg) ☒
Use this code for Vabomere.
CMS: 100-04,4,260.1; 100-04,4,260.1.1
AHA: 1Q,19; 4Q,18

J2210 Injection, methylergonovine maleate, up to 0.2 mg ☒ ☒ ☑
Use this code for Methergine.
CMS: 100-04,4,20.6.4
AHA: 4Q,18

J2212 Injection, methylnaltrexone, 0.1 mg ☒ ☒ ☑
Use this code for Relistor.
CMS: 100-02,15,50.5
AHA: 4Q,18

J2247 Injection, micafungin sodium (Par Pharm) not therapeutically equivalent to J2248, 1 mg
Use this code for micafungin sodium manufactured by Par Pharm.
AHA: 1Q,23

J2248 Injection, micafungin sodium, 1 mg ☒ ☒ ☑
Use this code for Mycamine.
AHA: 4Q,18

● **J2249** Injection, remimazolam, 1 mg
Use this code for Byfavo.
AHA: 3Q,23

J2250 Injection, midazolam HCl, per 1 mg ☒ ☒ ☑
Use this code for Versed.
CMS: 100-04,4,20.6.4
AHA: 4Q,18

J2251 Injection, midazolam HCl (WG Critical Care) not therapeutically equivalent to J2250, per 1 mg
Use this code for midazolam HCl manufactured by WG Critical Care.
AHA: 1Q,23

J2260 Injection, milrinone lactate, 5 mg ☒ ☒ ☑
Use this code for Primacor.
CMS: 100-04,20,180; 100-04,32,411.3; 100-04,4,20.6.4
AHA: 4Q,18

J2265 Injection, minocycline HCl, 1 mg ☒ ☒ ☑
Use this code for MINOCIN.
AHA: 4Q,18

J2270 Injection, morphine sulfate, up to 10 mg ☒ ☒ ☑
Use this code for Depodur, Infumorph.
CMS: 100-04,20,180; 100-04,4,20.6.4
AHA: 4Q,18

J2272 Injection, morphine sulfate (Fresenius Kabi) not therapeutically equivalent to J2270, up to 10 mg
Use this code for morphine sulfate manufactured by Fresenius Kabi.
AHA: 1Q,23

J2274 Injection, morphine sulfate, preservative free for epidural or intrathecal use, 10 mg ☒ ☒ ☑
Use this code for DepoDur, Astromorph PF, Durarmorph PF.
CMS: 100-04,20,180
AHA: 4Q,18

J2278 Injection, ziconotide, 1 mcg ☒ ☒ ☑
Use this code for Prialt.
CMS: 100-04,20,180
AHA: 4Q,18

J2280 Injection, moxifloxacin, 100 mg ☒ ☒ ☑
Use this code for Avelox.
CMS: 100-04,4,20.6.4
AHA: 4Q,18

J2281 Injection, moxifloxacin (Fresenius Kabi) not therapeutically equivalent to J2280, 100 mg
Use this code for moxifloxacin manufactured by Fresenius Kabi.
AHA: 1Q,23

J2300 Injection, nalbuphine HCl, per 10 mg ☒ ☒ ☑
Use this code for Nubain.
CMS: 100-04,4,20.6.4
AHA: 4Q,18

● **J2305** Injection, nitroglycerin, 5 mg
AHA: 3Q,23

J2310 Injection, naloxone HCl, per 1 mg ☒ ☒ ☑
Use this code for Narcan.
AHA: 4Q,18

J2311 Injection, naloxone HCl (Zimhi), 1 mg
Use this code for naloxone HCl (Zimhi) manufactured by Adamis.
AHA: 1Q,23

J2315 Injection, naltrexone, depot form, 1 mg ☒ ☒ ☑
Use this code for Vivitrol.
AHA: 4Q,18

J2320 Injection, nandrolone decanoate, up to 50 mg ☒ ☒ ☑
AHA: 4Q,18

J2323 Injection, natalizumab, 1 mg ☒ ☒ ☑
Use this code for Tysabri.
AHA: 4Q,18

J2325 Injection, nesiritide, 0.1 mg ☒ ☑
Use this code for Natrecor.
CMS: 100-03,200.1
AHA: 4Q,18

J2326 Injection, nusinersen, 0.1 mg ☒ ☒
Use this code for Spinraza.
AHA: 1Q,21; 1Q,20; 4Q,18; 1Q,18

J2327 Injection, risankizumab-rzaa, intravenous, 1 mg ☒
AHA: 1Q,23

● **J2329** Injection, ublituximab-xiiy, 1mg ☒
Use this code for Briumvi.
AHA: 3Q,23

Special Coverage Instructions   Noncovered by Medicare   Carrier Discretion   ☑ Quantity Alert ● New Code ○ Recycled/Reinstated ▲ Revised Code

☒ Age Edit   ☒ Maternity Edit   ♀ Female Only   ♂ Male Only   ☒-☒ OPPS Status Indicators   © 2023 Optum360, LLC

J2350	Injection, ocrelizumab, 1 mg	G K2
	Use this code for Ocrevus.	
	AHA: 4Q,18; 1Q,18	
J2353	Injection, octreotide, depot form for intramuscular injection, 1 mg	K K2 ☑
	Use this code for Sandostatin LAR.	
	AHA: 4Q,18	
J2354	Injection, octreotide, nondepot form for subcutaneous or intravenous injection, 25 mcg	N N1 ☑
	Use this code for Sandostatin.	
	CMS: 100-02,15,50.5	
	AHA: 4Q,18	
J2355	Injection, oprelvekin, 5 mg	K ☑
	Use this code for Neumega.	
	AHA: 4Q,18	
J2356	Injection, tezepelumab-ekko, 1 mg	K2
	Use this code for Tezspire.	
	AHA: 3Q,22	
J2357	Injection, omalizumab, 5 mg	K K2 ☑
	Use this code for Xolair.	
	AHA: 4Q,18	
J2358	Injection, olanzapine, long-acting, 1 mg	N N1 ☑
	Use this code for ŻYPREXA RELPREVV.	
	AHA: 4Q,10	
● **J2359**	Injection, olanzapine, 0.5 mg	N1
J2360	Injection, orphenadrine citrate, up to 60 mg	N N1 ☑
	Use this code for Norflex.	
	AHA: 4Q,18	
J2370	Injection, phenylephrine HCl, up to 1 ml	
● **J2371**	Injection, phenylephrine HCl, 20 mcg	
	AHA: 3Q,23	
● **J2372**	Injection, phenylephrine HCl (Biorphen), 20 mcg	
	AHA: 3Q,23	
J2401	Injection, chloroprocaine HCl, per 1 mg	
	AHA: 1Q,23	
J2402	Injection, chloroprocaine HCl (Clorotekal), per 1 mg	
	Use this code for chloroprocaine HCl (Clorotekal) manufactured by B. Braun.	
	AHA: 1Q,23	
● **J2403**	Chloroprocaine HCl ophthalmic, 3% gel, 1 mg	K2
	Use this code for Iheezo.	
	AHA: 2Q,23	
● **J2404**	Injection, nicardipine, 0.1 mg	
	Use this code for Cardene IV.	
J2405	Injection, ondansetron HCl, per 1 mg	N N1 ☑
	Use this code for Zofran.	
	AHA: 4Q,18	
J2406	Injection, oritavancin (Kimyrsa), 10 mg	K2
	AHA: 4Q,21	
J2407	Injection, oritavancin (Orbactiv), 10 mg	K K2 ☑
	Use this code for Orbactiv.	
	AHA: 4Q,18	
J2410	Injection, oxymorphone HCl, up to 1 mg	N ☑
	Use this code for Numorphan, Oxymorphone HCl.	
	AHA: 4Q,18	
J2425	Injection, palifermin, 50 mcg	K K2 ☑
	Use this code for Kepivance.	
	AHA: 4Q,18	

▲ **J2426**	Injection, paliperidone palmitate extended release (Invega Sustenna), 1 mg	K K2 ☑
	Use this code for INVEGA SUSTENNA.	
	AHA: 3Q,23; 4Q,18	
● **J2427**	Injection, paliperidone palmitate extended release (Invega Hafyera or Invega Trinza), 1 mg	K2
	AHA: 3Q,23	
J2430	Injection, pamidronate disodium, per 30 mg	N N1 ☑
	Use this code for Aredia.	
	AHA: 4Q,18	
J2440	Injection, papaverine HCl, up to 60 mg	N N1 ☑
	AHA: 4Q,18	
J2460	Injection, oxytetracycline HCl, up to 50 mg	EI ☑
	Use this code for Terramycin IM.	
	AHA: 4Q,18	
J2469	Injection, palonosetron HCl, 25 mcg	K N1 ☑
	Use this code for Aloxi.	
	AHA: 4Q,18	
J2501	Injection, paricalcitol, 1 mcg	N N1 ☑
	Use this code For Zemplar.	
	AHA: 4Q,18	
J2502	Injection, pasireotide long acting, 1 mg	K K2 ☑
	Use this code for Signifor LAR.	
	AHA: 4Q,18	
J2503	Injection, pegaptanib sodium, 0.3 mg	K ☑
	Use this code for Macugen.	
	AHA: 4Q,18	
J2504	Injection, pegademase bovine, 25 IU	K N1 ☑
	Use this code for Adagen.	
	AHA: 4Q,18	
J2506	Injection, pegfilgrastim, excludes biosimilar, 0.5 mg	K2
	Use this code for Neulasta.	
	AHA: 1Q,22	
J2507	Injection, pegloticase, 1 mg	K K2 ☑
	Use this code for KRYSTEXXA.	
	AHA: 4Q,18	
● **J2508**	Injection, pegunigalsidase alfa-iwxj, 1 mg	
	Use this code for Elfabrio.	
J2510	Injection, penicillin G procaine, aqueous, up to 600,000 units	N K2 ☑
	Use this code for Wycillin, Duracillin A.S., Pfizerpen A.S., Crysticillin 300 A.S., Crysticillin 600 A.S.	
	AHA: 4Q,18	
J2513	Injection, pentastarch, 10% solution, 100 ml	EI ☑
	AHA: 4Q,18	
J2515	Injection, pentobarbital sodium, per 50 mg	K K2 ☑
	Use this code for Nembutal Sodium Solution.	
	AHA: 4Q,18	
J2540	Injection, penicillin G potassium, up to 600,000 units	N N1 ☑
	Use this code for Pfizerpen.	
	AHA: 4Q,18	
J2543	Injection, piperacillin sodium/tazobactam sodium, 1 g/0.125 g (1.125 g)	N N1 ☑
	Use this code for Zosyn.	
	AHA: 4Q,18	
J2545	Pentamidine isethionate, inhalation solution, FDA-approved final product, noncompounded, administered through DME, unit dose form, per 300 mg	B ☑
	Use this code for Nebupent, Pentam 300.	

Special Coverage Instructions   Noncovered by Medicare   Carrier Discretion   ☑ Quantity Alert   ● New Code   ○ Recycled/Reinstated   ▲ Revised Code

J2547 Injection, peramivir, 1 mg K K2 ☑
Use this code for Rapivab.
AHA: 4Q,18

J2550 Injection, promethazine HCl, up to 50 mg N N1 ☑
Use this code for Phenergan.
AHA: 4Q,18

J2560 Injection, phenobarbital sodium, up to 120 mg N K2 ☑
AHA: 4Q,18

● **J2561** Injection, phenobarbital sodium (Sezaby), 1 mg
AHA: 3Q,23

J2562 Injection, plerixafor, 1 mg K K2 ☑
Use this code for Mozobil.
AHA: 4Q,18

J2590 Injection, oxytocin, up to 10 units N N1 ☑
Use this code for Pitocin, Syntocinon.
AHA: 4Q,18

J2597 Injection, desmopressin acetate, per 1 mcg K K2 ☑
Use this code for DDAVP.
AHA: 4Q,18

● **J2598** Injection, vasopressin, 1 unit
AHA: 3Q,23

● **J2599** Injection, vasopressin (American Regent) not therapeutically equivalent to J2598, 1 unit
Use this code for vasopressin manufactured by American Regent.
AHA: 3Q,23

J2650 Injection, prednisolone acetate, up to 1 ml N N1 ☑
AHA: 4Q,18

J2670 Injection, tolazoline HCl, up to 25 mg N ☑
AHA: 4Q,18

J2675 Injection, progesterone, per 50 mg N N1 ☑
Use this code for Gesterone, Gestrin.
AHA: 4Q,18

● **J2679** Injection, fluphenazine HCl, 1.25 mg

J2680 Injection, fluphenazine decanoate, up to 25 mg N N1 ☑
AHA: 4Q,18

J2690 Injection, procainamide HCl, up to 1 g N N1 ☑
Use this code for Pronestyl.
AHA: 4Q,18

J2700 Injection, oxacillin sodium, up to 250 mg N N1 ☑
Use this code for Bactocill
AHA: 4Q,18

J2704 Injection, propofol, 10 mg N N1 ☑
Use this code for Diprivan.
AHA: 4Q,18

J2710 Injection, neostigmine methylsulfate, up to 0.5 mg N N1 ☑
Use this code for Prostigmin.
AHA: 4Q,18

J2720 Injection, protamine sulfate, per 10 mg N N1 ☑
AHA: 4Q,18

J2724 Injection, protein C concentrate, intravenous, human, 10 IU K K2 ☑
AHA: 4Q,18

J2725 Injection, protirelin, per 250 mcg EI ☑
Use this code for Thyrel TRH.
AHA: 4Q,18

J2730 Injection, pralidoxime chloride, up to 1 g N N1 ☑
Use this code for Protopam Chloride.
AHA: 4Q,18

J2760 Injection, phentolamine mesylate, up to 5 mg K K2 ☑
Use this code for Regitine.
AHA: 4Q,18

J2765 Injection, metoclopramide HCl, up to 10 mg N N1 ☑
Use this code for Reglan.
AHA: 4Q,18

J2770 Injection, quinupristin/dalfopristin, 500 mg (150/350) K K2 ☑
Use this code for Synercid.
AHA: 4Q,18

J2777 Injection, faricimab-svoa, 0.1 mg K2
Use this code for Vabysmo.
AHA: 4Q,22

J2778 Injection, ranibizumab, 0.1 mg K K2 ☑
Use this code for Lucentis.
AHA: 4Q,18

J2779 Injection, ranibizumab, via intravitreal implant (Susvimo), 0.1 mg K2
AHA: 3Q,22

J2780 Injection, ranitidine HCl, 25 mg N N1 ☑
Use this code for Zantac.
AHA: 4Q,18

● **J2781** Injection, pegcetacoplan, intravitreal, 1 mg K2
Use this code for Syfovre.

J2783 Injection, rasburicase, 0.5 mg K K2 ☑
Use this code for Elitek.
AHA: 4Q,18

J2785 Injection, regadenoson, 0.1 mg N N1 ☑
Use this code for Lexiscan.
AHA: 4Q,18

J2786 Injection, reslizumab, 1 mg G K2 ☑
Use this code for Cinqair.
AHA: 4Q,18

J2787 Riboflavin 5'-phosphate, ophthalmic solution, up to 3 ml
Use this code for Photrexa Viscous.
CMS: 100-04,4,260.1; 100-04,4,260.1.1
AHA: 1Q,19

J2788 Injection, Rho D immune globulin, human, minidose, 50 mcg (250 IU) N N1 ☑
Use this code for RhoGam, MiCRhoGAM.
AHA: 4Q,18

J2790 Injection, Rho D immune globulin, human, full dose, 300 mcg (1500 IU) N N1 ☑
Use this code for RhoGam, HypRho SD.
AHA: 4Q,18

J2791 Injection, Rho D immune globulin (human), (Rhophylac), intramuscular or intravenous, 100 IU N N1 ☑
Use this for Rhophylac.
AHA: 4Q,18

J2792 Injection, Rho D immune globulin, intravenous, human, solvent detergent, 100 IU K K2 ☑
Use this code for WINRho SDF.
AHA: 4Q,18

J2793 Injection, rilonacept, 1 mg K ☑
Use this code for Arcalyst.
CMS: 100-02,15,50.5
AHA: 4Q,18

J2794 Injection, risperidone (RISPERDAL CONSTA), 0.5 mg K K2 ☑
AHA: 4Q,18

Special Coverage Instructions   Noncovered by Medicare   Carrier Discretion   ☑ Quantity Alert ● New Code ○ Recycled/Reinstated ▲ Revised Code

108 — J Codes   A Age Edit   M Maternity Edit   ♀ Female Only   ♂ Male Only   A-Y OPPS Status Indicators   © 2023 Optum360, LLC

J2795	Injection, ropivacaine HCl, 1 mg	N N1 ☑
	Use this code for Naropin.	
	AHA: 4Q,18	
J2796	Injection, romiplostim, 10 mcg	K K2 ☑
	Use this code for Nplate.	
	AHA: 4Q,18	
J2797	Injection, rolapitant, 0.5 mg	
	Use this code for Varubi.	
	AHA: 1Q,19; 4Q,18	
J2798	Injection, risperidone, (Perseris), 0.5 mg	K2
	AHA: 4Q,19	
● **J2799**	Injection, risperidone (Uzedy), 1 mg	
	Use this code for Uzedy.	
J2800	Injection, methocarbamol, up to 10 ml	N N1 ☑
	Use this code for Robaxin.	
	AHA: 4Q,18	
J2805	Injection, sincalide, 5 mcg	N N1 ☑
	Use this code for Kinevac.	
	AHA: 4Q,18	
● **J2806**	Injection, sincalide (MAIA) not therapeutically equivalent to J2805, 5 mcg	
	Use this code for sincalide manufactured by MAIA.	
	AHA: 3Q,23	
J2810	Injection, theophylline, per 40 mg	N N1 ☑
	AHA: 4Q,18	
J2820	Injection, sargramostim (GM-CSF), 50 mcg	K K2 ☑
	Use this code for Leukine.	
	AHA: 4Q,18	
J2840	Injection, sebelipase alfa, 1 mg	G K2 ☑
	Use this code for Kanuma.	
	AHA: 4Q,18	
J2850	Injection, secretin, synthetic, human, 1 mcg	K N1 ☑
	AHA: 4Q,18	
J2860	Injection, siltuximab, 10 mg	K K2 ☑
	Use this code for Sylvant.	
	AHA: 4Q,18	
J2910	Injection, aurothioglucose, up to 50 mg	E1 ☑
	Use this code for Solganal.	
	AHA: 4Q,18	
J2916	Injection, sodium ferric gluconate complex in sucrose injection, 12.5 mg	N N1 ☑
	CMS: 100-03,110.10	
	AHA: 4Q,18	
J2920	Injection, methylprednisolone sodium succinate, up to 40 mg	N N1 ☑
	Use this code for Solu-Medrol, A-methaPred.	
	AHA: 4Q,18	
J2930	Injection, methylprednisolone sodium succinate, up to 125 mg	N N1 ☑
	Use this code for Solu-Medrol, A-methaPred.	
	AHA: 4Q,18	
J2940	Injection, somatrem, 1 mg	F1 ☑
	Use this code for Protropin.	
	AHA: 4Q,18	
J2941	Injection, somatropin, 1 mg	K K2 ☑
	Use this code for Humatrope, Genotropin Nutropin, Biotropin, Genotropin, Genotropin Miniquick, Norditropin, Nutropin, Nutropin AQ, Saizen, Saizen Somatropin RDNA Origin, Serostim, Serostim RDNA Origin, Zorbtive.	
	CMS: 100-02,15,50.5	
	AHA: 4Q,18	
J2950	Injection, promazine HCl, up to 25 mg	N N1 ☑
	Use this code for Sparine, Prozine-50.	
	AHA: 4Q,18	
J2993	Injection, reteplase, 18.1 mg	K K2 ☑
	Use this code for Retavase.	
	AHA: 3Q,21; 4Q,18	
J2995	Injection, streptokinase, per 250,000 IU	N ☑
	Use this code for Streptase.	
	AHA: 3Q,21; 4Q,18	
J2997	Injection, alteplase recombinant, 1 mg	K K2 ☑
	Use this code for Activase, Cathflo.	
	AHA: 3Q,21; 4Q,18	
J2998	Injection, plasminogen, human-tvmh, 1 mg	K2
	Use this code for Ryplazim.	
	AHA: 3Q,22	
J3000	Injection, streptomycin, up to 1 g	N N1 ☑
	Use this code for Streptomycin Sulfate.	
	AHA: 4Q,18	
J3010	Injection, fentanyl citrate, 0.1 mg	N N1 ☑
	Use this code for Sublimaze.	
	CMS: 100-04,20,180; 100-04,32,411.3	
	AHA: 4Q,18	
J3030	Injection, sumatriptan succinate, 6 mg (code may be used for Medicare when drug administered under the direct supervision of a physician, not for use when drug is self-administered)	N N1 ☑
	Use this code for Imitrex.	
	CMS: 100-02,15,50.5	
	AHA: 4Q,18	
J3031	Injection, fremanezumab-vfrm, 1 mg (code may be used for Medicare when drug administered under the direct supervision of a physician, not for use when drug is self-administered)	K2
	Use this code for Ajovy.	
	AHA: 4Q,19	
J3032	Injection, eptinezumab-jjmr, 1 mg	K2
	Use this code for Vyepti.	
	AHA: 4Q,20	
J3060	Injection, taliglucerase alfa, 10 units	K K2 ☑
	Use this code for Elelyso.	
	AHA: 4Q,18	
J3070	Injection, pentazocine, 30 mg	K N1 ☑
	Use this code for Talwin.	
	AHA: 4Q,18	
J3090	Injection, tedizolid phosphate, 1 mg	K K2 ☑
	Use this code for Sivextro.	
	AHA: 4Q,18	
J3095	Injection, telavancin, 10 mg	K K2 ☑
	Use this code for VIBATIV.	
	AHA: 4Q,18	
J3101	Injection, tenecteplase, 1 mg	K K2 ☑
	Use this code for TNKase.	
	AHA: 3Q,21; 3Q,20; 4Q,18	
J3105	Injection, terbutaline sulfate, up to 1 mg	N N1 ☑
	For terbutaline in inhalation solution, see K0525 and K0526.	
	AHA: 4Q,18	
J3110	Injection, teriparatide, 10 mcg	B ☑
	Use this code for Forteo.	
	CMS: 100-02,15,50.5; 100-04,10,90.1	
	AHA: 4Q,18	

Special Coverage Instructions	Noncovered by Medicare	Carrier Discretion	☑ Quantity Alert ● New Code ○ Recycled/Reinstated ▲ Revised Code

Drugs Administered Other Than Oral Method

J3111 — J3370

J3111 Injection, romosozumab-aqqg, 1 mg ☒ K2
Use this code for Evenity.
CMS: 100-04,10,90.1

J3121 Injection, testosterone enanthate, 1 mg ☒N ☒N1 ☑
Use this code for Delatstryl.
AHA: 4Q,18

J3145 Injection, testosterone undecanoate, 1 mg ☒K ☒K2 ☑
Use this code for Aveed.
AHA: 4Q,18

J3230 Injection, chlorpromazine HCl, up to 50 mg ☒N ☒N1 ☑
Use this code for Thorazine.
AHA: 4Q,18

J3240 Injection, thyrotropin alpha, 0.9 mg, provided in 1.1 mg vial ☒K ☒K2 ☑
Use this code for Thyrogen.
AHA: 4Q,18

J3241 Injection, teprotumumab-trbw, 10 mg ☒ K2
Use this code for Tepezza.
AHA: 4Q,20

J3243 Injection, tigecycline, 1 mg ☒K ☒N1 ☑
Use this code for Tygacil.
AHA: 4Q,18

J3244 Injection, tigecycline (Accord) not therapeutically equivalent to J3243, 1 mg
Use this code for tigecycline manufactured by Accord.
AHA: 1Q,23

J3245 Injection, tildrakizumab, 1 mg ☒ K2
Use this code for Ilumya.
AHA: 4Q,18

J3246 Injection, tirofiban HCl, 0.25 mg ☒K ☒N1 ☑
Use this code for Aggrastat.
AHA: 4Q,18

J3250 Injection, trimethobenzamide HCl, up to 200 mg ☒N ☒N1 ☑
Use this code for Tigan, Tiject-20, Arrestin.
AHA: 4Q,18

J3260 Injection, tobramycin sulfate, up to 80 mg ☒N ☒N1 ☑
Use this code for Nebcin.
AHA: 4Q,18

J3262 Injection, tocilizumab, 1 mg ☒K ☒K2 ☑
Use this code for ACTEMRA.
AHA: 4Q,18

J3265 Injection, torsemide, 10 mg/ml ☒N ☑
Use this code for Demadex, Torsemide.
AHA: 4Q,18

J3280 Injection, thiethylperazine maleate, up to 10 mg ☒E1 ☑
AHA: 4Q,18

J3285 Injection, treprostinil, 1 mg ☒K ☒K2 ☑
Use this code for Remodulin.
CMS: 100-04,20,180; 100-04,32,411.3
AHA: 4Q,18

J3299 Injection, triamcinolone acetonide (Xipere), 1 mg ☒ K2
AHA: 3Q,22

J3300 Injection, triamcinolone acetonide, preservative free, 1 mg ☒K ☒N1 ☑
Use this code for TRIVARIS, TRIESENCE.
AHA: 4Q,18

J3301 Injection, triamcinolone acetonide, not otherwise specified, 10 mg ☒N ☒N1 ☑
Use this code for Kenalog-10, Kenalog-40, Tri-Kort, Kenaject-40, Cenacort A-40, Triam-A, Trilog.
AHA: 4Q,18; 3Q,17

J3302 Injection, triamcinolone diacetate, per 5 mg ☒N ☒N1 ☑
Use this code for Aristocort, Aristocort Intralesional, Aristocort Forte, Amcort, Trilone, Cenacort Forte.
AHA: 4Q,18

J3303 Injection, triamcinolone hexacetonide, per 5 mg ☒N ☒N1 ☑
Use this code for Aristospan Intralesional, Aristospan Intra-articular.
AHA: 4Q,18

J3304 Injection, triamcinolone acetonide, preservative-free, extended-release, microsphere formulation, 1 mg ☒ K2
Use this code for Zilretta.
AHA: 1Q,19; 4Q,18

J3305 Injection, trimetrexate glucuronate, per 25 mg ☒E1 ☑
Use this code for Neutrexin.
AHA: 4Q,18

J3310 Injection, perphenazine, up to 5 mg ☒N ☒N1 ☑
Use this code for Trilafon.
AHA: 4Q,18

J3315 Injection, triptorelin pamoate, 3.75 mg ♂ ☒K ☒K2 ☑
Use this code for Trelstar Depot, Trelstar Depot Plus Debioclip Kit, Trelstar LA.
AHA: 4Q,18

J3316 Injection, triptorelin, extended-release, 3.75 mg ☒ K2
Use this code for Triptodur.
AHA: 1Q,19; 4Q,18

J3320 Injection, spectinomycin dihydrochloride, up to 2 g ☒E1 ☑
Use this code for Trobicin.
AHA: 4Q,18

J3350 Injection, urea, up to 40 g ☒N ☑
AHA: 4Q,18

J3355 Injection, urofollitropin, 75 IU ☒E1 ☑
Use this code for Metrodin, Bravelle, Fertinex.
CMS: 100-02,15,50.5
AHA: 4Q,18

J3357 Ustekinumab, for subcutaneous injection, 1 mg ☒K ☒K2 ☑
Use this code for STELARA.
CMS: 100-02,15,50.5
AHA: 4Q,18; 1Q,17

J3358 Ustekinumab, for intravenous injection, 1 mg ☒G ☒K2
Use this code for Stelara.
AHA: 4Q,18; 1Q,18

J3360 Injection, diazepam, up to 5 mg ☒N ☒N1 ☑
Use this code for Diastat, Dizac, Valium.
CMS: 100-04,8,60.2.1
AHA: 4Q,18

J3364 Injection, urokinase, 5,000 IU vial ☒N ☒N1 ☑
Use this code for Kinlytic.
AHA: 3Q,21; 4Q,18

J3365 Injection, IV, urokinase, 250,000 IU vial ☒E1 ☑
Use this code for Kinlytic.
AHA: 3Q,21; 4Q,18

J3370 Injection, vancomycin HCl, 500 mg ☒N ☒N1 ☑
Use this code for Vancocin.
AHA: 4Q,18

Special Coverage Instructions   Noncovered by Medicare   Carrier Discretion   ☑ Quantity Alert ● New Code   ○ Recycled/Reinstated ▲ Revised Code

110 — J Codes   Ⓐ Age Edit   Ⓜ Maternity Edit   ♀ Female Only   ♂ Male Only   Ⓐ-Ⓨ OPPS Status Indicators   © 2023 Optum360, LLC

J3371   **Injection, vancomycin HCl (Mylan) not therapeutically equivalent to J3370, 500 mg**
Use this code for vancomycin HCl manufactured by Mylan.
AHA: 1Q,23

J3372   **Injection, vancomycin HCl (Xellia) not therapeutically equivalent to J3370, 500 mg**
Use this code for vancomycin HCl manufactured by Xellia.
AHA: 1Q,23

J3380   **Injection, vedolizumab, 1 mg**   K K2 ☑
Use this code for Entyvio.
AHA: 4Q,18

J3385   **Injection, velaglucerase alfa, 100 units**   K K2 ☑
Use this code for VPRIV.
AHA: 4Q,18

J3396   **Injection, verteporfin, 0.1 mg**   K K2 ☑
Use this code for Visudyne.
CMS: 100-03,80.2; 100-03,80.2.1; 100-03,80.3; 100-03,80.3.1; 100-04,32,300; 100-04,32,300.1; 100-04,32,300.2
AHA: 1Q,20; 4Q,18

J3397   **Injection, vestronidase alfa-vjbk, 1 mg**
Use this code for Mepsevii.
CMS: 100-04,4,260.1; 100-04,4,260.1.1
AHA: 1Q,19; 4Q,18

J3398   **Injection, voretigene neparvovec-rzyl, 1 billion vector genomes**   K2
Use this code for Luxturna.
AHA: 1Q,19; 4Q,18

J3399   **Injection, onasemnogene abeparvovec-xioi, per treatment, up to 5×10^{15} vector genomes**
Use this code for Zolgensma.
AHA: 2Q,20

J3400   **Injection, triflupromazine HCl, up to 20 mg**   EI ☑
AHA: 4Q,18

● **J3401**   **Beremagene geperpavec-svdt for topical administration, containing nominal 5×10^9 PFU/ml vector genomes, per 0.1 ml**
Use this code for Vyjuvek.

J3410   **Injection, hydroxyzine HCl, up to 25 mg**   N N1 ☑
Use this code for Vistaril, Vistaject-25, Hyzine, Hyzine-50.
AHA: 4Q,18

J3411   **Injection, thiamine HCl, 100 mg**   N N1 ☑
AHA: 4Q,18

J3415   **Injection, pyridoxine HCl, 100 mg**   N N1 ☑
AHA: 4Q,18

J3420   **Injection, vitamin B-12 cyanocobalamin, up to 1,000 mcg**   N N1 ☑
Use this code for Sytobex, Redisol, Rubramin PC, Betalin 12, Berubigen, Cobex, Cobal, Crystal B12, Cyano, Cyanocobalamin, Hydroxocobalamin, Hydroxycobal, Nutri-Twelve.
AHA: 4Q,18

● **J3425**   **Injection, hydroxocobalamin, 10 mcg**

J3430   **Injection, phytonadione (vitamin K), per 1 mg**   N N1 ☑
Use this code for AquaMephyton, Konakion, Menadione, Phytonadione.
AHA: 4Q,18

J3465   **Injection, voriconazole, 10 mg**   K N1 ☑
AHA: 4Q,18

J3470   **Injection, hyaluronidase, up to 150 units**   N N1 ☑
AHA: 4Q,18

J3471   **Injection, hyaluronidase, ovine, preservative free, per 1 USP unit (up to 999 USP units)**   N N1 ☑
AHA: 4Q,18

J3472   **Injection, hyaluronidase, ovine, preservative free, per 1,000 USP units**   N N1 ☑
AHA: 4Q,18

J3473   **Injection, hyaluronidase, recombinant, 1 USP unit**   N N1 ☑
AHA: 4Q,18

J3475   **Injection, magnesium sulfate, per 500 mg**   N N1 ☑
Use this code for Mag Sul, Sulfa Mag.
AHA: 4Q,18

J3480   **Injection, potassium chloride, per 2 mEq**   N N1 ☑
AHA: 4Q,18

J3485   **Injection, zidovudine, 10 mg**   N N1 ☑
Use this code for Retrovir, Zidovudine.
AHA: 4Q,18

J3486   **Injection, ziprasidone mesylate, 10 mg**   N N1 ☑
Use this code for Geodon.
AHA: 4Q,18

J3489   **Injection, zoledronic acid, 1 mg**   N N1 ☑
Use this code for Reclast and Zometa.
AHA: 4Q,18

J3490   **Unclassified drugs**   N N1 ☑
CMS: 100-02,15,50.5; 100-03,1,110.22; 100-03,110.22; 100-04,10,90.1; 100-04,32,280.1; 100-04,32,280.2; 100-04,32,400; 100-04,32,400.1; 100-04,32,400.2; 100-04,32,400.2.1; 100-04,32,400.2.2; 100-04,32,400.2.3; 100-04,32,400.2.3.1; 100-04,32,400.2.4; 100-04,32,400.2.5; 100-04,32,400.3; 100-04,32,400.4; 100-04,4,260.1; 100-04,4,260.1.1; 100-04,8,60.2.1.1; 100-04,8,60.2.3
AHA: 3Q,23; 3Q,21; 1Q,17

J3520   **Edetate disodium, per 150 mg**   EI ☑
Use this code for Endrate, Disotate, Meritate, Chealamide, E.D.T.A. This drug is used in chelation therapy, a treatment for atherosclerosis that is not covered by Medicare.

J3530   **Nasal vaccine inhalation**   N N1 ☑

J3535   **Drug administered through a metered dose inhaler**   EI ☑

J3570   **Laetrile, amygdalin, vitamin B-17**   EI ☑
The FDA has found Laetrile to have no safe or effective therapeutic purpose.

J3590   **Unclassified biologics**   N N1 ☑
CMS: 100-02,15,50.5; 100-03,1,110.22; 100-03,110.22; 100-04,10,90.1; 100-04,32,280.1; 100-04,32,280.2; 100-04,32,400; 100-04,32,400.1; 100-04,32,400.2; 100-04,32,400.2.1; 100-04,32,400.2.2; 100-04,32,400.2.3; 100-04,32,400.2.3.1; 100-04,32,400.2.4; 100-04,32,400.2.5; 100-04,32,400.3; 100-04,32,400.4
AHA: 3Q,23; 1Q,17

J3591   **Unclassified drug or biological used for ESRD on dialysis**
CMS: 100-04,4,260.1; 100-04,4,260.1.1; 100-04,8,20
AHA: 1Q,19

J7030   **Infusion, normal saline solution, 1,000 cc**   N N1 ☑

J7040   **Infusion, normal saline solution, sterile (500 ml=1 unit)**   N N1 ☑

J7042   **5% dextrose/normal saline (500 ml = 1 unit)**   N N1 ☑

J7050   **Infusion, normal saline solution, 250 cc**   N N1 ☑

J7060   **5% dextrose/water (500 ml = 1 unit)**   N N1 ☑

J7070   **Infusion, D-5-W, 1,000 cc**   N N1 ☑

J7100   **Infusion, dextran 40, 500 ml**   N N1 ☑
Use this code for Gentran, 10% LMD, Rheomacrodex.

Drugs Administered Other Than Oral Method

J3371 — J7100

Special Coverage Instructions   Noncovered by Medicare   Carrier Discretion   ☑ Quantity Alert   ● New Code   ○ Recycled/Reinstated   ▲ Revised Code

J7110 Infusion, dextran 75, 500 ml N M1 ☑
Use this code for Gentran 75.

J7120 Ringers lactate infusion, up to 1,000 cc N M1 ☑

J7121 5% dextrose in lactated ringers infusion, up to 1000 cc N M1 ☑

J7131 Hypertonic saline solution, 1 ml N M1 ☑

J7168 Prothrombin complex concentrate (human), Kcentra, per IU of Factor IX activity K2
AHA: 3Q,21

J7169 Injection, coagulation Factor Xa (recombinant), inactivated-zhzo (Andexxa), 10 mg K2
AHA: 2Q,20

J7170 Injection, emicizumab-kxwh, 0.5 mg K2
Use this code for Hemlibra.
AHA: 1Q,19; 4Q,18

J7175 Injection, Factor X, (human), 1 IU K K2 ☑
Use this code for Coagadex.
AHA: 4Q,18; 1Q,17

J7177 Injection, human fibrinogen concentrate (Fibryga), 1 mg K2
CMS: 100-04,4,260.1; 100-04,4,260.1.1
AHA: 1Q,19; 4Q,18

J7178 Injection, human fibrinogen concentrate, not otherwise specified, 1 mg K K2 ☑
Use this code for RiaSTAP.
AHA: 4Q,18

J7179 Injection, von Willebrand factor (recombinant), (Vonvendi), 1 IU VWF:RCo G K2 ☑
AHA: 4Q,18; 1Q,17

J7180 Injection, Factor XIII (antihemophilic factor, human), 1 IU K M1 ☑
Use this code for Corifact.
AHA: 4Q,18

J7181 Injection, Factor XIII A-subunit, (recombinant), per IU K M1 ☑
AHA: 4Q,18

J7182 Injection, Factor VIII, (antihemophilic factor, recombinant), (NovoEight), per IU K K2 ☑
AHA: 4Q,18

J7183 Injection, von Willebrand factor complex (human), Wilate, 1 IU VWF:RCO K K2 ☑
AHA: 4Q,18

J7185 Injection, Factor VIII (antihemophilic factor, recombinant) (Xyntha), per IU K K2 ☑
AHA: 4Q,18

J7186 Injection, antihemophilic Factor VIII/von Willebrand factor complex (human), per Factor VIII IU K K2 ☑
Use this code for Alphanate.
CMS: 100-04,17,80.4.1
AHA: 4Q,18

J7187 Injection, von Willebrand factor complex (Humate-P), per IU VWF:RCO K K2 ☑
CMS: 100-04,17,80.4.1
AHA: 4Q,18

J7188 Injection, Factor VIII (antihemophilic factor, recombinant) (Obizur), per IU K K2 ☑
AHA: 4Q,18

J7189 Factor VIIa (antihemophilic factor, recombinant), (NovoSeven RT), 1 mcg K K2 ☑
CMS: 100-04,17,80.4.1

J7190 Factor VIII (antihemophilic factor, human) per IU K K2 ☑
Use this code for Koate-DVI, Monarc-M, Monoclate-P.
CMS: 100-04,17,80.4; 100-04,17,80.4.1

J7191 Factor VIII (antihemophilic factor (porcine)), per IU EI ☑
CMS: 100-04,17,80.4; 100-04,17,80.4.1

J7192 Factor VIII (antihemophilic factor, recombinant) per IU, not otherwise specified K K2 ☑
Use this code for Advate rAHF-PFM, Antihemophilic Factor Human Method M Monoclonal Purified, Bioclate, Kogenate FS, Recombinate, Refacto.
CMS: 100-04,17,80.4; 100-04,17,80.4.1

J7193 Factor IX (antihemophilic factor, purified, nonrecombinant) per IU K K2 ☑
Use this code for AlphaNine SD, Mononine.
CMS: 100-04,17,80.4; 100-04,17,80.4.1

J7194 Factor IX complex, per IU K K2 ☑
Use this code for Konyne-80, Profilnine SD, Proplex T, Proplex T, Bebulin VH, factor IX+ complex, Profilnine SD.
CMS: 100-04,17,80.4; 100-04,17,80.4.1

J7195 Injection, Factor IX (antihemophilic factor, recombinant) per IU, not otherwise specified K K2 ☑
Use this code for Antithrombate III, Benefix, Thrombate III.
CMS: 100-04,17,80.4; 100-04,17,80.4.1
AHA: 4Q,18

J7196 Injection, antithrombin recombinant, 50 IU EI ☑
Use this code for ATryn.
AHA: 4Q,18

J7197 Antithrombin III (human), per IU K K2 ☑
Use this code for Thrombate III, ATnativ.
CMS: 100-04,17,80.4.1

J7198 Antiinhibitor, per IU K K2 ☑
Medicare jurisdiction: local contractor. Use this code for Autoplex T, Feiba VH AICC.
CMS: 100-03,110.3; 100-04,17,80.4; 100-04,17,80.4.1

J7199 Hemophilia clotting factor, not otherwise classified B ☑
Medicare jurisdiction: local contractor.
CMS: 100-04,17,80.4; 100-04,17,80.4.1

J7200 Injection, Factor IX, (antihemophilic factor, recombinant), Rixubis, per IU K K2 ☑
AHA: 4Q,18

J7201 Injection, Factor IX, Fc fusion protein, (recombinant), Alprolix, 1 IU K K2 ☑
AHA: 4Q,18

J7202 Injection, Factor IX, albumin fusion protein, (recombinant), Idelvion, 1 IU G K2 ☑
AHA: 4Q,18

J7203 Injection Factor IX, (antihemophilic factor, recombinant), glycoPEGylated, (Rebinyn), 1 IU K2
AHA: 1Q,19; 4Q,18

J7204 Injection, Factor VIII, antihemophilic factor (recombinant), (Esperoct), glycopegylated-exei, per IU K2
AHA: 2Q,20

J7205 Injection, Factor VIII Fc fusion protein (recombinant), per IU K K2 ☑
Use this code for Eloctate.
AHA: 4Q,18

J7207 Injection, Factor VIII, (antihemophilic factor, recombinant), PEGylated, 1 IU G K2 ☑
Use this code for Adynovate.
AHA: 4Q,18

Special Coverage Instructions   Noncovered by Medicare   Carrier Discretion   ☑ Quantity Alert   ● New Code   ○ Recycled/Reinstated   ▲ Revised Code

J7208 Injection, Factor VIII, (antihemophilic factor, recombinant), PEGylated-aucl, (Jivi), 1 IU K2
AHA: 3Q,19

J7209 Injection, Factor VIII, (antihemophilic factor, recombinant), (Nuwiq), 1 IU G K2 ☑
AHA: 4Q,18

J7210 Injection, Factor VIII, (antihemophilic factor, recombinant), (Afstyla), 1 IU G K2
AHA: 4Q,18; 1Q,18

J7211 Injection, Factor VIII, (antihemophilic factor, recombinant), (Kovaltry), 1 IU K K2
AHA: 4Q,18; 1Q,18

J7212 Factor VIIa (antihemophilic factor, recombinant)-jncw (Sevenfact), 1 mcg K2
AHA: 1Q,21

● **J7213** Injection, coagulation factor IX (recombinant), Ixinity, 1 IU K2
AHA: 3Q,23

● **J7214** Injection, Factor VIII/von Willebrand factor complex, recombinant (Altuviiio), per Factor VIII IU K2

J7294 Segesterone acetate and ethinyl estradiol 0.15 mg, 0.013 mg per 24 hours; yearly vaginal system, ea
Use this code for Annovera vaginal ring.
AHA: 4Q,21

J7295 Ethinyl estradiol and etonogestrel 0.015 mg, 0.12 mg per 24 hours; monthly vaginal ring, ea
Use this code for NuvaRing vaginal ring.
AHA: 4Q,21

J7296 Levonorgestrel-releasing intrauterine contraceptive system, (Kyleena), 19.5 mg ♀ EI
AHA: 1Q,18

J7297 Levonorgestrel-releasing intrauterine contraceptive system (Liletta), 52 mg M ♀ EI ☑

J7298 Levonorgestrel-releasing intrauterine contraceptive system (Mirena), 52 mg M ♀ EI ☑
AHA: 1Q,23

J7300 Intrauterine copper contraceptive EI ☑
Use this code for Paragard T380A.

J7301 Levonorgestrel-releasing intrauterine contraceptive system (Skyla), 13.5 mg M ♀ EI ☑

J7304 Contraceptive supply, hormone containing patch, each EI ☑

J7306 Levonorgestrel (contraceptive) implant system, including implants and supplies EI ☑

J7307 Etonogestrel (contraceptive) implant system, including implant and supplies EI ☑
Use this code for Implanon and Nexplanon.

J7308 Aminolevulinic acid HCl for topical administration, 20%, single unit dosage form (354 mg) K K2 ☑
Use this code for Levulan Kerastick.
AHA: 1Q,20

J7309 Methyl aminolevulinate (MAL) for topical administration, 16.8%, 1 g N ☑
Use this code for Metvixia.
AHA: 1Q,20

J7310 Ganciclovir, 4.5 mg, long-acting implant EI ☑
Use this code for Vitrasert.

J7311 Injection, fluocinolone acetonide, intravitreal implant (Retisert), 0.01 mg K K2 ☑

J7312 Injection, dexamethasone, intravitreal implant, 0.1 mg K K2 ☑
Use this code for OZURDEX.
AHA: 4Q,18

J7313 Injection, fluocinolone acetonide, intravitreal implant (Iluvien), 0.01 mg K K2 ☑
AHA: 4Q,18

J7314 Injection, fluocinolone acetonide, intravitreal implant (Yutiq), 0.01 mg K2
AHA: 4Q,19

J7315 Mitomycin, opthalmic, 0.2 mg N N1 ☑
Use this code for Mitosol.

J7316 Injection, ocriplasmin, 0.125 mg K K2 ☑
Use this code for Jetrea.
AHA: 4Q,18

J7318 Hyaluronan or derivative, Durolane, for intra-articular injection, 1 mg K2
AHA: 1Q,19; 4Q,18

J7320 Hyaluronan or derivative, GenVisc 850, for intra-articular injection, 1 mg K K2 ☑
AHA: 4Q,18

J7321 Hyaluronan or derivative, Hyalgan, Supartz or Visco-3, for intra-articular injection, per dose K M1 ☑
AHA: 1Q,21; 2Q,20; 4Q,18

J7322 Hyaluronan or derivative, Hymovis, for intra-articular injection, 1 mg G K2 ☑
AHA: 4Q,18

J7323 Hyaluronan or derivative, Euflexxa, for intra-articular injection, per dose K K2 ☑
AHA: 4Q,18

J7324 Hyaluronan or derivative, Orthovisc, for intra-articular injection, per dose K K2 ☑
AHA: 4Q,18

J7325 Hyaluronan or derivative, Synvisc or Synvisc-One, for intra-articular injection, 1 mg K K2 ☑
AHA: 4Q,18

J7326 Hyaluronan or derivative, Gel-One, for intra-articular injection, per dose K K2 ☑
AHA: 4Q,18

J7327 Hyaluronan or derivative, Monovisc, for intra-articular injection, per dose K K2 ☑
AHA: 4Q,18

J7328 Hyaluronan or derivative, GELSYN-3, for intra-articular injection, 0.1 mg G K2 ☑
AHA: 4Q,18

J7329 Hyaluronan or derivative, Trivisc, for intra-articular injection, 1 mg K2
CMS: 100-04,4,260.1; 100-04,4,260.1.1
AHA: 1Q,19; 4Q,18

J7330 Autologous cultured chondrocytes, implant B ☑
Medicare jurisdiction: local contractor. Use this code for Carticel.

J7331 Hyaluronan or derivative, SYNOJOYNT, for intra-articular injection, 1 mg K2
AHA: 4Q,19

J7332 Hyaluronan or derivative, Triluron, for intra-articular injection, 1 mg N1
AHA: 4Q,19

J7336 Capsaicin 8% patch, per sq cm K K2 ☑
Use this code for Qutenza.

Special Coverage Instructions   Noncovered by Medicare   Carrier Discretion   ☑ Quantity Alert ● New Code   ○ Recycled/Reinstated   ▲ Revised Code

J7340 Carbidopa 5 mg/levodopa 20 mg enteral suspension, 100 ml K K2 ☑
Use this code for Duopa.

J7342 Instillation, ciprofloxacin otic suspension, 6 mg G K2 ☑
Use this code for Otiprio.

J7345 Aminolevulinic acid HCl for topical administration, 10% gel, 10 mg G K2
Use this code for Ameluz.
AHA: 1Q,20; 1Q,18; 4Q,17

J7351 Injection, bimatoprost, intracameral implant, 1 mcg K2
Use this code for Durysta.
AHA: 4Q,20

J7352 Afamelanotide implant, 1 mg K2
Use this code for Scenesse.
AHA: 1Q,21

● **J7353** Anacaulase-bcdb, 8.8% gel, 1 gm N1
Use this code for Nexobrid.

J7402 Mometasone furoate sinus implant, (Sinuva), 10 mcg K2
AHA: 1Q,21

J7500 Azathioprine, oral, 50 mg N N1 ☑
Use this code for Azasan, Imuran.
CMS: 100-04,17,80.3

J7501 Azathioprine, parenteral, 100 mg K K2 ☑
CMS: 100-04,17,80.3

J7502 Cyclosporine, oral, 100 mg N N1 ☑
Use this code for Neoral, Sandimmune, Gengraf, Sangcya.
CMS: 100-04,17,80.3

J7503 Tacrolimus, extended release, (Envarsus XR), oral, 0.25 mg G N1 ☑

J7504 Lymphocyte immune globulin, antithymocyte globulin, equine, parenteral, 250 mg K K2 ☑
Use this code for Atgam.
CMS: 100-03,260.7; 100-04,17,80.3

J7505 Muromonab-CD3, parenteral, 5 mg K N1 ☑
Use this code for Orthoclone OKT3.
CMS: 100-04,17,80.3

J7507 Tacrolimus, immediate release, oral, 1 mg N N1 ☑
Use this code for Prograf.
CMS: 100-04,17,80.3

J7508 Tacrolimus, extended release, (Astagraf XL), oral, 0.1 mg N N1 ☑

J7509 Methylprednisolone, oral, per 4 mg N N1 ☑
Use this code for Medrol, Methylpred.
CMS: 100-04,17,80.3

J7510 Prednisolone, oral, per 5 mg N N1 ☑
Use this code for Delta-Cortef, Cotolone, Pediapred, Prednoral, Prelone.
CMS: 100-04,17,80.3

J7511 Lymphocyte immune globulin, antithymocyte globulin, rabbit, parenteral, 25 mg K K2 ☑
Use this code for Thymoglobulin.
CMS: 100-04,17,80.3

J7512 Prednisone, immediate release or delayed release, oral, 1 mg N N1 ☑

J7513 Daclizumab, parenteral, 25 mg E1 ☑
Use this code for Zenapax.
CMS: 100-04,17,80.3

J7515 Cyclosporine, oral, 25 mg N N1 ☑
Use this code for Neoral, Sandimmune, Gengraf, Sangcya.
CMS: 100-04,17,80.3

J7516 Cyclosporine, parenteral, 250 mg N N1 ☑
Use this code for Neoral, Sandimmune, Gengraf, Sangcya.
CMS: 100-04,17,80.3

J7517 Mycophenolate mofetil, oral, 250 mg N N1 ☑
Use this code for CellCept.
CMS: 100-04,17,80.3

J7518 Mycophenolic acid, oral, 180 mg N N1 ☑
Use this code for Myfortic Delayed Release.
CMS: 100-04,17,80.3.1

● **J7519** Injection, mycophenolate mofetil, 10 mg K2
Use this code for CellCept.

J7520 Sirolimus, oral, 1 mg N N1 ☑
Use this code for Rapamune.
CMS: 100-04,17,80.3

J7525 Tacrolimus, parenteral, 5 mg K K2 ☑
Use this code for Prograf.
CMS: 100-04,17,80.3

J7527 Everolimus, oral, 0.25 mg N N1 ☑
Use this code for Zortress, Afinitor.

J7599 Immunosuppressive drug, not otherwise classified N N1 ☑
Determine if an alternative HCPCS Level II or a CPT code better describes the service being reported. This code should be used only if a more specific code is unavailable.
CMS: 100-04,17,80.3

Inhalation Drugs

J7604 Acetylcysteine, inhalation solution, compounded product, administered through DME, unit dose form, per g M ☑

J7605 Arformoterol, inhalation solution, FDA-approved final product, noncompounded, administered through DME, unit dose form, 15 mcg M ☑
CMS: 100-02,15,50.5

J7606 Formoterol fumarate, inhalation solution, FDA-approved final product, noncompounded, administered through DME, unit dose form, 20 mcg M ☑
Use this code for PERFOROMIST.
CMS: 100-02,15,50.5

J7607 Levalbuterol, inhalation solution, compounded product, administered through DME, concentrated form, 0.5 mg M ☑
CMS: 100-03,200.2

J7608 Acetylcysteine, inhalation solution, FDA-approved final product, noncompounded, administered through DME, unit dose form, per g M ☑
Use this code for Acetadote, Mucomyst, Mucosil.

J7609 Albuterol, inhalation solution, compounded product, administered through DME, unit dose, 1 mg M ☑

J7610 Albuterol, inhalation solution, compounded product, administered through DME, concentrated form, 1 mg M ☑

J7611 Albuterol, inhalation solution, FDA-approved final product, noncompounded, administered through DME, concentrated form, 1 mg M ☑
Use this code for Accuneb, Proventil, Respirol, Ventolin.

J7612 Levalbuterol, inhalation solution, FDA-approved final product, noncompounded, administered through DME, concentrated form, 0.5 mg M ☑
Use this code for Xopenex HFA.
CMS: 100-03,200.2

J7613 Albuterol, inhalation solution, FDA-approved final product, noncompounded, administered through DME, unit dose, 1 mg M ☑
Use this code for Accuneb, Proventil, Respirol, Ventolin.

Special Coverage Instructions   Noncovered by Medicare   Carrier Discretion   ☑ Quantity Alert ● New Code ○ Recycled/Reinstated ▲ Revised Code

114 — J Codes   A Age Edit   M Maternity Edit   ♀ Female Only   ♂ Male Only   A-Y OPPS Status Indicators   © 2023 Optum360, LLC

J7614 Levalbuterol, inhalation solution, FDA-approved final product, noncompounded, administered through DME, unit dose, 0.5 mg ☑ M ☑
Use this code for Xopenex.
CMS: 100-03,200.2

J7615 Levalbuterol, inhalation solution, compounded product, administered through DME, unit dose, 0.5 mg ☑ M ☑
CMS: 100-03,200.2

J7620 Albuterol, up to 2.5 mg and ipratropium bromide, up to 0.5 mg, FDA-approved final product, noncompounded, administered through DME ☑ M ☑

J7622 Beclomethasone, inhalation solution, compounded product, administered through DME, unit dose form, per mg ☑ M ☑
Use this code for Beclovent, Beconase.

J7624 Betamethasone, inhalation solution, compounded product, administered through DME, unit dose form, per mg ☑ M ☑

J7626 Budesonide, inhalation solution, FDA-approved final product, noncompounded, administered through DME, unit dose form, up to 0.5 mg ☑ M ☑
Use this code for Pulmicort, Pulmicort Flexhaler, Pulmicort Respules, Vanceril.

J7627 Budesonide, inhalation solution, compounded product, administered through DME, unit dose form, up to 0.5 mg ☑ M ☑

J7628 Bitolterol mesylate, inhalation solution, compounded product, administered through DME, concentrated form, per mg ☑ M ☑

J7629 Bitolterol mesylate, inhalation solution, compounded product, administered through DME, unit dose form, per mg ☑ M ☑

J7631 Cromolyn sodium, inhalation solution, FDA-approved final product, noncompounded, administered through DME, unit dose form, per 10 mg ☑ M ☑
Use this code for Intal, Nasalcrom.

J7632 Cromolyn sodium, inhalation solution, compounded product, administered through DME, unit dose form, per 10 mg ☑ M ☑

J7633 Budesonide, inhalation solution, FDA-approved final product, noncompounded, administered through DME, concentrated form, per 0.25 mg ☑ M ☑
Use this code for Pulmicort, Pulmicort Flexhaler, Pulmicort Respules, Vanceril.

J7634 Budesonide, inhalation solution, compounded product, administered through DME, concentrated form, per 0.25 mg ☑ M ☑

J7635 Atropine, inhalation solution, compounded product, administered through DME, concentrated form, per mg ☑ M ☑

J7636 Atropine, inhalation solution, compounded product, administered through DME, unit dose form, per mg ☑ M ☑

J7637 Dexamethasone, inhalation solution, compounded product, administered through DME, concentrated form, per mg ☑ M ☑

J7638 Dexamethasone, inhalation solution, compounded product, administered through DME, unit dose form, per mg ☑ M ☑

J7639 Dornase alfa, inhalation solution, FDA-approved final product, noncompounded, administered through DME, unit dose form, per mg ☑ M ☑
Use this code for Pulmozyme.
CMS: 100-02,15,50.5

J7640 Formoterol, inhalation solution, compounded product, administered through DME, unit dose form, 12 mcg ☑ E1 ☑

J7641 Flunisolide, inhalation solution, compounded product, administered through DME, unit dose, per mg ☑ M ☑
Use this code for Aerobid, Flunisolide.

J7642 Glycopyrrolate, inhalation solution, compounded product, administered through DME, concentrated form, per mg ☑ M ☑

J7643 Glycopyrrolate, inhalation solution, compounded product, administered through DME, unit dose form, per mg ☑ M ☑

J7644 Ipratropium bromide, inhalation solution, FDA-approved final product, noncompounded, administered through DME, unit dose form, per mg ☑ M ☑
Use this code for Atrovent.

J7645 Ipratropium bromide, inhalation solution, compounded product, administered through DME, unit dose form, per mg ☑ M ☑

J7647 Isoetharine HCl, inhalation solution, compounded product, administered through DME, concentrated form, per mg ☑ M ☑

J7648 Isoetharine HCl, inhalation solution, FDA-approved final product, noncompounded, administered through DME, concentrated form, per mg ☑ M ☑
Use this code for Beta-2.

J7649 Isoetharine HCl, inhalation solution, FDA-approved final product, noncompounded, administered through DME, unit dose form, per mg ☑ M ☑

J7650 Isoetharine HCl, inhalation solution, compounded product, administered through DME, unit dose form, per mg ☑ M ☑

J7657 Isoproterenol HCl, inhalation solution, compounded product, administered through DME, concentrated form, per mg ☑ M ☑

J7658 Isoproterenol HCl, inhalation solution, FDA-approved final product, noncompounded, administered through DME, concentrated form, per mg ☑ M ☑
Use this code for Isuprel HCl.

J7659 Isoproterenol HCl, inhalation solution, FDA-approved final product, noncompounded, administered through DME, unit dose form, per mg ☑ M ☑
Use this code for Isuprel HCl.

J7660 Isoproterenol HCl, inhalation solution, compounded product, administered through DME, unit dose form, per mg ☑ M ☑

J7665 Mannitol, administered through an inhaler, 5 mg ☑ N III ☑
Use this code for ARIDOL.

J7667 Metaproterenol sulfate, inhalation solution, compounded product, concentrated form, per 10 mg ☑ M ☑

J7668 Metaproterenol sulfate, inhalation solution, FDA-approved final product, noncompounded, administered through DME, concentrated form, per 10 mg ☑ M ☑
Use this code for Alupent.

J7669 Metaproterenol sulfate, inhalation solution, FDA-approved final product, noncompounded, administered through DME, unit dose form, per 10 mg ☑ M ☑
Use this code for Alupent.

J7670 Metaproterenol sulfate, inhalation solution, compounded product, administered through DME, unit dose form, per 10 mg ☑ M ☑

J7674 Methacholine chloride administered as inhalation solution through a nebulizer, per 1 mg ☑ N III ☑

J7676 Pentamidine isethionate, inhalation solution, compounded product, administered through DME, unit dose form, per 300 mg ☑ M ☑

J7677 Revefenacin inhalation solution, FDA-approved final product, noncompounded, administered through DME, 1 mcg ☑
Use this code for Yupelri.

J7680 Terbutaline sulfate, inhalation solution, compounded product, administered through DME, concentrated form, per mg ☑ M ☑
Use this code for Brethine.

Special Coverage Instructions   Noncovered by Medicare   Carrier Discretion   ☑ Quantity Alert   ● New Code   ○ Recycled/Reinstated   ▲ Revised Code

© 2023 Optum360, LLC   A2-Z3 ASC Pmt   CMS: IOM   AHA: Coding Clinic   ⅋ DMEPOS Paid   ⊘ SNF Excluded   J Codes — 115

Chemotherapy Drugs

J7681 — J9025

Code	Description	Indicators
J7681	**Terbutaline sulfate, inhalation solution, compounded product, administered through DME, unit dose form, per mg**	M ☑
	Use this code for Brethine.	
J7682	**Tobramycin, inhalation solution, FDA-approved final product, noncompounded, unit dose form, administered through DME, per 300 mg**	M ☑
	Use this code for Tobi.	
	CMS: 100-02,15,50.5	
J7683	**Triamcinolone, inhalation solution, compounded product, administered through DME, concentrated form, per mg**	M ☑
	Use this code for Azmacort.	
J7684	**Triamcinolone, inhalation solution, compounded product, administered through DME, unit dose form, per mg**	M ☑
	Use this code for Azmacort.	
J7685	**Tobramycin, inhalation solution, compounded product, administered through DME, unit dose form, per 300 mg**	M ☑
J7686	**Treprostinil, inhalation solution, FDA-approved final product, noncompounded, administered through DME, unit dose form, 1.74 mg**	M ☑
	Use this code for Tyvaso.	
	CMS: 100-02,15,50.5	
J7699	**NOC drugs, inhalation solution administered through DME**	M ☑
	CMS: 100-02,15,50.5	
J7799	**NOC drugs, other than inhalation drugs, administered through DME**	N N1 ☑
	CMS: 100-04,20,180; 100-04,32,411.4; 100-04,32,411.5; 100-04,32,411.6	
J7999	**Compounded drug, not otherwise classified**	N N1 ☑
	CMS: 100-04,20,180; 100-04,32,411.4; 100-04,32,411.5; 100-04,32,411.6	
J8498	**Antiemetic drug, rectal/suppository, not otherwise specified**	B ☑
J8499	**Prescription drug, oral, nonchemotherapeutic, NOS**	E1 ☑
	CMS: 100-02,15,50.5	

J Codes Chemotherapy Drugs J8501-J9999

Oral Chemotherapy Drugs

Code	Description	Indicators
J8501	**Aprepitant, oral, 5 mg**	K N1 ☑
	Use this code for Emend.	
	CMS: 100-02,15,50.5.4; 100-03,110.18; 100-04,17,80.2.1; 100-04,17,80.2.4	
J8510	**Busulfan, oral, 2 mg**	N N1 ☑
	Use this code for Busulfex, Myleran.	
	CMS: 100-04,17,80.1.1	
J8515	**Cabergoline, oral, 0.25 mg**	E1 ☑
	Use this code for Dostinex.	
J8520	**Capecitabine, oral, 150 mg**	N N1 ☑
	Use this code for Xeloda.	
	CMS: 100-04,17,80.1.1	
J8521	**Capecitabine, oral, 500 mg**	N N1 ☑
	Use this code for Xeloda.	
	CMS: 100-04,17,80.1.1	
J8530	**Cyclophosphamide, oral, 25 mg**	N N1 ☑
	Use this code for Cytoxan.	
	CMS: 100-04,17,80.1.1	
J8540	**Dexamethasone, oral, 0.25 mg**	N N1 ☑
	Use this code for Decadron.	
J8560	**Etoposide, oral, 50 mg**	K K2 ☑
	Use this code for VePesid.	
	CMS: 100-04,17,80.1.1	

Code	Description	Indicators
J8562	**Fludarabine phosphate, oral, 10 mg**	E1 ☑
	Use this code for Oforta.	
J8565	**Gefitinib, oral, 250 mg**	E1 ☑
	Use this code for Iressa.	
	CMS: 100-04,17,80.1.1	
J8597	**Antiemetic drug, oral, not otherwise specified**	N N1 ☑
J8600	**Melphalan, oral, 2 mg**	N ☑
	Use this code for Alkeran.	
	CMS: 100-04,17,80.1.1	
J8610	**Methotrexate, oral, 2.5 mg**	N N1 ☑
	Use this code for Trexall, RHEUMATREX.	
	CMS: 100-04,17,80.1.1	
J8650	**Nabilone, oral, 1 mg**	E1 ☑
	Use this code for Cesamet.	
J8655	**Netupitant 300 mg and palonosetron 0.5 mg, oral**	K K2 ☑
	Use this code for Akynzeo.	
J8670	**Rolapitant, oral, 1 mg**	K K2 ☑
	Use this code for Varubi.	
J8700	**Temozolomide, oral, 5 mg**	N N1 ☑
	Use this code for Temodar.	
J8705	**Topotecan, oral, 0.25 mg**	K N1 ☑
	Use this code for Hycamtin.	
J8999	**Prescription drug, oral, chemotherapeutic, NOS**	B ☑
	Determine if an alternative HCPCS Level II or a CPT code better describes the service being reported. This code should be used only if a more specific code is unavailable.	
	CMS: 100-04,17,80.1.1; 100-04,17,80.1.2	

Injectable Chemotherapy Drugs

These codes cover the cost of the chemotherapy drug only, not the administration.

Code	Description	Indicators
J9000	**Injection, doxorubicin HCl, 10 mg**	N N1 ☑ ⊘
	Use this code for Adriamycin PFS, Adriamycin RDF, Rubex.	
	CMS: 100-04,20,180; 100-04,32,411.3	
	AHA: 4Q,18	
J9015	**Injection, aldesleukin, per single use vial**	K K2 ☑ ⊘
	Use this code for Proleukin, IL-2, Interleukin.	
	AHA: 4Q,18	
J9017	**Injection, arsenic trioxide, 1 mg**	K K2 ☑ ⊘
	Use this code for Trisenox.	
	AHA: 4Q,18	
J9019	**Injection, asparaginase (Erwinaze), 1,000 IU**	K K2 ☑
	AHA: 4Q,18	
J9020	**Injection, asparaginase, not otherwise specified, 10,000 units**	N ☑ ⊘
	Use this code for Elspar.	
	AHA: 4Q,18	
J9021	**Injection, asparaginase, recombinant, (Rylaze), 0.1 mg**	K2
	Use this code for Rylaze.	
	AHA: 1Q,22	
J9022	**Injection, atezolizumab, 10 mg**	G K2
	Use this code for Tecentriq.	
	AHA: 4Q,18; 1Q,18	
J9023	**Injection, avelumab, 10 mg**	G K2
	Use this code for Bavencio.	
	AHA: 4Q,18; 1Q,18	
J9025	**Injection, azacitidine, 1 mg**	K N1 ☑ ⊘
	Use this code for Vidaza.	
	AHA: 4Q,18	

Special Coverage Instructions   Noncovered by Medicare   Carrier Discretion   ☑ Quantity Alert   ● New Code   ○ Recycled/Reinstated   ▲ Revised Code

J9027 Injection, clofarabine, 1 mg K K2 ☑ ⊘
Use this code for Clolar.
AHA: 4Q,18

● **J9029** Injection, nadofaragene firadenovec-vncg, per therapeutic dose
Use this code for Adstiladrin.
AHA: 3Q,23

J9030 BCG live intravesical instillation, 1 mg N1
Use this code for Pacis, TICE BCG.
AHA: 3Q,19

J9032 Injection, belinostat, 10 mg K K2 ☑
Use this code for Beleodaq.
AHA: 4Q,18

J9033 Injection, bendamustine HCl (Treanda), 1 mg K K2 ☑ ⊘
AHA: 4Q,18

J9034 Injection, bendamustine HCl (Bendeka), 1 mg G K2 ☑
AHA: 4Q,18; 1Q,17

J9035 Injection, bevacizumab, 10 mg K K2 ☑ ⊘
Use this code for Avastin.
CMS: 100-03,110.17
AHA: 4Q,18

J9036 Injection, bendamustine HCl, (Belrapzo/bendamustine), 1 mg K2
AHA: 3Q,19

J9037 Injection, belantamab mafodotin-blmf, 0.5 mg K2
Use this code for Blenrep.
AHA: 1Q,21

J9039 Injection, blinatumomab, 1 mcg K K2 ☑
Use this code for Blincyto.
CMS: 100-04,20,180; 100-04,32,411.3
AHA: 4Q,18

J9040 Injection, bleomycin sulfate, 15 units N N1 ☑ ⊘
Use this code for Blenoxane.
CMS: 100-04,20,180; 100-04,32,411.3
AHA: 4Q,18

J9041 Injection, bortezomib, 0.1 mg K K2 ☑ ⊘
AHA: 1Q,23; 4Q,18

J9042 Injection, brentuximab vedotin, 1 mg K K2 ☑
Use this code for Adcentris.
AHA: 4Q,18

J9043 Injection, cabazitaxel, 1 mg K K2 ☑
Use this code for Jevtana.
AHA: 4Q,18

J9045 Injection, carboplatin, 50 mg N N1 ☑ ⊘
Use this code for Paraplatin.
AHA: 4Q,18

J9046 Injection, bortezomib (Dr. Reddy's), not therapeutically equivalent to J9041, 0.1 mg K2
Use this code for bortezomib manufactured by Dr. Reddy's.
AHA: 1Q,23

J9047 Injection, carfilzomib, 1 mg K K2 ☑
Use this code for Kyprolis.
AHA: 4Q,18

J9048 Injection, bortezomib (Fresenius Kabi), not therapeutically equivalent to J9041, 0.1 mg K2
Use this code for bortezomib manufactured by Fresenius Kabi.
AHA: 1Q,23

J9049 Injection, bortezomib (Hospira), not therapeutically equivalent to J9041, 0.1 mg K2
Use this code for bortezomib manufactured by Hospira.
AHA: 1Q,23

J9050 Injection, carmustine, 100 mg K K2 ☑ ⊘
Use this code for BiCNU.
AHA: 4Q,18

● **J9051** Injection, bortezomib (MAIA), not therapeutically equivalent to J9041, 0.1 mg

● **J9052** Injection, carmustine (Accord), not therapeutically equivalent to J9050, 100 mg

J9055 Injection, cetuximab, 10 mg K K2 ☑ ⊘
Use this code for Erbitux.
CMS: 100-03,110.17
AHA: 4Q,18

● **J9056** Injection, bendamustine HCl (Vivimusta), 1 mg K2
AHA: 3Q,23

J9057 Injection, copanlisib, 1 mg K2
Use this code for Aliqopa.
AHA: 1Q,19; 4Q,18

● **J9058** Injection, bendamustine HCl (Apotex), 1 mg K2
Use this code for bendamustine HCl manufactured by Apotex.
AHA: 3Q,23

● **J9059** Injection, bendamustine HCl (Baxter), 1 mg K2
Use this code for bendamustine HCl manufactured by Baxter.
AHA: 3Q,23

J9060 Injection, cisplatin, powder or solution, 10 mg N N1 ☑ ⊘
Use this code for Plantinol AQ.
AHA: 4Q,18

J9061 Injection, amivantamab-vmjw, 2 mg K2
Use this code for Rybrevant.
AHA: 1Q,22

● **J9063** Injection, mirvetuximab soravtansine-gynx, 1 mg K2
Use this code for Elahere.
AHA: 3Q,23

● **J9064** Injection, cabazitaxel (Sandoz), not therapeutically equivalent to J9043, 1 mg

J9065 Injection, cladribine, per 1 mg K K2 ☑ ⊘
Use this code for Leustatin.
CMS: 100-04,20,180; 100-04,32,411.3
AHA: 4Q,18

J9070 Cyclophosphamide, 100 mg K K2 ☑ ⊘
Use this code for Endoxan-Asta.
AHA: 4Q,18

J9071 Injection, cyclophosphamide, (AuroMedics), 5 mg K2
AHA: 2Q,22

● **J9072** Injection, cyclophosphamide, (Dr. Reddy's), 5 mg

J9098 Injection, cytarabine liposome, 10 mg K ☑ ⊘
Use this code for Depocyt.
AHA: 4Q,18

J9100 Injection, cytarabine, 100 mg N N1 ☑ ⊘
Use this code for Cytosar-U, Ara-C, Tarabin CFS.
CMS: 100-04,20,180; 100-04,32,411.3
AHA: 4Q,18

J9118 Injection, calaspargase pegol-mknl, 10 units
Use this code for Asparlas.
AHA: 4Q,19

Special Coverage Instructions   Noncovered by Medicare   Carrier Discretion   ☑ Quantity Alert ● New Code ○ Recycled/Reinstated ▲ Revised Code

© 2023 Optum360, LLC   A2-Z3 ASC Pmt   **CMS:** IOM   **AHA:** Coding Clinic   ⅋ DMEPOS Paid   ⊘ SNF Excluded   **J Codes — 117**

Chemotherapy Drugs

J9119 — J9213

J9119 Injection, cemiplimab-rwlc, 1 mg   K2
Use this code for Libtayo.
AHA: 4Q,19

J9120 Injection, dactinomycin, 0.5 mg   K K2 ☑ ⊘
Use this code for Cosmegen.
AHA: 4Q,18

J9130 Dacarbazine, 100 mg   N N1 ☑ ⊘
Use this code for DTIC-Dome.
AHA: 4Q,18

J9144 Injection, daratumumab, 10 mg and hyaluronidase-fihj   K2
Use this code for Darzalex Faspro.
AHA: 1Q,21

J9145 Injection, daratumumab, 10 mg   G K2 ☑
Use this code for Darzalex.
AHA: 4Q,18

J9150 Injection, daunorubicin, 10 mg   K K2 ☑ ⊘
Use this code for Cerubidine.
AHA: 4Q,18

J9151 Injection, daunorubicin citrate, liposomal formulation, 10
mg   EI ☑ ⊘
Use this code for Daunoxome.
AHA: 4Q,18

J9153 Injection, liposomal, 1 mg daunorubicin and 2.27 mg
cytarabine   K2
Use this code for Vyxeos.
AHA: 1Q,19; 4Q,18

J9155 Injection, degarelix, 1 mg   K K2 ☑
CMS: 100-02,15,50.5
AHA: 4Q,18

J9160 Injection, denileukin diftitox, 300 mcg

J9165 Injection, diethylstilbestrol diphosphate, 250 mg   EI ☑
AHA: 4Q,18

J9171 Injection, docetaxel, 1 mg   K N1 ☑ ⊘
Use this code for Taxotere.
AHA: 4Q,18

● **J9172** Injection, docetaxel (Ingenus), not therapeutically equivalent
to J9171, 1 mg

J9173 Injection, durvalumab, 10 mg   K2
Use this code for Imfinzi.
AHA: 1Q,19; 4Q,18

J9175 Injection, Elliotts' B solution, 1 ml   N N1 ☑
AHA: 4Q,18

J9176 Injection, elotuzumab, 1 mg   G K2 ☑
Use this code for Empliciti.
AHA: 4Q,18

J9177 Injection, enfortumab vedotin-ejfv, 0.25 mg   K2
Use this code for PADCEV.
AHA: 2Q,20

J9178 Injection, epirubicin HCl, 2 mg   N N1 ☑ ⊘
Use this code for Ellence.
AHA: 4Q,18

J9179 Injection, eribulin mesylate, 0.1 mg   K K2 ☑
Use this code for Halaven.
AHA: 4Q,18

J9181 Injection, etoposide, 10 mg   N N1 ☑ ⊘
Use this code for VePesid, Toposar.
AHA: 4Q,18

J9185 Injection, fludarabine phosphate, 50 mg   K K2 ☑ ⊘
Use this code for Fludara.
AHA: 4Q,18

J9190 Injection, fluorouracil, 500 mg   N N1 ☑
Use this code for Adrucil.
CMS: 100-04,20,180; 100-04,32,411.3
AHA: 4Q,18

● **J9196** Injection, gemcitabine HCl (Accord), not therapeutically
equivalent to J9201, 200 mg   N1
Use this code for gemcitabine HCl manufactured by Accord.
AHA: 2Q,23

J9198 Injection, gemcitabine HCl, (Infugem), 100 mg   K2
AHA: 2Q,20

J9200 Injection, floxuridine, 500 mg   N N1 ☑ ⊘
Use this code for FUDR.
CMS: 100-04,20,180
AHA: 4Q,18

J9201 Injection, gemcitabine HCl, not otherwise specified, 200
mg   N N1 ☑ ⊘
Use this code for Gemzar.
AHA: 4Q,18

J9202 Goserelin acetate implant, per 3.6 mg   K K2 ☑
Use this code for Zoladex.
AHA: 4Q,18

J9203 Injection, gemtuzumab ozogamicin, 0.1 mg   G K2
Use this code for Mylotarg.
AHA: 4Q,18; 1Q,18; 4Q,17

J9204 Injection, mogamulizumab-kpkc, 1 mg   K2
Use this code for Poteligeo.
AHA: 4Q,19

J9205 Injection, irinotecan liposome, 1 mg   G K2 ☑
Use this code for Onivyde.
AHA: 4Q,18

J9206 Injection, irinotecan, 20 mg   N N1 ☑ ⊘
Use this code for Camptosar.
CMS: 100-03,110.17
AHA: 4Q,18

J9207 Injection, ixabepilone, 1 mg   K K2 ☑ ⊘
Use this code for IXEMPRA.
AHA: 4Q,18

J9208 Injection, ifosfamide, 1 g   N N1 ☑ ⊘
Use this code for IFEX, Mitoxana.
AHA: 4Q,18

J9209 Injection, mesna, 200 mg   N N1 ☑
Use this code for Mesnex.
AHA: 4Q,18

J9210 Injection, emapalumab-lzsg, 1 mg   K2
Use this code for Gamifant.
AHA: 4Q,19

J9211 Injection, idarubicin HCl, 5 mg   K N1 ☑ ⊘
Use this code for Idamycin.
AHA: 4Q,18

J9212 Injection, interferon alfacon-1, recombinant, 1 mcg N ☑
Use this code for Infergen.
AHA: 4Q,18

J9213 Injection, interferon, alfa-2a, recombinant, 3 million
units   N ☑
Use this code for Roferon-A.
AHA: 4Q,18

Special Coverage Instructions | Noncovered by Medicare | Carrier Discretion | ☑ Quantity Alert ● New Code ○ Recycled/Reinstated ▲ Revised Code

J9214	**Injection, interferon, alfa-2b, recombinant, 1 million units** K $K2$ ☑
	Use this code for Intron A, Rebetron Kit.
	CMS: 100-02,15,50.5
	AHA: 4Q,18
J9215	**Injection, interferon, alfa-N3, (human leukocyte derived), 250,000 IU** $E1$ ☑
	Use this code for Alferon N.
	AHA: 4Q,18
J9216	**Injection, interferon, gamma 1-b, 3 million units** K ☑
	Use this code for Actimmune.
	CMS: 100-02,15,50.5
	AHA: 4Q,18
J9217	**Leuprolide acetate (for depot suspension), 7.5 mg** K $K2$ ☑
	Use this code for Lupron Depot, Eligard.
	AHA: 2Q,19; 4Q,18
J9218	**Leuprolide acetate, per 1 mg** K $K2$ ☑
	Use this code for Lupron.
	CMS: 100-02,15,50.5
	AHA: 2Q,19; 4Q,18
J9219	**Leuprolide acetate implant, 65 mg** $E1$ ☑
	Use this code for Lupron Implant, Viadur.
	AHA: 4Q,18
J9223	**Injection, lurbinectedin, 0.1 mg** $K2$
	Use this code for Zepzelca.
	AHA: 1Q,21
J9225	**Histrelin implant (Vantas), 50 mg** K $K2$ ☑ ⊘
	AHA: 4Q,18
J9226	**Histrelin implant (Supprelin LA), 50 mg** K $N1$ ☑
	AHA: 4Q,18
J9227	**Injection, isatuximab-irfc, 10 mg** $K2$
	Use this code for Sarclisa.
	AHA: 4Q,20
J9228	**Injection, ipilimumab, 1 mg** K $K2$ ☑
	Use this code for YERVOY.
	AHA: 4Q,18
J9229	**Injection, inotuzumab ozogamicin, 0.1 mg** $K2$
	Use this code for Besponsa.
	AHA: 1Q,19; 4Q,18
J9230	**Injection, mechlorethamine HCl, (nitrogen mustard), 10 mg** K $N1$ ☑ ⊘
	Use this code for Mustargen.
	AHA: 4Q,18
J9245	**Injection, melphalan HCl, not otherwise specified, 50 mg** K $K2$ ☑ ⊘
	AHA: 2Q,20; 4Q,18
J9246	**Injection, melphalan (Evomela), 1 mg** $K2$
	AHA: 2Q,20
J9247	**Injection, melphalan flufenamide, 1 mg** $K2$
	Use this code for Pepaxto.
	AHA: 4Q,21
J9250	**Methotrexate sodium, 5 mg** N $N1$ ☑
	Use this code for Folex, Folex PFS, Methotrexate LPF.
	AHA: 4Q,18
● **J9255**	**Injection, methotrexate (Accord), not therapeutically equivalent to J9250 and J9260, 50 mg**
● **J9258**	**Injection, paclitaxel protein-bound particles (Teva), not therapeutically equivalent to J9264, 1 mg**
● **J9259**	**Injection, paclitaxel protein-bound particles (American Regent) not therapeutically equivalent to J9264, 1 mg** $K2$
	Use this code for paclitaxel protein-bound particles manufactured by American Regent.
	AHA: 3Q,23
J9260	**Methotrexate sodium, 50 mg** N $N1$ ☑
	Use this code for Folex, Folex PFS, Methotrexate LPF.
	AHA: 4Q,18
J9261	**Injection, nelarabine, 50 mg** K $K2$ ☑ ⊘
	Use this code for Arranon.
	AHA: 4Q,18
J9262	**Injection, omacetaxine mepesuccinate, 0.01 mg** K $K2$ ☑
	Use this code for Synribo.
	CMS: 100-02,15,50.5
	AHA: 4Q,18
J9263	**Injection, oxaliplatin, 0.5 mg** N $N1$ ☑ ⊘
	Use this code for Eloxatin.
	AHA: 4Q,18
J9264	**Injection, paclitaxel protein-bound particles, 1 mg** K $K2$ ☑ ⊘
	Use this code for Abraxane.
	AHA: 4Q,18
J9266	**Injection, pegaspargase, per single dose vial** K $K2$ ☑ ⊘
	Use this code for Oncaspar.
	AHA: 4Q,18
J9267	**Injection, paclitaxel, 1 mg** N $N1$ ☑
	Use this code for Taxol.
	AHA: 4Q,18
J9268	**Injection, pentostatin, 10 mg** K $K2$ ☑ ⊘
	Use this code for Nipent.
	AHA: 4Q,18
J9269	**Injection, tagraxofusp-erzs, 10 mcg** $K2$
	Use this code for Elzonris.
	AHA: 4Q,19
J9270	**Injection, plicamycin, 2.5 mg** N $N1$ ☑ ⊘
	Use this code for Mithracin.
	AHA: 4Q,18
J9271	**Injection, pembrolizumab, 1 mg** K $K2$ ☑
	Use this code for Keytruda.
	AHA: 4Q,18
J9272	**Injection, dostarlimab-gxly, 10 mg** $K2$
	Use this code for Jemperli.
	AHA: 1Q,22
J9273	**Injection, tisotumab vedotin-tftv, 1 mg** $K2$
	Use this code for Tivdak.
	AHA: 2Q,22
J9274	**Injection, tebentafusp-tebn, 1 mcg** $K2$
	Use this code for Kimmtrak.
	AHA: 4Q,22
J9280	**Injection, mitomycin, 5 mg** K $K2$ ☑ ⊘
	Use this code for Mutamycin.
	AHA: 4Q,18; 4Q,17
J9281	**Mitomycin pyelocalyceal instillation, 1 mg** $K2$
	Use this code for Jelmyto.
	AHA: 1Q,21
J9285	**Injection, olaratumab, 10 mg** G $N1$
	Use this code for Lartruvo.
	AHA: 4Q,18; 1Q,18
● **J9286**	**Injection, glofitamab-gxbm, 2.5 mg**
	Use this code for Columvi.

Chemotherapy Drugs

J9214 — J9286

Special Coverage Instructions	Noncovered by Medicare	Carrier Discretion

☑ Quantity Alert ● New Code ○ Recycled/Reinstated ▲ Revised Code

J9293 Injection, mitoxantrone HCl, per 5 mg K K2 ☑ ⊘
Use this code for Novantrone.
AHA: 4Q,18

● **J9294** Injection, pemetrexed (Hospira), not therapeutically equivalent to J9305, 10 mg K2
Use this code for pemetrexed manufactured by Hospira.
AHA: 2Q,23

J9295 Injection, necitumumab, 1 mg G K2 ☑
Use this code for Portrazza.
AHA: 4Q,18

● **J9296** Injection, pemetrexed (Accord), not therapeutically equivalent to J9305, 10 mg K2
Use this code for pemetrexed manufactured by Accord.
AHA: 2Q,23

● **J9297** Injection, pemetrexed (Sandoz), not therapeutically equivalent to J9305, 10 mg K2
Use this code for pemetrexed manufactured by Sandoz.
AHA: 2Q,23

J9298 Injection, nivolumab and relatlimab-rmbw, 3 mg/1 mg K2
Use this code for Opdualag.
AHA: 4Q,22

J9299 Injection, nivolumab, 1 mg K K2 ☑
Use this code for Opdivo.
AHA: 4Q,18

J9301 Injection, obinutuzumab, 10 mg K K2 ☑
Use this code for Gazyva.
AHA: 4Q,18

J9302 Injection, ofatumumab, 10 mg K K2 ☑
Use this code for Arzerra.
AHA: 4Q,18

J9303 Injection, panitumumab, 10 mg K K2 ☑ ⊘
Use this code for Vectibix.
AHA: 4Q,18

J9304 Injection, pemetrexed (Pemfexy), 10 mg K2
AHA: 4Q,20

J9305 Injection, pemetrexed, NOS, 10 mg K K2 ☑ ⊘
AHA: 4Q,20; 4Q,18

J9306 Injection, pertuzumab, 1 mg K K2 ☑
Use this code for Perjeta.
AHA: 4Q,18

J9307 Injection, pralatrexate, 1 mg K K2 ☑
Use this code for FOLOTYN.
AHA: 4Q,18

J9308 Injection, ramucirumab, 5 mg K K2 ☑
Use this code for Cyramza.
AHA: 4Q,18

J9309 Injection, polatuzumab vedotin-piiq, 1 mg K2
Use this code for Polivy.

J9311 Injection, rituximab 10 mg and hyaluronidase K2
Use this code for Rituxan Hycela.
AHA: 1Q,19; 4Q,18

J9312 Injection, rituximab, 10 mg K2
Use this code for Rituxan.
AHA: 1Q,19; 4Q,18

J9313 Injection, moxetumomab pasudotox-tdfk, 0.01 mg K2
Use this code for Lumoxiti.
AHA: 4Q,19

J9314 Injection, pemetrexed (Teva) not therapeutically equivalent to J9305, 10 mg K2
Use this code for pemetrexed manufactured by Teva.
AHA: 2Q,23; 1Q,23

J9316 Injection, pertuzumab, trastuzumab, and hyaluronidase-zzxf, per 10 mg K2
Use this code for PHESGO.
AHA: 1Q,21

J9317 Injection, sacituzumab govitecan-hziy, 2.5 mg K2
Use this code for Trodelvy.
AHA: 1Q,21

J9318 Injection, romidepsin, nonlyophilized, 0.1 mg K2
AHA: 4Q,21

J9319 Injection, romidepsin, lyophilized, 0.1 mg K2
Use this code for Istodax.
AHA: 4Q,21

J9320 Injection, streptozocin, 1 g K K2 ☑ ⊘
Use this code for Zanosar.
AHA: 4Q,18

● **J9321** Injection, epcoritamab-bysp, 0.16 mg
Use this code for Epkinly.

● **J9322** Injection, pemetrexed (BluePoint) not therapeutically equivalent to J9305, 10 mg K2
Use this code for pemetrexed manufactured by BluePoint.
AHA: 3Q,23

● **J9323** Injection, pemetrexed ditromethamine, 10 mg K2
Use this code for pemetrexed manufactured by Hospira.
AHA: 3Q,23

● **J9324** Injection, pemetrexed (Pemrydi RTU), 10 mg

J9325 Injection, talimogene laherparepvec, per 1 million plaque forming units G K2 ☑
Use this code for Imlygic.
AHA: 2Q,19; 4Q,18

J9328 Injection, temozolomide, 1 mg K K2 ☑ ⊘
Use this code for Temodar.
AHA: 4Q,18

J9330 Injection, temsirolimus, 1 mg K K2 ☑ ⊘
Use this code for TORISEL.
AHA: 4Q,18

J9331 Injection, sirolimus protein-bound particles, 1 mg K2
AHA: 3Q,22

J9332 Injection, efgartigimod alfa-fcab, 2 mg K2
Use this code for Vyvgart.
AHA: 3Q,22

● **J9333** Injection, rozanolixizumab-noli, 1 mg
Use this code for Rystiggo.

● **J9334** Injection, efgartigimod alfa, 2 mg and hyaluronidase-qvfc
Use this code for Vyvgart.

J9340 Injection, thiotepa, 15 mg K K2 ☑ ⊘
Use this code for Thioplex.
AHA: 4Q,18

● **J9345** Injection, retifanlimab-dlwr, 1 mg K2
Use this code for Zynyz.

● **J9347** Injection, tremelimumab-actl, 1 mg K2
Use this code for Imjudo.
AHA: 3Q,23

J9348 Injection, naxitamab-gqgk, 1 mg K2
AHA: 3Q,21

Special Coverage Instructions Noncovered by Medicare Carrier Discretion ☑ Quantity Alert ● New Code ○ Recycled/Reinstated ▲ Revised Code

A Age Edit M Maternity Edit ♀ Female Only ♂ Male Only A-Y OPPS Status Indicators © 2023 Optum360, LLC

J9349 Injection, tafasitamab-cxix, 2 mg [K2]
Use this code for Monjuvi.
AHA: 1Q,21

○ **J9350** Injection, mosunetuzumab-axgb, 1 mg [K2]
Use this code for Lunsumio.
AHA: 3Q,23

J9351 Injection, topotecan, 0.1 mg [N] [N1] ☑
Use this code for Hycamtin.
AHA: 4Q,18

J9352 Injection, trabectedin, 0.1 mg [G] [K2] ☑
Use this code for Yondelis.
AHA: 4Q,18

J9353 Injection, margetuximab-cmkb, 5 mg [K2]
AHA: 3Q,21

J9354 Injection, ado-trastuzumab emtansine, 1 mg [K] [K2] ☑
Use this code for Kadcyla.
AHA: 4Q,18

J9355 Injection, trastuzumab, excludes biosimilar, 10 mg [K] [K2] ☑ ⊘
Use this code for Herceptin.
AHA: 3Q,19; 4Q,18

J9356 Injection, trastuzumab, 10 mg and hyaluronidase-oysk [K2]
Use this code for Herceptin Hylecta.
AHA: 3Q,19

J9357 Injection, valrubicin, intravesical, 200 mg [K] [K2] ☑ ⊘
Use this code for Valstar.
AHA: 4Q,18

J9358 Injection, fam-trastuzumab deruxtecan-nxki, 1 mg [K2]
Use this code for Enhertu.
AHA: 2Q,20

J9359 Injection, loncastuximab tesirine-lpyl, 0.075 mg [K2]
Use this code for Zylonta.
AHA: 2Q,22

J9360 Injection, vinblastine sulfate, 1 mg [N] [N1] ☑ ⊘
Use this code for Velban.
CMS: 100-04,20,100; 100-04,32,411.3
AHA: 4Q,18

J9370 Vincristine sulfate, 1 mg [N] [N1] ☑ ⊘
Use this code for Oncovin, Vincasar PFS.
CMS: 100-04,20,180; 100-04,32,411.3
AHA: 4Q,18

J9371 Injection, vincristine sulfate liposome, 1 mg [K] [K2] ☑
Use this code for Marqibo kit.
AHA: 4Q,18

○ **J9380** Injection, teclistamab-cqyv, 0.5 mg [K2]
Use this code for Tecvayli.
AHA: 3Q,23

● **J9381** Injection, teplizumab-mzwv, 5 mcg [K2]
Use this code for Tzield.
AHA: 3Q,23

J9390 Injection, vinorelbine tartrate, 10 mg [N] [N1] ☑ ⊘
Use this code for Navelbine.
AHA: 4Q,18

J9393 Injection, fulvestrant (Teva) not therapeutically equivalent to J9395, 25 mg [K2]
Use this code for fulvestrant manufactured by Teva.
AHA: 1Q,23

J9394 Injection, fulvestrant (Fresenius Kabi) not therapeutically equivalent to J9395, 25 mg [K2]
Use this code for fulvestrant manufactured by Fresenius Kabi.
AHA: 1Q,23

J9395 Injection, fulvestrant, 25 mg [K] [K2] ☑ ⊘
Use this code for Faslodex.
AHA: 4Q,18

J9400 Injection, ziv-aflibercept, 1 mg [K] [K2] ☑
Use this code for Zaltrap.
AHA: 4Q,18

J9600 Injection, porfimer sodium, 75 mg [K] [K2] ☑ ⊘
Use this code for Photofrin.
AHA: 1Q,20; 4Q,18

J9999 Not otherwise classified, antineoplastic drugs [N] [N1] ☑
Determine if an alternative HCPCS Level II or a CPT code better describes the service being reported. This code should be used only if a more specific code is unavailable.
CMS: 100-02,15,50.5; 100-04,32,400; 100-04,32,400.1; 100-04,32,400.2; 100-04,32,400.2.1; 100-04,32,400.2.2; 100-04,32,400.2.3; 100-04,32,400.2.3.1; 100-04,32,400.2.4; 100-04,32,400.2.5; 100-04,32,400.3; 100-04,32,400.4; 100-04,32,411.3; 100-04,4,260.1; 100-04,4,260.1.1

Special Coverage Instructions   Noncovered by Medicare   Carrier Discretion   ☑ Quantity Alert   ● New Code   ○ Recycled/Reinstated   ▲ Revised Code

© 2023 Optum360, LLC   [A2]-[Z4] ASC Pmt   **CMS:** IOM   **AHA:** Coding Clinic   ⅙ DMEPOS Paid   ⊘ SNF Excluded   J Codes — 121

Temporary Codes K0001-K1036

The K codes were established for use by the DME Medicare Administrative Contractors (DME MACs). The K codes are developed when the currently existing permanent national codes for supplies and certain product categories do not include the codes needed to implement a DME MAC medical review policy.

Wheelchairs and Accessories

Code	Description	Indicators
K0001	Standard wheelchair	☑ & (RR)
K0002	Standard hemi (low seat) wheelchair	☑ & (RR)
K0003	Lightweight wheelchair	☑ & (RR)
K0004	High strength, lightweight wheelchair	☑ & (RR)
K0005	Ultralightweight wheelchair	☑ & (NU, RR, UE)
K0006	Heavy-duty wheelchair	☑ & (RR)
K0007	Extra heavy-duty wheelchair	☑ & (RR)
K0008	Custom manual wheelchair/base	☑
K0009	Other manual wheelchair/base	☑ & (RR)
K0010	Standard-weight frame motorized/power wheelchair	☑ & (RR)
K0011	Standard-weight frame motorized/power wheelchair with programmable control parameters for speed adjustment, tremor dampening, acceleration control and braking	☑ & (RR)
	CMS: 100 04,20,30.9	
K0012	Lightweight portable motorized/power wheelchair	☑ & (RR)
K0013	Custom motorized/power wheelchair base	☑
K0014	Other motorized/power wheelchair base	☑
K0015	Detachable, nonadjustable height armrest, each	☑ ☑ & (RR)
K0017	Detachable, adjustable height armrest, base, replacement only, each	ⓘ ☑ & (NU, RR, UE)
K0018	Detachable, adjustable height armrest, upper portion, replacement only, each	☑ ☑ & (NU, RR, UE)
K0019	Arm pad, replacement only, each	☑ ☑ & (NU, RR, UE)
K0020	Fixed, adjustable height armrest, pair	☑ ☑ & (NU, RR, UE)
K0037	High mount flip-up footrest, each	☑ ☑ & (NU, RR, UE)
K0038	Leg strap, each	☑ ☑ & (NU, RR, UE)
K0039	Leg strap, H style, each	☑ ☑ & (NU, RR, UE)
K0040	Adjustable angle footplate, each	☑ ☑ & (NU, RR, UE)
K0041	Large size footplate, each	☑ ☑ & (NU, RR, UE)
K0042	Standard size footplate, replacement only, each	☑ ☑ & (NU, RR, UE)
K0043	Footrest, lower extension tube, replacement only, each	☑ ☑ & (NU, RR, UE)
K0044	Footrest, upper hanger bracket, replacement only, each	☑ ☑ & (NU, RR, UE)
K0045	Footrest, complete assembly, replacement only, each	☑ & (NU, RR, UE)
K0046	Elevating legrest, lower extension tube, replacement only, each	☑ ☑ & (NU, RR, UE)
K0047	Elevating legrest, upper hanger bracket, replacement only, each	☑ ☑ & (NU, RR, UE)
K0050	Ratchet assembly, replacement only	☑ & (NU, RR, UE)
K0051	Cam release assembly, footrest or legrest, replacement only, each	☑ ☑ & (NU, RR, UE)
K0052	Swingaway, detachable footrests, replacement only, each	☑ ☑ & (NU, RR, UE)
K0053	Elevating footrests, articulating (telescoping), each	☑ ☑ & (NU, RR, UE)
K0056	Seat height less than 17 in or equal to or greater than 21 in for a high-strength, lightweight, or ultralightweight wheelchair	☑ ☑ & (NU, RR, UE)
K0065	Spoke protectors, each	☑ ☑ & (NU, RR, UE)
K0069	Rear wheel assembly, complete, with solid tire, spokes or molded, replacement only, each	☑ ☑ & (NU, RR, UE)
K0070	Rear wheel assembly, complete, with pneumatic tire, spokes or molded, replacement only, each	☑ ☑ & (RR)
K0071	Front caster assembly, complete, with pneumatic tire, replacement only, each	☑ ☑ & (NU, RR, UE)
K0072	Front caster assembly, complete, with semi-pneumatic tire, replacement only, each	☑ ☑ & (NU, RR, UE)
K0073	Caster pin lock, each	☑ ☑ & (NU, RR, UE)
K0077	Front caster assembly, complete, with solid tire, replacement only, each	☑ ☑ & (NU, RR, UE)
K0098	Drive belt for power wheelchair, replacement only	☑ & (NU, RR, UE)
K0105	IV hanger, each	☑ ☑ & (NU, RR, UE)
K0108	Wheelchair component or accessory, not otherwise specified	☑
K0195	Elevating legrests, pair (for use with capped rental wheelchair base)	☑ & (RR)

Equipment, Replacement, Repair, Rental

Code	Description	Indicators
K0455	Infusion pump used for uninterrupted parenteral administration of medication, (e.g., epoprostenol or treprostinol)	☑ & (RR)
K0462	Temporary replacement for patient-owned equipment being repaired, any type	☑
	CMS: 100-04,20,40.1	
K0552	Supplies for external noninsulin drug infusion pump, syringe type cartridge, sterile, each	☑ ☑ &
K0601	Replacement battery for external infusion pump owned by patient, silver oxide, 1.5 volt, each	☑ ☑ & (NU)
K0602	Replacement battery for external infusion pump owned by patient, silver oxide, 3 volt, each	☑ ☑ & (NU)
K0603	Replacement battery for external infusion pump owned by patient, alkaline, 1.5 volt, each	☑ ☑ & (NU)
K0604	Replacement battery for external infusion pump owned by patient, lithium, 3.6 volt, each	☑ ☑ & (NU)
K0605	Replacement battery for external infusion pump owned by patient, lithium, 4.5 volt, each	☑ ☑ & (NU)
K0606	Automatic external defibrillator, with integrated electrocardiogram analysis, garment type	☑ (RR)
K0607	Replacement battery for automated external defibrillator, garment type only, each	☑ ☑ & (RR)
K0608	Replacement garment for use with automated external defibrillator, each	☑ ☑ & (NU, RR, UE)
K0609	Replacement electrodes for use with automated external defibrillator, garment type only, each	☑ ☑ & (KF)
K0669	Wheelchair accessory, wheelchair seat or back cushion, does not meet specific code criteria or no written coding verification from DME PDAC	☑
K0672	Addition to lower extremity orthotic, removable soft interface, all components, replacement only, each	Ⓐ ☑ &

Special Coverage Instructions   Noncovered by Medicare   Carrier Discretion   ☑ Quantity Alert   ● New Code   ○ Recycled/Reinstated   ▲ Revised Code

   A2-Z3 ASC Pmt   **CMS:** IOM   **AHA:** Coding Clinic   & DMEPOS Paid   ⊘ SNF Excluded

K0730	Controlled dose inhalation drug delivery system	☑ ♿ (RR)
K0733	Power wheelchair accessory, 12 to 24 amp hour sealed lead acid battery, each (e.g., gel cell, absorbed glassmat)	☑ ♿ (NU, RR, UE)
K0738	Portable gaseous oxygen system, rental; home compressor used to fill portable oxygen cylinders; includes portable containers, regulator, flowmeter, humidifier, cannula or mask, and tubing CMS: 100-04,20,130.6	☑ ♿ (RR)
K0739	Repair or nonroutine service for durable medical equipment other than oxygen equipment requiring the skill of a technician, labor component, per 15 minutes	☑ ☑
K0740	Repair or nonroutine service for oxygen equipment requiring the skill of a technician, labor component, per 15 minutes	EI ☑
K0743	Suction pump, home model, portable, for use on wounds	☑
K0744	Absorptive wound dressing for use with suction pump, home model, portable, pad size 16 sq in or less	A ☑
K0745	Absorptive wound dressing for use with suction pump, home model, portable, pad size more than 16 sq in but less than or equal to 48 sq in	A ☑
K0746	Absorptive wound dressing for use with suction pump, home model, portable, pad size greater than 48 sq in	A

Power Operated Vehicle and Accessories

K0800	Power operated vehicle, group 1 standard, patient weight capacity up to and including 300 pounds CMS: 100-04,12,30.6.15.4	☑ ♿ (NU, RR, UE)
K0801	Power operated vehicle, group 1 heavy-duty, patient weight capacity 301 to 450 pounds CMS: 100-04,12,30.6.15.4	☑ ♿ (NU, RR, UE)
K0802	Power operated vehicle, group 1 very heavy-duty, patient weight capacity 451 to 600 pounds CMS: 100-04,12,30.6.15.4	☑ ♿ (NU, RR, UE)
K0806	Power operated vehicle, group 2 standard, patient weight capacity up to and including 300 pounds CMS: 100-04,12,30.6.15.4	☑ ♿ (NU, RR, UE)
K0807	Power operated vehicle, group 2 heavy-duty, patient weight capacity 301 to 450 pounds CMS: 100-04,12,30.6.15.4	☑ ♿ (NU, RR, UE)
K0808	Power operated vehicle, group 2 very heavy-duty, patient weight capacity 451 to 600 pounds CMS: 100-04,12,30.6.15.4	☑ ♿ (NU, RR, UE)
K0812	Power operated vehicle, not otherwise classified CMS: 100-04,12,30.6.15.4	☑

Power Wheelchairs

K0813	Power wheelchair, group 1 standard, portable, sling/solid seat and back, patient weight capacity up to and including 300 pounds	☑ ♿ (RR)
K0814	Power wheelchair, group 1 standard, portable, captain's chair, patient weight capacity up to and including 300 pounds	☑ ♿ (RR)
K0815	Power wheelchair, group 1 standard, sling/solid seat and back, patient weight capacity up to and including 300 pounds	☑ ♿ (RR)
K0816	Power wheelchair, group 1 standard, captain's chair, patient weight capacity up to and including 300 pounds	☑ ♿ (RR)
K0820	Power wheelchair, group 2 standard, portable, sling/solid seat/back, patient weight capacity up to and including 300 pounds	☑ ♿ (RR)
K0821	Power wheelchair, group 2 standard, portable, captain's chair, patient weight capacity up to and including 300 pounds	☑ ♿ (RR)
K0822	Power wheelchair, group 2 standard, sling/solid seat/back, patient weight capacity up to and including 300 pounds	☑ ♿ (RR)
K0823	Power wheelchair, group 2 standard, captain's chair, patient weight capacity up to and including 300 pounds	☑ ♿ (RR)
K0824	Power wheelchair, group 2 heavy-duty, sling/solid seat/back, patient weight capacity 301 to 450 pounds	☑ ♿ (RR)
K0825	Power wheelchair, group 2 heavy-duty, captain's chair, patient weight capacity 301 to 450 pounds	☑ ♿ (RR)
K0826	Power wheelchair, group 2 very heavy-duty, sling/solid seat/back, patient weight capacity 451 to 600 pounds	☑ ♿ (RR)
K0827	Power wheelchair, group 2 very heavy-duty, captain's chair, patient weight capacity 451 to 600 pounds	☑ ♿ (RR)
K0828	Power wheelchair, group 2 extra heavy-duty, sling/solid seat/back, patient weight capacity 601 pounds or more	☑ ♿ (RR)
K0829	Power wheelchair, group 2 extra heavy-duty, captain's chair, patient weight 601 pounds or more	☑ ♿ (RR)
K0830	Power wheelchair, group 2 standard, seat elevator, sling/solid seat/back, patient weight capacity up to and including 300 pounds	☑
K0831	Power wheelchair, group 2 standard, seat elevator, captain's chair, patient weight capacity up to and including 300 pounds	☑
K0835	Power wheelchair, group 2 standard, single power option, sling/solid seat/back, patient weight capacity up to and including 300 pounds	☑ ♿ (RR)
K0836	Power wheelchair, group 2 standard, single power option, captain's chair, patient weight capacity up to and including 300 pounds	☑ ♿ (RR)
K0837	Power wheelchair, group 2 heavy-duty, single power option, sling/solid seat/back, patient weight capacity 301 to 450 pounds	☑ ♿ (RR)
K0838	Power wheelchair, group 2 heavy-duty, single power option, captain's chair, patient weight capacity 301 to 450 pounds	☑ ♿ (RR)
K0839	Power wheelchair, group 2 very heavy-duty, single power option sling/solid seat/back, patient weight capacity 451 to 600 pounds	☑ ♿ (RR)
K0840	Power wheelchair, group 2 extra heavy-duty, single power option, sling/solid seat/back, patient weight capacity 601 pounds or more	☑ ♿ (RR)
K0841	Power wheelchair, group 2 standard, multiple power option, sling/solid seat/back, patient weight capacity up to and including 300 pounds	☑ ♿ (RR)
K0842	Power wheelchair, group 2 standard, multiple power option, captain's chair, patient weight capacity up to and including 300 pounds	☑ ♿ (RR)
K0843	Power wheelchair, group 2 heavy-duty, multiple power option, sling/solid seat/back, patient weight capacity 301 to 450 pounds	☑ ♿ (RR)

Special Coverage Instructions | Noncovered by Medicare | Carrier Discretion | ☑ Quantity Alert | ● New Code | ○ Recycled/Reinstated | ▲ Revised Code

A Age Edit   M Maternity Edit   ♀ Female Only   ♂ Male Only   A-Y OPPS Status Indicators   © 2023 Optum360, LLC

K0848   Power wheelchair, group 3 standard, sling/solid seat/back, patient weight capacity up to and including 300 pounds   ☑ & (RR)
CMS: 100-04,20,30.9

K0849   Power wheelchair, group 3 standard, captain's chair, patient weight capacity up to and including 300 pounds   ☑ & (RR)
CMS: 100-04,20,30.9

K0850   Power wheelchair, group 3 heavy-duty, sling/solid seat/back, patient weight capacity 301 to 450 pounds   ☑ & (RR)
CMS: 100-04,20,30.9

K0851   Power wheelchair, group 3 heavy-duty, captain's chair, patient weight capacity 301 to 450 pounds   ☑ & (RR)
CMS: 100-04,20,30.9

K0852   Power wheelchair, group 3 very heavy-duty, sling/solid seat/back, patient weight capacity 451 to 600 pounds   ☑ & (RR)
CMS: 100-04,20,30.9

K0853   Power wheelchair, group 3 very heavy-duty, captain's chair, patient weight capacity 451 to 600 pounds   ☑ & (RR)
CMS: 100-04,20,30.9

K0854   Power wheelchair, group 3 extra heavy-duty, sling/solid seat/back, patient weight capacity 601 pounds or more   ☑ & (RR)
CMS: 100-04,20,30.9

K0855   Power wheelchair, group 3 extra heavy-duty, captain's chair, patient weight capacity 601 pounds or more   ☑ & (RR)
CMS: 100-04,20,30.9

K0856   Power wheelchair, group 3 standard, single power option, sling/solid seat/back, patient weight capacity up to and Including 300 pounds   ☑ & (RR)
CMS: 100-04,20,30.9

K0857   Power wheelchair, group 3 standard, single power option, captain's chair, patient weight capacity up to and including 300 pounds   ☑ & (RR)
CMS: 100-04,20,30.9

K0858   Power wheelchair, group 3 heavy-duty, single power option, sling/solid seat/back, patient weight 301 to 450 pounds   ☑ & (RR)
CMS: 100-04,20,30.9

K0859   Power wheelchair, group 3 heavy-duty, single power option, captain's chair, patient weight capacity 301 to 450 pounds   ☑ & (RR)
CMS: 100-04,20,30.9

K0860   Power wheelchair, group 3 very heavy-duty, single power option, sling/solid seat/back, patient weight capacity 451 to 600 pounds   ☑ & (RR)
CMS: 100-04,20,30.9

K0861   Power wheelchair, group 3 standard, multiple power option, sling/solid seat/back, patient weight capacity up to and including 300 pounds   ☑ & (RR)
CMS: 100-04,20,30.9

K0862   Power wheelchair, group 3 heavy-duty, multiple power option, sling/solid seat/back, patient weight capacity 301 to 450 pounds   ☑ & (RR)
CMS: 100-04,20,30.9

K0863   Power wheelchair, group 3 very heavy-duty, multiple power option, sling/solid seat/back, patient weight capacity 451 to 600 pounds   ☑ & (RR)
CMS: 100-04,20,30.9

K0864   Power wheelchair, group 3 extra heavy-duty, multiple power option, sling/solid seat/back, patient weight capacity 601 pounds or more   ☑ & (RR)
CMS: 100-04,20,30.9

K0868   Power wheelchair, group 4 standard, sling/solid seat/back, patient weight capacity up to and including 300 pounds   ☑

K0869   Power wheelchair, group 4 standard, captain's chair, patient weight capacity up to and including 300 pounds   ☑

K0870   Power wheelchair, group 4 heavy-duty, sling/solid seat/back, patient weight capacity 301 to 450 pounds   ☑

K0871   Power wheelchair, group 4 very heavy-duty, sling/solid seat/back, patient weight capacity 451 to 600 pounds   ☑

K0877   Power wheelchair, group 4 standard, single power option, sling/solid seat/back, patient weight capacity up to and including 300 pounds   ☑

K0878   Power wheelchair, group 4 standard, single power option, captain's chair, patient weight capacity up to and including 300 pounds   ☑

K0879   Power wheelchair, group 4 heavy-duty, single power option, sling/solid seat/back, patient weight capacity 301 to 450 pounds   ☑

K0880   Power wheelchair, group 4 very heavy-duty, single power option, sling/solid seat/back, patient weight capacity 451 to 600 pounds   ☑

K0884   Power wheelchair, group 4 standard, multiple power option, sling/solid seat/back, patient weight capacity up to and including 300 pounds   ☑

K0885   Power wheelchair, group 4 standard, multiple power option, captain's chair, patient weight capacity up to and including 300 pounds   ☑

K0886   Power wheelchair, group 4 heavy-duty, multiple power option, sling/solid seat/back, patient weight capacity 301 to 450 pounds   ☑

K0890   Power wheelchair, group 5 pediatric, single power option, sling/solid seat/back, patient weight capacity up to and including 125 pounds   ☑

K0891   Power wheelchair, group 5 pediatric, multiple power option, sling/solid seat/back, patient weight capacity up to and including 125 pounds   ☑

K0898   Power wheelchair, not otherwise classified   ☑

K0899   Power mobility device, not coded by DME PDAC or does not meet criteria   ☑
CMS: 100-04,12,30.6.15.4

Other DME

K0900   Customized durable medical equipment, other than wheelchair   ☑

K1001   ~~Electronic positional obstructive sleep apnea treatment, with sensor, includes all components and accessories, any type~~
To report, see ~E0530

K1002   ~~Cranial electrotherapy stimulation (CES) system, any type~~
To report, see ~E0732

K1003   ~~Whirlpool tub, walk in, portable~~
To report, see ~E1301

▲ K1004   Low frequency ultrasonic diathermy treatment device for home use

K1005   ~~Disposable collection and storage bag for breast milk, any size, any type, each~~
To report, see ~A4287

Special Coverage Instructions   Noncovered by Medicare   Carrier Discretion   ☑ Quantity Alert   ● New Code   ○ Recycled/Reinstated   ▲ Revised Code

© 2023 Optum360, LLC   A2-Z3 ASC Pmt   CMS: IOM   AHA: Coding Clinic   & DMEPOS Paid   ⊘ SNF Excluded   K Codes — 125

K1006 ~~Suction pump, home model, portable or stationary, electric, any type, for use with external urine management system~~
To report, see ~E2001

K1007 Bilateral hip, knee, ankle, foot (HKAFO) device, powered, includes pelvic component, single or double upright(s), knee joints any type, with or without ankle joints any type, includes all components and accessories, motors, microprocessors, sensors

K1009 ~~Speech volume modulation system, any type, including all components and accessories~~
To report, see ~E3000

K1013 ~~Enema tube, with or without adapter, any type, replacement only, each~~
To report, see ~A4457

K1014 ~~Addition, endoskeletal knee-shin system, 4 bar linkage or multiaxial, fluid swing and stance phase control~~
To report, see ~L5615

K1015 ~~Foot, adductus positioning device, adjustable~~
To report, see ~L3161

K1016 ~~Transcutaneous electrical nerve stimulator for electrical stimulation of the trigeminal nerve~~
To report, see ~E0733

K1017 ~~Monthly supplies for use of device coded at K1016~~
To report, see ~A4541

K1018 ~~External upper limb tremor stimulator of the peripheral nerves of the wrist~~
To report, see ~E0734

K1019 ~~Supplies and accessories for external upper limb tremor stimulator of the peripheral nerves of the wrist~~
To report, see ~A4542

K1020 Noninvasive vagus nerve stimulator
To report, see ~E0735

K1021 ~~Exsufflation belt, includes all supplies and accessories~~
To report, see ~A4468

K1022 ~~Addition to lower extremity prosthesis, endoskeletal, knee disarticulation, above knee, hip disarticulation, positional rotation unit, any type~~
To report, see ~L5926

K1023 ~~Distal transcutaneous electrical nerve stimulator, stimulates peripheral nerves of the upper arm~~
To report, see ~A4540

K1024 ~~Nonpneumatic compression controller with sequential calibrated gradient pressure~~
To report, see ~E0680-E0681

K1025 ~~Nonpneumatic sequential compression garment, full arm~~
To report, see ~E0682

K1026 ~~Mechanical allergen particle barrier/inhalation filter, cream, nasal, topical~~
To report, see ~A7023

K1027 Oral device/appliance used to reduce upper airway collapsibility, without fixed mechanical hinge, custom fabricated, includes fitting and adjustment

K1028 ~~Power source and control electronics unit for oral device/appliance for neuromuscular electrical stimulation of the tongue muscle, controlled by phone application~~
To report, see ~E0492-E0493

K1029 ~~Oral device/appliance for neuromuscular electrical stimulation of the tongue muscle, used in conjunction with the power source and control electronics unit, controlled by phone application, 90-day supply~~
To report, see ~E0492-E0493

K1030 External recharging system for battery (internal) for use with implanted cardiac contractility modulation generator, replacement only

K1031 ~~Nonpneumatic compression controller without calibrated gradient pressure~~
To report, see ~E0680-E0681

K1032 ~~Nonpneumatic sequential compression garment, full leg~~
To report, see ~E0678

K1033 ~~Nonpneumatic sequential compression garment, half leg~~
To report, see ~E0679

K1034 Provision of COVID-19 test, nonprescription self-administered and self-collected use, FDA approved, authorized or cleared, one test count
AHA: 3Q,22

● **K1035** Molecular diagnostic test reader, nonprescription self-administered and self-collected use, FDA approved, authorized or cleared
AHA: 2Q,23

● **K1036** Supplies and accessories (e.g., transducer) for low frequency ultrasonic diathermy treatment device, per month

Special Coverage Instructions | Noncovered by Medicare | Carrier Discretion | ☑ Quantity Alert | ● New Code | ○ Recycled/Reinstated | ▲ Revised Code

126 — K Codes | Ⓐ Age Edit | Ⓜ Maternity Edit | ♀ Female Only | ♂ Male Only | Ⓐ-Ⓨ OPPS Status Indicators | © 2023 Optum360, LLC

Orthotic Procedures and Devices L0112-L4631

L codes include orthotic and prosthetic procedures and devices, as well as scoliosis equipment, orthopedic shoes, and prosthetic implants.

Cervical

L0112 Cranial cervical orthosis, congenital torticollis type, with or without soft interface material, adjustable range of motion joint, custom fabricated Ⓐ ♿

L0113 Cranial cervical orthosis, torticollis type, with or without joint, with or without soft interface material, prefabricated, includes fitting and adjustment Ⓐ ♿

L0120 Cervical, flexible, nonadjustable, prefabricated, off-the-shelf (foam collar) Ⓐ ♿

L0130 Cervical, flexible, thermoplastic collar, molded to patient Ⓐ ♿

L0140 Cervical, semi-rigid, adjustable (plastic collar) Ⓐ ♿

L0150 Cervical, semi-rigid, adjustable molded chin cup (plastic collar with mandibular/occipital piece) Ⓐ ♿

L0160 Cervical, semi-rigid, wire frame occipital/mandibular support, prefabricated, off-the-shelf Ⓐ ♿

L0170 Cervical, collar, molded to patient model Ⓐ ♿

L0172 Cervical, collar, semi-rigid thermoplastic foam, two piece, prefabricated, off-the-shelf Ⓐ ♿

L0174 Cervical, collar, semi-rigid, thermoplastic foam, two piece with thoracic extension, prefabricated, off-the-shelf Ⓐ ♿

Multiple Post Collar

L0180 Cervical, multiple post collar, occipital/mandibular supports, adjustable Ⓐ ♿

L0190 Cervical, multiple post collar, occipital/mandibular supports, adjustable cervical bars (SOMI, Guilford, Taylor types) Ⓐ ♿

L0200 Cervical, multiple post collar, occipital/mandibular supports, adjustable cervical bars, and thoracic extension Ⓐ ♿

Thoracic

L0220 Thoracic, rib belt, custom fabricated Ⓐ ♿

L0450 Thoracic-lumbar-sacral orthosis (TLSO), flexible, provides trunk support, upper thoracic region, produces intracavitary pressure to reduce load on the intervertebral disks with rigid stays or panel(s), includes shoulder straps and closures, prefabricated, off-the-shelf Ⓐ ♿

TLSO brace with adjustable straps and pads (L0450). The model at right and similar devices such as the Boston brace are molded polymer over foam and may be bivalve (front and back components)

Thoracic lumbar sacral othosis (TLSO)

L0452 Thoracic-lumbar-sacral orthosis (TLSO), flexible, provides trunk support, upper thoracic region, produces intracavitary pressure to reduce load on the intervertebral disks with rigid stays or panel(s), includes shoulder straps and closures, custom fabricated Ⓐ ♿

L0454 Thoracic-lumbar-sacral orthosis (TLSO), flexible, provides trunk support, extends from sacrococcygeal junction to above T-9 vertebra, restricts gross trunk motion in the sagittal plane, produces intracavitary pressure to reduce load on the intervertebral disks with rigid stays or panel(s), includes shoulder straps and closures, prefabricated item that has been trimmed, bent, molded, assembled, or otherwise customized to fit a specific patient by an individual with expertise Ⓐ ♿

L0455 Thoracic-lumbar-sacral orthosis (TLSO), flexible, provides trunk support, extends from sacrococcygeal junction to above T-9 vertebra, restricts gross trunk motion in the sagittal plane, produces intracavitary pressure to reduce load on the intervertebral disks with rigid stays or panel(s), includes shoulder straps and closures, prefabricated, off-the-shelf Ⓐ ♿

L0456 Thoracic-lumbar-sacral orthosis (TLSO), flexible, provides trunk support, thoracic region, rigid posterior panel and soft anterior apron, extends from the sacrococcygeal junction and terminates just inferior to the scapular spine, restricts gross trunk motion in the sagittal plane, produces intracavitary pressure to reduce load on the intervertebral disks, includes straps and closures, prefabricated item that has been trimmed, bent, molded, assembled, or otherwise customized to fit a specific patient by an individual with expertise Ⓐ ♿

L0457 Thoracic-lumbar-sacral orthosis (TLSO), flexible, provides trunk support, thoracic region, rigid posterior panel and soft anterior apron, extends from the sacrococcygeal junction and terminates just inferior to the scapular spine, restricts gross trunk motion in the sagittal plane, produces intracavitary pressure to reduce load on the intervertebral disks, includes straps and closures, prefabricated, off-the-shelf Ⓐ ♿

Special Coverage Instructions   Noncovered by Medicare   Carrier Discretion   ☑ Quantity Alert   ● New Code   ○ Recycled/Reinstated   ▲ Revised Code

© 2023 Optum360, LLC   A2-Z3 ASC Pmt   **CMS:** IOM   **AHA:** Coding Clinic   ♿ DMEPOS Paid   ⊘ SNF Excluded   **L Codes — 127**

L0458 Thoracic-lumbar-sacral orthosis (TLSO), triplanar control, modular segmented spinal system, two rigid plastic shells, posterior extends from the sacrococcygeal junction and terminates just inferior to the scapular spine, anterior extends from the symphysis pubis to the xiphoid, soft liner, restricts gross trunk motion in the sagittal, coronal, and transverse planes, lateral strength is provided by overlapping plastic and stabilizing closures, includes straps and closures, prefabricated, includes fitting and adjustment Ⓐ ♿

L0460 Thoracic-lumbar-sacral orthosis (TLSO), triplanar control, modular segmented spinal system, two rigid plastic shells, posterior extends from the sacrococcygeal junction and terminates just inferior to the scapular spine, anterior extends from the symphysis pubis to the sternal notch, soft liner, restricts gross trunk motion in the sagittal, coronal, and transverse planes, lateral strength is provided by overlapping plastic and stabilizing closures, includes straps and closures, prefabricated item that has been trimmed, bent, molded, assembled, or otherwise customized to fit a specific patient by an individual with expertise Ⓐ ♿

L0462 Thoracic-lumbar-sacral orthosis (TLSO), triplanar control, modular segmented spinal system, three rigid plastic shells, posterior extends from the sacrococcygeal junction and terminates just inferior to the scapular spine, anterior extends from the symphysis pubis to the sternal notch, soft liner, restricts gross trunk motion in the sagittal, coronal, and transverse planes, lateral strength is provided by overlapping plastic and stabilizing closures, includes straps and closures, prefabricated, includes fitting and adjustment Ⓐ ♿

L0464 Thoracic-lumbar-sacral orthosis (TLSO), triplanar control, modular segmented spinal system, four rigid plastic shells, posterior extends from sacrococcygeal junction and terminates just inferior to scapular spine, anterior extends from symphysis pubis to the sternal notch, soft liner, restricts gross trunk motion in sagittal, coronal, and transverse planes, lateral strength is provided by overlapping plastic and stabilizing closures, includes straps and closures, prefabricated, includes fitting and adjustment Ⓐ ♿

L0466 Thoracic-lumbar-sacral orthosis (TLSO), sagittal control, rigid posterior frame and flexible soft anterior apron with straps, closures and padding, restricts gross trunk motion in sagittal plane, produces intracavitary pressure to reduce load on intervertebral disks, prefabricated item that has been trimmed, bent, molded, assembled, or otherwise customized to fit a specific patient by an individual with expertise Ⓐ ♿

L0467 Thoracic-lumbar-sacral orthosis (TLSO), sagittal control, rigid posterior frame and flexible soft anterior apron with straps, closures and padding, restricts gross trunk motion in sagittal plane, produces intracavitary pressure to reduce load on intervertebral disks, prefabricated, off-the-shelf Ⓐ ♿

L0468 Thoracic-lumbar-sacral orthosis (TLSO), sagittal-coronal control, rigid posterior frame and flexible soft anterior apron with straps, closures and padding, extends from sacrococcygeal junction over scapulae, lateral strength provided by pelvic, thoracic, and lateral frame pieces, restricts gross trunk motion in sagittal, and coronal planes, produces intracavitary pressure to reduce load on intervertebral disks, prefabricated item that has been trimmed, bent, molded, assembled, or otherwise customized to fit a specific patient by an individual with expertise Ⓐ ♿

L0469 Thoracic-lumbar-sacral orthosis (TLSO), sagittal-coronal control, rigid posterior frame and flexible soft anterior apron with straps, closures and padding, extends from sacrococcygeal junction over scapulae, lateral strength provided by pelvic, thoracic, and lateral frame pieces, restricts gross trunk motion in sagittal and coronal planes, produces intracavitary pressure to reduce load on intervertebral disks, prefabricated, off-the-shelf Ⓐ ♿

L0470 Thoracic-lumbar-sacral orthosis (TLSO), triplanar control, rigid posterior frame and flexible soft anterior apron with straps, closures and padding extends from sacrococcygeal junction to scapula, lateral strength provided by pelvic, thoracic, and lateral frame pieces, rotational strength provided by subclavicular extensions, restricts gross trunk motion in sagittal, coronal, and transverse planes, provides intracavitary pressure to reduce load on the intervertebral disks, includes fitting and shaping the frame, prefabricated, includes fitting and adjustment Ⓐ ♿

L0472 Thoracic-lumbar-sacral orthosis (TLSO), triplanar control, hyperextension, rigid anterior and lateral frame extends from symphysis pubis to sternal notch with two anterior components (one pubic and one sternal), posterior and lateral pads with straps and closures, limits spinal flexion, restricts gross trunk motion in sagittal, coronal, and transverse planes, includes fitting and shaping the frame, prefabricated, includes fitting and adjustment Ⓐ ♿

L0480 Thoracic-lumbar-sacral orthosis (TLSO), triplanar control, one-piece rigid plastic shell without interface liner, with multiple straps and closures, posterior extends from sacrococcygeal junction and terminates just inferior to scapular spine, anterior extends from symphysis pubis to sternal notch, anterior or posterior opening, restricts gross trunk motion in sagittal, coronal, and transverse planes, includes a carved plaster or CAD-CAM model, custom fabricated Ⓐ ♿

L0482 Thoracic-lumbar-sacral orthosis (TLSO), triplanar control, one-piece rigid plastic shell with interface liner, multiple straps and closures, posterior extends from sacrococcygeal junction and terminates just inferior to scapular spine, anterior extends from symphysis pubis to sternal notch, anterior or posterior opening, restricts gross trunk motion in sagittal, coronal, and transverse planes, includes a carved plaster or CAD-CAM model, custom fabricated Ⓐ ♿

L0484 Thoracic-lumbar-sacral orthosis (TLSO), triplanar control, two-piece rigid plastic shell without interface liner, with multiple straps and closures, posterior extends from sacrococcygeal junction and terminates just inferior to scapular spine, anterior extends from symphysis pubis to sternal notch, lateral strength is enhanced by overlapping plastic, restricts gross trunk motion in the sagittal, coronal, and transverse planes, includes a carved plaster or CAD-CAM model, custom fabricated Ⓐ ♿

L0486 Thoracic-lumbar-sacral orthosis (TLSO), triplanar control, two-piece rigid plastic shell with interface liner, multiple straps and closures, posterior extends from sacrococcygeal junction and terminates just inferior to scapular spine, anterior extends from symphysis pubis to sternal notch, lateral strength is enhanced by overlapping plastic, restricts gross trunk motion in the sagittal, coronal, and transverse planes, includes a carved plaster or CAD-CAM model, custom fabricated Ⓐ ♿

L0488 Thoracic-lumbar-sacral orthosis (TLSO), triplanar control, one-piece rigid plastic shell with interface liner, multiple straps and closures, posterior extends from sacrococcygeal junction and terminates just inferior to scapular spine, anterior extends from symphysis pubis to sternal notch, anterior or posterior opening, restricts gross trunk motion in sagittal, coronal, and transverse planes, prefabricated, includes fitting and adjustment Ⓐ ♿

L0490 Thoracic-lumbar-sacral orthosis (TLSO), sagittal-coronal control, one-piece rigid plastic shell, with overlapping reinforced anterior, with multiple straps and closures, posterior extends from sacrococcygeal junction and terminates at or before the T-9 vertebra, anterior extends from symphysis pubis to xiphoid, anterior opening, restricts gross trunk motion in sagittal and coronal planes, prefabricated, includes fitting and adjustment Ⓐ ♿

Special Coverage Instructions Noncovered by Medicare Carrier Discretion ☑ Quantity Alert ● New Code ○ Recycled/Reinstated ▲ Revised Code

128 — L Codes Ⓐ Age Edit Ⓜ Maternity Edit ♀ Female Only ♂ Male Only Ⓐ-Ⓨ OPPS Status Indicators © 2023 Optum360, LLC

L0491 Thoracic-lumbar-sacral orthosis (TLSO), sagittal-coronal control, modular segmented spinal system, two rigid plastic shells, posterior extends from the sacrococcygeal junction and terminates just inferior to the scapular spine, anterior extends from the symphysis pubis to the xiphoid, soft liner, restricts gross trunk motion in the sagittal and coronal planes, lateral strength is provided by overlapping plastic and stabilizing closures, includes straps and closures, prefabricated, includes fitting and adjustment Ⓐ ♿

L0492 Thoracic-lumbar-sacral orthosis (TLSO), sagittal-coronal control, modular segmented spinal system, three rigid plastic shells, posterior extends from the sacrococcygeal junction and terminates just inferior to the scapular spine, anterior extends from the symphysis pubis to the xiphoid, soft liner, restricts gross trunk motion in the sagittal and coronal planes, lateral strength is provided by overlapping plastic and stabilizing closures, includes straps and closures, prefabricated, includes fitting and adjustment Ⓐ ♿

Cervical-Thoracic-Lumbar-Sacral Orthoses

L0621 Sacroiliac orthosis (SO), flexible, provides pelvic-sacral support, reduces motion about the sacroiliac joint, includes straps, closures, may include pendulous abdomen design, prefabricated, off-the-shelf Ⓐ ♿

L0622 Sacroiliac orthosis (SO), flexible, provides pelvic-sacral support, reduces motion about the sacroiliac joint, includes straps, closures, may include pendulous abdomen design, custom fabricated Ⓐ ♿

L0623 Sacroiliac orthosis (SO), provides pelvic-sacral support, with rigid or semi-rigid panels over the sacrum and abdomen, reduces motion about the sacroiliac joint, includes straps, closures, may include pendulous abdomen design, prefabricated, off-the-shelf Ⓐ ♿

L0624 Sacroiliac orthosis (SO), provides pelvic-sacral support, with rigid or semi-rigid panels placed over the sacrum and abdomen, reduces motion about the sacroiliac joint, includes straps, closures, may include pendulous abdomen design, custom fabricated Ⓐ ♿

L0625 Lumbar orthosis (LO), flexible, provides lumbar support, posterior extends from L-1 to below L-5 vertebra, produces intracavitary pressure to reduce load on the intervertebral discs, includes straps, closures, may include pendulous abdomen design, shoulder straps, stays, prefabricated, off-the-shelf Ⓐ ♿

L0626 Lumbar orthosis (LO), sagittal control, with rigid posterior panel(s), posterior extends from L-1 to below L-5 vertebra, produces intracavitary pressure to reduce load on the intervertebral discs, includes straps, closures, may include padding, stays, shoulder straps, pendulous abdomen design, prefabricated item that has been trimmed, bent, molded, assembled, or otherwise customized to fit a specific patient by an individual with expertise Ⓐ ♿

L0627 Lumbar orthosis (LO), sagittal control, with rigid anterior and posterior panels, posterior extends from L-1 to below L-5 vertebra, produces intracavitary pressure to reduce load on the intervertebral discs, includes straps, closures, may include padding, shoulder straps, pendulous abdomen design, prefabricated item that has been trimmed, bent, molded, assembled, or otherwise customized to fit a specific patient by an individual with expertise Ⓐ ♿

L0628 Lumbar-sacral orthosis (LSO), flexible, provides lumbo-sacral support, posterior extends from sacrococcygeal junction to T-9 vertebra, produces intracavitary pressure to reduce load on the intervertebral discs, includes straps, closures, may include stays, shoulder straps, pendulous abdomen design, prefabricated, off-the-shelf Ⓐ ♿

L0629 Lumbar-sacral orthosis (LSO), flexible, provides lumbo-sacral support, posterior extends from sacrococcygeal junction to T-9 vertebra, produces intracavitary pressure to reduce load on the intervertebral discs, includes straps, closures, may include stays, shoulder straps, pendulous abdomen design, custom fabricated Ⓐ ♿

L0630 Lumbar-sacral orthosis (LSO), sagittal control, with rigid posterior panel(s), posterior extends from sacrococcygeal junction to T-9 vertebra, produces intracavitary pressure to reduce load on the intervertebral discs, includes straps, closures, may include padding, stays, shoulder straps, pendulous abdomen design, prefabricated item that has been trimmed, bent, molded, assembled, or otherwise customized to fit a specific patient by an individual with expertise Ⓐ ♿

L0631 Lumbar-sacral orthosis (LSO), sagittal control, with rigid anterior and posterior panels, posterior extends from sacrococcygeal junction to T-9 vertebra, produces intracavitary pressure to reduce load on the intervertebral discs, includes straps, closures, may include padding, shoulder straps, pendulous abdomen design, prefabricated item that has been trimmed, bent, molded, assembled, or otherwise customized to fit a specific patient by an individual with expertise Ⓐ ♿

L0632 Lumbar-sacral orthosis (LSO), sagittal control, with rigid anterior and posterior panels, posterior extends from sacrococcygeal junction to T-9 vertebra, produces intracavitary pressure to reduce load on the intervertebral discs, includes straps, closures, may include padding, shoulder straps, pendulous abdomen design, custom fabricated Ⓐ ♿

L0633 Lumbar-sacral orthosis (LSO), sagittal-coronal control, with rigid posterior frame/panel(s), posterior extends from sacrococcygeal junction to T-9 vertebra, lateral strength provided by rigid lateral frame/panels, produces intracavitary pressure to reduce load on intervertebral discs, includes straps, closures, may include padding, stays, shoulder straps, pendulous abdomen design, prefabricated item that has been trimmed, bent, molded, assembled, or otherwise customized to fit a specific patient by an individual with expertise Ⓐ ♿

L0634 Lumbar-sacral orthosis (LSO), sagittal-coronal control, with rigid posterior frame/panel(s), posterior extends from sacrococcygeal junction to T-9 vertebra, lateral strength provided by rigid lateral frame/panel(s), produces intracavitary pressure to reduce load on intervertebral discs, includes straps, closures, may include padding, stays, shoulder straps, pendulous abdomen design, custom fabricated Ⓐ ♿

L0635 Lumbar-sacral orthosis (LSO), sagittal-coronal control, lumbar flexion, rigid posterior frame/panel(s), lateral articulating design to flex the lumbar spine, posterior extends from sacrococcygeal junction to T-9 vertebra, lateral strength provided by rigid lateral frame/panel(s), produces intracavitary pressure to reduce load on intervertebral discs, includes straps, closures, may include padding, anterior panel, pendulous abdomen design, prefabricated, includes fitting and adjustment Ⓐ ♿

L0636 Lumbar-sacral orthosis (LSO), sagittal-coronal control, lumbar flexion, rigid posterior frame/panels, lateral articulating design to flex the lumbar spine, posterior extends from sacrococcygeal junction to T-9 vertebra, lateral strength provided by rigid lateral frame/panels, produces intracavitary pressure to reduce load on intervertebral discs, includes straps, closures, may include padding, anterior panel, pendulous abdomen design, custom fabricated Ⓐ ♿

Special Coverage Instructions   Noncovered by Medicare   Carrier Discretion   ☑ Quantity Alert   ● New Code   ↻ Recycled/Reinstated   ▲ Revised Code

© 2023 Optum360, LLC   Ⓐ²⁻Ⓩ³ ASC Pmt   **CMS:** IOM   **AHA:** Coding Clinic   ♿ DMEPOS Paid   ⊘ SNF Excluded   L Codes — 129

Orthotic Devices and Procedures

L0637 — L0999

L0637 Lumbar-sacral orthosis (LSO), sagittal-coronal control, with rigid anterior and posterior frame/panels, posterior extends from sacrococcygeal junction to T-9 vertebra, lateral strength provided by rigid lateral frame/panels, produces intracavitary pressure to reduce load on intervertebral discs, includes straps, closures, may include padding, shoulder straps, pendulous abdomen design, prefabricated item that has been trimmed, bent, molded, assembled, or otherwise customized to fit a specific patient by an individual with expertise ⒶⅭ

L0638 Lumbar-sacral orthosis (LSO), sagittal-coronal control, with rigid anterior and posterior frame/panels, posterior extends from sacrococcygeal junction to T-9 vertebra, lateral strength provided by rigid lateral frame/panels, produces intracavitary pressure to reduce load on intervertebral discs, includes straps, closures, may include padding, shoulder straps, pendulous abdomen design, custom fabricated ⒶⅭ

L0639 Lumbar-sacral orthosis (LSO), sagittal-coronal control, rigid shell(s)/panel(s), posterior extends from sacrococcygeal junction to T-9 vertebra, anterior extends from symphysis pubis to xyphoid, produces intracavitary pressure to reduce load on the intervertebral discs, overall strength is provided by overlapping rigid material and stabilizing closures, includes straps, closures, may include soft interface, pendulous abdomen design, prefabricated item that has been trimmed, bent, molded, assembled, or otherwise customized to fit a specific patient by an individual with expertise ⒶⅭ

L0640 Lumbar-sacral orthosis (LSO), sagittal-coronal control, rigid shell(s)/panel(s), posterior extends from sacrococcygeal junction to T-9 vertebra, anterior extends from symphysis pubis to xyphoid, produces intracavitary pressure to reduce load on the intervertebral discs, overall strength is provided by overlapping rigid material and stabilizing closures, includes straps, closures, may include soft interface, pendulous abdomen design, custom fabricated ⒶⅭ

L0641 Lumbar orthosis (LO), sagittal control, with rigid posterior panel(s), posterior extends from L-1 to below L-5 vertebra, produces intracavitary pressure to reduce load on the intervertebral discs, includes straps, closures, may include padding, stays, shoulder straps, pendulous abdomen design, prefabricated, off-the-shelf ⒶⅭ

L0642 Lumbar orthosis (LO), sagittal control, with rigid anterior and posterior panels, posterior extends from L-1 to below L-5 vertebra, produces intracavitary pressure to reduce load on the intervertebral discs, includes straps, closures, may include padding, shoulder straps, pendulous abdomen design, prefabricated, off-the-shelf ⒶⅭ

L0643 Lumbar-sacral orthosis (LSO), sagittal control, with rigid posterior panel(s), posterior extends from sacrococcygeal junction to T-9 vertebra, produces intracavitary pressure to reduce load on the intervertebral discs, includes straps, closures, may include padding, stays, shoulder straps, pendulous abdomen design, prefabricated, off-the-shelf ⒶⅭ

L0648 Lumbar-sacral orthosis (LSO), sagittal control, with rigid anterior and posterior panels, posterior extends from sacrococcygeal junction to T-9 vertebra, produces intracavitary pressure to reduce load on the intervertebral discs, includes straps, closures, may include padding, shoulder straps, pendulous abdomen design, prefabricated, off-the-shelf ⒶⅭ

L0649 Lumbar-sacral orthosis (LSO), sagittal-coronal control, with rigid posterior frame/panel(s), posterior extends from sacrococcygeal junction to T-9 vertebra, lateral strength provided by rigid lateral frame/panels, produces intracavitary pressure to reduce load on intervertebral discs, includes straps, closures, may include padding, stays, shoulder straps, pendulous abdomen design, prefabricated, off-the-shelf ⒶⅭ

L0650 Lumbar-sacral orthosis (LSO), sagittal-coronal control, with rigid anterior and posterior frame/panel(s), posterior extends from sacrococcygeal junction to T-9 vertebra, lateral strength provided by rigid lateral frame/panel(s), produces intracavitary pressure to reduce load on intervertebral discs, includes straps, closures, may include padding, shoulder straps, pendulous abdomen design, prefabricated, off-the-shelf ⒶⅭ

L0651 Lumbar-sacral orthosis (LSO), sagittal-coronal control, rigid shell(s)/panel(s), posterior extends from sacrococcygeal junction to T-9 vertebra, anterior extends from symphysis pubis to xyphoid, produces intracavitary pressure to reduce load on the intervertebral discs, overall strength is provided by overlapping rigid material and stabilizing closures, includes straps, closures, may include soft interface, pendulous abdomen design, prefabricated, off-the-shelf ⒶⅭ

L0700 Cervical-thoracic-lumbar-sacral orthosis (CTLSO), anterior-posterior-lateral control, molded to patient model, (Minerva type) ⒶⅭ

L0710 Cervical-thoracic-lumbar-sacral orthosis (CTLSO), anterior-posterior-lateral control, molded to patient model, with interface material, (Minerva type) ⒶⅭ

Halo Procedure

L0810 Halo procedure, cervical halo incorporated into jacket vest ⒶⅭ

L0820 Halo procedure, cervical halo incorporated into plaster body jacket ⒶⅭ

L0830 Halo procedure, cervical halo incorporated into Milwaukee type orthotic ⒶⅭ

L0859 Addition to halo procedure, magnetic resonance image compatible systems, rings and pins, any material ⒶⅭ

L0861 Addition to halo procedure, replacement liner/interface material ⒶⅭ

Additions to Spinal Orthoses

L0970 Thoracic-lumbar-sacral orthosis (TLSO), corset front ⒶⅭ

L0972 Lumbar-sacral orthosis (LSO), corset front ⒶⅭ

L0974 Thoracic-lumbar-sacral orthosis (TLSO), full corset ⒶⅭ

L0976 Lumbar-sacral orthosis (LSO), full corset ⒶⅭ

L0978 Axillary crutch extension ⒶⅭ

L0980 Peroneal straps, prefabricated, off-the-shelf, pair Ⓐ☑Ⅽ

L0982 Stocking supporter grips, prefabricated, off-the-shelf, set of four (4) Ⓐ☑Ⅽ

L0984 Protective body sock, prefabricated, off-the-shelf, each Ⓐ☑Ⅽ

L0999 Addition to spinal orthosis, not otherwise specified Ⓐ

Determine if an alternative HCPCS Level II or a CPT code better describes the service being reported. This code should be used only if a more specific code is unavailable.

Orthotic Devices - Scoliosis Procedures

The orthotic care of scoliosis differs from other orthotic care in that the treatment is more dynamic in nature and uses continual modification of the orthosis to the patient's changing condition. This coding structure uses the proper names - or eponyms - of the procedures because they have historic and universal acceptance in the profession. It should be recognized that variations to the basic procedures described by the founders/developers are accepted in various medical and orthotic practices throughout the country. All procedures include model of patient when indicated.

Special Coverage Instructions Noncovered by Medicare Carrier Discretion ☑ Quantity Alert ● New Code ○ Recycled/Reinstated ▲ Revised Code

130 — L Codes Ⓐ Age Edit Ⓜ Maternity Edit ♀ Female Only ♂ Male Only Ⓐ-Ⓨ OPPS Status Indicators © 2023 Optum360, LLC

L1000 Cervical-thoracic-lumbar-sacral orthosis (CTLSO) (Milwaukee), inclusive of furnishing initial orthotic, including model Ⓐ &

A variety of configurations are available for the Milwaukee brace (L1000)

Cervical component

Axilla sling (L1010)

Thoracic component

Lumbar-sacral component

Milwaukee-style braces, cervical thoracic lumbar sacral orthosis (CTSLO)

L1001 Cervical-thoracic-lumbar-sacral orthosis (CTLSO), immobilizer, infant size, prefabricated, includes fitting and adjustment Ⓐ Ⓐ &

L1005 Tension based scoliosis orthosis and accessory pads, includes fitting and adjustment Ⓐ &

L1010 Addition to cervical-thoracic-lumbar-sacral orthosis (CTLSO) or scoliosis orthosis, axilla sling Ⓐ &

L1020 Addition to cervical-thoracic-lumbar-sacral orthosis (CTLSO) or scoliosis orthosis, kyphosis pad Ⓐ &

L1025 Addition to cervical-thoracic-lumbar-sacral orthosis (CTLSO) or scoliosis orthosis, kyphosis pad, floating Ⓐ &

L1030 Addition to cervical-thoracic-lumbar-sacral orthosis (CTLSO) or scoliosis orthosis, lumbar bolster pad Ⓐ &

L1040 Addition to cervical-thoracic-lumbar-sacral orthosis (CTLSO) or scoliosis orthosis, lumbar or lumbar rib pad Ⓐ &

L1050 Addition to cervical-thoracic-lumbar-sacral orthosis (CTLSO) or scoliosis orthosis, sternal pad Ⓐ &

L1060 Addition to cervical-thoracic-lumbar-sacral orthosis (CTLSO) or scoliosis orthosis, thoracic pad Ⓐ &

L1070 Addition to cervical-thoracic-lumbar-sacral orthosis (CTLSO) or scoliosis orthosis, trapezius sling Ⓐ &

L1080 Addition to cervical-thoracic-lumbar-sacral orthosis (CTLSO) or scoliosis orthosis, outrigger Ⓐ &

L1085 Addition to cervical-thoracic-lumbar-sacral orthosis (CTLSO) or scoliosis orthosis, outrigger, bilateral with vertical extensions Ⓐ &

L1090 Addition to cervical-thoracic-lumbar-sacral orthosis (CTLSO) or scoliosis orthosis, lumbar sling Ⓐ &

L1100 Addition to cervical-thoracic-lumbar-sacral orthosis (CTLSO) or scoliosis orthosis, ring flange, plastic or leather Ⓐ &

L1110 Addition to cervical-thoracic-lumbar-sacral orthosis (CTLSO) or scoliosis orthosis, ring flange, plastic or leather, molded to patient model Ⓐ &

L1120 Addition to cervical-thoracic-lumbar-sacral orthosis (CTLSO), scoliosis orthosis, cover for upright, each Ⓐ ☑ &

Thoracic-Lumbar-Sacral Orthosis (TLSO) (Low Profile)

L1200 Thoracic-lumbar-sacral orthosis (TLSO), inclusive of furnishing initial orthosis only Ⓐ &

L1210 Addition to thoracic-lumbar-sacral orthosis (TLSO), (low profile), lateral thoracic extension Ⓐ &

L1220 Addition to thoracic-lumbar-sacral orthosis (TLSO), (low profile), anterior thoracic extension Ⓐ &

L1230 Addition to thoracic-lumbar-sacral orthosis (TLSO), (low profile), Milwaukee type superstructure Ⓐ &

L1240 Addition to thoracic-lumbar-sacral orthosis (TLSO), (low profile), lumbar derotation pad Ⓐ &

L1250 Addition to thoracic-lumbar-sacral orthosis (TLSO), (low profile), anterior ASIS pad Ⓐ &

L1260 Addition to thoracic-lumbar-sacral orthosis (TLSO), (low profile), anterior thoracic derotation pad Ⓐ &

L1270 Addition to thoracic-lumbar-sacral orthosis (TLSO), (low profile), abdominal pad Ⓐ &
AHA: 2Q,19

L1280 Addition to thoracic-lumbar-sacral orthosis (TLSO), (low profile), rib gusset (elastic), each Ⓐ ☑ &

L1290 Addition to thoracic-lumbar-sacral orthosis (TLSO), (low profile), lateral trochanteric pad Ⓐ &

Other Scoliosis Procedures

L1300 Other scoliosis procedure, body jacket molded to patient model Ⓐ &

L1310 Other scoliosis procedure, postoperative body jacket Ⓐ &

L1499 Spinal orthosis, not otherwise specified Ⓐ
Determine if an alternative HCPCS Level II or a CPT code better describes the service being reported. This code should be used only if a more specific code is unavailable.

Hip Orthoses (HO) - Flexible

L1600 Hip orthosis (HO), abduction control of hip joints, flexible, Frejka type with cover, prefabricated item that has been trimmed, bent, molded, assembled, or otherwise customized to fit a specific patient by an individual with expertise Ⓐ &

L1610 Hip orthosis (HO), abduction control of hip joints, flexible, (Frejka cover only), prefabricated item that has been trimmed, bent, molded, assembled, or otherwise customized to fit a specific patient by an individual with expertise Ⓐ &

L1620 Hip orthosis (HO), abduction control of hip joints, flexible, (Pavlik harness), prefabricated item that has been trimmed, bent, molded, assembled, or otherwise customized to fit a specific patient by an individual with expertise Ⓐ &

L1630 Hip orthosis (HO), abduction control of hip joints, semi-flexible (Von Rosen type), custom fabricated Ⓐ &

L1640 Hip orthosis (HO), abduction control of hip joints, static, pelvic band or spreader bar, thigh cuffs, custom fabricated Ⓐ &

L1650 Hip orthosis (HO), abduction control of hip joints, static, adjustable, (Ilfled type), prefabricated, includes fitting and adjustment Ⓐ &

L1652 Hip orthosis (HO), bilateral thigh cuffs with adjustable abductor spreader bar, adult size, prefabricated, includes fitting and adjustment, any type Ⓐ &

L1660 Hip orthosis (HO), abduction control of hip joints, static, plastic, prefabricated, includes fitting and adjustment Ⓐ &

Special Coverage Instructions   Noncovered by Medicare   Carrier Discretion   ☑ Quantity Alert   ● New Code   ○ Recycled/Reinstated   ▲ Revised Code

© 2023 Optum360, LLC   A2-Z3 ASC Pmt   CMS: IOM   AHA: Coding Clinic   & DMEPOS Paid   ⊘ SNF Excluded   L Codes — 131

Orthotic Devices and Procedures

L1680 — L1920

L1680 Hip orthosis (HO), abduction control of hip joints, dynamic, pelvic control, adjustable hip motion control, thigh cuffs (Rancho hip action type), custom fabricated Ⓐ�&

● **L1681** Hip orthosis (HO), bilateral hip joints and thigh cuffs, adjustable flexion, extension, abduction control of hip joint, postoperative hip abduction type, prefabricated item that has been trimmed, bent, molded, assembled, or otherwise customized to fit a specific patient by an individual with expertise

L1685 Hip orthosis (HO), abduction control of hip joint, postoperative hip abduction type, custom fabricated Ⓐ&

L1686 Hip orthosis (HO), abduction control of hip joint, postoperative hip abduction type, prefabricated, includes fitting and adjustment Ⓐ&

L1690 Combination, bilateral, lumbo-sacral, hip, femur orthosis providing adduction and internal rotation control, prefabricated, includes fitting and adjustment Ⓐ&

Legg Perthes

L1700 Legg Perthes orthosis, (Toronto type), custom fabricated Ⓐ&

L1710 Legg Perthes orthosis, (Newington type), custom fabricated Ⓐ&

L1720 Legg Perthes orthosis, trilateral, (Tachdijan type), custom fabricated Ⓐ&

L1730 Legg Perthes orthosis, (Scottish Rite type), custom fabricated Ⓐ&

L1755 Legg Perthes orthosis, (Patten bottom type), custom fabricated Ⓐ&

Knee Orthosis

L1810 Knee orthosis (KO), elastic with joints, prefabricated item that has been trimmed, bent, molded, assembled, or otherwise customized to fit a specific patient by an individual with expertise Ⓐ&

L1812 Knee orthosis (KO), elastic with joints, prefabricated, off-the-shelf Ⓐ&

L1820 Knee orthosis (KO), elastic with condylar pads and joints, with or without patellar control, prefabricated, includes fitting and adjustment Ⓐ&

L1830 Knee orthosis (KO), immobilizer, canvas longitudinal, prefabricated, off-the-shelf Ⓐ&

L1831 Knee orthosis (KO), locking knee joint(s), positional orthosis, prefabricated, includes fitting and adjustment Ⓐ&

L1832 Knee orthosis (KO), adjustable knee joints (unicentric or polycentric), positional orthosis, rigid support, prefabricated item that has been trimmed, bent, molded, assembled, or otherwise customized to fit a specific patient by an individual with expertise Ⓐ&

L1833 Knee orthosis (KO), adjustable knee joints (unicentric or polycentric), positional orthosis, rigid support, prefabricated, off-the shelf Ⓐ&

L1834 Knee orthosis (KO), without knee joint, rigid, custom fabricated Ⓐ&

L1836 Knee orthosis (KO), rigid, without joint(s), includes soft interface material, prefabricated, off-the-shelf Ⓐ&

L1840 Knee orthosis (KO), derotation, medial-lateral, anterior cruciate ligament, custom fabricated Ⓐ&

L1843 Knee orthosis (KO), single upright, thigh and calf, with adjustable flexion and extension joint (unicentric or polycentric), medial-lateral and rotation control, with or without varus/valgus adjustment, prefabricated item that has been trimmed, bent, molded, assembled, or otherwise customized to fit a specific patient by an individual with expertise Ⓐ&

L1844 Knee orthosis (KO), single upright, thigh and calf, with adjustable flexion and extension joint (unicentric or polycentric), medial-lateral and rotation control, with or without varus/valgus adjustment, custom fabricated Ⓐ&

L1845 Knee orthosis (KO), double upright, thigh and calf, with adjustable flexion and extension joint (unicentric or polycentric), medial-lateral and rotation control, with or without varus/valgus adjustment, prefabricated item that has been trimmed, bent, molded, assembled, or otherwise customized to fit a specific patient by an individual with expertise Ⓐ&

L1846 Knee orthosis (KO), double upright, thigh and calf, with adjustable flexion and extension joint (unicentric or polycentric), medial-lateral and rotation control, with or without varus/valgus adjustment, custom fabricated Ⓐ&

L1847 Knee orthosis (KO), double upright with adjustable joint, with inflatable air support chamber(s), prefabricated item that has been trimmed, bent, molded, assembled, or otherwise customized to fit a specific patient by an individual with expertise Ⓐ&

L1848 Knee orthosis (KO), double upright with adjustable joint, with inflatable air support chamber(s), prefabricated, off-the-shelf Ⓐ&

L1850 Knee orthosis (KO), Swedish type, prefabricated, off-the-shelf Ⓐ&

L1851 Knee orthosis (KO), single upright, thigh and calf, with adjustable flexion and extension joint (unicentric or polycentric), medial-lateral and rotation control, with or without varus/valgus adjustment, prefabricated, off-the-shelf Ⓐ&

L1852 Knee orthosis (KO), double upright, thigh and calf, with adjustable flexion and extension joint (unicentric or polycentric), medial-lateral and rotation control, with or without varus/valgus adjustment, prefabricated, off-the-shelf Ⓐ&

L1860 Knee orthosis (KO), modification of supracondylar prosthetic socket, custom fabricated (SK) Ⓐ&

Ankle-Foot Orthosis (AFO)

L1900 Ankle-foot orthosis (AFO), spring wire, dorsiflexion assist calf band, custom fabricated Ⓐ&

L1902 Ankle orthosis (AO), ankle gauntlet or similar, with or without joints, prefabricated, off-the-shelf Ⓐ&

L1904 Ankle orthosis (AO), ankle gauntlet or similar, with or without joints, custom fabricated Ⓐ&

L1906 Ankle foot orthosis (AFO), multiligamentous ankle support, prefabricated, off-the-shelf Ⓐ&

L1907 Ankle orthosis (AO), supramalleolar with straps, with or without interface/pads, custom fabricated Ⓐ&

L1910 Ankle-foot orthosis (AFO), posterior, single bar, clasp attachment to shoe counter, prefabricated, includes fitting and adjustment Ⓐ&

L1920 Ankle-foot orthosis (AFO), single upright with static or adjustable stop (Phelps or Perlstein type), custom fabricated Ⓐ&

Special Coverage Instructions   Noncovered by Medicare   Carrier Discretion   ☑ Quantity Alert   ● New Code   ○ Recycled/Reinstated   ▲ Revised Code

132 — L Codes   Ⓐ Age Edit   Ⓜ Maternity Edit   ♀ Female Only   ♂ Male Only   Ⓐ-Ⓨ OPPS Status Indicators   © 2023 Optum360, LLC

L1930 Ankle-foot orthosis (AFO), plastic or other material, prefabricated, includes fitting and adjustment   A &

Ankle foot orthotic (AFO), plastic or other material (L1930)

Flexible carbon component

Foot component may fit inside shoe

L1932 Ankle-foot orthosis (AFO), rigid anterior tibial section, total carbon fiber or equal material, prefabricated, includes fitting and adjustment   A &

L1940 Ankle-foot orthosis (AFO), plastic or other material, custom fabricated   A &

L1945 Ankle-foot orthosis (AFO), plastic, rigid anterior tibial section (floor reaction), custom fabricated   A &

Rigid tibial anterior floor reaction; ankle-foot orthosis (AFO) (L1945)

Spiral; ankle foot orthosis (AFO) (L1950)

L1950 Ankle-foot orthosis (AFO), spiral, (Institute of Rehabilitative Medicine type), plastic, custom fabricated   A &

L1951 Ankle-foot orthosis (AFO), spiral, (Institute of rehabilitative Medicine type), plastic or other material, prefabricated, includes fitting and adjustment   A &

L1960 Ankle-foot orthosis (AFO), posterior solid ankle, plastic, custom fabricated   A &

L1970 Ankle-foot orthosis (AFO), plastic with ankle joint, custom fabricated   A &

L1971 Ankle-foot orthosis (AFO), plastic or other material with ankle joint, prefabricated, includes fitting and adjustment   A &

L1980 Ankle-foot orthosis (AFO), single upright free plantar dorsiflexion, solid stirrup, calf band/cuff (single bar 'BK' orthosis), custom fabricated   A &

L1990 Ankle-foot orthosis (AFO), double upright free plantar dorsiflexion, solid stirrup, calf band/cuff (double bar 'BK' orthosis), custom fabricated   A &

Knee-Ankle-Foot Orthosis (KAFO) - Or Any Combination

L2000 Knee-ankle-foot orthosis (KAFO), single upright, free knee, free ankle, solid stirrup, thigh and calf bands/cuffs (single bar 'AK' orthosis), custom fabricated   A &

L2005 Knee-ankle-foot orthosis (KAFO), any material, single or double upright, stance control, automatic lock and swing phase release, any type activation, includes ankle joint, any type, custom fabricated   A &

L2006 Knee ankle foot device, any material, single or double upright, swing and stance phase microprocessor control with adjustability, includes all components (e.g., sensors, batteries, charger), any type activation, with or without ankle joint(s), custom fabricated   A &

L2010 Knee-ankle-foot orthosis (KAFO), single upright, free ankle, solid stirrup, thigh and calf bands/cuffs (single bar 'AK' orthosis), without knee joint, custom fabricated   A &

L2020 Knee-ankle-foot orthosis (KAFO), double upright, free ankle, solid stirrup, thigh and calf bands/cuffs (double bar 'AK' orthosis), custom fabricated   A &

L2030 Knee-ankle-foot orthosis (KAFO), double upright, free ankle, solid stirrup, thigh and calf bands/cuffs, (double bar 'AK' orthosis), without knee joint, custom fabricated   A &

L2034 Knee-ankle-foot orthosis (KAFO), full plastic, single upright, with or without free motion knee, medial-lateral rotation control, with or without free motion ankle, custom fabricated   A &

L2035 Knee-ankle-foot orthosis (KAFO), full plastic, static (pediatric size), without free motion ankle, prefabricated, includes fitting and adjustment   A &

L2036 Knee-ankle-foot orthosis (KAFO), full plastic, double upright, with or without free motion knee, with or without free motion ankle, custom fabricated   A &

L2037 Knee-ankle-foot orthosis (KAFO), full plastic, single upright, with or without free motion knee, with or without free motion ankle, custom fabricated   A &

L2038 Knee-ankle-foot orthosis (KAFO), full plastic, with or without free motion knee, multi-axis ankle, custom fabricated   A &

Torsion Control: Hip-Knee-Ankle-Foot Orthosis (HKAFO)

L2040 Hip-knee-ankle-foot orthosis (HKAFO), torsion control, bilateral rotation straps, pelvic band/belt, custom fabricated   A &

L2050 Hip-knee-ankle-foot orthosis (HKAFO), torsion control, bilateral torsion cables, hip joint, pelvic band/belt, custom fabricated   A &

L2060 Hip-knee-ankle-foot orthosis (HKAFO), torsion control, bilateral torsion cables, ball bearing hip joint, pelvic band/ belt, custom fabricated   A &

L2070 Hip-knee-ankle-foot orthosis (HKAFO), torsion control, unilateral rotation straps, pelvic band/belt, custom fabricated   A &

L2080 Hip-knee-ankle-foot orthosis (HKAFO), torsion control, unilateral torsion cable, hip joint, pelvic band/belt, custom fabricated   A &

L2090 Hip-knee-ankle-foot orthosis (HKAFO), torsion control, unilateral torsion cable, ball bearing hip joint, pelvic band/ belt, custom fabricated   A &

L2106 Ankle-foot orthosis (AFO), fracture orthosis, tibial fracture cast orthosis, thermoplastic type casting material, custom fabricated   A &

Special Coverage Instructions   Noncovered by Medicare   Carrier Discretion   ☑ Quantity Alert   ● New Code   ○ Recycled/Reinstated   ▲ Revised Code

© 2023 Optum360, LLC   A2-Z3 ASC Pmt   **CMS:** IOM   **AHA:** Coding Clinic   & DMEPOS Paid   ⊘ SNF Excluded   **L Codes — 133**

L2108	Ankle-foot orthosis (AFO), fracture orthosis, tibial fracture cast orthosis, custom fabricated 🅰 ♿
L2112	Ankle-foot orthosis (AFO), fracture orthosis, tibial fracture orthosis, soft, prefabricated, includes fitting and adjustment 🅰 ♿
L2114	Ankle-foot orthosis (AFO), fracture orthosis, tibial fracture orthosis, semi-rigid, prefabricated, includes fitting and adjustment 🅰 ♿
L2116	Ankle-foot orthosis (AFO), fracture orthosis, tibial fracture orthosis, rigid, prefabricated, includes fitting and adjustment 🅰 ♿
L2126	Knee-ankle-foot orthosis (KAFO), fracture orthosis, femoral fracture cast orthosis, thermoplastic type casting material, custom fabricated 🅰 ♿
L2128	Knee-ankle-foot orthosis (KAFO), fracture orthosis, femoral fracture cast orthosis, custom fabricated 🅰 ♿
L2132	Knee-ankle-foot orthosis (KAFO), fracture orthosis, femoral fracture cast orthosis, soft, prefabricated, includes fitting and adjustment 🅰 ♿
L2134	Knee-ankle-foot orthosis (KAFO), fracture orthosis, femoral fracture cast orthosis, semi-rigid, prefabricated, includes fitting and adjustment 🅰 ♿
L2136	Knee-ankle-foot orthosis (KAFO), fracture orthosis, femoral fracture cast orthosis, rigid, prefabricated, includes fitting and adjustment 🅰 ♿

Additions to Fracture Orthosis

L2180	Addition to lower extremity fracture orthosis, plastic shoe insert with ankle joints 🅰 ♿
L2182	Addition to lower extremity fracture orthosis, drop lock knee joint 🅰 ♿
L2184	Addition to lower extremity fracture orthosis, limited motion knee joint 🅰 ♿
L2186	Addition to lower extremity fracture orthosis, adjustable motion knee joint, Lerman type 🅰 ♿
L2188	Addition to lower extremity fracture orthosis, quadrilateral brim 🅰 ♿
L2190	Addition to lower extremity fracture orthosis, waist belt 🅰 ♿
L2192	Addition to lower extremity fracture orthosis, hip joint, pelvic band, thigh flange, and pelvic belt 🅰 ♿

Additions to Lower Extremity Orthosis: Shoe-Ankle-Shin-Knee

L2200	Addition to lower extremity, limited ankle motion, each joint 🅰 ☑ ♿
L2210	Addition to lower extremity, dorsiflexion assist (plantar flexion resist), each joint 🅰 ☑ ♿
L2220	Addition to lower extremity, dorsiflexion and plantar flexion assist/resist, each joint 🅰 ☑ ♿
L2230	Addition to lower extremity, split flat caliper stirrups and plate attachment 🅰 ♿
L2232	Addition to lower extremity orthosis, rocker bottom for total contact ankle-foot orthosis (AFO), for custom fabricated orthosis only 🅰 ♿
L2240	Addition to lower extremity, round caliper and plate attachment 🅰 ♿
L2250	Addition to lower extremity, foot plate, molded to patient model, stirrup attachment 🅰 ♿

L2260	Addition to lower extremity, reinforced solid stirrup (Scott-Craig type) 🅰 ♿
L2265	Addition to lower extremity, long tongue stirrup 🅰 ♿
L2270	Addition to lower extremity, varus/valgus correction (T) strap, padded/lined or malleolus pad 🅰 ♿
L2275	Addition to lower extremity, varus/valgus correction, plastic modification, padded/lined 🅰 ♿
L2280	Addition to lower extremity, molded inner boot 🅰 ♿
L2300	Addition to lower extremity, abduction bar (bilateral hip involvement), jointed, adjustable 🅰 ♿
L2310	Addition to lower extremity, abduction bar, straight 🅰 ♿
L2320	Addition to lower extremity, nonmolded lacer, for custom fabricated orthosis only 🅰 ♿
L2330	Addition to lower extremity, lacer molded to patient model, for custom fabricated orthosis only 🅰 ♿
L2335	Addition to lower extremity, anterior swing band 🅰 ♿
L2340	Addition to lower extremity, pretibial shell, molded to patient model 🅰 ♿
L2350	Addition to lower extremity, prosthetic type, (BK) socket, molded to patient model, (used for PTB, AFO orthoses) 🅰 ♿
L2360	Addition to lower extremity, extended steel shank 🅰 ♿
L2370	Addition to lower extremity, Patten bottom 🅰 ♿
L2375	Addition to lower extremity, torsion control, ankle joint and half solid stirrup 🅰 ♿
L2380	Addition to lower extremity, torsion control, straight knee joint, each joint 🅰 ☑ ♿
L2385	Addition to lower extremity, straight knee joint, heavy-duty, each joint 🅰 ☑ ♿
L2387	Addition to lower extremity, polycentric knee joint, for custom fabricated knee-ankle-foot orthosis (KAFO), each joint 🅰 ☑ ♿
L2390	Addition to lower extremity, offset knee joint, each joint 🅰 ☑ ♿
L2395	Addition to lower extremity, offset knee joint, heavy-duty, each joint 🅰 ☑ ♿
L2397	Addition to lower extremity orthosis, suspension sleeve 🅰 ♿

Additions to Straight Knee or Offset Knee Joints

L2405	Addition to knee joint, drop lock, each 🅰 ☑ ♿
L2415	Addition to knee lock with integrated release mechanism (bail, cable, or equal), any material, each joint 🅰 ☑ ♿
L2425	Addition to knee joint, disc or dial lock for adjustable knee flexion, each joint 🅰 ☑ ♿
L2430	Addition to knee joint, ratchet lock for active and progressive knee extension, each joint 🅰 ☑ ♿
L2492	Addition to knee joint, lift loop for drop lock ring 🅰 ♿

Additions: Thigh/Weight Bearing - Gluteal/Ischial Weight Bearing

L2500	Addition to lower extremity, thigh/weight bearing, gluteal/ischial weight bearing, ring 🅰 ♿
L2510	Addition to lower extremity, thigh/weight bearing, quadri-lateral brim, molded to patient model 🅰 ♿
L2520	Addition to lower extremity, thigh/weight bearing, quadri-lateral brim, custom fitted 🅰 ♿
L2525	Addition to lower extremity, thigh/weight bearing, ischial containment/narrow M-L brim molded to patient model 🅰 ♿

Special Coverage Instructions   Noncovered by Medicare   Carrier Discretion   ☑ Quantity Alert ● New Code   ○ Recycled/Reinstated ▲ Revised Code

134 — L Codes   🅰 Age Edit   Ⓜ Maternity Edit   ♀ Female Only   ♂ Male Only   🅰-Ⓨ OPPS Status Indicators   © 2023 Optum360, LLC

L2526	Addition to lower extremity, thigh/weight bearing, ischial containment/narrow M-L brim, custom fitted 〔A〕⅊
L2530	Addition to lower extremity, thigh/weight bearing, lacer, nonmolded 〔A〕⅊
L2540	Addition to lower extremity, thigh/weight bearing, lacer, molded to patient model 〔A〕⅊
L2550	Addition to lower extremity, thigh/weight bearing, high roll cuff 〔A〕⅊

Additions: Pelvic and Thoracic Control

L2570	Addition to lower extremity, pelvic control, hip joint, Clevis type two-position joint, each 〔A〕☑⅊
L2580	Addition to lower extremity, pelvic control, pelvic sling 〔A〕⅊
L2600	Addition to lower extremity, pelvic control, hip joint, Clevis type, or thrust bearing, free, each 〔A〕☑⅊
L2610	Addition to lower extremity, pelvic control, hip joint, Clevis or thrust bearing, lock, each 〔A〕☑⅊
L2620	Addition to lower extremity, pelvic control, hip joint, heavy-duty, each 〔A〕☑⅊
L2622	Addition to lower extremity, pelvic control, hip joint, adjustable flexion, each 〔A〕☑⅊
L2624	Addition to lower extremity, pelvic control, hip joint, adjustable flexion, extension, abduction control, each 〔A〕☑⅊
L2627	Addition to lower extremity, pelvic control, plastic, molded to patient model, reciprocating hip joint and cables 〔A〕⅊
L2628	Addition to lower extremity, pelvic control, metal frame, reciprocating hip joint and cables 〔A〕⅊
L2630	Addition to lower extremity, pelvic control, band and belt, unilateral 〔A〕⅊
L2640	Addition to lower extremity, pelvic control, band and belt, bilateral 〔A〕⅊
L2650	Addition to lower extremity, pelvic and thoracic control, gluteal pad, each 〔A〕⅊
L2660	Addition to lower extremity, thoracic control, thoracic band 〔A〕⅊
L2670	Addition to lower extremity, thoracic control, paraspinal uprights 〔A〕⅊
L2680	Addition to lower extremity, thoracic control, lateral support uprights 〔A〕⅊

Additions: General

L2750	Addition to lower extremity orthosis, plating chrome or nickel, per bar 〔A〕☑⅊
L2755	Addition to lower extremity orthosis, high strength, lightweight material, all hybrid lamination/prepreg composite, per segment, for custom fabricated orthosis only 〔A〕⅊
L2760	Addition to lower extremity orthosis, extension, per extension, per bar (for lineal adjustment for growth) 〔A〕☑⅊
L2768	Orthotic side bar disconnect device, per bar 〔A〕☑⅊
L2780	Addition to lower extremity orthosis, noncorrosive finish, per bar 〔A〕☑⅊
L2785	Addition to lower extremity orthosis, drop lock retainer, each 〔A〕☑⅊
L2795	Addition to lower extremity orthosis, knee control, full kneecap 〔A〕⅊

L2800	Addition to lower extremity orthosis, knee control, knee cap, medial or lateral pull, for use with custom fabricated orthosis only 〔A〕⅊
L2810	Addition to lower extremity orthosis, knee control, condylar pad 〔A〕⅊
L2820	Addition to lower extremity orthosis, soft interface for molded plastic, below knee section 〔A〕⅊
L2830	Addition to lower extremity orthosis, soft interface for molded plastic, above knee section 〔A〕⅊
L2840	Addition to lower extremity orthosis, tibial length sock, fracture or equal, each 〔A〕☑⅊
L2850	Addition to lower extremity orthosis, femoral length sock, fracture or equal, each 〔A〕☑⅊
L2861	Addition to lower extremity joint, knee or ankle, concentric adjustable torsion style mechanism for custom fabricated orthotics only, each 〔E〕☑
L2999	Lower extremity orthoses, not otherwise specified 〔A〕 Determine if an alternative HCPCS Level II or a CPT code better describes the service being reported. This code should be used only if a more specific code is unavailable.

Orthopedic Footwear

Inserts

L3000	Foot insert, removable, molded to patient model, UCB type, Berkeley shell, each 〔A〕☑⅊
L3001	Foot, insert, removable, molded to patient model, Spenco, each 〔A〕☑⅊
L3002	Foot insert, removable, molded to patient model, Plastazote or equal, each 〔A〕☑⅊
L3003	Foot insert, removable, molded to patient model, silicone gel, each 〔A〕☑⅊
L3010	Foot insert, removable, molded to patient model, longitudinal arch support, each 〔A〕☑⅊
L3020	Foot insert, removable, molded to patient model, longitudinal/metatarsal support, each 〔A〕☑⅊
L3030	Foot insert, removable, formed to patient foot, each 〔A〕☑⅊
L3031	Foot, insert/plate, removable, addition to lower extremity orthosis, high strength, lightweight material, all hybrid lamination/prepreg composite, each 〔A〕☑⅊

Arch Support, Removable, Premolded

L3040	Foot, arch support, removable, premolded, longitudinal, each 〔A〕☑⅊
L3050	Foot, arch support, removable, premolded, metatarsal, each 〔A〕☑⅊
L3060	Foot, arch support, removable, premolded, longitudinal/metatarsal, each 〔A〕☑⅊

Arch Support, Nonremovable, Attached to Shoe

L3070	Foot, arch support, nonremovable, attached to shoe, longitudinal, each 〔A〕☑⅊
L3080	Foot, arch support, nonremovable, attached to shoe, metatarsal, each 〔A〕☑⅊
L3090	Foot, arch support, nonremovable, attached to shoe, longitudinal/metatarsal, each 〔A〕☑⅊
L3100	Hallus-valgus night dynamic splint, prefabricated, off-the-shelf 〔A〕⅊

Special Coverage Instructions   Noncovered by Medicare   Carrier Discretion   ☑ Quantity Alert   ● New Code   ○ Recycled/Reinstated   ▲ Revised Code

© 2023 Optum360, LLC   〔A2〕-〔Z3〕 ASC Pmt   CMS: IOM   AHA: Coding Clinic   ⅊ DMEPOS Paid   ⊘ SNF Excluded   L Codes — 135

Orthotic Devices and Procedures

L3140 — L3500

Abduction and Rotation Bars

L3140   Foot, abduction rotation bar, including shoes   Ⓐ ♿

A Denis-Browne style splint is a bar that can be applied by a strap or mounted on a shoe. This type of splint generally corrects congenital conditions such as genu varus

The angle may be adjusted on a plate on the sole of the shoe

Denis-Browne splint

L3150   Foot, abduction rotation bar, without shoes   Ⓐ ♿

L3160   Foot, adjustable shoe-styled positioning device   Ⓐ

● **L3161**   Foot, adductus positioning device, adjustable

L3170   Foot, plastic, silicone or equal, heel stabilizer, prefabricated, off-the-shelf, each   Ⓐ ☑ ♿

Orthopedic Shoes and Boots

L3201   Orthopedic shoe, Oxford with supinator or pronator, infant   Ⓐ Ⓐ

L3202   Orthopedic shoe, Oxford with supinator or pronator, child   Ⓐ Ⓐ

L3203   Orthopedic shoe, Oxford with supinator or pronator, junior   Ⓐ Ⓐ

L3204   Orthopedic shoe, hightop with supinator or pronator, infant   Ⓐ Ⓐ

L3206   Orthopedic shoe, hightop with supinator or pronator, child   Ⓐ Ⓐ

L3207   Orthopedic shoe, hightop with supinator or pronator, junior   Ⓐ Ⓐ

L3208   Surgical boot, each, infant   Ⓐ Ⓐ ☑

L3209   Surgical boot, each, child   Ⓐ Ⓐ ☑

L3211   Surgical boot, each, junior   Ⓐ Ⓐ ☑

L3212   Benesch boot, pair, infant   Ⓐ Ⓐ ☑

L3213   Benesch boot, pair, child   Ⓐ Ⓐ ☑

L3214   Benesch boot, pair, junior   Ⓐ Ⓐ ☑

L3215   Orthopedic footwear, ladies shoe, Oxford, each   Ⓐ ♀ Ⓔ ☑

L3216   Orthopedic footwear, ladies shoe, depth inlay, each   Ⓐ ♀ Ⓔ ☑

L3217   Orthopedic footwear, ladies shoe, hightop, depth inlay, each   Ⓐ ♀ Ⓔ ☑

L3219   Orthopedic footwear, mens shoe, Oxford, each   Ⓐ ♂ Ⓔ ☑

L3221   Orthopedic footwear, mens shoe, depth inlay, each   Ⓐ ♂ Ⓔ ☑

L3222   Orthopedic footwear, mens shoe, hightop, depth inlay, each   Ⓐ ♂ Ⓔ ☑

L3224   Orthopedic footwear, woman's shoe, Oxford, used as an integral part of a brace (orthosis)   ♀ Ⓐ ♿

L3225   Orthopedic footwear, man's shoe, Oxford, used as an integral part of a brace (orthosis)   ♂ Ⓐ ♿

L3230   Orthopedic footwear, custom shoe, depth inlay, each   Ⓐ ☑

L3250   Orthopedic footwear, custom molded shoe, removable inner mold, prosthetic shoe, each   Ⓐ ☑

L3251   Foot, shoe molded to patient model, silicone shoe, each   Ⓐ ☑

L3252   Foot, shoe molded to patient model, Plastazote (or similar), custom fabricated, each   Ⓐ ☑

L3253   Foot, molded shoe, Plastazote (or similar), custom fitted, each   Ⓐ ☑

L3254   Nonstandard size or width   Ⓐ

L3255   Nonstandard size or length   Ⓐ

L3257   Orthopedic footwear, additional charge for split size   Ⓐ

L3260   Surgical boot/shoe, each   Ⓔ ☑

L3265   Plastazote sandal, each   Ⓐ ☑

Shoe Modification - Lifts

L3300   Lift, elevation, heel, tapered to metatarsals, per in   Ⓐ ☑ ♿

L3310   Lift, elevation, heel and sole, neoprene, per in   Ⓐ ☑ ♿

L3320   Lift, elevation, heel and sole, cork, per in   Ⓐ ☑

L3330   Lift, elevation, metal extension (skate)   Ⓐ ♿

L3332   Lift, elevation, inside shoe, tapered, up to one-half in   Ⓐ ☑ ♿

L3334   Lift, elevation, heel, per in   Ⓐ ☑ ♿

Shoe Modification - Wedges

L3340   Heel wedge, SACH   Ⓐ ♿

L3350   Heel wedge   Ⓐ ♿

L3360   Sole wedge, outside sole   Ⓐ ♿

L3370   Sole wedge, between sole   Ⓐ ♿

L3380   Clubfoot wedge   Ⓐ ♿

L3390   Outflare wedge   Ⓐ ♿

L3400   Metatarsal bar wedge, rocker   Ⓐ ♿

L3410   Metatarsal bar wedge, between sole   Ⓐ ♿

L3420   Full sole and heel wedge, between sole   Ⓐ ♿

Shoe Modifications - Heels

L3430   Heel, counter, plastic reinforced   Ⓐ ♿

L3440   Heel, counter, leather reinforced   Ⓐ ♿

L3450   Heel, SACH cushion type   Ⓐ ♿

L3455   Heel, new leather, standard   Ⓐ ♿

L3460   Heel, new rubber, standard   Ⓐ ♿

L3465   Heel, Thomas with wedge   Ⓐ ♿

L3470   Heel, Thomas extended to ball   Ⓐ ♿

L3480   Heel, pad and depression for spur   Ⓐ ♿

L3485   Heel, pad, removable for spur   Ⓐ

Miscellaneous Shoe Additions

L3500   Orthopedic shoe addition, insole, leather   Ⓐ ♿

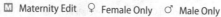

Special Coverage Instructions   Noncovered by Medicare   Carrier Discretion   ☑ Quantity Alert ● New Code   ○ Recycled/Reinstated   ▲ Revised Code

136 — L Codes   Ⓐ Age Edit   Ⓜ Maternity Edit   ♀ Female Only   ♂ Male Only   Ⓐ–Ⓨ OPPS Status Indicators   © 2023 Optum360, LLC

L3510	Orthopedic shoe addition, insole, rubber	A &
L3520	Orthopedic shoe addition, insole, felt covered with leather	A &
L3530	Orthopedic shoe addition, sole, half	A &
L3540	Orthopedic shoe addition, sole, full	A &
L3550	Orthopedic shoe addition, toe tap, standard	A &
L3560	Orthopedic shoe addition, toe tap, horseshoe	A &
L3570	Orthopedic shoe addition, special extension to instep (leather with eyelets)	A &
L3580	Orthopedic shoe addition, convert instep to Velcro closure	A &
L3590	Orthopedic shoe addition, convert firm shoe counter to soft counter	A &
L3595	Orthopedic shoe addition, March bar	A &

Transfer or Replacement

L3600	Transfer of an orthosis from one shoe to another, caliper plate, existing	A &
L3610	Transfer of an orthosis from one shoe to another, caliper plate, new	A &
L3620	Transfer of an orthosis from one shoe to another, solid stirrup, existing	A &
L3630	Transfer of an orthosis from one shoe to another, solid stirrup, new	A &
L3640	Transfer of an orthosis from one shoe to another, Dennis Browne splint (Riveton), both shoes	A &
L3649	Orthopedic shoe, modification, addition or transfer, not otherwise specified	A

Determine if an alternative HCPCS Level II or a CPT code better describes the service being reported. This code should be used only if a more specific code is unavailable.

Shoulder Orthosis (SO)

L3650	Shoulder orthosis (SO), figure of eight design abduction restrainer, prefabricated, off-the-shelf	A &
L3660	Shoulder orthosis (SO), figure of eight design abduction restrainer, canvas and webbing, prefabricated, off-the-shelf	A &
L3670	Shoulder orthosis (SO), acromio/clavicular (canvas and webbing type), prefabricated, off-the-shelf	A &
L3671	Shoulder orthosis (SO), shoulder joint design, without joints, may include soft interface, straps, custom fabricated, includes fitting and adjustment	A &
L3674	Shoulder orthosis (SO), abduction positioning (airplane design), thoracic component and support bar, with or without nontorsion joint/turnbuckle, may include soft interface, straps, custom fabricated, includes fitting and adjustment	A &
L3675	Shoulder orthosis (SO), vest type abduction restrainer, canvas webbing type or equal, prefabricated, off-the-shelf	A &
L3677	Shoulder orthosis (SO), shoulder joint design, without joints, may include soft interface, straps, prefabricated item that has been trimmed, bent, molded, assembled, or otherwise customized to fit a specific patient by an individual with expertise	A
L3678	Shoulder orthosis (SO), shoulder joint design, without joints, may include soft interface, straps, prefabricated, off-the-shelf	A

Elbow Orthosis (EO)

L3702	Elbow orthosis (EO), without joints, may include soft interface, straps, custom fabricated, includes fitting and adjustment	A &
L3710	Elbow orthosis (EO), elastic with metal joints, prefabricated, off-the-shelf	A &
L3720	Elbow orthosis (EO), double upright with forearm/arm cuffs, free motion, custom fabricated	A &
L3730	Elbow orthosis (EO), double upright with forearm/arm cuffs, extension/ flexion assist, custom fabricated	A &
L3740	Elbow orthosis (EO), double upright with forearm/arm cuffs, adjustable position lock with active control, custom fabricated	A &
L3760	Elbow orthosis (EO), with adjustable position locking joint(s), prefabricated, item that has been trimmed, bent, molded, assembled, or otherwise customized to fit a specific patient by an individual with expertise	A &
L3761	Elbow orthosis (EO), with adjustable position locking joint(s), prefabricated, off-the-shelf	A &
L3762	Elbow orthosis (EO), rigid, without joints, includes soft interface material, prefabricated, off-the-shelf	A &
L3763	Elbow wrist-hand orthosis (EWHO), rigid, without joints, may include soft interface, straps, custom fabricated, includes fitting and adjustment	A &
L3764	Elbow-wrist-hand orthosis (EWHO), includes one or more nontorsion joints, elastic bands, turnbuckles, may include soft interface, straps, custom fabricated, includes fitting and adjustment	A &
L3765	Elbow-wrist-hand-finger orthosis (EWHFO), rigid, without joints, may include soft interface, straps, custom fabricated, includes fitting and adjustment	A &
L3766	Elbow-wrist-hand-finger orthosis (EWHFO), includes one or more nontorsion joints, elastic bands, turnbuckles, may include soft interface, straps, custom fabricated, includes fitting and adjustment	A &

Wrist-Hand-Finger Orthosis (WHFO)

L3806	Wrist-hand-finger orthosis (WHFO), includes one or more nontorsion joint(s), turnbuckles, elastic bands/springs, may include soft interface material, straps, custom fabricated, includes fitting and adjustment	A &
L3807	Wrist-hand-finger orthosis (WHFO), without joint(s), prefabricated item that has been trimmed, bent, molded, assembled, or otherwise customized to fit a specific patient by an individual with expertise	A &
L3808	Wrist-hand-finger orthosis (WHFO), rigid without joints, may include soft interface material; straps, custom fabricated, includes fitting and adjustment	A &
L3809	Wrist-hand-finger orthosis (WHFO), without joint(s), prefabricated, off-the-shelf, any type	A &

Additions to Upper Extremity Orthosis

L3891	Addition to upper extremity joint, wrist or elbow, concentric adjustable torsion style mechanism for custom fabricated orthotics only, each	E ☑

Dynamic Flexor Hinge, Reciprocal Wrist Extension/Flexion, Finger Flexion/Extension

L3900	Wrist-hand-finger orthosis (WHFO), dynamic flexor hinge, reciprocal wrist extension/ flexion, finger flexion/extension, wrist or finger driven, custom fabricated	A &

Special Coverage Instructions   Noncovered by Medicare   Carrier Discretion   ☑ Quantity Alert ● New Code   ○ Recycled/Reinstated   ▲ Revised Code

© 2023 Optum360, LLC   A2-Z3 ASC Pmt   CMS: IOM   AHA: Coding Clinic   & DMEPOS Paid   ⊘ SNF Excluded   L Codes — 137

L3901 Wrist-hand-finger orthosis (WHFO), dynamic flexor hinge, reciprocal wrist extension/ flexion, finger flexion/extension, cable driven, custom fabricated 🅰 ♿

External Power

L3904 Wrist-hand-finger orthosis (WHFO), external powered, electric, custom fabricated 🅰 ♿

Other Upper Extremity Orthoses

L3905 Wrist-hand orthosis (WHO), includes one or more nontorsion joints, elastic bands, turnbuckles, may include soft interface, straps, custom fabricated, includes fitting and adjustment 🅰 ♿

L3906 Wrist-hand orthosis (WHO), without joints, may include soft interface, straps, custom fabricated, includes fitting and adjustment 🅰 ♿

L3908 Wrist-hand orthosis (WHO), wrist extension control cock-up, nonmolded, prefabricated, off-the-shelf 🅰 ♿

L3912 Hand-finger orthosis (HFO), flexion glove with elastic finger control, prefabricated, off-the-shelf 🅰 ♿

L3913 Hand-finger orthosis (HFO), without joints, may include soft interface, straps, custom fabricated, includes fitting and adjustment 🅰 ♿

L3915 Wrist-hand orthosis (WHO), includes one or more nontorsion joint(s), elastic bands, turnbuckles, may include soft interface, straps, prefabricated item that has been trimmed, bent, molded, assembled, or otherwise customized to fit a specific patient by an individual with expertise 🅰 ♿

L3916 Wrist-hand orthosis (WHO), includes one or more nontorsion joint(s), elastic bands, turnbuckles, may include soft interface, straps, prefabricated, off-the-shelf 🅰 ♿

L3917 Hand orthosis (HO), metacarpal fracture orthosis, prefabricated item that has been trimmed, bent, molded, assembled, or otherwise customized to fit a specific patient by an individual with expertise 🅰 ♿

L3918 Hand orthosis (HO), metacarpal fracture orthosis, prefabricated, off-the-shelf 🅰 ♿

L3919 Hand orthosis (HO), without joints, may include soft interface, straps, custom fabricated, includes fitting and adjustment 🅰 ♿

L3921 Hand-finger orthosis (HFO), includes one or more nontorsion joints, elastic bands, turnbuckles, may include soft interface, straps, custom fabricated, includes fitting and adjustment 🅰 ♿

L3923 Hand-finger orthosis (HFO), without joints, may include soft interface, straps, prefabricated item that has been trimmed, bent, molded, assembled, or otherwise customized to fit a specific patient by an individual with expertise 🅰 ♿

L3924 Hand-finger orthosis (HFO), without joints, may include soft interface, straps, prefabricated, off-the-shelf 🅰 ♿

L3925 Finger orthosis (FO), proximal interphalangeal (PIP)/distal interphalangeal (DIP), nontorsion joint/spring, extension/flexion, may include soft interface material, prefabricated, off-the-shelf 🅰 ♿

L3927 Finger orthosis (FO), proximal interphalangeal (PIP)/distal interphalangeal (DIP), without joint/spring, extension/flexion (e.g., static or ring type), may include soft interface material, prefabricated, off-the-shelf 🅰 ♿

L3929 Hand-finger orthosis (HFO), includes one or more nontorsion joint(s), turnbuckles, elastic bands/springs, may include soft interface material, straps, prefabricated item that has been trimmed, bent, molded, assembled, or otherwise customized to fit a specific patient by an individual with expertise 🅰 ♿

L3930 Hand-finger orthosis (HFO), includes one or more nontorsion joint(s), turnbuckles, elastic bands/springs, may include soft interface material, straps, prefabricated, off-the-shelf 🅰 ♿

L3931 Wrist-hand-finger orthosis (WHFO), includes one or more nontorsion joint(s), turnbuckles, elastic bands/springs, may include soft interface material, straps, prefabricated, includes fitting and adjustment 🅰 ♿

L3933 Finger orthosis (FO), without joints, may include soft interface, straps, custom fabricated, includes fitting and adjustment 🅰 ♿

L3935 Finger orthosis (FO), nontorsion joint, may include soft interface, straps, custom fabricated, includes fitting and adjustment 🅰 ♿

L3956 Addition of joint to upper extremity orthosis, any material; per joint 🅰 ☑ ♿

Shoulder, Elbow, Wrist, Hand Orthosis

L3960 Shoulder-elbow-wrist-hand orthosis (SEWHO), abduction positioning, airplane design, prefabricated, includes fitting and adjustment 🅰 ♿

L3961 Shoulder-elbow-wrist-hand orthosis (SEWHO), shoulder cap design, without joints, may include soft interface, straps, custom fabricated, includes fitting and adjustment 🅰 ♿

L3962 Shoulder-elbow-wrist-hand orthosis (SEWHO), abduction positioning, Erb's palsy design, prefabricated, includes fitting and adjustment 🅰 ♿

L3967 Shoulder-elbow-wrist-hand orthosis (SEWHO), abduction positioning (airplane design), thoracic component and support bar, without joints, may include soft interface, straps, custom fabricated, includes fitting and adjustment 🅰 ♿

Additions to Mobile Arm Supports

L3971 Shoulder-elbow-wrist-hand orthotic (SEWHO), shoulder cap design, includes one or more nontorsion joints, elastic bands, turnbuckles, may include soft interface, straps, custom fabricated, includes fitting and adjustment 🅰 ♿

L3973 Shoulder-elbow-wrist-hand orthosis (SEWHO), abduction positioning (airplane design), thoracic component and support bar, includes one or more nontorsion joints, elastic bands, turnbuckles, may include soft interface, straps, custom fabricated, includes fitting and adjustment 🅰 ♿

L3975 Shoulder-elbow-wrist-hand-finger orthosis (SEWHO), shoulder cap design, without joints, may include soft interface, straps, custom fabricated, includes fitting and adjustment 🅰 ♿

L3976 Shoulder-elbow-wrist-hand-finger orthosis (SEWHO), abduction positioning (airplane design), thoracic component and support bar, without joints, may include soft interface, straps, custom fabricated, includes fitting and adjustment 🅰 ♿

L3977 Shoulder-elbow-wrist-hand-finger orthosis (SEWHO), shoulder cap design, includes one or more nontorsion joints, elastic bands, turnbuckles, may include soft interface, straps, custom fabricated, includes fitting and adjustment 🅰 ♿

L3978 Shoulder-elbow-wrist-hand-finger orthosis (SEWHO), abduction positioning (airplane design), thoracic component and support bar, includes one or more nontorsion joints, elastic bands, turnbuckles, may include soft interface, straps, custom fabricated, includes fitting and adjustment 🅰 ♿

Special Coverage Instructions   Noncovered by Medicare   Carrier Discretion   ☑ Quantity Alert   ● New Code   ○ Recycled/Reinstated   ▲ Revised Code

138 — L Codes   🅰 Age Edit   Ⓜ Maternity Edit   ♀ Female Only   ♂ Male Only   🅰-Ⓨ OPPS Status Indicators   © 2023 Optum360, LLC

Fracture Orthotic

L3980 Upper extremity fracture orthosis, humeral, prefabricated, includes fitting and adjustment Ⓐ ♿

L3981 Upper extremity fracture orthosis, humeral, prefabricated, includes shoulder cap design, with or without joints, forearm section, may include soft interface, straps, includes fitting and adjustments Ⓐ ♿

L3982 Upper extremity fracture orthosis, radius/ulnar, prefabricated, includes fitting and adjustment Ⓐ ♿

L3984 Upper extremity fracture orthosis, wrist, prefabricated, includes fitting and adjustment Ⓐ ♿

L3995 Addition to upper extremity orthosis, sock, fracture or equal, each Ⓐ ☑ ♿

L3999 Upper limb orthosis, not otherwise specified Ⓐ

Repairs

L4000 Replace girdle for spinal orthosis (cervical-thoracic-lumbar-sacral orthosis (CTLSO) or spinal orthosis SO) Ⓐ ♿

L4002 Replacement strap, any orthosis, includes all components, any length, any type Ⓐ ♿

L4010 Replace trilateral socket brim Ⓐ ♿

L4020 Replace quadrilateral socket brim, molded to patient model Ⓐ ♿

L4030 Replace quadrilateral socket brim, custom fitted Ⓐ ♿

L4040 Replace molded thigh lacer, for custom fabricated orthosis only Ⓐ ♿

L4045 Replace nonmolded thigh lacer, for custom fabricated orthosis only Ⓐ ♿

L4050 Replace molded calf lacer, for custom fabricated orthosis only Ⓐ ♿

L4055 Replace nonmolded calf lacer, for custom fabricated orthosis only Ⓐ ♿

L4060 Replace high roll cuff Ⓐ ♿

L4070 Replace proximal and distal upright for KAFO Ⓐ ♿

L4080 Replace metal bands KAFO, proximal thigh Ⓐ ♿

L4090 Replace metal bands KAFO-AFO, calf or distal thigh Ⓐ ♿

L4100 Replace leather cuff KAFO, proximal thigh Ⓐ ♿

L4110 Replace leather cuff KAFO-AFO, calf or distal thigh Ⓐ ♿

L4130 Replace pretibial shell Ⓐ ♿

L4205 Repair of orthotic device, labor component, per 15 minutes Ⓐ ☑

L4210 Repair of orthotic device, repair or replace minor parts Ⓐ

Miscellaneous Lower Limb Supports

L4350 Ankle control orthosis, stirrup style, rigid, includes any type interface (e.g., pneumatic, gel), prefabricated, off-the-shelf Ⓐ ♿

L4360 Walking boot, pneumatic and/or vacuum, with or without joints, with or without interface material, prefabricated item that has been trimmed, bent, molded, assembled, or otherwise customized to fit a specific patient by an individual with expertise Ⓐ ♿

L4361 Walking boot, pneumatic and/or vacuum, with or without joints, with or without interface material, prefabricated, off-the-shelf Ⓐ ♿

L4370 Pneumatic full leg splint, prefabricated, off-the-shelf Ⓐ ♿

L4386 Walking boot, nonpneumatic, with or without joints, with or without interface material, prefabricated item that has been trimmed, bent, molded, assembled, or otherwise customized to fit a specific patient by an individual with expertise Ⓐ ♿

L4387 Walking boot, nonpneumatic, with or without joints, with or without interface material, prefabricated, off-the-shelf Ⓐ ♿

L4392 Replacement, soft interface material, static AFO Ⓐ ♿

L4394 Replace soft interface material, foot drop splint Ⓐ ♿

L4396 Static or dynamic ankle foot orthosis, including soft interface material, adjustable for fit, for positioning, may be used for minimal ambulation, prefabricated item that has been trimmed, bent, molded, assembled, or otherwise customized to fit a specific patient by an individual with expertise Ⓐ ♿

L4397 Static or dynamic ankle foot orthosis, including soft interface material, adjustable for fit, for positioning, may be used for minimal ambulation, prefabricated, off-the-shelf Ⓐ ♿

L4398 Foot drop splint, recumbent positioning device, prefabricated, off-the-shelf Ⓐ ♿

L4631 Ankle-foot orthosis (AFO), walking boot type, varus/valgus correction, rocker bottom, anterior tibial shell, soft interface, custom arch support, plastic or other material, includes straps and closures, custom fabricated Ⓐ ♿

Prosthetic Procedures L5000-L9900

The codes in this section are considered as "base" or "basic procedures or prosthetics" and may be modified by listing items/procedures or special materials from the "additions" sections and adding them to the base procedure.

Partial Foot

L5000 Partial foot, shoe insert with longitudinal arch, toe filler Ⓐ ♿

L5010 Partial foot, molded socket, ankle height, with toe filler Ⓐ ♿

L5020 Partial foot, molded socket, tibial tubercle height, with toe filler Ⓐ ♿

Ankle

L5050 Ankle, Symes, molded socket, SACH foot Ⓐ ⊘ ♿

L5060 Ankle, Symes, metal frame, molded leather socket, articulated ankle/foot (SACH) Ⓐ ⊘ ♿

Below Knee

L5100 Below knee (BK), molded socket, shin, SACH foot Ⓐ ⊘ ♿

L5105 Below knee (BK), plastic socket, joints and thigh lacer, SACH foot Ⓐ ⊘ ♿

Knee Disarticulation

L5150 Knee disarticulation (or through knee), molded socket, external knee joints, shin, SACH foot Ⓐ ⊘ ♿

L5160 Knee disarticulation (or through knee), molded socket, bent knee configuration, external knee joints, shin, SACH foot Ⓐ ⊘ ♿

Above Knee

L5200 Above knee (AK), molded socket, single axis constant friction knee, shin, SACH foot Ⓐ ⊘ ♿

L5210 Above knee (AK), short prosthesis, no knee joint (stubbies), with foot blocks, no ankle joints, each Ⓐ ☑ ⊘ ♿

L5220 Above knee (AK), short prosthesis, no knee joint (stubbies), with articulated ankle/foot, dynamically aligned, each Ⓐ ☑ ⊘ ♿

L5230 Above knee (AK), for proximal femoral focal deficiency, constant friction knee, shin, SACH foot Ⓐ ⊘ ♿

Special Coverage Instructions   Noncovered by Medicare   Carrier Discretion   ☑ Quantity Alert   ● New Code   ○ Recycled/Reinstated   ▲ Revised Code

© 2023 Optum360, LLC   A2-Z3 ASC Pmt   CMS: IOM   AHA: Coding Clinic   ♿ DMEPOS Paid   ⊘ SNF Excluded   L Codes — 139

Prosthetic Devices and Procedures

Hip Disarticulation

L5250 Hip disarticulation, Canadian type; molded socket, hip joint, single axis constant friction knee, shin, SACH foot　A ⊘ &

L5270 Hip disarticulation, tilt table type; molded socket, locking hip joint, single axis constant friction knee, shin, SACH foot　A ⊘ &

Hemipelvectomy

L5280 Hemipelvectomy, Canadian type; molded socket, hip joint, single axis constant friction knee, shin, SACH foot　A ⊘ &

L5301 Below knee (BK), molded socket, shin, SACH foot, endoskeletal system　A ⊘ &

L5312 Knee disarticulation (or through knee), molded socket, single axis knee, pylon, SACH foot, endoskeletal system　A &

L5321 Above knee (AK), molded socket, open end, SACH foot, endoskeletal system, single axis knee　A ⊘ &

L5331 Hip disarticulation, Canadian type, molded socket, endoskeletal system, hip joint, single axis knee, SACH foot　A ⊘ &

L5341 Hemipelvectomy, Canadian type, molded socket, endoskeletal system, hip joint, single axis knee, SACH foot　A ⊘ &

Immediate Postsurgical or Early Fitting Procedures

L5400 Immediate postsurgical or early fitting, application of initial rigid dressing, including fitting, alignment, suspension, and one cast change, below knee (BK)　A ☑ &

Above-the-knee test socket

Below-the-knee early fitting rigid dressing (L5400)

Test sockets are often made of clear plastic so the prosthetist can visualize the fit against the residual limb

L5410 Immediate postsurgical or early fitting, application of initial rigid dressing, including fitting, alignment and suspension, below knee (BK), each additional cast change and realignment　A ☑ &

L5420 Immediate postsurgical or early fitting, application of initial rigid dressing, including fitting, alignment and suspension and one cast change above knee (AK) or knee disarticulation　A ☑ &

L5430 Immediate postsurgical or early fitting, application of initial rigid dressing, including fitting, alignment and suspension, above knee (AK) or knee disarticulation, each additional cast change and realignment　A ☑ &

L5450 Immediate postsurgical or early fitting, application of nonweight bearing rigid dressing, below knee (BK)　A &

L5460 Immediate postsurgical or early fitting, application of nonweight bearing rigid dressing, above knee (AK)　A &

Initial Prosthesis

L5500 Initial, below knee (BK) PTB type socket, nonalignable system, pylon, no cover, SACH foot, plaster socket, direct formed　A ⊘ &

L5505 Initial, above knee (AK), knee disarticulation, ischial level socket, nonalignable system, pylon, no cover, SACH foot, plaster socket, direct formed　A ⊘ &

Preparatory Prosthesis

L5510 Preparatory, below knee (BK) PTB type socket, nonalignable system, pylon, no cover, SACH foot, plaster socket, molded to model　A ⊘ &

L5520 Preparatory, below knee (BK) PTB type socket, nonalignable system, pylon, no cover, SACH foot, thermoplastic or equal, direct formed　A ⊘ &

L5530 Preparatory, below knee (BK) PTB type socket, nonalignable system, pylon, no cover, SACH foot, thermoplastic or equal, molded to model　A ⊘ &

L5535 Preparatory, below knee (BK) PTB type socket, nonalignable system, no cover, SACH foot, prefabricated, adjustable open end socket　A ⊘ &

L5540 Preparatory, below knee (BK) PTB type socket, nonalignable system, pylon, no cover, SACH foot, laminated socket, molded to model　A ⊘ &

L5560 Preparatory, above knee (AK), knee disarticulation, ischial level socket, nonalignable system, pylon, no cover, SACH foot, plaster socket, molded to model　A ⊘ &

L5570 Preparatory, above knee (AK), knee disarticulation, ischial level socket, nonalignable system, pylon, no cover, SACH foot, thermoplastic or equal, direct formed　A ⊘ &

L5580 Preparatory, above knee (AK), knee disarticulation, ischial level socket, nonalignable system, pylon, no cover, SACH foot, thermoplastic or equal, molded to model　A ⊘ &

L5585 Preparatory, above knee (AK), knee disarticulation, ischial level socket, nonalignable system, pylon, no cover, SACH foot, prefabricated adjustable open end socket　A ⊘ &

L5590 Preparatory, above knee (AK), knee disarticulation, ischial level socket, nonalignable system, pylon, no cover, SACH foot, laminated socket, molded to model　A ⊘ &

L5595 Preparatory, hip disarticulation/hemipelvectomy, pylon, no cover, SACH foot, thermoplastic or equal, molded to patient model　A ⊘ &

L5600 Preparatory, hip disarticulation/hemipelvectomy, pylon, no cover, SACH foot, laminated socket, molded to patient model　A ⊘ &

Additions

Additions: Lower Extremity

L5610 Addition to lower extremity, endoskeletal system, above knee (AK), hydracadence system　A ⊘ &

L5611 Addition to lower extremity, endoskeletal system, above knee (AK), knee disarticulation, four-bar linkage, with friction swing phase control　A ⊘ &

L5613 Addition to lower extremity, endoskeletal system, above knee (AK), knee disarticulation, four-bar linkage, with hydraulic swing phase control　A ⊘ &

L5614 Addition to lower extremity, exoskeletal system, above knee (AK), knee disarticulation, four-bar linkage, with pneumatic swing phase control　A ⊘ &

● **L5615** Addition, endoskeletal knee-shin system, 4 bar linkage or multiaxial, fluid swing and stance phase control

Special Coverage Instructions　　Noncovered by Medicare　　Carrier Discretion　　☑ Quantity Alert　● New Code　○ Recycled/Reinstated　▲ Revised Code

140 — L Codes　　A Age Edit　M Maternity Edit　♀ Female Only　♂ Male Only　A-Y OPPS Status Indicators　© 2023 Optum360, LLC

L5616 Addition to lower extremity, endoskeletal system, above knee (AK), universal multiplex system, friction swing phase control A ⊘ &

L5617 Addition to lower extremity, quick change self-aligning unit, above knee (AK) or below knee (BK), each A ☑ ⊘ &

Additions: Test Sockets

L5618 Addition to lower extremity, test socket, Symes A ⊘ &

L5620 Addition to lower extremity, test socket, below knee (BK) A ⊘ &

L5622 Addition to lower extremity, test socket, knee disarticulation A ⊘ &

L5624 Addition to lower extremity, test socket, above knee (AK) A ⊘ &

L5626 Addition to lower extremity, test socket, hip disarticulation A ⊘ &

L5628 Addition to lower extremity, test socket, hemipelvectomy A ⊘ &

L5629 Addition to lower extremity, below knee, acrylic socket A ⊘ &

Additions: Socket Variations

L5630 Addition to lower extremity, Symes type, expandable wall socket A ⊘ &

L5631 Addition to lower extremity, above knee (AK) or knee disarticulation, acrylic socket A ⊘ &

L5632 Addition to lower extremity, Symes type, PTB brim design socket A ⊘ &

L5634 Addition to lower extremity, Symes type, posterior opening (Canadian) socket A ⊘ &

L5636 Addition to lower extremity, Symes type, medial opening socket A ⊘ &

L5637 Addition to lower extremity, below knee (BK), total contact A ⊘ &

L5638 Addition to lower extremity, below knee (BK), leather socket A ⊘ &

L5639 Addition to lower extremity, below knee (BK), wood socket A ⊘ &

L5640 Addition to lower extremity, knee disarticulation, leather socket A ⊘ &

L5642 Addition to lower extremity, above knee (AK), leather socket A ⊘ &

L5643 Addition to lower extremity, hip disarticulation, flexible inner socket, external frame A ⊘ &

L5644 Addition to lower extremity, above knee (AK), wood socket A ⊘ &

L5645 Addition to lower extremity, below knee (BK), flexible inner socket, external frame A ⊘ &

L5646 Addition to lower extremity, below knee (BK), air, fluid, gel or equal, cushion socket A ⊘ &

L5647 Addition to lower extremity, below knee (BK), suction socket A ⊘ &

L5648 Addition to lower extremity, above knee (AK), air, fluid, gel or equal, cushion socket A ⊘ &

L5649 Addition to lower extremity, ischial containment/narrow M-L socket A ⊘ &

L5650 Additions to lower extremity, total contact, above knee (AK) or knee disarticulation socket A ⊘ &

L5651 Addition to lower extremity, above knee (AK), flexible inner socket, external frame A ⊘ &

L5652 Addition to lower extremity, suction suspension, above knee (AK) or knee disarticulation socket A ⊘ &

L5653 Addition to lower extremity, knee disarticulation, expandable wall socket A ⊘ &

Additions: Socket Insert and Suspension

L5654 Addition to lower extremity, socket insert, Symes, (Kemblo, Pelite, Aliplast, Plastazote or equal) A ⊘ &

L5655 Addition to lower extremity, socket insert, below knee (BK) (Kemblo, Pelite, Aliplast, Plastazote or equal) A ⊘ &

L5656 Addition to lower extremity, socket insert, knee disarticulation (Kemblo, Pelite, Aliplast, Plastazote or equal) A ⊘ &

L5658 Addition to lower extremity, socket insert, above knee (AK) (Kemblo, Pelite, Aliplast, Plastazote or equal) A ⊘ &

L5661 Addition to lower extremity, socket insert, multidurometer Symes A ⊘ &

L5665 Addition to lower extremity, socket insert, multidurometer, below knee (BK) A ⊘ &

L5666 Addition to lower extremity, below knee (BK), cuff suspension A ⊘ &

L5668 Addition to lower extremity, below knee (BK), molded distal cushion A ⊘ &

L5670 Addition to lower extremity, below knee (BK), molded supracondylar suspension (PTS or similar) A ⊘ &

As the suspension sleeve is donned, air is driven out through a valve

The valve is closed upon donning and a suction fit is formed around the residual limb

Residual limb

Sealing membrane

Sleeve

Open valve

Closed valve

L5671 Addition to lower extremity, below knee (BK)/above knee (AK) suspension locking mechanism (shuttle, lanyard, or equal), excludes socket insert A ⊘ &

L5672 Addition to lower extremity, below knee (BK), removable medial brim suspension A ⊘ &

L5673 Addition to lower extremity, below knee (BK)/above knee (AK), custom fabricated from existing mold or prefabricated, socket insert, silicone gel, elastomeric or equal, for use with locking mechanism A ⊘ &

L5676 Additions to lower extremity, below knee (BK), knee joints, single axis, pair A ☑ ⊘ &

Special Coverage Instructions   Noncovered by Medicare   Carrier Discretion   ☑ Quantity Alert ● New Code   ◯ Recycled/Reinstated   ▲ Revised Code

© 2023 Optum360, LLC   A2-A3 ASC Pmt   CMS: IOM   AHA: Coding Clinic   & DMEPOS Paid   ⊘ SNF Excluded   L Codes — 141

Prosthetic Devices and Procedures

L5677 — L5824

L5677 Additions to lower extremity, below knee (BK), knee joints, polycentric, pair ☒ ☑ ⊘ ♿

L5678 Additions to lower extremity, below knee (BK), joint covers, pair ☒ ☑ ⊘ ♿

L5679 Addition to lower extremity, below knee (BK)/above knee (AK), custom fabricated from existing mold or prefabricated, socket insert, silicone gel, elastomeric or equal, not for use with locking mechanism ☒ ⊘ ♿

L5680 Addition to lower extremity, below knee (BK), thigh lacer, nonmolded ☒ ⊘ ♿

L5681 Addition to lower extremity, below knee (BK)/above knee (AK), custom fabricated socket insert for congenital or atypical traumatic amputee, silicone gel, elastomeric or equal, for use with or without locking mechanism, initial only (for other than initial, use code L5673 or L5679) ☒ ⊘ ♿

L5682 Addition to lower extremity, below knee (BK), thigh lacer, gluteal/ischial, molded ☒ ⊘ ♿

L5683 Addition to lower extremity, below knee (BK)/above knee (AK), custom fabricated socket insert for other than congenital or atypical traumatic amputee, silicone gel, elastomeric or equal, for use with or without locking mechanism, initial only (for other than initial, use code L5673 or L5679) ☒ ⊘ ♿

L5684 Addition to lower extremity, below knee, fork strap ☒ ⊘ ♿

L5685 Addition to lower extremity prosthesis, below knee, suspension/sealing sleeve, with or without valve, any material, each ☒ ⊘ ♿

L5686 Addition to lower extremity, below knee (BK), back check (extension control) ☒ ⊘ ♿

L5688 Addition to lower extremity, below knee (BK), waist belt, webbing ☒ ⊘ ♿

L5690 Addition to lower extremity, below knee (BK), waist belt, padded and lined ☒ ⊘ ♿

L5692 Addition to lower extremity, above knee (AK), pelvic control belt, light ☒ ⊘ ♿

L5694 Addition to lower extremity, above knee (AK), pelvic control belt, padded and lined ☒ ⊘ ♿

L5695 Addition to lower extremity, above knee (AK), pelvic control, sleeve suspension, neoprene or equal, each ☒ ☑ ⊘ ♿

L5696 Addition to lower extremity, above knee (AK) or knee disarticulation, pelvic joint ☒ ⊘ ♿

L5697 Addition to lower extremity, above knee (AK) or knee disarticulation, pelvic band ☒ ⊘ ♿

L5698 Addition to lower extremity, above knee (AK) or knee disarticulation, Silesian bandage ☒ ⊘ ♿

L5699 All lower extremity prostheses, shoulder harness ☒ ⊘ ♿

Replacements

L5700 Replacement, socket, below knee (BK), molded to patient model ☒ ⊘ ♿

L5701 Replacement, socket, above knee (AK)/knee disarticulation, including attachment plate, molded to patient model ☒ ⊘ ♿

L5702 Replacement, socket, hip disarticulation, including hip joint, molded to patient model ☒ ⊘ ♿

L5703 Ankle, Symes, molded to patient model, socket without solid ankle cushion heel (SACH) foot, replacement only ☒ ⊘ ♿

L5704 Custom shaped protective cover, below knee (BK) ☒ ⊘ ♿

L5705 Custom shaped protective cover, above knee (AK) ☒ ⊘ ♿

L5706 Custom shaped protective cover, knee disarticulation ☒ ⊘ ♿

L5707 Custom shaped protective cover, hip disarticulation ☒ ⊘ ♿

Additions: Exoskeletal Knee-Shin System

L5710 Addition, exoskeletal knee-shin system, single axis, manual lock ☒ ⊘ ♿

L5711 Additions exoskeletal knee-shin system, single axis, manual lock, ultra-light material ☒ ⊘ ♿

L5712 Addition, exoskeletal knee-shin system, single axis, friction swing and stance phase control (safety knee) ☒ ⊘ ♿

L5714 Addition, exoskeletal knee-shin system, single axis, variable friction swing phase control ☒ ⊘ ♿

L5716 Addition, exoskeletal knee-shin system, polycentric, mechanical stance phase lock ☒ ⊘ ♿

L5718 Addition, exoskeletal knee-shin system, polycentric, friction swing and stance phase control ☒ ⊘ ♿

L5722 Addition, exoskeletal knee-shin system, single axis, pneumatic swing, friction stance phase control ☒ ⊘ ♿

L5724 Addition, exoskeletal knee-shin system, single axis, fluid swing phase control ☒ ⊘ ♿

L5726 Addition, exoskeletal knee-shin system, single axis, external joints, fluid swing phase control ☒ ⊘ ♿

L5728 Addition, exoskeletal knee-shin system, single axis, fluid swing and stance phase control ☒ ⊘ ♿

L5780 Addition, exoskeletal knee-shin system, single axis, pneumatic/hydra pneumatic swing phase control ☒ ⊘ ♿

L5781 Addition to lower limb prosthesis, vacuum pump, residual limb volume management and moisture evacuation system ☒ ⊘ ♿

L5782 Addition to lower limb prosthesis, vacuum pump, residual limb volume management and moisture evacuation system, heavy-duty ☒ ⊘ ♿

Component Modification

L5785 Addition, exoskeletal system, below knee (BK), ultra-light material (titanium, carbon fiber or equal) ☒ ⊘ ♿

L5790 Addition, exoskeletal system, above knee (AK), ultra-light material (titanium, carbon fiber or equal) ☒ ⊘ ♿

L5795 Addition, exoskeletal system, hip disarticulation, ultra-light material (titanium, carbon fiber or equal) ☒ ⊘ ♿

Additions: Endoskeletal Knee-Shin System

L5810 Addition, endoskeletal knee-shin system, single axis, manual lock ☒ ⊘ ♿

L5811 Addition, endoskeletal knee-shin system, single axis, manual lock, ultra-light material ☒ ⊘ ♿

L5812 Addition, endoskeletal knee-shin system, single axis, friction swing and stance phase control (safety knee) ☒ ⊘ ♿

L5814 Addition, endoskeletal knee-shin system, polycentric, hydraulic swing phase control, mechanical stance phase lock ☒ ⊘ ♿

L5816 Addition, endoskeletal knee-shin system, polycentric, mechanical stance phase lock ☒ ⊘ ♿

L5818 Addition, endoskeletal knee-shin system, polycentric, friction swing and stance phase control ☒ ⊘ ♿

L5822 Addition, endoskeletal knee-shin system, single axis, pneumatic swing, friction stance phase control ☒ ⊘ ♿

L5824 Addition, endoskeletal knee-shin system, single axis, fluid swing phase control ☒ ⊘ ♿

Special Coverage Instructions   Noncovered by Medicare   Carrier Discretion   ☑ Quantity Alert ● New Code   ○ Recycled/Reinstated ▲ Revised Code

L5826 Addition, endoskeletal knee-shin system, single axis, hydraulic swing phase control, with miniature high activity frame Ⓐ Ⓝ ♿

L5828 Addition, endoskeletal knee-shin system, single axis, fluid swing and stance phase control Ⓐ ♿

L5830 Addition, endoskeletal knee-shin system, single axis, pneumatic/swing phase control Ⓐ Ⓝ ♿

L5840 Addition, endoskeletal knee-shin system, four-bar linkage or multiaxial, pneumatic swing phase control Ⓐ Ⓝ ♿

L5845 Addition, endoskeletal knee-shin system, stance flexion feature, adjustable Ⓐ Ⓝ ♿

L5848 Addition to endoskeletal knee-shin system, fluid stance extension, dampening feature, with or without adjustability Ⓐ Ⓝ ♿

L5850 Addition, endoskeletal system, above knee (AK) or hip disarticulation, knee extension assist Ⓐ Ⓝ ♿

L5855 Addition, endoskeletal system, hip disarticulation, mechanical hip extension assist Ⓐ Ⓝ ♿

L5856 Addition to lower extremity prosthesis, endoskeletal knee-shin system, microprocessor control feature, swing and stance phase, includes electronic sensor(s), any type Ⓐ Ⓝ ♿

L5857 Addition to lower extremity prosthesis, endoskeletal knee-shin system, microprocessor control feature, swing phase only, includes electronic sensor(s), any type Ⓐ Ⓝ ♿

L5858 Addition to lower extremity prosthesis, endoskeletal knee-shin system, microprocessor control feature, stance phase only, includes electronic sensor(s), any type Ⓐ Ⓝ ♿

L5859 Addition to lower extremity prosthesis, endoskeletal knee-shin system, powered and programmable flexion/extension assist control, includes any type motor(s) Ⓐ ♿

L5910 Addition, endoskeletal system, below knee (BK), alignable system Ⓐ Ⓝ ♿

L5920 Addition, endoskeletal system, above knee (AK) or hip disarticulation, alignable system Ⓐ Ⓝ ♿

L5925 Addition, endoskeletal system, above knee (AK), knee disarticulation or hip disarticulation, manual lock Ⓐ Ⓝ ♿

● **L5926** Addition to lower extremity prosthesis, endoskeletal, knee disarticulation, above knee, hip disarticulation, positional rotation unit, any type

L5930 Addition, endoskeletal system, high activity knee control frame Ⓐ Ⓝ ♿

L5940 Addition, endoskeletal system, below knee (BK), ultra-light material (titanium, carbon fiber or equal) Ⓐ Ⓝ ♿

L5950 Addition, endoskeletal system, above knee (AK), ultra-light material (titanium, carbon fiber or equal) Ⓐ Ⓝ ♿

L5960 Addition, endoskeletal system, hip disarticulation, ultra-light material (titanium, carbon fiber or equal) Ⓐ Ⓝ ♿

L5961 Addition, endoskeletal system, polycentric hip joint, pneumatic or hydraulic control, rotation control, with or without flexion and/or extension control Ⓐ ♿

L5962 Addition, endoskeletal system, below knee (BK), flexible protective outer surface covering system Ⓐ Ⓝ ♿

L5964 Addition, endoskeletal system, above knee (AK), flexible protective outer surface covering system Ⓐ Ⓝ ♿

L5966 Addition, endoskeletal system, hip disarticulation, flexible protective outer surface covering system Ⓐ Ⓝ ♿

L5968 Addition to lower limb prosthesis, multiaxial ankle with swing phase active dorsiflexion feature Ⓐ Ⓝ ♿

L5969 Addition, endoskeletal ankle-foot or ankle system, power assist, includes any type motor(s) Ⓐ

L5970 All lower extremity prostheses, foot, external keel, SACH foot Ⓐ Ⓝ ♿

L5971 All lower extremity prostheses, solid ankle cushion heel (SACH) foot, replacement only Ⓐ Ⓝ ♿

L5972 All lower extremity prostheses, foot, flexible keel Ⓐ Ⓝ ♿

L5973 Endoskeletal ankle foot system, microprocessor controlled feature, dorsiflexion and/or plantar flexion control, includes power source Ⓐ Ⓝ ♿

L5974 All lower extremity prostheses, foot, single axis ankle/foot Ⓐ Ⓝ ♿

Foot prosthesis (L5974)

Energy storing foot (L5976)

Carbon

L5975 All lower extremity prostheses, combination single axis ankle and flexible keel foot Ⓐ Ⓝ ♿

L5976 All lower extremity prostheses, energy storing foot (Seattle Carbon Copy II or equal) Ⓐ Ⓝ ♿

L5978 All lower extremity prostheses, foot, multiaxial ankle/foot Ⓐ Ⓝ ♿

Foot prosthesis, multi-axial ankle (L5978)

L5979 All lower extremity prostheses, multiaxial ankle, dynamic response foot, one-piece system Ⓐ Ⓝ ♿

L5980 All lower extremity prostheses, flex-foot system Ⓐ Ⓝ ♿

L5981 All lower extremity prostheses, flex-walk system or equal Ⓐ Ⓝ ♿

L5982 All exoskeletal lower extremity prostheses, axial rotation unit Ⓐ Ⓝ ♿

L5826 — L5982

Special Coverage Instructions   Noncovered by Medicare   Carrier Discretion   ☑ Quantity Alert   ● New Code   ○ Recycled/Reinstated   ▲ Revised Code

© 2023 Optum360, LLC   Ⓐ²–Ⓩ³ ASC Pmt   **CMS:** IOM   **AHA:** Coding Clinic   ♿ DMEPOS Paid   Ⓝ SNF Excluded   **L Codes — 143**

Prosthetic Devices and Procedures

L5984 — L6588

Code	Description	
L5984	All endoskeletal lower extremity prostheses, axial rotation unit, with or without adjustability	Ⓐ ⊘ ♿
L5985	All endoskeletal lower extremity prostheses, dynamic prosthetic pylon	Ⓐ ⊘ ♿
L5986	All lower extremity prostheses, multiaxial rotation unit (MCP or equal)	Ⓐ ♿
L5987	All lower extremity prostheses, shank foot system with vertical loading pylon	Ⓐ ♿
L5988	Addition to lower limb prosthesis, vertical shock reducing pylon feature	Ⓐ ⊘ ♿
L5990	Addition to lower extremity prosthesis, user adjustable heel height	Ⓐ ⊘ ♿
● L5991	Addition to lower extremity prostheses, osseointegrated external prosthetic connector	
L5999	Lower extremity prosthesis, not otherwise specified	Ⓐ
	Determine if an alternative HCPCS Level II or a CPT code better describes the service being reported. This code should be used only if a more specific code is unavailable.	

Partial Hand

Code	Description	
L6000	Partial hand, thumb remaining	Ⓐ ♿
L6010	Partial hand, little and/or ring finger remaining	Ⓐ ♿
L6020	Partial hand, no finger remaining	Ⓐ ♿
L6026	Transcarpal/metacarpal or partial hand disarticulation prosthesis, external power, self-suspended, inner socket with removable forearm section, electrodes and cables, two batteries, charger, myoelectric control of terminal device, excludes terminal device(s)	Ⓐ ♿

Wrist Disarticulation

Code	Description	
L6050	Wrist disarticulation, molded socket, flexible elbow hinges, triceps pad	Ⓐ ⊘ ♿
L6055	Wrist disarticulation, molded socket with expandable interface, flexible elbow hinges, triceps pad	Ⓐ ⊘ ♿

Below Elbow

Code	Description	
L6100	Below elbow, molded socket, flexible elbow hinge, triceps pad	Ⓐ ⊘ ♿
L6110	Below elbow, molded socket (Muenster or Northwestern suspension types)	Ⓐ ⊘ ♿
L6120	Below elbow, molded double wall split socket, step-up hinges, half cuff	Ⓐ ⊘ ♿
L6130	Below elbow, molded double wall split socket, stump activated locking hinge, half cuff	Ⓐ ⊘ ♿

Elbow Disarticulation

L6200	Elbow disarticulation, molded socket, outside locking hinge, forearm	Ⓐ ⊘ ♿
L6205	Elbow disarticulation, molded socket with expandable interface, outside locking hinges, forearm	Ⓐ ⊘ ♿

Above Elbow

Code	Description	
L6250	Above elbow, molded double wall socket, internal locking elbow, forearm	Ⓐ ⊘ ♿

Shoulder Disarticulation

Code	Description	
L6300	Shoulder disarticulation, molded socket, shoulder bulkhead, humeral section, internal locking elbow, forearm	Ⓐ ♿
L6310	Shoulder disarticulation, passive restoration (complete prosthesis)	Ⓐ ⊘ ♿
L6320	Shoulder disarticulation, passive restoration (shoulder cap only)	Ⓐ ⊘ ♿

Interscapular Thoracic

Code	Description	
L6350	Interscapular thoracic, molded socket, shoulder bulkhead, humeral section, internal locking elbow, forearm	Ⓐ ♿
L6360	Interscapular thoracic, passive restoration (complete prosthesis)	Ⓐ ⊘ ♿
L6370	Interscapular thoracic, passive restoration (shoulder cap only)	Ⓐ ⊘ ♿

Immediate and Early Postsurgical Procedures

Code	Description	
L6380	Immediate postsurgical or early fitting, application of initial rigid dressing, including fitting alignment and suspension of components, and one cast change, wrist disarticulation or below elbow	Ⓐ ♿
L6382	Immediate postsurgical or early fitting, application of initial rigid dressing including fitting alignment and suspension of components, and one cast change, elbow disarticulation or above elbow	Ⓐ ☑ ♿
L6384	Immediate postsurgical or early fitting, application of initial rigid dressing including fitting alignment and suspension of components, and one cast change, shoulder disarticulation or interscapular thoracic	Ⓐ ☑ ♿
L6386	Immediate postsurgical or early fitting, each additional cast change and realignment	Ⓐ ☑ ♿
L6388	Immediate postsurgical or early fitting, application of rigid dressing only	Ⓐ ♿

Molded Socket

Code	Description	
L6400	Below elbow, molded socket, endoskeletal system, including soft prosthetic tissue shaping	Ⓐ ⊘ ♿
L6450	Elbow disarticulation, molded socket, endoskeletal system, including soft prosthetic tissue shaping	Ⓐ ⊘ ♿
L6500	Above elbow, molded socket, endoskeletal system, including soft prosthetic tissue shaping	Ⓐ ⊘ ♿
L6550	Shoulder disarticulation, molded socket, endoskeletal system, including soft prosthetic tissue shaping	Ⓐ ⊘ ♿
L6570	Interscapular thoracic, molded socket, endoskeletal system, including soft prosthetic tissue shaping	Ⓐ ⊘ ♿

Preparatory Socket

Code	Description	
L6580	Preparatory, wrist disarticulation or below elbow, single wall plastic socket, friction wrist, flexible elbow hinges, figure of eight harness, humeral cuff, Bowden cable control, USMC or equal pylon, no cover, molded to patient model	Ⓐ ⊘ ♿
L6582	Preparatory, wrist disarticulation or below elbow, single wall socket, friction wrist, flexible elbow hinges, figure of eight harness, humeral cuff, Bowden cable control, USMC or equal pylon, no cover, direct formed	Ⓐ ⊘ ♿
L6584	Preparatory, elbow disarticulation or above elbow, single wall plastic socket, friction wrist, locking elbow, figure of eight harness, fair lead cable control, USMC or equal pylon, no cover, molded to patient model	Ⓐ ⊘ ♿
L6586	Preparatory, elbow disarticulation or above elbow, single wall socket, friction wrist, locking elbow, figure of eight harness, fair lead cable control, USMC or equal pylon, no cover, direct formed	Ⓐ ⊘ ♿
L6588	Preparatory, shoulder disarticulation or interscapular thoracic, single wall plastic socket, shoulder joint, locking elbow, friction wrist, chest strap, fair lead cable control, USMC or equal pylon, no cover, molded to patient model	Ⓐ ⊘ ♿

Special Coverage Instructions   Noncovered by Medicare   Carrier Discretion   ☑ Quantity Alert   ● New Code   ○ Recycled/Reinstated   ▲ Revised Code

144 — L Codes   Ⓐ Age Edit   Ⓜ Maternity Edit   ♀ Female Only   ♂ Male Only   Ⓐ-Ⓨ OPPS Status Indicators   © 2023 Optum360, LLC

L6590 Preparatory, shoulder disarticulation or interscapular thoracic, single wall socket, shoulder joint, locking elbow, friction wrist, chest strap, fair lead cable control, USMC or equal pylon, no cover, direct formed A ⊘ &

Additions: Upper Limb

The following procedures/modifications/components may be added to other base procedures. The items in this section should reflect the additional complexity of each modification procedure, in addition to the base procedure, at the time of the original order.

L6600 Upper extremity additions, polycentric hinge, pair A ☑ ⊘ &

L6605 Upper extremity additions, single pivot hinge, pair A ☑ ⊘ &

L6610 Upper extremity additions, flexible metal hinge, pair A ☑ ⊘ &

L6611 Addition to upper extremity prosthesis, external powered, additional switch, any type A ⊘ &

L6615 Upper extremity addition, disconnect locking wrist unit A ⊘ &

L6616 Upper extremity addition, additional disconnect insert for locking wrist unit, each A ☑ ⊘ &

L6620 Upper extremity addition, flexion/extension wrist unit, with or without friction A ⊘ &

L6621 Upper extremity prosthesis addition, flexion/extension wrist with or without friction, for use with external powered terminal device A ⊘ &

L6623 Upper extremity addition, spring assisted rotational wrist unit with latch release A ⊘ &

L6624 Upper extremity addition, flexion/extension and rotation wrist unit A ⊘ &

L6625 Upper extremity addition, rotation wrist unit with cable lock A ⊘ &

L6628 Upper extremity addition, quick disconnect hook adapter, Otto Bock or equal A ⊘ &

L6629 Upper extremity addition, quick disconnect lamination collar with coupling piece, Otto Bock or equal A ⊘ &

L6630 Upper extremity addition, stainless steel, any wrist A ⊘ &

L6632 Upper extremity addition, latex suspension sleeve, each A ☑ ⊘ &

L6635 Upper extremity addition, lift assist for elbow A ⊘ &

L6637 Upper extremity addition, nudge control elbow lock A ⊘ &

L6638 Upper extremity addition to prosthesis, electric locking feature, only for use with manually powered elbow A ⊘ &

L6640 Upper extremity additions, shoulder abduction joint, pair A ☑ ⊘ &

L6641 Upper extremity addition, excursion amplifier, pulley type A ⊘ &

L6642 Upper extremity addition, excursion amplifier, lever type A ⊘ &

L6645 Upper extremity addition, shoulder flexion-abduction joint, each A ☑ ⊘ &

L6646 Upper extremity addition, shoulder joint, multipositional locking, flexion, adjustable abduction friction control, for use with body powered or external powered system A ⊘ &

L6647 Upper extremity addition, shoulder lock mechanism, body powered actuator A ⊘ &

L6648 Upper extremity addition, shoulder lock mechanism, external powered actuator A ⊘ &

L6650 Upper extremity addition, shoulder universal joint, each A ☑ &

L6655 Upper extremity addition, standard control cable, extra A ⊘ &

L6660 Upper extremity addition, heavy-duty control cable • A ⊘ &

L6665 Upper extremity addition, Teflon, or equal, cable lining A ⊘ &

L6670 Upper extremity addition, hook to hand, cable adapter A ⊘ &

L6672 Upper extremity addition, harness, chest or shoulder, saddle type A ⊘ &

L6675 Upper extremity addition, harness, (e.g., figure of eight type), single cable design A ⊘ &

L6676 Upper extremity addition, harness, (e.g., figure of eight type), dual cable design A ⊘ &

L6677 Upper extremity addition, harness, triple control, simultaneous operation of terminal device and elbow A ⊘ &

L6680 Upper extremity addition, test socket, wrist disarticulation or below elbow A ⊘ &

L6682 Upper extremity addition, test socket, elbow disarticulation or above elbow A ⊘ &

L6684 Upper extremity addition, test socket, shoulder disarticulation or interscapular thoracic A ⊘ &

L6686 Upper extremity addition, suction socket A ⊘ &

L6687 Upper extremity addition, frame type socket, below elbow or wrist disarticulation A ⊘ &

L6688 Upper extremity addition, frame type socket, above elbow or elbow disarticulation A ⊘ &

L6689 Upper extremity addition, frame type socket, shoulder disarticulation A ⊘ &

L6690 Upper extremity addition, frame type socket, interscapular-thoracic A ⊘ &

L6691 Upper extremity addition, removable insert, each A ☑ ⊘ &

L6692 Upper extremity addition, silicone gel insert or equal, each A ☑ ⊘ &

L6693 Upper extremity addition, locking elbow, forearm counterbalance A ⊘ &

L6694 Addition to upper extremity prosthesis, below elbow/above elbow, custom fabricated from existing mold or prefabricated, socket insert, silicone gel, elastomeric or equal, for use with locking mechanism A ⊘ &

L6695 Addition to upper extremity prosthesis, below elbow/above elbow, custom fabricated from existing mold or prefabricated, socket insert, silicone gel, elastomeric or equal, not for use with locking mechanism A ⊘ &

L6696 Addition to upper extremity prosthesis, below elbow/above elbow, custom fabricated socket insert for congenital or atypical traumatic amputee, silicone gel, elastomeric or equal, for use with or without locking mechanism, initial only (for other than initial, use code L6694 or L6695) A ⊘ &

L6697 Addition to upper extremity prosthesis, below elbow/above elbow, custom fabricated socket insert for other than congenital or atypical traumatic amputee, silicone gel, elastomeric or equal, for use with or without locking mechanism, initial only (for other than initial, use code L6694 or L6695) A ⊘ &

L6698 Addition to upper extremity prosthesis, below elbow/above elbow, lock mechanism, excludes socket insert A ⊘ &

Special Coverage Instructions Noncovered by Medicare Carrier Discretion ☑ Quantity Alert ● New Code ○ Recycled/Reinstated ▲ Revised Code

© 2023 Optum360, LLC A2-A3 ASC Pmt CMS: IOM AHA: Coding Clinic & DMEPOS Paid ⊘ SNF Excluded L Codes — 145

Prosthetic Devices and Procedures

L6703 — L6975

Terminal Device

L6703 Terminal device, passive hand/mitt, any material, any size [A]⊘&

L6704 Terminal device, sport/recreational/work attachment, any material, any size [A]⊘&

L6706 Terminal device, hook, mechanical, voluntary opening, any material, any size, lined or unlined [A]⊘&

L6707 Terminal device, hook, mechanical, voluntary closing, any material, any size, lined or unlined [A]⊘&

L6708 Terminal device, hand, mechanical, voluntary opening, any size [A]⊘&

L6709 Terminal device, hand, mechanical, voluntary closing, any size [A]⊘&

L6711 Terminal device, hook, mechanical, voluntary opening, any material, any size, lined or unlined, pediatric [A]&

L6712 Terminal device, hook, mechanical, voluntary closing, any material, any size, lined or unlined, pediatric [A]&

L6713 Terminal device, hand, mechanical, voluntary opening, any material, any size, pediatric [A]&

L6714 Terminal device, hand, mechanical, voluntary closing, any material, any size, pediatric [A]&

L6715 Terminal device, multiple articulating digit, includes motor(s), initial issue or replacement [A]&

L6721 Terminal device, hook or hand, heavy-duty, mechanical, voluntary opening, any material, any size, lined or unlined [A]&

L6722 Terminal device, hook or hand, heavy-duty, mechanical, voluntary closing, any material, any size, lined or unlined [A]&

Addition to Terminal Device

L6805 Addition to terminal device, modifier wrist unit [A]⊘&

L6810 Addition to terminal device, precision pinch device [A]⊘&

L6880 Electric hand, switch or myoelectric controlled, independently articulating digits, any grasp pattern or combination of grasp patterns, includes motor(s) [A]&

L6881 Automatic grasp feature, addition to upper limb electric prosthetic terminal device [A]⊘&

L6882 Microprocessor control feature, addition to upper limb prosthetic terminal device [A]⊘&

Replacement Socket

L6883 Replacement socket, below elbow/wrist disarticulation, molded to patient model, for use with or without external power [A]⊘&

L6884 Replacement socket, above elbow/elbow disarticulation, molded to patient model, for use with or without external power [A]⊘&

L6885 Replacement socket, shoulder disarticulation/interscapular thoracic, molded to patient model, for use with or without external power [A]⊘&

Hand Restoration

L6890 Addition to upper extremity prosthesis, glove for terminal device, any material, prefabricated, includes fitting and adjustment [A]&

L6895 Addition to upper extremity prosthesis, glove for terminal device, any material, custom fabricated [A]&

L6900 Hand restoration (casts, shading and measurements included), partial hand, with glove, thumb or one finger remaining [A]&

L6905 Hand restoration (casts, shading and measurements included), partial hand, with glove, multiple fingers remaining [A]&

L6910 Hand restoration (casts, shading and measurements included), partial hand, with glove, no fingers remaining [A]&

L6915 Hand restoration (shading and measurements included), replacement glove for above [A]&

External Power

L6920 Wrist disarticulation, external power, self-suspended inner socket, removable forearm shell, Otto Bock or equal switch, cables, two batteries and one charger, switch control of terminal device [A]⊘&

L6925 Wrist disarticulation, external power, self-suspended inner socket, removable forearm shell, Otto Bock or equal electrodes, cables, two batteries and one charger, myoelectronic control of terminal device [A]⊘&

L6930 Below elbow, external power, self-suspended inner socket, removable forearm shell, Otto Bock or equal switch, cables, two batteries and one charger, switch control of terminal device [A]⊘&

L6935 Below elbow, external power, self-suspended inner socket, removable forearm shell, Otto Bock or equal electrodes, cables, two batteries and one charger, myoelectronic control of terminal device [A]⊘&

L6940 Elbow disarticulation, external power, molded inner socket, removable humeral shell, outside locking hinges, forearm, Otto Bock or equal switch, cables, two batteries and one charger, switch control of terminal device [A]⊘&

L6945 Elbow disarticulation, external power, molded inner socket, removable humeral shell, outside locking hinges, forearm, Otto Bock or equal electrodes, cables, two batteries and one charger, myoelectronic control of terminal device [A]⊘&

L6950 Above elbow, external power, molded inner socket, removable humeral shell, internal locking elbow, forearm, Otto Bock or equal switch, cables, two batteries and one charger, switch control of terminal device [A]⊘&

L6955 Above elbow, external power, molded inner socket, removable humeral shell, internal locking elbow, forearm, Otto Bock or equal electrodes, cables, two batteries and one charger, myoelectronic control of terminal device [A]⊘&

L6960 Shoulder disarticulation, external power, molded inner socket, removable shoulder shell, shoulder bulkhead, humeral section, mechanical elbow, forearm, Otto Bock or equal switch, cables, two batteries and one charger, switch control of terminal device [A]⊘&

L6965 Shoulder disarticulation, external power, molded inner socket, removable shoulder shell, shoulder bulkhead, humeral section, mechanical elbow, forearm, Otto Bock or equal electrodes, cables, two batteries and one charger, myoelectronic control of terminal device [A]⊘&

L6970 Interscapular-thoracic, external power, molded inner socket, removable shoulder shell, shoulder bulkhead, humeral section, mechanical elbow, forearm, Otto Bock or equal switch, cables, two batteries and one charger, switch control of terminal device [A]⊘&

L6975 Interscapular-thoracic, external power, molded inner socket, removable shoulder shell, shoulder bulkhead, humeral section, mechanical elbow, forearm, Otto Bock or equal electrodes, cables, two batteries and one charger, myoelectronic control of terminal device [A]⊘&

Special Coverage Instructions | Noncovered by Medicare | Carrier Discretion | ☑ Quantity Alert ● New Code ○ Recycled/Reinstated ▲ Revised Code

[A] Age Edit [M] Maternity Edit ♀ Female Only ♂ Male Only [A]-[Y] OPPS Status Indicators © 2023 Optum360, LLC

Electric Hand and Accessories

L7007 Electric hand, switch or myoelectric controlled, adult 　　Ⓐ Ⓐ ⊘ ও

L7008 Electric hand, switch or myoelectric, controlled, pediatric 　　Ⓐ Ⓐ ⊘ ও

L7009 Electric hook, switch or myoelectric controlled, adult 　　Ⓐ Ⓐ ⊘ ও

L7040 Prehensile actuator, switch controlled 　　Ⓐ ⊘ ও

L7045 Electric hook, switch or myoelectric controlled, pediatric 　　Ⓐ ⊘ ও

Electronic Elbow and Accessories

L7170 Electronic elbow, Hosmer or equal, switch controlled 　　Ⓐ ⊘ ও

L7180 Electronic elbow, microprocessor sequential control of elbow and terminal device 　　Ⓐ ⊘ ও

L7181 Electronic elbow, microprocessor simultaneous control of elbow and terminal device 　　Ⓐ ⊘ ও

L7185 Electronic elbow, adolescent, Variety Village or equal, switch controlled 　　Ⓐ ⊘ ও

L7186 Electronic elbow, child, Variety Village or equal, switch controlled 　　Ⓐ ⊘ ও

L7190 Electronic elbow, adolescent, Variety Village or equal, myoelectronically controlled 　　Ⓐ ⊘ ও

L7191 Electronic elbow, child, Variety Village or equal, myoelectronically controlled 　　Ⓐ ⊘ ও

Electronic Wrist and Accessories

L7259 Electronic wrist rotator, any type 　　Ⓐ ও

Battery Components

L7360 Six volt battery, each 　　Ⓐ ☑ ও

L7362 Battery charger, six volt, each 　　Ⓐ ☑ ⊘ ও

L7364 Twelve volt battery, each 　　Ⓐ ☑ ⊘ ও

L7366 Battery charger, 12 volt, each 　　Ⓐ ☑ ⊘ ও

L7367 Lithium ion battery, rechargeable, replacement 　　Ⓐ ⊘ ও

L7368 Lithium ion battery charger, replacement only 　　Ⓐ ⊘ ও

Additions to Upper Extremity Prosthesis

L7400 Addition to upper extremity prosthesis, below elbow/wrist disarticulation, ultra-light material (titanium, carbon fiber or equal) 　　Ⓐ ও

L7401 Addition to upper extremity prosthesis, above elbow disarticulation, ultra-light material (titanium, carbon fiber or equal) 　　Ⓐ ⊘ ও

L7402 Addition to upper extremity prosthesis, shoulder disarticulation/interscapular thoracic, ultra-light material (titanium, carbon fiber or equal) 　　Ⓐ ⊘ ও

L7403 Addition to upper extremity prosthesis, below elbow/wrist disarticulation, acrylic material 　　Ⓐ ⊘ ও

L7404 Addition to upper extremity prosthesis, above elbow disarticulation, acrylic material 　　Ⓐ ⊘ ও

L7405 Addition to upper extremity prosthesis, shoulder disarticulation/interscapular thoracic, acrylic material 　　Ⓐ ⊘ ও

L7499 Upper extremity prosthesis, not otherwise specified 　　Ⓐ

Repairs

L7510 Repair of prosthetic device, repair or replace minor parts 　　Ⓐ
Medicare jurisdiction: local contractor if repair of implanted prosthetic device.

L7520 Repair prosthetic device, labor component, per 15 minutes 　　Ⓐ ☑
Medicare jurisdiction: local contractor if repair of implanted prosthetic device.

Prosthesis Supplies

L7600 Prosthetic donning sleeve, any material, each 　　Ⓔ ☑

L7700 Gasket or seal, for use with prosthetic socket insert, any type, each 　　Ⓐ ও

Male Prosthetic

L7900 Male vacuum erection system 　　♂ Ⓔ

L7902 Tension ring, for vacuum erection device, any type, replacement only, each 　　♂ Ⓔ

Breast Prosthesis

L8000 Breast prosthesis, mastectomy bra, without integrated breast prosthesis form, any size, any type 　　♀ Ⓐ ও

L8001 Breast prosthesis, mastectomy bra, with integrated breast prosthesis form, unilateral, any size, any type 　　♀ Ⓐ ও

L8002 Breast prosthesis, mastectomy bra, with integrated breast prosthesis form, bilateral, any size, any type 　　♀ Ⓐ ও

L8010 Breast prosthesis, mastectomy sleeve 　　♀ Ⓐ

L8015 External breast prosthesis garment, with mastectomy form, post mastectomy 　　♀ Ⓐ ও

L8020 Breast prosthesis, mastectomy form 　　♀ Ⓐ ও

L8030 Breast prosthesis, silicone or equal, without integral adhesive 　　♀ Ⓐ ও

L8031 Breast prosthesis, silicone or equal, with integral adhesive 　　Ⓐ ও

L8032 Nipple prosthesis, prefabricated, reusable, any type, each 　　Ⓐ ☑ ও

L8033 Nipple prosthesis, custom fabricated, reusable, any material, any type, each

L8035 Custom breast prosthesis, post mastectomy, molded to patient model 　　♀ Ⓐ

L8039 Breast prosthesis, not otherwise specified 　　♀ Ⓐ

Prosthetic Devices and Procedures

L8040 — L8600

Face and Ear Prosthesis

L8040   Nasal prosthesis, provided by a nonphysician   Ⓐ & (KM, KN)
CMS: 100-04,20,30.9

Nasal prosthesis (L8040)

Orbital and midfacial prosthesis (L8041–L8042)

Prosthesis ▭

Frontal bone
Nasal bone
Maxilla ■
Zygoma ▨
(L8043–L8044)

Facial prosthetics are typically custom manufactured from polymers and carefully matched to the original features. The maxilla, zygoma, frontal, and nasal bones are often involved, either singly or in combination (L8040-L8044)

L8041   Midfacial prosthesis, provided by a nonphysician   Ⓐ & (KM, KN)
CMS: 100-04,20,30.9

L8042   Orbital prosthesis, provided by a nonphysician   Ⓐ & (KM, KN)
CMS: 100-04,20,30.9

L8043   Upper facial prosthesis, provided by a nonphysician   Ⓐ & (KM, KN)
CMS: 100-04,20,30.9

L8044   Hemi-facial prosthesis, provided by a nonphysician   Ⓐ & (KM, KN)
CMS: 100-04,20,30.9

L8045   Auricular prosthesis, provided by a nonphysician   Ⓐ & (KM, KN)
CMS: 100-04,20,30.9

L8046   Partial facial prosthesis, provided by a nonphysician   Ⓐ & (KM, KN)
CMS: 100-04,20,30.9

L8047   Nasal septal prosthesis, provided by a nonphysician   Ⓐ & (KM, KN)
CMS: 100-04,20,30.9

L8048   Unspecified maxillofacial prosthesis, by report, provided by a nonphysician   Ⓐ

L8049   Repair or modification of maxillofacial prosthesis, labor component, 15 minute increments, provided by a nonphysician   Ⓐ

Trusses

L8300   Truss, single with standard pad   Ⓐ &

L8310   Truss, double with standard pads   Ⓐ &

L8320   Truss, addition to standard pad, water pad   Ⓐ &

L8330   Truss, addition to standard pad, scrotal pad   ♂ Ⓐ &

Prosthetic Socks

L8400   Prosthetic sheath, below knee, each   Ⓐ ☑ &

L8410   Prosthetic sheath, above knee, each   Ⓐ ☑ &

L8415   Prosthetic sheath, upper limb, each   Ⓐ ☑ &

L8417   Prosthetic sheath/sock, including a gel cushion layer, below knee (BK) or above knee (AK), each   Ⓐ ☑ &

L8420   Prosthetic sock, multiple ply, below knee (BK), each   Ⓐ ☑ &

L8430   Prosthetic sock, multiple ply, above knee (AK), each   Ⓐ ☑ &

L8435   Prosthetic sock, multiple ply, upper limb, each   Ⓐ ☑ &

L8440   Prosthetic shrinker, below knee (BK), each   Ⓐ ☑ &

L8460   Prosthetic shrinker, above knee (AK), each   Ⓐ ☑ &

L8465   Prosthetic shrinker, upper limb, each   Ⓐ ☑ &

L8470   Prosthetic sock, single ply, fitting, below knee (BK), each   Ⓐ ☑ &

L8480   Prosthetic sock, single ply, fitting, above knee (AK), each   Ⓐ ☑ &

L8485   Prosthetic sock, single ply, fitting, upper limb, each   Ⓐ ☑ &

L8499   Unlisted procedure for miscellaneous prosthetic services   Ⓐ
Determine if an alternative HCPCS Level II or a CPT code better describes the service being reported. This code should be used only if a more specific code is unavailable.

Larynx and Trachea Prothetics and Accessories

L8500   Artificial larynx, any type   Ⓐ &

L8501   Tracheostomy speaking valve   Ⓐ &

L8505   Artificial larynx replacement battery/accessory, any type   Ⓐ

L8507   Tracheo-esophageal voice prosthesis, patient inserted, any type, each   Ⓐ ☑ &

L8509   Tracheo-esophageal voice prosthesis, inserted by a licensed health care provider, any type   Ⓐ &

L8510   Voice amplifier   Ⓐ &

L8511   Insert for indwelling tracheo-esophageal prosthesis, with or without valve, replacement only, each   Ⓐ ☑ &

L8512   Gelatin capsules or equivalent, for use with tracheo-esophageal voice prosthesis, replacement only, per 10   Ⓐ ☑ &

L8513   Cleaning device used with tracheoesophageal voice prosthesis, pipet, brush, or equal, replacement only, each   Ⓐ ☑ &

L8514   Tracheo-esophageal puncture dilator, replacement only, each   Ⓐ ☑ &

L8515   Gelatin capsule, application device for use with tracheo-esophageal voice prosthesis, each   Ⓐ ☑ &

Breast Implant

L8600   Implantable breast prosthesis, silicone or equal   ♀ Ⓜ Ⓝ &
Medicare covers implants inserted in post-mastectomy reconstruction in a breast cancer patient. Always report concurrent to the implant procedure.
CMS: 100-04,4,190

Pectoralis muscle
Rib bones
Prosthesis
Gel-type prosthesis

Special Coverage Instructions   Noncovered by Medicare   Carrier Discretion   ☑ Quantity Alert   ● New Code   ○ Recycled/Reinstated   ▲ Revised Code

Ⓐ Age Edit   Ⓜ Maternity Edit   ♀ Female Only   ♂ Male Only   Ⓐ-Ⓨ OPPS Status Indicators   © 2023 Optum360, LLC

Bulking Agents

L8603 Injectable bulking agent, collagen implant, urinary tract, 2.5 ml syringe, includes shipping and necessary supplies [N] [N1] [☑] [&]
CMS: 100-04,4,190

L8604 Injectable bulking agent, dextranomer/hyaluronic acid copolymer implant, urinary tract, 1 ml, includes shipping and necessary supplies [N] [N1] [☑]

L8605 Injectable bulking agent, dextranomer/hyaluronic acid copolymer implant, anal canal, 1 ml, includes shipping and necessary supplies [N] [N1] [&]

L8606 Injectable bulking agent, synthetic implant, urinary tract, 1 ml syringe, includes shipping and necessary supplies [N] [N1] [☑] [&]

L8607 Injectable bulking agent for vocal cord medialization, 0.1 ml, includes shipping and necessary supplies [N] [N1] [&]

Eye and Ear Implants and Accessories

L8608 Miscellaneous external component, supply or accessory for use with the Argus II Retinal Prosthesis System

L8609 Artificial cornea [N] [N1] [&]

L8610 Ocular implant [N] [N1] [&]
CMS: 100-04,4,190

L8612 Aqueous shunt [N] [N1] [&]
CMS: 100-04,4,190

L8613 Ossicula implant [N] [N1] [&]
CMS: 100-04,4,190

L8614 Cochlear device, includes all internal and external components [N] [N1] [&]
A cochlear implant is covered by Medicare when the patient has bilateral sensorineural deafness.
CMS: 100-04,11,40.8; 100-04,4,100; 100-04,4,60.4.3

L8615 Headset/headpiece for use with cochlear implant device, replacement [A] [&]

L8616 Microphone for use with cochlear implant device, replacement [A] [&]

L8617 Transmitting coil for use with cochlear implant device, replacement [A] [&]

L8618 Transmitter cable for use with cochlear implant device or auditory osseointegrated device, replacement [A] [&]

L8619 Cochlear implant, external speech processor and controller, integrated system, replacement [A] [&]
Medicare jurisdiction: local contractor.

L8621 Zinc air battery for use with cochlear implant device and auditory osseointegrated sound processors, replacement, each [A] [☑] [&]

L8622 Alkaline battery for use with cochlear implant device, any size, replacement, each [A] [☑] [&]

L8623 Lithium ion battery for use with cochlear implant device speech processor, other than ear level, replacement, each [A] [☑] [&]

L8624 Lithium ion battery for use with cochlear implant or auditory osseointegrated device speech processor, ear level, replacement, each [A] [☑] [&]

L8625 External recharging system for battery for use with cochlear implant or auditory osseointegrated device, replacement only, each [A] [&]

L8627 Cochlear implant, external speech processor, component, replacement [A] [&]

L8628 Cochlear implant, external controller component, replacement [A] [&]

L8629 Transmitting coil and cable, integrated, for use with cochlear implant device, replacement [A] [&]

Upper Extremity Implants

L8630 Metacarpophalangeal joint implant [N] [N1] [&]
CMS: 100-04,4,190

Bone is cut at the MP joint (arthroplasty)

Bone may be hollowed out in both metacarpal and phalangeal sides in preparation for a prosthesis

Prosthetic joint implant

Prosthesis in place

Metacarpophalangeal prosthetic implant

L8631 Metacarpal phalangeal joint replacement, two or more pieces, metal (e.g., stainless steel or cobalt chrome), ceramic-like material (e.g., pyrocarbon), for surgical implantation (all sizes, includes entire system) [N] [N1] [&]

Lower Extremity Implants

L8641 Metatarsal joint implant [N] [N1] [&]
CMS: 100-04,4,190

L8642 Hallux implant [N] [N1] [&]
CMS: 100-04,4,190

Interphalangeal Implants

L8658 Interphalangeal joint spacer, silicone or equal, each [N] [N1] [☑] [&]
CMS: 100-04,4,190

L8659 Interphalangeal finger joint replacement, two or more pieces, metal (e.g., stainless steel or cobalt chrome), ceramic-like material (e.g., pyrocarbon) for surgical implantation, any size [N] [N1] [&]

Cardiovascular Implant

L8670 Vascular graft material, synthetic, implant [N] [N1] [&]
CMS: 100-04,4,190

Neurostimulator and Accessories

● **L8678** Electrical stimulator supplies (external) for use with implantable neurostimulator, per month [N1]
AHA: 2Q,23

L8679 Implantable neurostimulator, pulse generator, any type [N] [N1] [&]

L8603 — L8679

Special Coverage Instructions | Noncovered by Medicare | Carrier Discretion | ☑ Quantity Alert | ● New Code | ◯ Recycled/Reinstated | ▲ Revised Code

© 2023 Optum360, LLC | [A2]-[Z3] ASC Pmt | CMS: IOM | AHA: Coding Clinic | & DMEPOS Paid | ◯ SNF Excluded | L Codes — 149

L8680 Implantable neurostimulator electrode, each   EI ☑

L8681 Patient programmer (external) for use with implantable programmable neurostimulator pulse generator, replacement only   A &

L8682 Implantable neurostimulator radiofrequency receiver   N M &

L8683 Radiofrequency transmitter (external) for use with implantable neurostimulator radiofrequency receiver   A &

L8684 Radiofrequency transmitter (external) for use with implantable sacral root neurostimulator receiver for bowel and bladder management, replacement   A &

L8685 Implantable neurostimulator pulse generator, single array, rechargeable, includes extension   EI

L8686 Implantable neurostimulator pulse generator, single array, nonrechargeable, includes extension   EI

L8687 Implantable neurostimulator pulse generator, dual array, rechargeable, includes extension   EI

L8688 Implantable neurostimulator pulse generator, dual array, nonrechargeable, includes extension   EI

L8689 External recharging system for battery (internal) for use with implantable neurostimulator, replacement only   A &

Miscellaneous Prosthetics and Accessories

L8690 Auditory osseointegrated device, includes all internal and external components   N M &
CMS: 100-04,14,40.8; 100-04,4,60.4.2

L8691 Auditory osseointegrated device, external sound processor, excludes transducer/actuator, replacement only, each   A &

L8692 Auditory osseointegrated device, external sound processor, used without osseointegration, body worn, includes headband or other means of external attachment   EI

L8693 Auditory osseointegrated device abutment, any length, replacement only   A &

L8694 Auditory osseointegrated device, transducer/actuator, replacement only, each   A &

L8695 External recharging system for battery (external) for use with implantable neurostimulator, replacement only   A &

L8696 Antenna (external) for use with implantable diaphragmatic/phrenic nerve stimulation device, replacement, each   A &

L8698 Miscellaneous component, supply or accessory for use with total artificial heart system

L8699 Prosthetic implant, not otherwise specified   N M
Determine if an alternative HCPCS Level II or a CPT code better describes the service being reported. This code should be used only if a more specific code is unavailable.
CMS: 100-04,4,190

L8701 Powered upper extremity range of motion assist device, elbow, wrist, hand with single or double upright(s), includes microprocessor, sensors, all components and accessories, custom fabricated

L8702 Powered upper extremity range of motion assist device, elbow, wrist, hand, finger, single or double upright(s), includes microprocessor, sensors, all components and accessories, custom fabricated

L9900 Orthotic and prosthetic supply, accessory, and/or service component of another HCPCS L code   N M

Special Coverage Instructions   Noncovered by Medicare   Carrier Discretion   ☑ Quantity Alert ● New Code ○ Recycled/Reinstated ▲ Revised Code

150 — L Codes   A Age Edit   M Maternity Edit   ♀ Female Only   ♂ Male Only   A-Y OPPS Status Indicators   © 2023 Optum360, LLC

MIPS Value Pathways M0001-M0010

M0001 Advancing Cancer Care MIPS Value Pathways

M0002 Optimal Care for Kidney Health MIPS Value Pathways

M0003 Optimal Care for Patients with Episodic Neurological Conditions MIPS Value Pathways

M0004 Supportive Care for Neurodegenerative Conditions MIPS Value Pathways

▲ **M0005** Value in primary care MIPS value pathway

● **M0010** Enhancing oncology model (EOM) monthly enhanced oncology services (MEOS) payment for EOM enhanced services
AHA: 2Q,23

Medical Services M0075-M0301

Other Medical Services

M codes include office services, cellular therapy, prolotherapy, intragastric hypothermia, IV chelation therapy, and fabric wrapping of an abdominal aneurysm.

M0075 Cellular therapy [EI]
The therapeutic efficacy of injecting foreign proteins has not been established.

M0076 Prolotherapy [EI]
The therapeutic efficacy of prolotherapy and joint sclerotherapy has not been established.

M0100 Intragastric hypothermia using gastric freezing [EI]
Code with caution: This procedure is considered obsolete.

▲ **M0201** Administration of pneumococcal, influenza, hepatitis B, and/or COVID-19 vaccine inside a patient's home; reported only once per individual home per date of service when such vaccine administration(s) are performed at the patient's home
AHA: 3Q,21

M0220 Injection, tixagevimab and cilgavimab, for the pre-exposure prophylaxis only, for certain adults and pediatric individuals (12 years of age and older weighing at least 40kg) with no known SARS-CoV-2 exposure, who either have moderate to severely compromised immune systems or for whom vaccination with any available COVID-19 vaccine is not recommended due to a history of severe adverse reaction to a COVID-19 vaccine(s) and/or COVID-19 vaccine component(s), includes injection and post administration monitoring
AHA: 2Q,22

M0221 Injection, tixagevimab and cilgavimab, for the pre-exposure prophylaxis only, for certain adults and pediatric individuals (12 years of age and older weighing at least 40kg) with no known SARS-CoV-2 exposure, who either have moderate to severely compromised immune systems or for whom vaccination with any available COVID-19 vaccine is not recommended due to a history of severe adverse reaction to a COVID-19 vaccine(s) and/or COVID-19 vaccine component(s), includes injection and post administration monitoring in the home or residence; this includes a beneficiary's home that has been made provider-based to the hospital during the COVID-19 public health emergency
AHA: 2Q,22

M0222 Intravenous injection, bebtelovimab, includes injection and post administration monitoring
AHA: 2Q,22

M0223 Intravenous injection, bebtelovimab, includes injection and post administration monitoring in the home or residence; this includes a beneficiary's home that has been made provider-based to the hospital during the COVID-19 public health emergency
AHA: 2Q,22

M0240 Intravenous infusion or subcutaneous injection, casirivimab and imdevimab, includes infusion or injection and post administration monitoring, subsequent repeat doses
Use this code for casirivimab and imdevimab 600 mg administered as post exposure prophylaxis. Report also Q0240 for drug.
AHA: 4Q,21; 3Q,21

M0241 Intravenous infusion or subcutaneous injection, casirivimab and imdevimab, includes infusion or injection, and post administration monitoring in the home or residence. This includes a beneficiary's home that has been made provider-based to the hospital during the covid-19 public health emergency, subsequent repeat doses
Use this code for casirivimab and imdevimab 600 mg administered as post exposure prophylaxis. Report also Q0240 for drug.
AHA: 4Q,21; 3Q,21

M0243 Intravenous infusion or subcutaneous injection, casirivimab and imdevimab, includes infusion or injection, and post administration monitoring
Use this code for administration of Casirivimab and Imdevimab (REGN-COV2), Regeneron. Report also Q0243 for drug.
AHA: 2Q,22; 1Q,21; 4Q,20

M0244 Intravenous infusion or subcutaneous injection, casirivimab and imdevimab, includes infusion or injection and post administration monitoring in the home or residence; this includes a beneficiary's home that has been made provider-based to the hospital during the COVID-19 public health emergency
Use this code for administration of casirivimab and imdevimab in the home setting. Report also Q0243 for drug.
AHA: 3Q,21

M0245 Intravenous infusion, bamlanivimab and etesevimab, includes infusion and post administration monitoring
Use this code for administration of bamlanivimab (LY-CoV555) and etesevimab (LY-CoV016). Report also Q0245 for drug.
AHA: 1Q,21

M0246 Intravenous infusion, bamlanivimab and etesevimab, includes infusion and post administration monitoring in the home or residence; this includes a beneficiary's home that has been made provider-based to the hospital during the COVID-19 public health emergency
Use this code for administration of bamlanivimab and etesevimab in the home setting. Report also Q0245 for drug.
AHA: 3Q,21

M0247 Intravenous infusion, sotrovimab, includes infusion and post administration monitoring
AHA: 3Q,21

M0248 Intravenous infusion, sotrovimab, includes infusion and post administration monitoring in the home or residence; this includes a beneficiary's home that has been made provider-based to the hospital during the COVID-19 public health emergency
AHA: 3Q,21

M0249 Intravenous infusion, tocilizumab, for hospitalized adults and pediatric patients (2 years of age and older) with COVID-19 who are receiving systemic corticosteroids and require supplemental oxygen, non-invasive or invasive mechanical ventilation, or extracorporeal membrane oxygenation (ECMO) only, includes infusion and post administration monitoring, first dose
AHA: 4Q,21

M0250 Intravenous infusion, tocilizumab, for hospitalized adults and pediatric patients (2 years of age and older) with COVID-19 who are receiving systemic corticosteroids and require supplemental oxygen, non-invasive or invasive mechanical ventilation, or extracorporeal membrane oxygenation (ECMO) only, includes infusion and post administration monitoring, second dose
AHA: 4Q,21

Special Coverage Instructions   Noncovered by Medicare   Carrier Discretion   ☑ Quantity Alert ● New Code   ○ Recycled/Reinstated   ▲ Revised Code

© 2023 Optum360, LLC   A2-Z3 ASC Pmt   **CMS:** IOM   **AHA:** Coding Clinic   ⚒ DMEPOS Paid   ⊘ SNF Excluded   **M Codes — 151**

Cardiovascular Services

M0300 IV chelation therapy (chemical endarterectomy)   [E]
Chelation therapy is considered experimental in the United States.
CMS: 100-03*; 100-03,20.22

M0301 Fabric wrapping of abdominal aneurysm   [E]
Code with caution: This procedure has largely been replaced with more effective treatment modalities. Submit documentation.

Quality Measures M1003-M1370

Quality Measures

M1003 TB screening performed and results interpreted within 12 months prior to initiation of first-time biologic and/or immune response modifier therapy

M1004 Documentation of medical reason for not screening for TB or interpreting results (i.e., patient positive for TB and documentation of past treatment; patient who has recently completed a course of anti-TB therapy)

M1005 TB screening not performed or results not interpreted, reason not given

M1006 Disease activity not assessed, reason not given

M1007 >=50% of total number of a patient's outpatient RA encounters assessed

M1008 <50% of total number of a patient's outpatient RA encounters assessed

M1009 Discharge/discontinuation of the episode of care documented in the medical record

M1010 Discharge/discontinuation of the episode of care documented in the medical record

M1011 Discharge/discontinuation of the episode of care documented in the medical record

M1012 Discharge/discontinuation of the episode of care documented in the medical record

M1013 Discharge/discontinuation of the episode of care documented in the medical record

M1014 Discharge/discontinuation of the episode of care documented in the medical record

M1016 Female patients unable to bear children

M1018 Patients with an active diagnosis or history of cancer (except basal cell and squamous cell skin carcinoma), patients who are heavy tobacco smokers, lung cancer screening patients

M1019 Adolescent patients 12 to 17 years of age with major depression or dysthymia who reached remission at 12 months as demonstrated by a 12 month (+/-60 days) PHQ-9 or PHQ-9M score of less than 5

M1020 Adolescent patients 12 to 17 years of age with major depression or dysthymia who did not reach remission at 12 months as demonstrated by a 12 month (+/-60 days) PHQ-9 or PHQ-9M score of less than 5. Either PHQ-9 or PHQ-9M score was not assessed or is greater than or equal to 5

M1021 Patient had only urgent care visits during the performance period

M1027 Imaging of the head (CT or MRI) was obtained

M1028 Documentation of patients with primary headache diagnosis and imaging other than CT or MRI obtained

M1029 Imaging of the head (CT or MRI) was not obtained, reason not given

M1032 Adults currently taking pharmacotherapy for OUD

M1034 Adults who have at least 180 days of continuous pharmacotherapy with a medication prescribed for OUD without a gap of more than seven days

M1035 Adults who are deliberately phased out of medication assisted treatment (MAT) prior to 180 days of continuous treatment

M1036 Adults who have not had at least 180 days of continuous pharmacotherapy with a medication prescribed for OUD without a gap of more than seven days

M1037 Patients with a diagnosis of lumbar spine region cancer at the time of the procedure

M1038 Patients with a diagnosis of lumbar spine region fracture at the time of the procedure

M1039 Patients with a diagnosis of lumbar spine region infection at the time of the procedure

M1040 Patients with a diagnosis of lumbar idiopathic or congenital scoliosis

M1041 Patient had cancer, acute fracture or infection related to the lumbar spine or patient had neuromuscular, idiopathic or congenital lumbar scoliosis

M1043 Functional status was not measured by the Oswestry Disability Index (ODI version 2.1a) at 1 year (9 to 15 months) postoperatively

M1045 Functional status measured by the Oxford Knee Score (OKS) at one year (9 to 15 months) postoperatively was greater than or equal to 37 or knee injury and osteoarthritis outcome score joint replacement (KOOS, JR.) was greater than or equal to 71

M1046 Functional status measured by the Oxford Knee Score (OKS) at one year (9 to 15 months) postoperatively was less than 37 or the knee injury and osteoarthritis outcome score joint replacement (KOOS, JR.) was less than 71 postoperatively

M1049 Functional status was not measured by the Oswestry Disability Index (ODI version 2.1a) at 3 months (6 to 20 weeks) postoperatively

M1051 Patient had cancer, acute fracture or infection related to the lumbar spine or patient had neuromuscular, idiopathic or congenital lumbar scoliosis

M1052 Leg pain was not measured by the visual analog scale (VAS) or numeric pain scale at one year (9 to 15 months) postoperatively

M1054 Patient had only urgent care visits during the performance period

M1055 Aspirin or another antiplatelet therapy used

M1056 Prescribed anticoagulant medication during the performance period, history of GI bleeding, history of intracranial bleeding, bleeding disorder and specific provider documented reasons: allergy to aspirin or antiplatelets, use of nonsteroidal antiinflammatory agents, drug-drug interaction, uncontrolled hypertension > 180/110 mm Hg or gastroesophageal reflux disease

M1057 Aspirin or another antiplatelet therapy not used, reason not given

M1058 Patient was a permanent nursing home resident at any time during the performance period

M1059 Patient was in hospice or receiving palliative care at any time during the performance period

M1060 Patient died prior to the end of the performance period

M1067 Hospice services for patient provided any time during the measurement period

M1068 Adults who are not ambulatory

M1069 Patient screened for future fall risk

M1070 Patient not screened for future fall risk, reason not given

M1106 The start of an episode of care documented in the medical record

Special Coverage Instructions   Noncovered by Medicare   Carrier Discretion   ☑ Quantity Alert   ● New Code   ○ Recycled/Reinstated   ▲ Revised Code

152 — M Codes   [A] Age Edit   [M] Maternity Edit   ♀ Female Only   ♂ Male Only   [A]-[Y] OPPS Status Indicators   © 2023 Optum360, LLC

M1107	Documentation stating patient has a diagnosis of a degenerative neurological condition such as ALS, MS, or Parkinson's diagnosed at any time before or during the episode of care
M1108	Ongoing care not clinically indicated because the patient needed a home program only, referral to another provider or facility, or consultation only, as documented in the medical record
M1109	Ongoing care not medically possible because the patient was discharged early due to specific medical events, documented in the medical record, such as the patient became hospitalized or scheduled for surgery
M1110	Ongoing care not possible because the patient self-discharged early (e.g., financial or insurance reasons, transportation problems, or reason unknown)
M1111	The start of an episode of care documented in the medical record
M1112	Documentation stating patient has a diagnosis of a degenerative neurological condition such as ALS, MS, or Parkinson's diagnosed at any time before or during the episode of care
M1113	Ongoing care not clinically indicated because the patient needed a home program only, referral to another provider or facility, or consultation only, as documented in the medical record
M1114	Ongoing care not medically possible because the patient was discharged early due to specific medical events, documented in the medical record, such as the patient became hospitalized or scheduled for surgery
M1115	Ongoing care not possible because the patient self-discharged early (e.g., financial or insurance reasons, transportation problems, or reason unknown)
M1116	The start of an episode of care documented in the medical record
M1117	Documentation stating patient has a diagnosis of a degenerative neurological condition such as ALS, MS, or Parkinson's diagnosed at any time before or during the episode of care
M1118	Ongoing care not clinically indicated because the patient needed a home program only, referral to another provider or facility, or consultation only, as documented in the medical record
M1119	Ongoing care not medically possible because the patient was discharged early due to specific medical events, documented in the medical record, such as the patient became hospitalized or scheduled for surgery
M1120	Ongoing care not possible because the patient self-discharged early (e.g., financial or insurance reasons, transportation problems, or reason unknown)
M1121	The start of an episode of care documented in the medical record
M1122	Documentation stating patient has a diagnosis of a degenerative neurological condition such as ALS, MS, or Parkinson's diagnosed at any time before or during the episode of care
M1123	Ongoing care not clinically indicated because the patient needed a home program only, referral to another provider or facility, or consultation only, as documented in the medical record
M1124	Ongoing care not medically possible because the patient was discharged early due to specific medical events, documented in the medical record, such as the patient became hospitalized or scheduled for surgery
M1125	Ongoing care not possible because the patient self-discharged early (e.g., financial or insurance reasons, transportation problems, or reason unknown)
M1126	The start of an episode of care documented in the medical record
M1127	Documentation stating patient has a diagnosis of a degenerative neurological condition such as ALS, MS, or Parkinson's diagnosed at any time before or during the episode of care
M1128	Ongoing care not clinically indicated because the patient needed a home program only, referral to another provider or facility, or consultation only, as documented in the medical record
M1129	Ongoing care not medically possible because the patient was discharged early due to specific medical events, documented in the medical record, such as the patient became hospitalized or scheduled for surgery
M1130	Ongoing care not possible because the patient self-discharged early (e.g., financial or insurance reasons, transportation problems, or reason unknown)
M1131	Documentation stating patient has a diagnosis of a degenerative neurological condition such as ALS, MS, or Parkinson's diagnosed at any time before or during the episode of care
M1132	Ongoing care not clinically indicated because the patient needed a home program only, referral to another provider or facility, or consultation only, as documented in the medical record
M1133	Ongoing care not medically possible because the patient was discharged early due to specific medical events, documented in the medical record, such as the patient became hospitalized or scheduled for surgery
M1134	Ongoing care not possible because the patient self-discharged early (e.g., financial or insurance reasons, transportation problems, or reason unknown)
M1135	The start of an episode of care documented in the medical record
M1141	Functional status was not measured by the Oxford Knee Score (OKS) or the knee injury and osteoarthritis outcome score joint replacement (KOOS, JR.) at one year (9 to 15 months) postoperatively
M1142	Emergent cases
M1143	Initiated episode of rehabilitation therapy, medical, or chiropractic care for neck impairment
M1146	Ongoing care not clinically indicated because the patient needed a home program only, referral to another provider or facility, or consultation only, as documented in the medical record
M1147	Ongoing care not medically possible because the patient was discharged early due to specific medical events, documented in the medical record, such as the patient became hospitalized or scheduled for surgery
M1148	Ongoing care not possible because the patient self-discharged early (e.g., financial or insurance reasons, transportation problems, or reason unknown)
M1149	Patient unable to complete the neck FS PROM at initial evaluation and/or discharge due to blindness, illiteracy, severe mental incapacity or language incompatibility, and an adequate proxy is not available
M1150	Left ventricular ejection fraction (LVEF) less than or equal to 40% or documentation of moderately or severely depressed left ventricular systolic function
M1151	Patients with a history of heart transplant or with a left ventricular assist device (LVAD)
M1152	Patients with a history of heart transplant or with a left ventricular assist device (LVAD)
M1153	Patient with diagnosis of osteoporosis on date of encounter
M1154	Hospice services provided to patient any time during the measurement period
M1155	Patient had anaphylaxis due to the pneumococcal vaccine any time during or before the measurement period

Special Coverage Instructions   Noncovered by Medicare   Carrier Discretion   ☑ Quantity Alert   ● New Code   ○ Recycled/Reinstated   ▲ Revised Code

© 2023 Optum360, LLC   A2–Z3 ASC Pmt   CMS: IOM   AHA: Coding Clinic   ⅋ DMEPOS Paid   ⊘ SNF Excluded   M Codes — 153

Medical Services

M1159 — M1199

M1156 Patient received active chemotherapy any time during the measurement period

M1157 Patient received bone marrow transplant any time during the measurement period

M1158 Patient had history of immunocompromising conditions prior to or during the measurement period

M1159 Hospice services provided to patient any time during the measurement period

M1160 Patient had anaphylaxis due to the meningococcal vaccine any time on or before the patient's 13th birthday

M1161 Patient had anaphylaxis due to the tetanus, diphtheria or pertussis vaccine any time on or before the patient's 13th birthday

M1162 Patient had encephalitis due to the tetanus, diphtheria or pertussis vaccine any time on or before the patient's 13th birthday

M1163 Patient had anaphylaxis due to the HPV vaccine any time on or before the patient's 13th birthday

M1164 Patients with dementia any time during the patient's history through the end of the measurement period

M1165 Patients who use hospice services any time during the measurement period

M1166 Pathology report for tissue specimens produced from wide local excisions or re-excisions

M1167 In hospice or using hospice services during the measurement period

M1168 Patient received an influenza vaccine on or between July 1 of the year prior to the measurement period and June 30 of the measurement period

M1169 Documentation of medical reason(s) for not administering influenza vaccine (e.g., prior anaphylaxis due to the influenza vaccine)

M1170 Patient did not receive an influenza vaccine on or between July 1 of the year prior to the measurement period and June 30 of the measurement period

M1171 Patient received at least 1 TD vaccine or 1 TDaP vaccine between 9 years prior to the encounter and the end of the measurement period

M1172 Documentation of medical reason(s) for not administering TD or TDaP vaccine (e.g., prior anaphylaxis due to the TD or TDaP vaccine or history of encephalopathy within 7 days after a previous dose of a TD-containing vaccine)

M1173 Patient did not receive at least 1 TD vaccine or 1 TDaP vaccine between 9 years prior to the encounter and the end of the measurement oneperiod

▲ M1174 Patient received at least two doses of the herpes zoster recombinant vaccine (at least 28 days apart) anytime on or after the patient's 50th birthday before or during the measurement period

M1175 Documentation of medical reason(s) for not administering zoster vaccine (e.g., prior anaphylaxis due to the zoster vaccine)

▲ M1176 Patient did not receive at least two doses of the herpes zoster recombinant vaccine (at least 28 days apart) anytime on or after the patient's 50th birthday before or during the measurement period

M1177 Patient received any pneumococcal conjugate or polysaccharide vaccine on or after their 60th birthday and before the end of the measurement period

M1178 Documentation of medical reason(s) for not administering pneumococcal vaccine (e.g., prior anaphylaxis due to the pneumococcal vaccine)

M1179 Patient did not receive any pneumococcal conjugate or polysaccharide vaccine, on or after their 60th birthday and before or during measurement period

M1180 Patients on immune checkpoint inhibitor therapy

M1181 Grade 2 or above diarrhea and/or Grade 2 or above colitis

M1182 Patients not eligible due to pre-existing inflammatory bowel disease (IBD) (e.g., ulcerative colitis, Crohn's disease)

M1183 Documentation of immune checkpoint inhibitor therapy held and corticosteroids or immunosuppressants prescribed or administered

M1184 Documentation of medical reason(s) for not prescribing or administering corticosteroid or immunosuppressant treatment (e.g., allergy, intolerance, infectious etiology, pancreatic insufficiency, hyperthyroidism, prior bowel surgical interventions, celiac disease, receiving other medication, awaiting diagnostic workup results for alternative etiologies, other medical reasons/contraindication)

M1185 Documentation of immune checkpoint inhibitor therapy not held and/or corticosteroids or immunosuppressants prescribed or administered was not performed, reason not given

M1186 Patients who have an order for or are receiving hospice or palliative care

M1187 Patients with a diagnosis of end stage renal disease (ESRD)

M1188 Patients with a diagnosis of chronic kidney disease (CKD) Stage 5

M1189 Documentation of a kidney health evaluation defined by an estimated glomerular filtration rate (EGFR) and urine albumin-creatinine ratio (UACR) performed

M1190 Documentation of a kidney health evaluation was not performed or defined by an estimated glomerular filtration rate (EGFR) and urine albumin-creatinine ratio (UACR)

M1191 Hospice services provided to patient any time during the measurement period

M1192 Patients with an existing diagnosis of squamous cell carcinoma of the esophagus

M1193 Surgical pathology reports that contain impression or conclusion of or recommendation for testing of MMR by immunohistochemistry, MSI by DNA-based testing status, or both

M1194 Documentation of medical reason(s) surgical pathology reports did not contain impression or conclusion of or recommendation for testing of MMR by immunohistochemistry, MSI by DNA-based testing status, or both tests were not included (e.g., patient will not be treated with checkpoint inhibitor therapy, no residual carcinoma is present in the sample [tissue exhausted or status post neoadjuvant treatment], insufficient tumor for testing)

M1195 Surgical pathology reports that do not contain impression or conclusion of or recommendation for testing of MMR by immunohistochemistry, MSI by DNA-based testing status, or both, reason not given

M1196 Initial (index visit) numeric rating scale (NRS), visual rating scale (VRS), or ItchyQuant assessment score of greater than or equal to 4

▲ M1197 Itch severity assessment score is reduced by three or more points from the initial (index) assessment score to the follow-up visit score

▲ M1198 Itch severity assessment score was not reduced by at least three points from initial (index) score to the follow-up visit score or assessment was not completed during the follow-up encounter

M1199 Patients receiving RRT

Special Coverage Instructions   Noncovered by Medicare   Carrier Discretion   ☑ Quantity Alert ● New Code ○ Recycled/Reinstated ▲ Revised Code

M1200	Ace inhibitor (ACE-I) or ARB therapy prescribed during the measurement period
M1201	Documentation of medical reason(s) for not prescribing ACE inhibitor (ACE-I) or ARB therapy during the measurement period (e.g., pregnancy, history of angioedema to ACE-I, other allergy to ACE-I and ARB, hyperkalemia or history of hyperkalemia while on ACE-I or ARB therapy, acute kidney injury due to ACE-I or ARB therapy), other medical reasons)
M1202	Documentation of patient reason(s) for not prescribing ACE inhibitor or ARB therapy during the measurement period, (e.g., patient declined, other patient reasons)
M1203	Ace inhibitor or ARB therapy not prescribed during the measurement period, reason not given
M1204	Initial (index visit) numeric rating scale (NRS), visual rating scale (VRS), or ItchyQuant assessment score of greater than or equal to 4
▲ **M1205**	Itch severity assessment score is reduced by three or more points from the initial (index) assessment score to the follow-up visit score
▲ **M1206**	Itch severity assessment score was not reduced by at least three points from initial (index) score to the follow-up visit score or assessment was not completed during the follow-up encounter
▲ **M1207**	Patient is screened for food insecurity, housing instability, transportation needs, utility difficulties, and interpersonal safety
▲ **M1208**	Patient is not screened for food insecurity, housing instability, transportation needs, utility difficulties, and interpersonal safety
M1209	At least two orders for high-risk medications from the same drug class, (Table 4), without appropriate diagnoses AIIA. 20,23
M1210	At least two orders for high-risk medications from the same drug class, (Table 4), not ordered
● **M1211**	Most recent hemoglobin A1c level > 9.0%
● **M1212**	Hemoglobin A1c level is missing, or was not performed during the measurement period (12 months)
● **M1213**	No history of spirometry results with confirmed airflow obstruction (FEV1/FVC < 70%) and present spirometry is >= 70%
● **M1214**	Spirometry results with confirmed airflow obstruction (FEV1/FVC < 70%) documented and reviewed
● **M1215**	Documentation of medical reason(s) for not documenting and reviewing spirometry results (e.g., patients with dementia or tracheostomy)
● **M1216**	No spirometry results with confirmed airflow obstruction FEV1/FVC < 70%) documented and/or no spirometry performed with results documented during the encounter
● **M1217**	Documentation of system reason(s) for not documenting and reviewing spirometry results (e.g., spirometry equipment not available at the time of the encounter)
● **M1218**	Patient has COPD symptoms (e.g., dyspnea, cough/sputum, wheezing)
● **M1219**	Anaphylaxis due to the vaccine on or before the date of the encounter
● **M1220**	Dilated retinal eye exam with interpretation by an ophthalmologist or optometrist or artificial intelligence (AI) interpretation documented and reviewed; with evidence of retinopathy
● **M1221**	Dilated retinal eye exam with interpretation by an ophthalmologist or optometrist or artificial intelligence (AI) interpretation documented and reviewed; without evidence of retinopathy
● **M1222**	Glaucoma plan of care not documented, reason not otherwise specified
● **M1223**	Glaucoma plan of care documented
● **M1224**	Intraocular pressure (IOP) reduced by a value less than 20% from the pre-intervention level
● **M1225**	Intraocular pressure (IOP) reduced by a value of greater than or equal to 20% from the pre-intervention level
● **M1226**	IOP measurement not documented, reason not otherwise specified
● **M1227**	Evidence-based therapy was prescribed
● **M1228**	Patient, who has a reactive HCV antibody test, and has a follow up HCV viral test that detected HCV viremia, has HCV treatment initiated within 3 months of the reactive HCV antibody test
● **M1229**	Patient, who has a reactive HCV antibody test, and has a follow up HCV viral test that detected HCV viremia, is referred within 1 month of the reactive HCV antibody test to a clinician who treats HCV infection
● **M1230**	Patient has a reactive HCV antibody test and does not have a follow-up HCV viral test, or patient has a reactive HCV antibody test and has a follow-up HCV viral test that detects HCV viremia and is not referred to a clinician who treats HCV infection within 1 month and does not have HCV treatment initiated within 3 months of the reactive HCV antibody test, reason not given
● **M1231**	Patient receives HCV antibody test with nonreactive result
● **M1232**	Patient receives HCV antibody test with reactive result
● **M1233**	Patient does not receive HCV antibody test or patient does receive HCV antibody test but results not documented, reason not given
● **M1234**	Patient has a reactive HCV antibody test, and has a follow-up HCV viral test that does not detect HCV viremia
● **M1235**	Documentation or patient report of HCV antibody test or HCV RNA test which occurred prior to the performance period
● **M1236**	Baseline MRS > 2
● **M1237**	Patient reason for not screening for food insecurity, housing instability, transportation needs, utility difficulties, and interpersonal safety (e.g., patient declined or other patient reasons)
● **M1238**	Documentation that administration of second recombinant zoster vaccine could not occur during the performance period due to the recommended 2 to 6 month interval between doses (i.e, first dose received after October 31)
● **M1239**	Patient did not respond to the question of "Patient felt heard and understood by this provider and team"
● **M1240**	Patient did not respond to the question of "Patient felt this provider and team put my best interests first when making recommendations about my care"
● **M1241**	Patient did not respond to the question of "Patient felt this provider and team saw me as a person, not just someone with a medical problem"
● **M1242**	Patient did not respond to the question of "Patient felt this provider and team understood what is important to me in my life"
● **M1243**	Patient provided a response other than "completely true" for the question of "Patient felt heard and understood by this provider and team"

Special Coverage Instructions   Noncovered by Medicare   Carrier Discretion   ☑ Quantity Alert   ● New Code   ○ Recycled/Reinstated   ▲ Revised Code

● **M1244** Patient provided a response other than "completely true" for the question of "Patient felt this provider and team put my best interests first when making recommendations about my care"

● **M1245** Patient provided a response other than "completely true" for the question of "Patient felt this provider and team saw me as a person, not just someone with a medical problem"

● **M1246** Patient provided a response other than "completely true" for the question of "Patient felt this provider and team understood what is important to me in my life"

● **M1247** Patient responded "completely true" for the question of "Patient felt this provider and team put my best interests first when making recommendations about my care"

● **M1248** Patient responded "completely true" for the question of "Patient felt this provider and team saw me as a person, not just someone with a medical problem"

● **M1249** Patient responded "completely true" for the question of "Patient felt this provider and team understood what is important to me in my life"

● **M1250** Patient responded as "completely true" for the question of "Patient felt heard and understood by this provider and team"

● **M1251** Patients for whom a proxy completed the entire HU survey on their behalf for any reason (no patient involvement)

● **M1252** Patients who did not complete at least one of the four patient experience HU survey items and return the HU survey within 60 days of the ambulatory palliative care visit

● **M1253** Patients who respond on the patient experience HU survey that they did not receive care by the listed ambulatory palliative care provider in the last 60 days (disavowal)

● **M1254** Patients who were deceased when the HU survey reached them

● **M1255** Patients who have another reason for visiting the clinic [not prenatal or postpartum care] and have a positive pregnancy test but have not established the clinic as an OB provider (e.g., plan to terminate the pregnancy or seek prenatal services elsewhere)

● **M1256** Prior history of known CVD

● **M1257** CVD risk assessment not performed or incomplete (e.g., CVD risk assessment was not documented), reason not otherwise specified

● **M1258** CVD risk assessment performed, have a documented calculated risk score

● **M1259** Patients listed on the kidney-pancreas transplant waitlist or who received a living donor transplant within the first year following initiation of dialysis

● **M1260** Patients who were not listed on the kidney-pancreas transplant waitlist or patients who did not receive a living donor transplant within the first year following initiation of dialysis

● **M1261** Patients who were on the kidney or kidney-pancreas waitlist prior to initiation of dialysis

● **M1262** Patients who had a transplant prior to initiation of dialysis

● **M1263** Patients in hospice on their initiation of dialysis date or during the month of evaluation

● **M1264** Patients age 75 or older on their initiation of dialysis date

● **M1265** CMS Medical Evidence Form 2728 for dialysis patients: initial form completed

● **M1266** Patients admitted to a skilled nursing facility (SNF)

● **M1267** Patients not on any kidney or kidney-pancreas transplant waitlist or is not in active status on any kidney or kidney-pancreas transplant waitlist as of the last day of each month during the measurement period

● **M1268** Patients on active status on any kidney or kidney-pancreas transplant waitlist as of the last day of each month during the measurement period

● **M1269** Receiving ESRD MCP dialysis services by the provider on the last day of the reporting month

● **M1270** Patients not on any kidney or kidney-pancreas transplant waitlist as of the last day of each month during the measurement period

● **M1271** Patients with dementia at any time prior to or during the month

● **M1272** Patients on any kidney or kidney-pancreas transplant waitlist as of the last day of each month during the measurement period

● **M1273** Patients who were admitted to a skilled nursing facility (SNF) within 1 year of dialysis initiation according to the CMS-2728 Form

● **M1274** Patients who were admitted to a skilled nursing facility (SNF) during the month of evaluation were excluded from that month

● **M1275** Patients determined to be in hospice were excluded from month of evaluation and the remainder of reporting period

● **M1276** BMI documented outside normal parameters, no follow-up plan documented, no reason given

● **M1277** Colorectal cancer screening results documented and reviewed

● **M1278** Elevated or hypertensive blood pressure reading documented, and the indicated follow-up is documented

● **M1279** Elevated or hypertensive blood pressure reading documented, indicated follow-up not documented, reason not given

● **M1280** Women who had a bilateral mastectomy or who have a history of a bilateral mastectomy or for whom there is evidence of a right and a left unilateral mastectomy

● **M1281** Blood pressure reading not documented, reason not given

● **M1282** Patient screened for tobacco use and identified as a tobacco non-user

● **M1283** Patient screened for tobacco use and identified as a tobacco user

● **M1284** Patients age 66 or older in institutional special needs plans (SNP) or residing in long-term care with POS code 32, 33, 34, 54, or 56 for more than 90 consecutive days during the measurement period

● **M1285** Screening, diagnostic, film, digital or digital breast tomosynthesis (3D) mammography results were not documented and reviewed, reason not otherwise specified

● **M1286** BMI is documented as being outside of normal parameters, follow-up plan is not completed for documented medical reason

● **M1287** BMI is documented below normal parameters and a follow-up plan is documented

● **M1288** Documented reason for not screening or recommending a follow-up for high blood pressure

● **M1289** Patient identified as tobacco user did not receive tobacco cessation intervention during the measurement period or in the 6 months prior to the measurement period (counseling and/or pharmacotherapy)

● **M1290** Patient not eligible due to active diagnosis of hypertension

---

Special Coverage Instructions   Noncovered by Medicare   Carrier Discretion   ☑ Quantity Alert ● New Code ○ Recycled/Reinstated ▲ Revised Code

156 — M Codes   Ⓐ Age Edit   Ⓜ Maternity Edit   ♀ Female Only   ♂ Male Only   Ⓐ-Ⓨ OPPS Status Indicators   © 2023 Optum360, LLC

● M1291 Patients 66 years of age and older with at least one claim/encounter for frailty during the measurement period and a dispensed medication for dementia during the measurement period or the year prior to the measurement period

● M1292 Patients 66 years of age and older with at least one claim/encounter for frailty during the measurement period and either one acute inpatient encounter with a diagnosis of advanced illness or two outpatient, observation, ED or nonacute inpatient encounters on different dates of service with an advanced illness diagnosis during the measurement period or the year prior to the measurement period

● M1293 BMI is documented above normal parameters and a follow-up plan is documented

● M1294 Normal blood pressure reading documented, follow-up not required

● M1295 Patients with a diagnosis or past history of total colectomy or colorectal cancer

● M1296 BMI is documented within normal parameters and no follow-up plan is required

● M1297 BMI not documented due to medical reason or patient refusal of height or weight measurement

● M1298 Documentation of patient pregnancy anytime during the measurement period prior to and including the current encounter

● M1299 Influenza immunization administered or previously received

● M1300 Influenza immunization was not administered for reasons documented by clinician (e.g., patient allergy or other medical reasons, patient declined or other patient reasons, vaccine not available or other system reasons)

● M1301 Patient identified as a tobacco user received tobacco cessation intervention during the measurement period or in the 6 months prior to the measurement period (counseling and/or pharmacotherapy)

● M1302 Screening, diagnostic, film digital or digital breast tomosynthesis (3D) mammography results documented and reviewed

● M1303 Hospice services provided to patient any time during the measurement period

● M1304 Patient did not receive any pneumococcal conjugate or polysaccharide vaccine on or after their 19th birthday and before the end of the measurement period

● M1305 Patient received any pneumococcal conjugate or polysaccharide vaccine on or after their 19th birthday and before the end of the measurement period

● M1306 Patient had anaphylaxis due to the pneumococcal vaccine any time during or before the measurement period

● M1307 Documentation stating the patient has received or is currently receiving palliative or hospice care

● M1308 Influenza immunization was not administered, reason not given

● M1309 Palliative care services provided to patient any time during the measurement period

● M1310 Patient screened for tobacco use and received tobacco cessation intervention during the measurement period or in the 6 months prior to the measurement period (counseling, pharmacotherapy, or both), if identified as a tobacco user

● M1311 Anaphylaxis due to the vaccine on or before the date of the encounter

● M1312 Patient not screened for tobacco use

● M1313 Tobacco screening not performed or tobacco cessation intervention not provided during the measurement period or in the 6 months prior to the measurement period

● M1314 BMI not documented and no reason is given

● M1315 Colorectal cancer screening results were not documented and reviewed; reason not otherwise specified

● M1316 Current tobacco non-user

● M1317 Patients who are counseled on connection with a CSP and explicitly opt out

● M1318 Patients who did not have documented contact with a CSP for at least one of their screened positive HRSNS within 60 days after screening or documentation that there was no contact with a CSP

● M1319 Patients who had documented contact with a CSP for at least one of their screened positive HRSNS within 60 days after screening

● M1320 Patients who screened positive for at least 1 of the 5 HRSNS

● M1321 Patients who were not seen within 7 weeks following the date of injection for follow-up or who did not have a documented IOP or no plan of care documented if the IOP was >25 mm Hg

● M1322 Patients seen within 7 weeks following the date of injection and are screened for elevated intraocular pressure (IOP) with tonometry with documented IOP =<25 mm Hg for injected eye

● M1323 Patients seen within 7 weeks following the date of injection and are screened for elevated intraocular pressure (IOP) with tonometry with documented IOP >25 mm Hg and a plan of care was documented

● M1324 Patients who had an intravitreal or periocular corticosteroid injection (e.g., triamcinolone, preservative-free triamcinolone, dexamethasone, dexamethasone intravitreal implant, or fluocinolone intravitreal implant)

● M1325 Patients who were not seen for reasons documented by clinician for patient or medical reasons (e.g., inadequate time for follow-up, patients who received a prior intravitreal or periocular steroid injection within the last 6 months and had a subsequent IOP evaluation with IOP <25mm Hg within 7 weeks of treatment)

● M1326 Patients with a diagnosis of hypotony

● M1327 Patients who were not appropriately evaluated during the initial exam and/or who were not re-evaluated within 8 weeks

● M1328 Patients with a diagnosis of acute vitreous hemorrhage

● M1329 Patients with a post-operative encounter of the eye with the acute PVD within 2 weeks before the initial encounter or 8 weeks after initial acute PVD encounter

● M1330 Documentation of patient reason(s) for not having a follow-up exam (e.g., inadequate time for follow-up)

● M1331 Patients who were appropriately evaluated during the initial exam and were re-evaluated no later than 8 weeks from initial exam

● M1332 Patients who were not appropriately evaluated during the initial exam and/or who were not re-evaluated within 2 weeks

● M1333 Acute vitreous hemorrhage

● M1334 Patients with a post-operative encounter of the eye with the acute PVD within 2 weeks before the initial encounter or 2 weeks after initial acute PVD encounter

● M1335 Documentation of patient reason(s) for not having a follow-up exam (e.g., inadequate time for follow-up)

● M1336 Patients who were appropriately evaluated during the initial exam and were re-evaluated no later than 2 weeks

● M1337 Acute PVD

Special Coverage Instructions   Noncovered by Medicare   Carrier Discretion   ☑ Quantity Alert ● New Code   ○ Recycled/Reinstated   ▲ Revised Code

© 2023 Optum360, LLC   A2-Z3 ASC Pmt   CMS: IOM   AHA: Coding Clinic   ᴧ DMEPOS Paid   ⊘ SNF Excluded   M Codes — 157

● **M1338** Patients who had follow-up assessment 30 to 180 days after the index assessment who did not demonstrate positive improvement or maintenance of functioning scores during the performance period

● **M1339** Patients who had follow-up assessment 30 to 180 days after the index assessment who demonstrated positive improvement or maintenance of functioning scores during the performance period

● **M1340** Index assessment completed using the 12-item WHODAS 2.0 or SDS during the denominator identification period

● **M1341** Patients who did not have a follow-up assessment or did not have an assessment within 30 to 180 days after the index assessment during the performance period

● **M1342** Patients who died during the performance period

● **M1343** Patients who are at PAM level 4 at baseline or patients who are flagged with extreme straight line response sets on the PAM

● **M1344** Patients who did not have a baseline PAM score and/or a second score within 6 to 12 month of baseline PAM score

● **M1345** Patients who had a baseline PAM score and a second score within 6 to 12 month of baseline PAM score

● **M1346** Patients who did not have a net increase in PAM score of at least 6 points within a 6 to 12 month period

● **M1347** Patients who achieved a net increase in PAM score of at least 3 points in a 6 to 12 month period (passing)

● **M1348** Patients who achieved a net increase in PAM score of at least 6 points in a 6 to 12 month period (excellent)

● **M1349** Patients who did not have a net increase in PAM score of at least 3 points within 6 to 12 month period

● **M1350** Patients who had a completed suicide safety plan initiated, reviewed, or updated in collaboration with their clinician (concurrent or within 24 hours of the index clinical encounter)

● **M1351** Patients who had a suicide safety plan initiated, reviewed, or updated and reviewed and updated in collaboration with the patient and their clinician (concurrent or within 24 hours of clinical encounter and within 120 days after initiation)

● **M1352** Suicidal ideation and/or behavior symptoms based on the C-SSRS or equivalent assessment

● **M1353** Patients who did not have a completed suicide safety plan initiated, reviewed, or updated in collaboration with their clinician (concurrent or within 24 hours of the index clinical encounter)

● **M1354** Patients who did not have a suicide safety plan initiated, reviewed, or updated or reviewed and updated in collaboration with the patient and their clinician (concurrent or within 24 hours of clinical encounter and within 120 days after initiation)

● **M1355** Suicide risk based on their clinician's evaluation or a clinician-rated tool

● **M1356** Patients who died during the measurement period

● **M1357** Patients who had a reduction in suicidal ideation and/or behavior upon follow-up assessment within 120 days of index assessment

● **M1358** Patients who did not have a reduction in suicidal ideation and/or behavior upon follow-up assessment within 120 days of index assessment

● **M1359** Index assessment during the denominator period when the suicidal ideation and/or behavior symptoms or increased suicide risk by clinician determination occurs and a non-zero C-SSRS score is obtained

● **M1360** Suicidal ideation and/or behavior symptoms based on the C-SSRS

● **M1361** Suicide risk based on their clinician's evaluation or a clinician-rated tool

● **M1362** Patients who died during the measurement period

● **M1363** Patients who did not have a follow-up assessment within 120 days of the index assessment

● **M1364** Calculated 10-year ASCVD risk score of >=20 percent during the performance period

● **M1365** Patient encounter during the performance period with hospice and palliative care specialty code 17

● **M1366** Focusing on women's health MIPS value pathway

● **M1367** Quality care for the treatment of ear, nose, and throat disorders MIPS value pathway

● **M1368** Prevention and treatment of infectious disorders including hepatitis C and HIV MIPS value pathway

● **M1369** Quality care in mental health and substance use disorders MIPS value pathway

● **M1370** Rehabilitative support for musculoskeletal care MIPS value pathway

Special Coverage Instructions   Noncovered by Medicare   Carrier Discretion   ☑ Quantity Alert ● New Code ○ Recycled/Reinstated ▲ Revised Code

158 — M Codes   Ⓐ Age Edit Ⓜ Maternity Edit ♀ Female Only ♂ Male Only Ⓐ-Ⓨ OPPS Status Indicators   © 2023 Optum360, LLC

Pathology and Laboratory Services P2028-P9615

P codes include chemistry, toxicology, and microbiology tests, screening Papanicolaou procedures, and various blood products.

Chemistry and Toxicology Tests

P2028   **Cephalin flocculation, blood**   A

Code with caution: This test is considered obsolete. Submit documentation.

P2029   **Congo red, blood**   A

Code with caution: This test is considered obsolete. Submit documentation.

P2031   **Hair analysis (excluding arsenic)**   E

P2033   **Thymol turbidity, blood**   A

Code with caution: This test is considered obsolete. Submit documentation.

P2038   **Mucoprotein, blood (seromucoid) (medical necessity procedure)**   A

Code with caution: This test is considered obsolete. Submit documentation.

Pathology Screening Tests

P3000   **Screening Papanicolaou smear, cervical or vaginal, up to three smears, by technician under physician supervision**   A ♀ A

One Pap test is covered by Medicare every two years, unless the physician suspects cervical abnormalities and shortens the interval. See also G0123-G0124.

CMS: 100-02,15,280.4; 100-03,210.2.1; 100-04,18,1.2; 100-04,18,30.2.1; 100-04,18,30.5; 100-04,18,30.6

P3001   **Screening Papanicolaou smear, cervical or vaginal, up to three smears, requiring interpretation by physician**   A ♀ B ⊘

One Pap test is covered by Medicare every two years, unless the physician suspects cervical abnormalities and shortens the interval. See also G0123 G0124.

CMS: 100-02,15,280.4; 100-03,210.2.1; 100-04,18,1.2; 100-04,18,30.2.1; 100-04,18,30.5; 100-04,18,30.6

Microbiology Tests

P7001   **Culture, bacterial, urine; quantitative, sensitivity study**   E

Miscellaneous

P9010   **Blood (whole), for transfusion, per unit**   R ☑

CMS: 100-01,3,20.5; 100-01,3,20.5.2; 100-01,3,20.5.3; 100-02,1,10; 100-04,3,40.2.2

P9011   **Blood, split unit**   R ☑

CMS: 100 01,3,20.5; 100 01,3,20.5.2; 100 01,3,20.5.3; 100 02,1,10; 100-04,3,40.2.2; 100-04,4,231.4

P9012   **Cryoprecipitate, each unit**   R ☑

CMS: 100-02,1,10; 100-04,3,40.2.2

P9016   **Red blood cells, leukocytes reduced, each unit**   R ☑

CMS: 100-02,1,10; 100-04,3,40.2.2

P9017   **Fresh frozen plasma (single donor), frozen within 8 hours of collection, each unit**   R ☑

CMS: 100-02,1,10; 100-04,3,40.2.2

P9019   **Platelets, each unit**   R ☑

CMS: 100-02,1,10; 100-04,3,40.2.2

P9020   **Platelet rich plasma, each unit**   R ☑

CMS: 100-04,3,40.2.2

P9021   **Red blood cells, each unit**   R ☑

CMS: 100-01,3,20.5; 100-01,3,20.5.2; 100-01,3,20.5.3; 100-02,1,10; 100-04,3,40.2.2

P9022   **Red blood cells, washed, each unit**   R ☑

CMS: 100-01,3,20.5; 100-01,3,20.5.2; 100-01,3,20.5.3; 100-02,1,10; 100-04,3,40.2.2

P9023   **Plasma, pooled multiple donor, solvent/detergent treated, frozen, each unit**   R ☑

CMS: 100-02,1,10; 100-04,3,40.2.2

P9025   **Plasma, cryoprecipitate reduced, pathogen reduced, each unit**

AHA: 4Q,21

P9026   **Cryoprecipitated fibrinogen complex, pathogen reduced, each unit**

AHA: 4Q,21

P9031   **Platelets, leukocytes reduced, each unit**   R ☑

CMS: 100-02,1,10; 100-04,3,40.2.2

P9032   **Platelets, irradiated, each unit**   R ☑

CMS: 100-02,1,10; 100-04,3,40.2.2

P9033   **Platelets, leukocytes reduced, irradiated, each unit**   R ☑

CMS: 100-02,1,10; 100-04,3,40.2.2

P9034   **Platelets, pheresis, each unit**   R ☑

CMS: 100-02,1,10; 100-04,3,40.2.2

P9035   **Platelets, pheresis, leukocytes reduced, each unit**   R ☑

CMS: 100-02,1,10; 100-04,3,40.2.2

P9036   **Platelets, pheresis, irradiated, each unit**   R ☑

CMS: 100-02,1,10; 100-04,3,40.2.2

P9037   **Platelets, pheresis, leukocytes reduced, irradiated, each unit**   R ☑

CMS: 100-02,1,10; 100-04,3,40.2.2

P9038   **Red blood cells, irradiated, each unit**   R ☑

CMS: 100-01,3,20.5; 100-01,3,20.5.2; 100-01,3,20.5.3; 100-02,1,10; 100-04,3,40.2.2

P9039   **Red blood cells, deglycerolized, each unit**   R ☑

CMS: 100-02,1,10; 100-04,3,40.2.2

P9040   **Red blood cells, leukocytes reduced, irradiated, each unit**   R ☑

CMS: 100-02,1,10; 100-04,3,40.2.2

P9041   **Infusion, albumin (human), 5%, 50 ml**   K K2 ☑

CMS: 100-02,1,10; 100-04,3,40.2.2

P9043   **Infusion, plasma protein fraction (human), 5%, 50 ml**   N ☑

CMS: 100-02,1,10; 100-04,3,40.2.2

P9044   **Plasma, cryoprecipitate reduced, each unit**   R ☑

CMS: 100-02,1,10; 100-04,3,40.2.2

P9045   **Infusion, albumin (human), 5%, 250 ml**   K K2 ☑

CMS: 100-02,1,10; 100-04,3,40.2.2

P9046   **Infusion, albumin (human), 25%, 20 ml**   K K2 ☑

CMS: 100-02,1,10; 100-04,3,40.2.2

P9047   **Infusion, albumin (human), 25%, 50 ml**   K K2 ☑

CMS: 100-02,1,10; 100-04,3,40.2.2

P9048   **Infusion, plasma protein fraction (human), 5%, 250 ml**   R ☑

CMS: 100-02,1,10; 100-04,3,40.2.2

P9050   **Granulocytes, pheresis, each unit**   E ☑

CMS: 100-02,1,10; 100-03,110.5; 100-04,3,40.2.2

P9051   **Whole blood or red blood cells, leukocytes reduced, CMV-negative, each unit**   R ☑

CMS: 100-02,1,10; 100-04,3,40.2.2

P9052   **Platelets, HLA-matched leukocytes reduced, apheresis/pheresis, each unit**   R ☑

CMS: 100-02,1,10; 100-04,3,40.2.2

P9053   **Platelets, pheresis, leukocytes reduced, CMV-negative, irradiated, each unit**   R ☑

CMS: 100-02,1,10; 100-04,3,40.2.2

P9054   **Whole blood or red blood cells, leukocytes reduced, frozen, deglycerol, washed, each unit**   R ☑

CMS: 100-02,1,10; 100-04,3,40.2.2

☐ Special Coverage Instructions   ☐ Noncovered by Medicare   Carrier Discretion   ☑ Quantity Alert   ● New Code   ○ Recycled/Reinstated   ▲ Revised Code

© 2023 Optum360, LLC   A2-Z6 ASC Pmt   **CMS:** IOM   **AHA:** Coding Clinic   ⅄ DMEPOS Paid   ⊘ SNF Excluded

P9055 Platelets, leukocytes reduced, CMV-negative, apheresis/pheresis, each unit R ☑
CMS: 100-02,1,10; 100-04,3,40.2.2

P9056 Whole blood, leukocytes reduced, irradiated, each unit R ☑
CMS: 100-02,1,10; 100-04,3,40.2.2

P9057 Red blood cells, frozen/deglycerolized/washed, leukocytes reduced, irradiated, each unit R ☑
CMS: 100-02,1,10; 100-04,3,40.2.2

P9058 Red blood cells, leukocytes reduced, CMV-negative, irradiated, each unit R ☑
CMS: 100-02,1,10; 100-04,3,40.2.2

P9059 Fresh frozen plasma between 8-24 hours of collection, each unit R ☑
CMS: 100-02,1,10; 100-04,3,40.2.2

P9060 Fresh frozen plasma, donor retested, each unit R ☑
CMS: 100-02,1,10; 100-04,3,40.2.2

P9070 Plasma, pooled multiple donor, pathogen reduced, frozen, each unit R

P9071 Plasma (single donor), pathogen reduced, frozen, each unit R

P9073 Platelets, pheresis, pathogen-reduced, each unit R
AHA: 1Q,18

P9099 Blood component or product not otherwise classified

P9100 Pathogen(s) test for platelets S
AHA: 1Q,18

P9603 Travel allowance, one way in connection with medically necessary laboratory specimen collection drawn from homebound or nursing homebound patient; prorated miles actually travelled A ☑
CMS: 100-04,16,60; 100-04,16,60.2

P9604 Travel allowance, one way in connection with medically necessary laboratory specimen collection drawn from homebound or nursing homebound patient; prorated trip charge A ☑
CMS: 100-04,16,60; 100-04,16,60.2

P9612 Catheterization for collection of specimen, single patient, all places of service A
CMS: 100-04,16,60; 100-04,16,60.1.2

P9615 Catheterization for collection of specimen(s) (multiple patients) N
CMS: 100-04,16,60; 100-04,16,60.1.2; 100-04,16,60.1.4

Special Coverage Instructions   Noncovered by Medicare   Carrier Discretion   ☑ Quantity Alert   ● New Code   ○ Recycled/Reinstated   ▲ Revised Code

160 — P Codes   A Age Edit   M Maternity Edit   ♀ Female Only   ♂ Male Only   A-Y OPPS Status Indicators   © 2023 Optum360, LLC

Q Codes (Temporary) Q0035-Q9992

Temporary Q codes are used to pay health care providers for supplies, drugs, and biologicals to which no permanent code has been assigned.

Q0035 Cardiokymography
Covered only in conjunction with electrocardiographic stress testing in male patients with atypical angina or nonischemic chest pain, or female patients with angina.

Q0081 Infusion therapy, using other than chemotherapeutic drugs, per visit

Q0083 Chemotherapy administration by other than infusion technique only (e.g., subcutaneous, intramuscular, push), per visit

Q0084 Chemotherapy administration by infusion technique only, per visit

Q0085 Chemotherapy administration by both infusion technique and other technique(s) (e.g. subcutaneous, intramuscular, push), per visit

Q0091 Screening Papanicolaou smear; obtaining, preparing and conveyance of cervical or vaginal smear to laboratory
One pap test is covered by Medicare every two years for low risk patients and every one year for high risk patients. Q0091 can be reported with an E/M code when a separately identifiable E/M service is provided.
CMS: 100-02,13,220; 100-02,13,220.1; 100-02,13,220.3; 100-02,15,280.4; 100-03,210.2.1; 100-04,18,1.2; 100-04,18,30.2.1; 100-04,18,30.5; 100-04,18,30.6; 1004-04,13,220.1

Q0092 Set-up portable x-ray equipment
CMS: 100-04,13,90.4

Q0111 Wet mounts, including preparations of vaginal, cervical or skin specimens

Q0112 All potassium hydroxide (KOH) preparations

Q0113 Pinworm examinations

Q0114 Fern test

Q0115 Postcoital direct, qualitative examinations of vaginal or cervical mucous

Q0138 Injection, ferumoxytol, for treatment of iron deficiency anemia, 1 mg (non-ESRD use)
Use this code for Feraheme.

Q0139 Injection, ferumoxytol, for treatment of iron deficiency anemia, 1 mg (for ESRD on dialysis)
Use this code for Feraheme.

Q0144 Azithromycin dihydrate, oral, capsules/powder, 1 g
Use this code for Zithromax, Zithromax Z-PAK.

Q0161 Chlorpromazine HCl, 5 mg, oral, FDA-approved prescription antiemetic, for use as a complete therapeutic substitute for an IV antiemetic at the time of chemotherapy treatment, not to exceed a 48-hour dosage regimen
CMS: 100-02,15,50.5.4; 100-03,110.18; 100-04,17,80.2.1

Q0162 Ondansetron 1 mg, oral, FDA-approved prescription antiemetic, for use as a complete therapeutic substitute for an IV antiemetic at the time of chemotherapy treatment, not to exceed a 48-hour dosage regimen
Use this code for Zofran, Zuplenz.
CMS: 100-02,15,50.5.4; 100-03,110.18; 100-04,17,80.2.1

Q0163 Diphenhydramine HCl, 50 mg, oral, FDA-approved prescription antiemetic, for use as a complete therapeutic substitute for an IV antiemetic at time of chemotherapy treatment not to exceed a 48-hour dosage regimen
See also J1200. Medicare covers at the time of chemotherapy if regimen doesn't exceed 48 hours. Submit on the same claim as the chemotherapy. Use this code for Truxadryl.
CMS: 100-02,15,50.5.4; 100-03,110.18; 100-04,17,80.2.1
AHA: 4Q,19

Q0164 Prochlorperazine maleate, 5 mg, oral, FDA-approved prescription antiemetic, for use as a complete therapeutic substitute for an IV antiemetic at the time of chemotherapy treatment, not to exceed a 48-hour dosage regimen
Medicare covers at the time of chemotherapy if regimen doesn't exceed 48 hours. Submit on the same claim as the chemotherapy. Use this code for Compazine.
CMS: 100-02,15,50.5.4; 100-03,110.18; 100-04,17,80.2.1

Q0166 Granisetron HCl, 1 mg, oral, FDA-approved prescription antiemetic, for use as a complete therapeutic substitute for an IV antiemetic at the time of chemotherapy treatment, not to exceed a 24-hour dosage regimen
Medicare covers at the time of chemotherapy if regimen doesn't exceed 48 hours. Submit on the same claim as the chemotherapy. Use this code for Kytril.
CMS: 100-02,15,50.5.4; 100-03,110.18; 100-04,17,80.2.1

Q0167 Dronabinol, 2.5 mg, oral, FDA-approved prescription antiemetic, for use as a complete therapeutic substitute for an IV antiemetic at the time of chemotherapy treatment, not to exceed a 48-hour dosage regimen
Medicare covers at the time of chemotherapy if regimen doesn't exceed 48 hours. Submit on the same claim as the chemotherapy. Use this code for Marinol.
CMS: 100-02,15,50.5.4; 100-03,110.18; 100-04,17,80.2.1

Q0169 Promethazine HCl, 12.5 mg, oral, FDA-approved prescription antiemetic, for use as a complete therapeutic substitute for an IV antiemetic at the time of chemotherapy treatment, not to exceed a 48-hour dosage regimen
Medicare covers at the time of chemotherapy if regimen doesn't exceed 48 hours. Submit on the same claim as the chemotherapy. Use this code for Phenergan.
CMS: 100-02,15,50.5.4; 100-03,110.18; 100-04,17,80.2.1

Q0173 Trimethobenzamide HCl, 250 mg, oral, FDA-approved prescription antiemetic, for use as a complete therapeutic substitute for an IV antiemetic at the time of chemotherapy treatment, not to exceed a 48-hour dosage regimen
Medicare covers at the time of chemotherapy if regimen doesn't exceed 48 hours. Submit on the same claim as the chemotherapy. Use this code for Tebamide, T-Gen, Ticon, Tigan, Triban, Trimazide.
CMS: 100-02,15,50.5.4; 100-03,110.18; 100-04,17,80.2.1

Q0174 Thiethylperazine maleate, 10 mg, oral, FDA-approved prescription antiemetic, for use as a complete therapeutic substitute for an IV antiemetic at the time of chemotherapy treatment, not to exceed a 48-hour dosage regimen
Medicare covers at the time of chemotherapy if regimen doesn't exceed 48 hours. Submit on the same claim as the chemotherapy.
CMS: 100-02,15,50.5.4; 100-03,110.18; 100-04,17,80.2.1

Q0175 Perphenazine, 4 mg, oral, FDA-approved prescription antiemetic, for use as a complete therapeutic substitute for an IV antiemetic at the time of chemotherapy treatment, not to exceed a 48-hour dosage regimen
Medicare covers at the time of chemotherapy if regimen doesn't exceed 48 hours. Submit on the same claim as the chemotherapy. Use this code for Trilifon.
CMS: 100-02,15,50.5.4; 100-03,110.18; 100-04,17,80.2.1

Q0177 Hydroxyzine pamoate, 25 mg, oral, FDA-approved prescription antiemetic, for use as a complete therapeutic substitute for an IV antiemetic at the time of chemotherapy treatment, not to exceed a 48-hour dosage regimen ☑ N M ☑

Medicare covers at the time of chemotherapy if regimen doesn't exceed 48 hours. Submit on the same claim as the chemotherapy. Use this code for Vistaril.

CMS: 100-02,15,50.5.4; 100-03,110.18; 100-04,17,80.2.1

Q0180 Dolasetron mesylate, 100 mg, oral, FDA-approved prescription antiemetic, for use as a complete therapeutic substitute for an IV antiemetic at the time of chemotherapy treatment, not to exceed a 24-hour dosage regimen N M ☑

Medicare covers at the time of chemotherapy if regimen doesn't exceed 24 hours. Submit on the same claim as the chemotherapy. Use this code for Anzemet.

CMS: 100-02,15,50.5.4; 100-03,110.18; 100-04,17,80.2.1

Q0181 Unspecified oral dosage form, FDA-approved prescription antiemetic, for use as a complete therapeutic substitute for an IV antiemetic at the time of chemotherapy treatment, not to exceed a 48-hour dosage regimen N M ☑

Medicare covers at the time of chemotherapy if regimen doesn't exceed 48-hours. Submit on the same claim as the chemotherapy.

CMS: 100-02,15,50.5.4; 100-03,110.18; 100-04,17,80.2.1

AHA: 4Q,19

Q0220 Injection, tixagevimab and cilgavimab, for the pre-exposure prophylaxis only, for certain adults and pediatric individuals (12 years of age and older weighing at least 40kg) with no known SARS-CoV-2 exposure, who either have moderate to severely compromised immune systems or for whom vaccination with any available COVID-19 vaccine is not recommended due to a history of severe adverse reaction to a COVID-19 vaccine(s) and/or COVID-19 vaccine component(s), 300 mg L1

Use this code for tixagevimab and cilgavimab (Evusheld) 300 mg administered as pre-exposure prophylaxis. Report also M0220 or M0221 for administration.

Q0221 Injection, tixagevimab and cilgavimab, for the pre-exposure prophylaxis only, for certain adults and pediatric individuals (12 years of age and older weighing at least 40kg) with no known SARS-CoV-2 exposure, who either have moderate to severely compromised immune systems or for whom vaccination with any available COVID-19 vaccine is not recommended due to a history of severe adverse reaction to a COVID-19 vaccine(s) and/or COVID-19 vaccine component(s), 600 mg L1

AHA: 2Q,22

Q0222 Injection, bebtelovimab, 175 mg L1

AHA: 2Q,22

Q0240 Injection, casirivimab and imdevimab, 600 mg L1

Use this code for casirivimab and imdevimab 600 mg administered as post exposure prophylaxis. Report also M0240 or M0241 for administration.

AHA: 4Q,21; 3Q,21

Q0243 Injection, casirivimab and imdevimab, 2400 mg L1

Use this code for Casirivimab and Imdevimab (REGN-COV2), Regeneron.

AHA: 1Q,21; 4Q,20

Q0244 Injection, casirivimab and imdevimab, 1200 mg L1

AHA: 4Q,21

Q0245 Injection, bamlanivimab and etesevimab, 2100 mg L1

Use this code for Eli Lilly's bamlanivimab (LY-CoV555) 700 mg and etesevimab (LY-CoV016) 1400 mg, administered together.

AHA: 1Q,21

Q0247 Injection, sotrovimab, 500 mg L1

AHA: 3Q,21

Q0249 Injection, tocilizumab, for hospitalized adults and pediatric patients (2 years of age and older) with COVID-19 who are receiving systemic corticosteroids and require supplemental oxygen, non-invasive or invasive mechanical ventilation, or extracorporeal membrane oxygenation (ECMO) only, 1 mg L1

AHA: 4Q,21

Q0477 Power module patient cable for use with electric or electric/pneumatic ventricular assist device, replacement only A �&

Q0478 Power adapter for use with electric or electric/pneumatic ventricular assist device, vehicle type A �&

Q0479 Power module for use with electric or electric/pneumatic ventricular assist device, replacement only A �&

Q0480 Driver for use with pneumatic ventricular assist device, replacement only A �&

CMS: 100-04,32,320.3.4

Q0481 Microprocessor control unit for use with electric ventricular assist device, replacement only A �&

CMS: 100-04,32,320.3.4

Q0482 Microprocessor control unit for use with electric/pneumatic combination ventricular assist device, replacement only A �&

CMS: 100-04,32,320.3.4

Q0483 Monitor/display module for use with electric ventricular assist device, replacement only A �&

CMS: 100-04,32,320.3.4

Q0484 Monitor/display module for use with electric or electric/pneumatic ventricular assist device, replacement only A �&

CMS: 100-04,32,320.3.4

Q0485 Monitor control cable for use with electric ventricular assist device, replacement only A �&

CMS: 100-04,32,320.3.4

Q0486 Monitor control cable for use with electric/pneumatic ventricular assist device, replacement only A �&

CMS: 100-04,32,320.3.4

Q0487 Leads (pneumatic/electrical) for use with any type electric/pneumatic ventricular assist device, replacement only A �&

CMS: 100-04,32,320.3.4

Q0488 Power pack base for use with electric ventricular assist device, replacement only A

CMS: 100-04,32,320.3.4

Q0489 Power pack base for use with electric/pneumatic ventricular assist device, replacement only A �&

CMS: 100-04,32,320.3.4

Q0490 Emergency power source for use with electric ventricular assist device, replacement only A �&

CMS: 100-04,32,320.3.4

Q0491 Emergency power source for use with electric/pneumatic ventricular assist device, replacement only A �&

CMS: 100-04,32,320.3.4

Q0492 Emergency power supply cable for use with electric ventricular assist device, replacement only A �&

CMS: 100-04,32,320.3.4

Q0493 Emergency power supply cable for use with electric/pneumatic ventricular assist device, replacement only A �&

CMS: 100-04,32,320.3.4

Q0494 Emergency hand pump for use with electric or electric/pneumatic ventricular assist device, replacement only A �&

CMS: 100-04,32,320.3.4

Special Coverage Instructions   Noncovered by Medicare   Carrier Discretion   ☑ Quantity Alert ● New Code   ○ Recycled/Reinstated ▲ Revised Code

162 — Q Codes (Temporary)   A Age Edit   M Maternity Edit   ♀ Female Only   ♂ Male Only   A-Y OPPS Status Indicators   © 2023 Optum360, LLC

Q0495   Battery/power pack charger for use with electric or electric/pneumatic ventricular assist device, replacement only   A ♿
CMS: 100-04,32,320.3.4

Q0496   Battery, other than lithium-ion, for use with electric or electric/pneumatic ventricular assist device, replacement only   A ♿
CMS: 100-04,32,320.3.4

Q0497   Battery clips for use with electric or electric/pneumatic ventricular assist device, replacement only   A ♿
CMS: 100-04,32,320.3.4

Q0498   Holster for use with electric or electric/pneumatic ventricular assist device, replacement only   A ♿
CMS: 100-04,32,320.3.4

Q0499   Belt/vest/bag for use to carry external peripheral components of any type ventricular assist device, replacement only   A ♿
CMS: 100-04,32,320.3.4

Q0500   Filters for use with electric or electric/pneumatic ventricular assist device, replacement only   A ☑ ♿
The base unit for this code is for each filter.
CMS: 100-04,32,320.3.4

Q0501   Shower cover for use with electric or electric/pneumatic ventricular assist device, replacement only   A ♿
CMS: 100-04,32,320.3.4

Q0502   Mobility cart for pneumatic ventricular assist device, replacement only   A ♿
CMS: 100-04,32,320.3.4

Q0503   Battery for pneumatic ventricular assist device, replacement only, each   A ☑ ♿
CMS: 100-04,32,320.3.4

Q0504   Power adapter for pneumatic ventricular assist device, replacement only, vehicle type   A ♿
CMS: 100-04,32,320.3.4

Q0506   Battery, lithium-ion, for use with electric or electric/pneumatic ventricular assist device, replacement only   A ♿
CMS: 100-04,32,320.3.4

Q0507   Miscellaneous supply or accessory for use with an external ventricular assist device   A
CMS: 100-04,32,320.3.4

Q0508   Miscellaneous supply or accessory for use with an implanted ventricular assist device   A
CMS: 100-04,32,320.3.4

Q0509   Miscellaneous supply or accessory for use with any implanted ventricular assist device for which payment was not made under Medicare Part A   A
CMS: 100-04,32,320.3.4

Q0510   Pharmacy supply fee for initial immunosuppressive drug(s), first month following transplant   B ☑

Q0511   Pharmacy supply fee for oral anticancer, oral antiemetic, or immunosuppressive drug(s); for the first prescription in a 30-day period   B ☑

Q0512   Pharmacy supply fee for oral anticancer, oral antiemetic, or immunosuppressive drug(s); for a subsequent prescription in a 30-day period   B ☑

Q0513   Pharmacy dispensing fee for inhalation drug(s); per 30 days   B ☑

Q0514   Pharmacy dispensing fee for inhalation drug(s); per 90 days   B ☑

Q0515   Injection, sermorelin acetate, 1 mcg   E1 ☑

● Q0516   Pharmacy supplying fee for HIV pre-exposure prophylaxis FDA-approved prescription drug, per 30-days

● Q0517   Pharmacy supplying fee for HIV pre-exposure prophylaxis FDA-approved prescription drug, per 60-days

● Q0518   Pharmacy supplying fee for HIV pre-exposure prophylaxis FDA-approved prescription drug, per 90-days

Q1004   New technology, intraocular lens, category 4 as defined in Federal Register notice   E1

Q1005   New technology, intraocular lens, category 5 as defined in Federal Register notice   E1

Q2004   Irrigation solution for treatment of bladder calculi, for example renacidin, per 500 ml   N N1 ☑

Q2009   Injection, fosphenytoin, 50 mg phenytoin equivalent   K N1 ☑
Use this code for Cerebyx.

Q2017   Injection, teniposide, 50 mg   K N1 ☑
Use this code for Vumon.

Q2026   Injection, Radiesse, 0.1 ml   E1 K2 ☑
CMS: 100-03,250.5; 100-04,32,260.1; 100-04,32,260.1.1; 100-04,32,260.2.1; 100-04,32,260.2.2

Q2028   Injection, sculptra, 0.5 mg   E1 K2 ☑
CMS: 100-04,32,260.1.1; 100-04,32,260.2.2

Q2034   Influenza virus vaccine, split virus, for intramuscular use (Agriflu)   L L1 ☑

Q2035   Influenza virus vaccine, split virus, when administered to individuals 3 years of age and older, for intramuscular use (AFLURIA)   A L L1 ☑
CMS: 100-02,15,50.4.4.2

Q2036   Influenza virus vaccine, split virus, when administered to individuals 3 years of age and older, for intramuscular use (FLULAVAL)   A L L1 ☑
CMS: 100-02,15,50.4.4.2

Q2037   Influenza virus vaccine, split virus, when administered to individuals 3 years of age and older, for intramuscular use (FLUVIRIN)   A L L1 ☑
CMS: 100-02,15,50.4.4.2

Q2038   Influenza virus vaccine, split virus, when administered to individuals 3 years of age and older, for intramuscular use (Fluzone)   A L L1 ☑
CMS: 100-02,15,50.4.4.2

Q2039   Influenza virus vaccine, not otherwise specified   A L L1 ☑
CMS: 100-02,15,50.4.4.2

Q2041   Axicabtagene ciloleucel, up to 200 million autologous anti-CD19 CAR positive T cells, including leukapheresis and dose preparation procedures, per therapeutic dose   G
Use this code for Yescarta.
CMS: 100-04,32,400; 100-04,32,400.1; 100-04,32,400.2; 100-04,32,400.2.1; 100-04,32,400.2.2; 100-04,32,400.2.3; 100-04,32,400.2.3.1; 100-04,32,400.2.4; 100-04,32,400.2.5; 100-04,32,400.3; 100-04,32,400.4; 100-04,32,66.2
AHA: 2Q,19; 2Q,18; 1Q,18

Q2042   Tisagenlecleucel, up to 600 million CAR-positive viable T cells, including leukapheresis and dose preparation procedures, per therapeutic dose
Use this code for Kymriah.
CMS: 100-04,32,400; 100-04,32,400.1; 100-04,32,400.2; 100-04,32,400.2.1; 100-04,32,400.2.2; 100-04,32,400.2.3; 100-04,32,400.2.3.1; 100-04,32,400.2.4; 100-04,32,400.2.5; 100-04,32,400.3; 100-04,32,400.4; 100-04,32,66.2
AHA: 2Q,19; 1Q,19

Special Coverage Instructions   Noncovered by Medicare   Carrier Discretion   ☑ Quantity Alert   ● New Code   ↻ Recycled/Reinstated   ▲ Revised Code

Q2043 Sipuleucel-T, minimum of 50 million autologous CD54+ cells activated with PAP-GM-CSF, including leukapheresis and all other preparatory procedures, per infusion ♂ K K2 ☑
Use this code for PROVENGE.
CMS: 100-03,1,110.22; 100-03,110.22; 100-04,32,280.1; 100-04,32,280.2; 100-04,32,280.4; 100-04,32,280.5

Q2049 Injection, doxorubicin HCl, liposomal, imported Lipodox, 10 mg K K2 ☑

Q2050 Injection, doxorubicin HCl, liposomal, not otherwise specified, 10 mg K K2 ☑ ⊘

Q2052 Services, supplies and accessories used in the home under the Medicare intravenous immune globulin (IVIG) demonstration EI ☑

Q2053 Brexucabtagene autoleucel, up to 200 million autologous anti-CD19 CAR positive viable T cells, including leukapheresis and dose preparation procedures, per therapeutic dose
Use this code for Tecartus.
CMS: 100-04,32,400; 100-04,32,400.1; 100-04,32,400.2; 100-04,32,400.2.1; 100-04,32,400.2.2; 100-04,32,400.2.3; 100-04,32,400.2.3.1; 100-04,32,400.2.4; 100-04,32,400.2.5; 100-04,32,400.3; 100-04,32,400.4
AHA: 1Q,21

Q2054 Lisocabtagene maraleucel, up to 110 million autologous anti-CD19 CAR-positive viable T cells, including leukapheresis and dose preparation procedures, per therapeutic dose
Use this code for Breyanzi.
CMS: 100-04,32,400; 100-04,32,400.1; 100-04,32,400.2; 100-04,32,400.2.2; 100-04,32,400.2.3; 100-04,32,400.2.3.1; 100-04,32,400.2.4; 100-04,32,400.2.5; 100-04,32,400.3; 100-04,32,400.4
AHA: 4Q,21

Q2055 Idecabtagene vicleucel, up to 460 million autologous B-cell maturation antigen (BCMA) directed CAR-positive T cells, including leukapheresis and dose preparation procedures, per therapeutic dose
Use this code for Abecma.
CMS: 100-04,32,400; 100-04,32,400.1; 100-04,32,400.2; 100-04,32,400.2.2; 100-04,32,400.2.3; 100-04,32,400.2.3.1; 100-04,32,400.2.4; 100-04,32,400.2.5; 100-04,32,400.3; 100-04,32,400.4
AHA: 1Q,22

Q2056 Ciltacabtagene autoleucel, up to 100 million autologous B-cell maturation antigen (BCMA) directed CAR-positive T cells, including leukapheresis and dose preparation procedures, per therapeutic dose
Use this code for Carvykti.
CMS: 100-04,32,400; 100-04,32,400.1; 100-04,32,400.2; 100-04,32,400.2.2; 100-04,32,400.2.3; 100-04,32,400.2.3.1; 100-04,32,400.2.4; 100-04,32,400.2.5; 100-04,32,400.3; 100-04,32,400.4
AHA: 4Q,22

Q3001 Radioelements for brachytherapy, any type, each B ☑ ⊘

Q3014 Telehealth originating site facility fee A ⊘
CMS: 100-04,12,190.5; 100-04,12,190.6; 100-04,39,30.5

Q3027 Injection, interferon beta-1a, 1 mcg for intramuscular use K K2 ☑
Use this code for Avonex.
CMS: 100-02,15,50.5

Q3028 Injection, interferon beta-1a, 1 mcg for subcutaneous use EI ☑
Use this code for Rebif.
CMS: 100-02,15,50.5

Q3031 Collagen skin test N NI

Q4001 Casting supplies, body cast adult, with or without head, plaster A B ♿
CMS: 100-04,20,170

Q4002 Cast supplies, body cast adult, with or without head, fiberglass A B ♿
CMS: 100-04,20,170

Q4003 Cast supplies, shoulder cast, adult (11 years +), plaster A B ♿
CMS: 100-04,20,170

Q4004 Cast supplies, shoulder cast, adult (11 years +), fiberglass A B ♿
CMS: 100-04,20,170

Q4005 Cast supplies, long arm cast, adult (11 years +), plaster A B ♿
CMS: 100-04,20,170

Q4006 Cast supplies, long arm cast, adult (11 years +), fiberglass A B ♿
CMS: 100-04,20,170

Q4007 Cast supplies, long arm cast, pediatric (0-10 years), plaster A B ♿
CMS: 100-04,20,170

Q4008 Cast supplies, long arm cast, pediatric (0-10 years), fiberglass A B ♿
CMS: 100-04,20,170

Q4009 Cast supplies, short arm cast, adult (11 years +), plaster A B ♿
CMS: 100-04,20,170

Q4010 Cast supplies, short arm cast, adult (11 years +), fiberglass A B ♿
CMS: 100-04,20,170

Q4011 Cast supplies, short arm cast, pediatric (0-10 years), plaster A B ♿
CMS: 100-04,20,170

Q4012 Cast supplies, short arm cast, pediatric (0-10 years), fiberglass A B ♿
CMS: 100-04,20,170

Q4013 Cast supplies, gauntlet cast (includes lower forearm and hand), adult (11 years +), plaster A B ♿
CMS: 100-04,20,170

Q4014 Cast supplies, gauntlet cast (includes lower forearm and hand), adult (11 years +), fiberglass A B ♿
CMS: 100-04,20,170

Q4015 Cast supplies, gauntlet cast (includes lower forearm and hand), pediatric (0-10 years), plaster A B ♿
CMS: 100-04,20,170

Q4016 Cast supplies, gauntlet cast (includes lower forearm and hand), pediatric (0-10 years), fiberglass A B ♿
CMS: 100-04,20,170

Q4017 Cast supplies, long arm splint, adult (11 years +), plaster A B ♿
CMS: 100-04,20,170

Q4018 Cast supplies, long arm splint, adult (11 years +), fiberglass A B ♿
CMS: 100-04,20,170

Q4019 Cast supplies, long arm splint, pediatric (0-10 years), plaster A B ♿
CMS: 100-04,20,170

Q4020 Cast supplies, long arm splint, pediatric (0-10 years), fiberglass A B ♿
CMS: 100-04,20,170

Special Coverage Instructions　Noncovered by Medicare　Carrier Discretion　☑ Quantity Alert　● New Code　○ Recycled/Reinstated　▲ Revised Code

164 — Q Codes (Temporary)　A Age Edit　M Maternity Edit　♀ Female Only　♂ Male Only　A-Y OPPS Status Indicators　© 2023 Optum360, LLC

Q4021   Cast supplies, short arm splint, adult (11 years +), plaster   Ⓐ Ⓑ ⓓ
CMS: 100-04,20,170

Q4022   Cast supplies, short arm splint, adult (11 years +), fiberglass   Ⓐ Ⓑ ⓓ
CMS: 100-04,20,170

Q4023   Cast supplies, short arm splint, pediatric (0-10 years), plaster   Ⓐ Ⓑ ⓓ
CMS: 100-04,20,170

Q4024   Cast supplies, short arm splint, pediatric (0-10 years), fiberglass   Ⓐ Ⓑ ⓓ
CMS: 100-04,20,170

Q4025   Cast supplies, hip spica (one or both legs), adult (11 years +), plaster   Ⓐ Ⓑ ⓓ
CMS: 100-04,20,170

Q4026   Cast supplies, hip spica (one or both legs), adult (11 years +), fiberglass   Ⓐ Ⓑ ⓓ
CMS: 100-04,20,170

Q4027   Cast supplies, hip spica (one or both legs), pediatric (0-10 years), plaster   Ⓐ Ⓑ ⓓ
CMS: 100-04,20,170

Q4028   Cast supplies, hip spica (one or both legs), pediatric (0-10 years), fiberglass   Ⓐ Ⓑ ⓓ
CMS: 100-04,20,170

Q4029   Cast supplies, long leg cast, adult (11 years +), plaster   Ⓐ Ⓑ ⓓ
CMS: 100-04,20,170

Q4030   Cast supplies, long leg cast, adult (11 years +), fiberglass   Ⓐ Ⓑ ⓓ
CMS: 100-04,20,170

Q4031   Cast supplies, long leg cast, pediatric (0-10 years), plaster   Ⓐ Ⓓ ⓓ
CMS: 100-04,20,170

Q4032   Cast supplies, long leg cast, pediatric (0-10 years), fiberglass   Ⓐ Ⓑ ⓓ
CMS: 100-04,20,170

Q4033   Cast supplies, long leg cylinder cast, adult (11 years +), plaster   Ⓐ Ⓑ ⓓ
CMS: 100-04,20,170

Q4034   Cast supplies, long leg cylinder cast, adult (11 years +), fiberglass   Ⓐ Ⓑ ⓓ
CMS: 100-04,20,170

Q4035   Cast supplies, long leg cylinder cast, pediatric (0-10 years), plaster   Ⓐ Ⓑ ⓓ
CMS: 100-04,20,170

Q4036   Cast supplies, long leg cylinder cast, pediatric (0-10 years), fiberglass   Ⓐ Ⓑ ⓓ
CMS: 100-04,20,170

Q4037   Cast supplies, short leg cast, adult (11 years +), plaster   Ⓐ Ⓑ ⓓ
CMS: 100-04,20,170

Q4038   Cast supplies, short leg cast, adult (11 years +), fiberglass   Ⓐ Ⓑ ⓓ
CMS: 100-04,20,170

Q4039   Cast supplies, short leg cast, pediatric (0-10 years), plaster   Ⓐ Ⓑ ⓓ
CMS: 100-04,20,170

Q4040   Cast supplies, short leg cast, pediatric (0-10 years), fiberglass   Ⓐ Ⓑ ⓓ
CMS: 100-04,20,170

Q4041   Cast supplies, long leg splint, adult (11 years +), plaster   Ⓐ Ⓑ ⓓ
CMS: 100-04,20,170

Q4042   Cast supplies, long leg splint, adult (11 years +), fiberglass   Ⓐ Ⓑ ⓓ
CMS: 100-04,20,170

Q4043   Cast supplies, long leg splint, pediatric (0-10 years), plaster   Ⓐ Ⓑ ⓓ
CMS: 100-04,20,170

Q4044   Cast supplies, long leg splint, pediatric (0-10 years), fiberglass   Ⓐ Ⓑ ⓓ
CMS: 100-04,20,170

Q4045   Cast supplies, short leg splint, adult (11 years +), plaster   Ⓐ Ⓑ ⓓ
CMS: 100-04,20,170

Q4046   Cast supplies, short leg splint, adult (11 years +), fiberglass   Ⓐ Ⓑ ⓓ
CMS: 100-04,20,170

Q4047   Cast supplies, short leg splint, pediatric (0-10 years), plaster   Ⓐ Ⓑ ⓓ
CMS: 100-04,20,170

Q4048   Cast supplies, short leg splint, pediatric (0-10 years), fiberglass   Ⓐ Ⓟ ⓓ
CMS: 100-04,20,170

Q4049   Finger splint, static   Ⓑ ⓓ
CMS: 100-04,20,170

Q4050   Cast supplies, for unlisted types and materials of casts   Ⓑ
CMS: 100-04,20,170

Q4051   Splint supplies, miscellaneous (includes thermoplastics, strapping, fasteners, padding and other supplies)   Ⓑ
CMS: 100-04,20,170

Q4074   Iloprost, inhalation solution, FDA-approved final product, noncompounded, administered through DME, unit dose form, up to 20 mcg   Ⓨ ☑
CMS: 100-02,15,50.5

Q4081   Injection, epoetin alfa, 100 units (for ESRD on dialysis)   Ⓝ ☑
CMS: 100-04,8,60.4; 100-04,8,60.4.1; 100-04,8,60.4.2; 100-04,8,60.4.4; 100-04,8,60.4.4.1; 100-04,8,60.4.4.2; 100-04,8,60.4.5.1

Q4082   Drug or biological, not otherwise classified, Part B drug competitive acquisition program (CAP)   Ⓑ ☑

Q4100   Skin substitute, not otherwise specified   Ⓝ Ⓝ1 ☑
CMS: 100-04,4,260.1; 100-04,4,260.1.1
AHA: 2Q,22; 2Q,18

Q4101   Apligraf, per sq cm   Ⓝ Ⓝ1 ☑
CMS: 100-04,4,260.1; 100-04,4,260.1.1

Q4102   Oasis wound matrix, per sq cm   Ⓝ Ⓝ1 ☑
CMS: 100-04,4,260.1; 100-04,4,260.1.1

Q4103   Oasis burn matrix, per sq cm   Ⓝ Ⓝ1 ☑
CMS: 100-04,4,260.1; 100-04,4,260.1.1

Q4104   Integra bilayer matrix wound dressing (BMWD), per sq cm   Ⓝ Ⓝ1 ☑
CMS: 100-04,4,260.1; 100-04,4,260.1.1

Q4105   Integra dermal regeneration template (DRT) or Integra Omnigraft dermal regeneration matrix, per sq cm   Ⓝ Ⓝ1 ☑
CMS: 100-04,4,260.1; 100-04,4,260.1.1

Q4106   Dermagraft, per sq cm   Ⓝ Ⓝ1 ☑
CMS: 100-04,4,260.1; 100-04,4,260.1.1

Special Coverage Instructions   Noncovered by Medicare   Carrier Discretion   ☑ Quantity Alert   ● New Code   ○ Recycled/Reinstated   ▲ Revised Code

Q4107	**GRAFTJACKET, per sq cm**	N NI ☑
	CMS: 100-04,4,260.1; 100-04,4,260.1.1	
Q4108	**Integra matrix, per sq cm**	N NI ☑
	CMS: 100-04,4,260.1; 100-04,4,260.1.1	
Q4110	**PriMatrix, per sq cm**	N NI ☑
	CMS: 100-04,4,260.1; 100-04,4,260.1.1	
Q4111	**GammaGraft, per sq cm**	N NI ☑
	CMS: 100-04,4,260.1; 100-04,4,260.1.1	
Q4112	**Cymetra, injectable, 1 cc**	N NI ☑
Q4113	**GRAFTJACKET XPRESS, injectable, 1 cc**	N NI ☑
Q4114	**Integra flowable wound matrix, injectable, 1 cc**	N NI ☑
Q4115	**AlloSkin, per sq cm**	N NI ☑
	CMS: 100-04,4,260.1; 100-04,4,260.1.1	
Q4116	**AlloDerm, per sq cm**	N NI ☑
	CMS: 100-04,4,260.1; 100-04,4,260.1.1	
Q4117	**HYALOMATRIX, per sq cm**	N NI ☑
	CMS: 100-04,4,260.1; 100-04,4,260.1.1	
Q4118	**MatriStem micromatrix, 1 mg**	N NI ☑
Q4121	**TheraSkin, per sq cm**	N NI ☑
	CMS: 100-04,4,260.1; 100-04,4,260.1.1	
Q4122	**DermACELL, DermACELL AWM or DermACELL AWM Porous, per sq cm**	N NI ☑
	CMS: 100-04,4,260.1; 100-04,4,260.1.1	
Q4123	**AlloSkin RT, per sq cm**	N NI ☑
	CMS: 100-04,4,260.1; 100-04,4,260.1.1	
Q4124	**OASIS ultra tri-layer wound matrix, per sq cm**	N NI ☑
	CMS: 100-04,4,260.1; 100-04,4,260.1.1	
Q4125	**ArthroFlex, per sq cm**	N NI ☑
Q4126	**MemoDerm, DermaSpan, TranZgraft or InteguPly, per sq cm**	N NI ☑
	CMS: 100-04,4,260.1; 100-04,4,260.1.1	
Q4127	**Talymed, per sq cm**	N NI ☑
	CMS: 100-04,4,260.1; 100-04,4,260.1.1	
Q4128	**FlexHD, or AllopatchHD, per sq cm**	N NI ☑
	CMS: 100-04,4,260.1; 100-04,4,260.1.1	
	AHA: 4Q,22	
Q4130	**Strattice™, per sq cm**	N NI ☑
Q4132	**Grafix Core and GrafixPL Core, per sq cm**	N NI ☑
	CMS: 100-04,4,260.1; 100-04,4,260.1.1	
Q4133	**Grafix PRIME, GrafixPL PRIME, Stravix and StravixPL, per sq cm**	N NI ☑
	CMS: 100-04,4,260.1; 100-04,4,260.1.1	
Q4134	**HMatrix, per sq cm**	N NI ☑
	CMS: 100-04,4,260.1; 100-04,4,260.1.1	
Q4135	**Mediskin, per sq cm**	N NI ☑
	CMS: 100-04,4,260.1; 100-04,4,260.1.1	
Q4136	**E-Z Derm, per sq cm**	N NI ☑
	CMS: 100-04,4,260.1; 100-04,4,260.1.1	
Q4137	**AmnioExcel, AmnioExcel Plus or BioDExcel, per sq cm**	N NI ☑
	CMS: 100-04,4,260.1; 100-04,4,260.1.1	
Q4138	**BioDFence DryFlex, per sq cm**	N NI ☑
	CMS: 100-04,4,260.1; 100-04,4,260.1.1	
Q4139	**AmnioMatrix or BioDMatrix, injectable, 1 cc**	N NI ☑
Q4140	**BioDFence, per sq cm**	N NI ☑
	CMS: 100-04,4,260.1; 100-04,4,260.1.1	
Q4141	**AlloSkin AC, per sq cm**	N NI ☑
	CMS: 100-04,4,260.1; 100-04,4,260.1.1	
Q4142	**XCM biologic tissue matrix, per sq cm**	N NI ☑
Q4143	**Repriza, per sq cm**	N NI ☑
	CMS: 100-04,4,260.1; 100-04,4,260.1.1	
Q4145	**EpiFix, injectable, 1 mg**	N NI ☑
Q4146	**Tensix, per sq cm**	N NI ☑
	CMS: 100-04,4,260.1; 100-04,4,260.1.1	
Q4147	**Architect, Architect PX, or Architect FX, extracellular matrix, per sq cm**	N NI ☑
	CMS: 100-04,4,260.1; 100-04,4,260.1.1	
Q4148	**Neox Cord 1K, Neox Cord RT, or Clarix Cord 1K, per sq cm**	N NI ☑
	CMS: 100-04,4,260.1; 100-04,4,260.1.1	
Q4149	**Excellagen, 0.1 cc**	N NI ☑
Q4150	**AlloWrap DS or dry, per sq cm**	N NI ☑
	CMS: 100-04,4,260.1; 100-04,4,260.1.1	
Q4151	**AmnioBand or Guardian, per sq cm**	N NI ☑
	CMS: 100-04,4,260.1; 100-04,4,260.1.1	
Q4152	**DermaPure, per sq cm**	N NI ☑
	CMS: 100-04,4,260.1; 100-04,4,260.1.1	
Q4153	**Dermavest and Plurivest, per sq cm**	N NI ☑
	CMS: 100-04,4,260.1; 100-04,4,260.1.1	
Q4154	**Biovance, per sq cm**	N NI ☑
	CMS: 100-04,4,260.1; 100-04,4,260.1.1	
Q4155	**Neox Flo or Clarix Flo 1 mg**	N NI ☑
Q4156	**Neox 100 or Clarix 100, per sq cm**	N NI ☑
	CMS: 100-04,4,260.1; 100-04,4,260.1.1	
Q4157	**Revitalon, per sq cm**	N NI ☑
	CMS: 100-04,4,260.1; 100-04,4,260.1.1	
Q4158	**Kerecis Omega3, per sq cm**	N NI ☑
	CMS: 100-04,4,260.1; 100-04,4,260.1.1	
Q4159	**Affinity, per sq cm**	N NI ☑
	CMS: 100-04,4,260.1; 100-04,4,260.1.1	
Q4160	**Nushield, per sq cm**	N NI ☑
	CMS: 100-04,4,260.1; 100-04,4,260.1.1	
Q4161	**bio-ConneKt wound matrix, per sq cm**	N NI ☑
	CMS: 100-04,4,260.1; 100-04,4,260.1.1	
Q4162	**WoundEx Flow, BioSkin Flow, 0.5 cc**	N NI ☑
Q4163	**WoundEx, BioSkin, per sq cm**	N NI ☑
	CMS: 100-04,4,260.1; 100-04,4,260.1.1	
Q4164	**Helicoll, per sq cm**	N NI ☑
	CMS: 100-04,4,260.1; 100-04,4,260.1.1	
Q4165	**Keramatrix or Kerasorb, per sq cm**	N NI ☑
	CMS: 100-04,4,260.1; 100-04,4,260.1.1	
Q4166	**Cytal, per sq cm**	N NI ☑
	CMS: 100-04,4,260.1; 100-04,4,260.1.1	
Q4167	**Truskin, per sq cm**	N NI ☑
	CMS: 100-04,4,260.1; 100-04,4,260.1.1	
Q4168	**AmnioBand, 1 mg**	N NI ☑
Q4169	**Artacent wound, per sq cm**	N NI ☑
	CMS: 100-04,4,260.1; 100-04,4,260.1.1	

Special Coverage Instructions   Noncovered by Medicare   Carrier Discretion   ☑ Quantity Alert ● New Code   ○ Recycled/Reinstated ▲ Revised Code

Q4170	Cygnus, per sq cm	N N1 ☑
	CMS: 100-04,4,260.1; 100-04,4,260.1.1	
Q4171	Interfyl, 1 mg	N N1 ☑
Q4173	PalinGen or PalinGen XPlus, per sq cm	N N1 ☑
	CMS: 100-04,4,260.1; 100-04,4,260.1.1	
Q4174	PalinGen or ProMatrX, 0.36 mg per 0.25 cc	N N1 ☑
Q4175	Miroderm, per sq cm	N N1 ☑
	CMS: 100-04,4,260.1; 100-04,4,260.1.1	
Q4176	Neopatch or therion, per square centimeter	N N1
	CMS: 100-04,4,260.1; 100-04,4,260.1.1	
	AHA: 2Q,20; 1Q,18	
Q4177	FlowerAmnioFlo, 0.1 cc	N N1
	AHA: 1Q,18	
Q4178	FlowerAmnioPatch, per sq cm	N N1
	CMS: 100-04,4,260.1; 100-04,4,260.1.1	
	AHA: 1Q,18	
Q4179	FlowerDerm, per sq cm	N N1
	CMS: 100-04,4,260.1; 100-04,4,260.1.1	
	AHA: 1Q,18	
Q4180	Revita, per sq cm	N N1
	CMS: 100-04,4,260.1; 100-04,4,260.1.1	
	AHA: 1Q,18	
Q4181	Amnio Wound, per sq cm	N N1
	CMS: 100-04,4,260.1; 100-04,4,260.1.1	
	AHA: 1Q,18	
Q4182	Transcyte, per sq cm	N N1
	CMS: 100-04,4,260.1; 100-04,4,260.1.1	
	AHA: 1Q,18	
Q4183	Surgigraft, per sq cm	N1
	CMS: 100-04,4,260.1; 100-04,4,260.1.1	
	AHA: 1Q,19	
Q4184	Cellesta or Cellesta Duo, per sq cm	N1
	CMS: 100-04,4,260.1; 100-04,4,260.1.1	
	AHA: 1Q,19	
Q4185	Cellesta Flowable Amnion (25 mg per cc); per 0.5 cc	N1
	CMS: 100-04,4,260.1; 100-04,4,260.1.1	
	AHA: 1Q,19	
Q4186	Epifix, per sq cm	N1
	CMS: 100-04,4,260.1; 100-04,4,260.1.1	
	AHA: 1Q,19	
Q4187	Epicord, per sq cm	N1
	CMS: 100-04,4,260.1; 100-04,4,260.1.1	
	AHA: 1Q,19	
Q4188	AmnioArmor, per sq cm	N1
	CMS: 100-04,4,260.1; 100-04,4,260.1.1	
	AHA: 1Q,19	
Q4189	Artacent AC, 1 mg	N1
	CMS: 100-04,4,260.1; 100-04,4,260.1.1	
	AHA: 1Q,19	
Q4190	Artacent AC, per sq cm	N1
	CMS: 100-04,4,260.1; 100-04,4,260.1.1	
	AHA: 1Q,19	
Q4191	Restorigin, per sq cm	N1
	CMS: 100-04,4,260.1; 100-04,4,260.1.1	
	AHA: 1Q,19	
Q4192	Restorigin, 1 cc	N1
	CMS: 100-04,4,260.1; 100-04,4,260.1.1	
	AHA: 1Q,19	
Q4193	Coll-e-Derm, per sq cm	N1
	CMS: 100-04,4,260.1; 100-04,4,260.1.1	
	AHA: 1Q,19	
Q4194	Novachor, per sq cm	N1
	CMS: 100-04,4,260.1; 100-04,4,260.1.1	
	AHA: 1Q,19	
Q4195	PuraPly, per sq cm	N1
	CMS: 100-04,4,260.1; 100-04,4,260.1.1	
	AHA: 1Q,19	
Q4196	PuraPly AM, per sq cm	N1
	CMS: 100-04,4,260.1; 100-04,4,260.1.1	
	AHA: 1Q,19	
Q4197	PuraPly XT, per sq cm	N1
	CMS: 100-04,4,260.1; 100-04,4,260.1.1	
	AHA: 1Q,19	
Q4198	Genesis Amniotic Membrane, per sq cm	N1
	CMS: 100-04,4,260.1; 100-04,4,260.1.1	
	AHA: 1Q,19	
Q4199	Cygnus matrix, per sq cm	N1
	AHA: 1Q,22	
Q4200	SkinTE, per sq cm	N1
	CMS: 100-04,4,260.1; 100-04,4,260.1.1	
	AHA: 1Q,19	
Q4201	Matrion, per sq cm	N1
	CMS: 100-04,4,260.1; 100-04,4,260.1.1	
	AHA: 1Q,19	
Q4202	Keroxx (2.5 g/cc), 1 cc	N1
	CMS: 100-04,4,260.1; 100-04,4,260.1.1	
	AHA: 1Q,19	
Q4203	Derma-Gide, per sq cm	N1
	CMS: 100-04,4,260.1; 100-04,4,260.1.1	
	AHA: 1Q,19	
Q4204	XWRAP, per sq cm	N1
	CMS: 100-04,4,260.1; 100-04,4,260.1.1	
	AHA: 1Q,19	
Q4205	Membrane Graft or Membrane Wrap, per sq cm	N1
	AHA: 4Q,19	
Q4206	Fluid Flow or Fluid GF, 1 cc	N1
	AHA: 4Q,19	
Q4208	Novafix, per sq cm	N1
	AHA: 4Q,19	
Q4209	SurGraft, per sq cm	N1
	AHA: 4Q,19	
Q4210	Axolotl Graft or Axolotl DualGraft, per sq cm	N1
	AHA: 4Q,19	
Q4211	Amnion Bio or AxoBioMembrane, per sq cm	N1
	AHA: 4Q,19	
Q4212	AlloGen, per cc	
	AHA: 4Q,19	
Q4213	Ascent, 0.5 mg	
	AHA: 4Q,19	
Q4214	Cellesta Cord, per sq cm	N1
	AHA: 4Q,19	
Q4215	Axolotl Ambient or Axolotl Cryo, 0.1 mg	
	AHA: 4Q,19	
Q4216	Artacent Cord, per sq cm	N1
	AHA: 4Q,19	

Special Coverage Instructions   Noncovered by Medicare   Carrier Discretion   ☑ Quantity Alert   ● New Code   ◯ Recycled/Reinstated   ▲ Revised Code

Q4217	WoundFix, BioWound, WoundFix Plus, BioWound Plus, WoundFix Xplus or BioWound Xplus, per sq cm	N1
	AHA: 4Q,19	
Q4218	SurgiCORD, per sq cm	N1
	AHA: 4Q,19	
Q4219	SurgiGRAFT-DUAL, per sq cm	N1
	AHA: 4Q,19	
Q4220	BellaCell HD or Surederm, per sq cm	N1
	AHA: 4Q,19	
Q4221	Amnio Wrap2, per sq cm	N1
	AHA: 4Q,19	
Q4222	ProgenaMatrix, per sq cm	N1
	AHA: 4Q,19	
Q4224	Human Health Factor 10 Amniotic Patch (HHF10-P), per sq cm	N1
	AHA: 2Q,22	
▲ Q4225	AmnioBind or DermaBind TL, per sq cm	N1
	AHA: 2Q,22	
Q4226	MyOwn Skin, includes harvesting and preparation procedures, per sq cm	N1
	AHA: 4Q,19	
Q4227	AmnioCore™, per sq cm	N1
	AHA: 2Q,20	
Q4229	Cogenex Amniotic Membrane, per sq cm	N1
	AHA: 2Q,20	
Q4230	Cogenex Flowable Amnion, per 0.5 cc	N1
	AHA: 2Q,20	
Q4231	Corplex P, per cc	N1
	AHA: 2Q,20	
Q4232	Corplex, per sq cm	N1
	AHA: 2Q,20	
Q4233	SurFactor or NuDyn, per 0.5 cc	N1
	AHA: 2Q,20	
Q4234	XCellerate, per sq cm	N1
	AHA: 2Q,20	
Q4235	AMNIOREPAIR or AltiPly, per sq cm	N1
	AHA: 2Q,20	
Q4236	carePATCH, per sq cm	N1
	AHA: 4Q,21; 2Q,20	
Q4237	Cryo-Cord, per sq cm	N1
	AHA: 2Q,20	
Q4238	Derm-Maxx, per sq cm	N1
	AHA: 2Q,20	
Q4239	Amnio-Maxx or Amnio-Maxx Lite, per sq cm	N1
	AHA: 2Q,20	
Q4240	CoreCyte, for topical use only, per 0.5 cc	N1
	AHA: 2Q,20	
Q4241	PolyCyte, for topical use only, per 0.5 cc	N1
	AHA: 2Q,20	
Q4242	AmnioCyte Plus, per 0.5 cc	N1
	AHA: 2Q,20	
Q4244	Procenta, per 200 mg	N1
	AHA: 2Q,20	
Q4245	AmnioText, per cc	N1
	AHA: 2Q,20	

Q4246	CoreText or ProText, per cc	N1
	AHA: 2Q,20	
Q4247	Amniotext patch, per sq cm	N1
	AHA: 2Q,20	
Q4248	Dermacyte Amniotic Membrane Allograft, per sq cm	N1
	AHA: 2Q,20	
Q4249	AMNIPLY, for topical use only, per sq cm	N1
	AHA: 4Q,20	
Q4250	AmnioAmp-MP, per sq cm	N1
	AHA: 4Q,20	
Q4251	Vim, per sq cm	N1
	AHA: 4Q,21	
Q4252	Vendaje, per sq cm	N1
	AHA: 4Q,21	
Q4253	Zenith Amniotic Membrane, per sq cm	N1
	AHA: 4Q,21	
Q4254	Novafix DL, per sq cm	N1
	AHA: 4Q,20	
Q4255	REGUaRD, for topical use only, per sq cm	N1
	AHA: 4Q,20	
Q4256	MLG-Complete, per sq cm	N1
	AHA: 2Q,22	
Q4257	Relese, per sq cm	N1
	AHA: 2Q,22	
Q4258	Enverse, per sq cm	N1
	AHA: 2Q,22	
Q4259	Celera Dual Layer or Celera Dual Membrane, per sq cm	N1
	AHA: 3Q,22	
Q4260	Signature APatch, per sq cm	N1
	AHA: 3Q,22	
Q4261	TAG, per sq cm	N1
	AHA: 3Q,22	
Q4262	Dual Layer Impax Membrane, per sq cm	N1
	AHA: 1Q,23	
Q4263	SurGraft TL, per sq cm	N1
	AHA: 1Q,23	
Q4264	Cocoon Membrane, per sq cm	N1
	AHA: 1Q,23	
● Q4265	NeoStim TL, per sq cm	N1
	AHA: 2Q,23	
● Q4266	NeoStim Membrane, per sq cm	N1
	AHA: 2Q,23	
● Q4267	NeoStim DL, per sq cm	N1
	AHA: 2Q,23	
● Q4268	SurGraft FT, per sq cm	N1
	AHA: 2Q,23	
● Q4269	SurGraft XT, per sq cm	N1
	AHA: 2Q,23	
● Q4270	Complete SL, per sq cm	N1
	AHA: 2Q,23	
● Q4271	Complete FT, per sq cm	N1
	AHA: 2Q,23	
● Q4272	Esano A, per sq cm	N1
	AHA: 3Q,23	

Special Coverage Instructions   Noncovered by Medicare   Carrier Discretion   ☑ Quantity Alert ● New Code   ○ Recycled/Reinstated ▲ Revised Code

● **Q4273** Esano AAA, per sq cm N1
AHA: 3Q,23

● **Q4274** Esano AC, per sq cm N1
AHA: 3Q,23

● **Q4275** Esano ACA, per sq cm N1
AHA: 3Q,23

● **Q4276** ORION, per sq cm N1
AHA: 3Q,23

● **Q4277** WoundPlus membrane or E-Graft, per sq cm N1
AHA: 3Q,23

● **Q4278** EPIEFFECT, per sq cm N1
AHA: 3Q,23

● **Q4279** Vendaje AC, per sq cm

● **Q4280** Xcell Amnio Matrix, per sq cm N1
AHA: 3Q,23

● **Q4281** Barrera SL or Barrera DL, per sq cm N1
AHA: 3Q,23

● **Q4282** Cygnus Dual, per sq cm N1
AHA: 3Q,23

● **Q4283** Biovance Tri-Layer or Biovance 3L, per sq cm N1
AHA: 3Q,23

● **Q4284** DermaBind SL, per sq cm N1
AHA: 3Q,23

● **Q4285** NuDYN DL or NuDYN DL MESH, per sq cm N1

● **Q4286** NuDYN SL or NuDYN SL W, per sq cm N1

● **Q4287** DermaBind DL, per sq cm

● **Q4288** DermaBind CH, per sq cm

● **Q4289** RevoShield+ Amniotic Barrier, per sq cm

● **Q4290** Membrane Wrap-Hydro™, per sq cm

● **Q4291** Lamellas XT, per sq cm

● **Q4292** Lamellas, per sq cm

● **Q4293** Acesso DL, per sq cm

● **Q4294** Amnio Quad-Core, per sq cm

● **Q4295** Amnio Tri-Core Amniotic, per sq cm

● **Q4296** Rebound Matrix, per sq cm

● **Q4297** Emerge Matrix, per sq cm

● **Q4298** AmniCore Pro, per sq cm

● **Q4299** AmniCore Pro+, per sq cm

● **Q4300** Acesso TL, per sq cm

● **Q4301** Activate Matrix, per sq cm

● **Q4302** Complete ACA, per sq cm

● **Q4303** Complete AA, per sq cm

● **Q4304** GRAFIX PLUS, per sq cm

Q5001 Hospice or home health care provided in patient's home/residence B
CMS: 100-01,3,30.3; 100-04,10,40.2; 100-04,11,10; 100-04,11,130.1; 100-04,11,30.3

Q5002 Hospice or home health care provided in assisted living facility B
CMS: 100-01,3,30.3; 100-04,10,40.2; 100-04,11,10; 100-04,11,130.1; 100-04,11,30.3

Q5003 Hospice care provided in nursing long-term care facility (LTC) or nonskilled nursing facility (NF) B
CMS: 100-01,3,30.3; 100-04,11,10; 100-04,11,130.1; 100-04,11,30.3

Q5004 Hospice care provided in skilled nursing facility (SNF) B
CMS: 100-01,3,30.3; 100-04,11,10; 100-04,11,130.1; 100-04,11,30.3

Q5005 Hospice care provided in inpatient hospital B
CMS: 100-01,3,30.3; 100-04,11,10; 100-04,11,130.1; 100-04,11,30.3

Q5006 Hospice care provided in inpatient hospice facility B
CMS: 100-01,3,30.3; 100-04,11,10; 100-04,11,130.1; 100-04,11,30.3

Q5007 Hospice care provided in long-term care facility B
CMS: 100-01,3,30.3; 100-04,11,10; 100-04,11,130.1; 100-04,11,30.3

Q5008 Hospice care provided in inpatient psychiatric facility B
CMS: 100-01,3,30.3; 100-04,11,10; 100-04,11,130.1; 100-04,11,30.3

Q5009 Hospice or home health care provided in place not otherwise specified (NOS) B
CMS: 100-01,3,30.3; 100-04,10,40.2; 100-04,11,10; 100-04,11,130.1; 100-04,11,30.3

Q5010 Hospice home care provided in a hospice facility B
CMS: 100-01,3,30.3; 100-04,11,10; 100-04,11,130.1; 100-04,11,30.3

Q5101 Injection, filgrastim-sndz, biosimilar, (Zarxio), 1 mcg G N1
AHA: 4Q,18; 2Q,18; 1Q,18

Q5103 Injection, infliximab-dyyb, biosimilar, (Inflectra), 10 mg G K2
AHA: 4Q,18; 2Q,18; 1Q,18

Q5104 Injection, infliximab-abda, biosimilar, (Renflexis), 10 mg G K2
AHA: 4Q,18; 2Q,18; 1Q,18

Q5105 Injection, epoetin alfa-epbx, biosimilar, (Retacrit) (for ESRD on dialysis), 100 units N1
CMS: 100-04,8,60.4.2
AHA: 4Q,18; 2Q,18

Q5106 Injection, epoetin alfa-epbx, biosimilar, (Retacrit) (for non-ESRD use), 1000 units K2
AHA: 4Q,18; 2Q,18

Q5107 Injection, bevacizumab-awwb, biosimilar, (Mvasi), 10 mg K2
CMS: 100-04,4,260.1; 100-04,4,260.1.1
AHA: 4Q,19; 1Q,19; 4Q,18

▲ **Q5108** Injection, pegfilgrastim-jmdb (Fulphila), biosimilar, 0.5 mg K2
CMS: 100-04,4,260.1; 100-04,4,260.1.1
AHA: 2Q,23; 1Q,19; 4Q,18; 3Q,18

Q5109 Injection, infliximab-qbtx, biosimilar, (Ixifi), 10 mg
CMS: 100-04,4,260.1; 100-04,4,260.1.1
AHA: 1Q,19; 4Q,18

Q5110 Injection, filgrastim-aafi, biosimilar, (Nivestym), 1 mcg K2
CMS: 100-04,4,260.1; 100-04,4,260.1.1
AHA: 1Q,19; 4Q,18; 3Q,18

▲ **Q5111** Injection, pegfilgrastim-cbqv (Udenyca), biosimilar, 0.5 mg K2
CMS: 100-04,4,260.1; 100-04,4,260.1.1
AHA: 2Q,23; 1Q,19; 4Q,18

Q5112 Injection, trastuzumab-dttb, biosimilar, (Ontruzant), 10 mg K2
AHA: 3Q,19

Q5113 Injection, trastuzumab-pkrb, biosimilar, (Herzuma), 10 mg K2
AHA: 3Q,19

Q5114 Injection, Trastuzumab-dkst, biosimilar, (Ogivri), 10 mg K2
AHA: 3Q,19

Q5115 Injection, rituximab-abbs, biosimilar, (Truxima), 10 mg K2
AHA: 3Q,19

Q5116 Injection, trastuzumab-qyyp, biosimilar, (Trazimera), 10 mg K2
AHA: 4Q,19

Special Coverage Instructions Noncovered by Medicare Carrier Discretion ☑ Quantity Alert ● New Code ○ Recycled/Reinstated ▲ Revised Code

© 2023 Optum360, LLC A2-Z3 ASC Pmt CMS: IOM AHA: Coding Clinic ⅃ DMEPOS Paid ⊘ SNF Excluded Q Codes (Temporary) — 169

Q Codes (Temporary)

Q5117 — Q9992

Q5117 Injection, trastuzumab-anns, biosimilar, (Kanjinti), 10 mg `K2`
AHA: 4Q,19

Q5118 Injection, bevacizumab-bvzr, biosimilar, (Zirabev), 10 mg `K2`
AHA: 4Q,19

Q5119 Injection, rituximab-pvvr, biosimilar, (RUXIENCE), 10 mg `K2`
AHA: 2Q,20

▲ **Q5120** Injection, pegfilgrastim-bmez (ZIEXTENZO), biosimilar, 0.5 mg `K2`
AHA: 2Q,23; 2Q,20

Q5121 Injection, infliximab-axxq, biosimilar, (AVSOLA), 10 mg `K2`
AHA: 2Q,20

▲ **Q5122** Injection, pegfilgrastim-apgf (Nyvepria), biosimilar, 0.5 mg `K2`
AHA: 2Q,23; 1Q,21

Q5123 Injection, rituximab-arrx, biosimilar, (Riabni), 10 mg `K2`
AHA: 3Q,21

Q5124 Injection, ranibizumab-nuna, biosimilar, (Byooviz), 0.1 mg `K2`
AHA: 2Q,22

Q5125 Injection, filgrastim-ayow, biosimilar, (Releuko), 1 mcg `K2`
AHA: 4Q,22

Q5126 Injection, bevacizumab-maly, biosimilar, (Alymsys), 10 mg `K2`
AHA: 1Q,23

● **Q5127** Injection, pegfilgrastim-fpgk (Stimufend), biosimilar, 0.5 mg `K2`
Use this code for Stimufend.
AHA: 2Q,23

● **Q5128** Injection, ranibizumab-eqrn (Cimerli), biosimilar, 0.1 mg `K2`
Use this code for Cimerli.
AHA: 2Q,23

● **Q5129** Injection, bevacizumab-adcd (Vegzelma), biosimilar, 10 mg `K2`
Use this code for Vegzelma.
AHA: 2Q,23

● **Q5130** Injection, pegfilgrastim-pbbk (Fylnetra), biosimilar, 0.5 mg `K2`
Use this code for Fylnetra.
AHA: 2Q,23

● **Q5131** Injection, adalimumab-aacf (Idacio), biosimilar, 20 mg `K2`
AHA: 3Q,23

● **Q5132** Injection, adalimumab-afzb (Abrilada), biosimilar, 10 mg

Q9001 Assessment by chaplain services
AHA: 4Q,22

Q9002 Counseling, individual, by chaplain services
AHA: 4Q,22

Q9003 Counseling, group, by chaplain services
AHA: 4Q,22

Q9004 Department of Veterans Affairs Whole Health Partner Services

Q9950 Injection, sulfur hexafluoride lipid microspheres, per ml `N` `M1`
Use this code for Lumason.
CMS: 100-03,1,220.2

Q9951 Low osmolar contrast material, 400 or greater mg/ml iodine concentration, per ml `N` `M1` ☑
CMS: 100-03,1,220.2

Q9953 Injection, iron-based magnetic resonance contrast agent, per ml `N` `M1` ☑
CMS: 100-03,1,220.2

Q9954 Oral magnetic resonance contrast agent, per 100 ml `N` `M1` ☑
CMS: 100-03,1,220.2

Q9955 Injection, perflexane lipid microspheres, per ml `N` `M1` ☑

Q9956 Injection, octafluoropropane microspheres, per ml `N` `M1` ☑
Use this code for Optison.

Q9957 Injection, perflutren lipid microspheres, per ml `N` `M1` ☑
Use this code for Definity.

Q9958 High osmolar contrast material, up to 149 mg/ml iodine concentration, per ml `N` `M1` ☑
CMS: 100-03,1,220.2

Q9959 High osmolar contrast material, 150-199 mg/ml iodine concentration, per ml `N` `M1` ☑
CMS: 100-03,1,220.2

Q9960 High osmolar contrast material, 200-249 mg/ml iodine concentration, per ml `N` `M1` ☑
CMS: 100-03,1,220.2

Q9961 High osmolar contrast material, 250-299 mg/ml iodine concentration, per ml `N` `M1` ☑
CMS: 100-03,1,220.2

Q9962 High osmolar contrast material, 300-349 mg/ml iodine concentration, per ml `N` `M1` ☑
CMS: 100-03,1,220.2

Q9963 High osmolar contrast material, 350-399 mg/ml iodine concentration, per ml `N` `M1` ☑
CMS: 100-03,1,220.2

Q9964 High osmolar contrast material, 400 or greater mg/ml iodine concentration, per ml `N` `M1` ☑
CMS: 100-03,1,220.2

Q9965 Low osmolar contrast material, 100-199 mg/ml iodine concentration, per ml `N` `M1` ☑
Use this code for Omnipaque 140, Omnipaque 180, Optiray 160, Optiray 140, ULTRAVIST 150.
CMS: 100-03,1,220.2

Q9966 Low osmolar contrast material, 200-299 mg/ml iodine concentration, per ml `N` `M1` ☑
Use this code for Omnipaque 240, Optiray 240, ULTRAVIST 240.
CMS: 100-03,1,220.2

Q9967 Low osmolar contrast material, 300-399 mg/ml iodine concentration, per ml `N` `M1` ☑
Use this code for Omnipaque 300, Omnipaque 350, Optiray, Optiray 300, Optiray 320, Oxilan 300, Oxilan 350, ULTRAVIST 300, ULTRAVIST 370.
CMS: 100-03,1,220.2

Q9968 Injection, nonradioactive, noncontrast, visualization adjunct (e.g., methylene blue, isosulfan blue), 1 mg `K` `K2` ☑

Q9969 Tc-99m from nonhighly enriched uranium source, full cost recovery add-on, per study dose `K` ☑

Q9982 Flutemetamol F18, diagnostic, per study dose, up to 5 mCi `G` `M1`
Use this code for Vizamyl.
CMS: 100-04,13,60.12; 100-04,32,60.12

Q9983 Florbetaben F18, diagnostic, per study dose, up to 8.1 mCi `G` `M1`
Use this code for Neuraceq.
CMS: 100-04,13,60.12; 100-04,32,60.12

Q9991 Injection, buprenorphine extended-release (Sublocade), less than or equal to 100 mg `K2`
AHA: 2Q,18

Q9992 Injection, buprenorphine extended-release (Sublocade), greater than 100 mg `K2`
AHA: 2Q,18

Special Coverage Instructions   Noncovered by Medicare   Carrier Discretion   ☑ Quantity Alert ● New Code   ○ Recycled/Reinstated ▲ Revised Code

Diagnostic Radiology Services R0070-R0076

R codes are used for the transportation of portable x-ray and/or EKG equipment.

R0070 **Transportation of portable x-ray equipment and personnel to home or nursing home, per trip to facility or location, one patient seen** ☑ ☑

Only a single, reasonable transportation charge is allowed for each trip the portable x-ray supplier makes to a location. When more than one patient is x-rayed at the same location, prorate the single allowable transport charge among all patients.

CMS: 100-04,13,90.3

R0075 **Transportation of portable x-ray equipment and personnel to home or nursing home, per trip to facility or location, more than one patient seen** ☑ ☑

Only a single, reasonable transportation charge is allowed for each trip the portable x-ray supplier makes to a location. When more than one patient is x-rayed at the same location, prorate the single allowable transport charge among all patients.

CMS: 100-04,13,90.3

R0076 **Transportation of portable EKG to facility or location, per patient** ☑ ☑

Only a single, reasonable transportation charge is allowed for each trip the portable EKG supplier makes to a location. When more than one patient is tested at the same location, prorate the single allowable transport charge among all patients.

CMS: 100-04,13,90.3; 100-04,6,20.3

Special Coverage Instructions   Noncovered by Medicare   Carrier Discretion   ☑ Quantity Alert   ● New Code   ◯ Recycled/Reinstated   ▲ Revised Code

© 2023 Optum360, LLC   A2-Z3 ASC Pmt   **CMS:** IOM   **AHA:** Coding Clinic   & DMEPOS Paid   ⊘ SNF Excluded   **R Codes — 171**

Temporary National Codes (Non-Medicare) S0012-S9999

The S codes are used by the Blue Cross/Blue Shield Association (BCBSA) and the Health Insurance Association of America (HIAA) to report drugs, services, and supplies for which there are no national codes but for which codes are needed by the private sector to implement policies, programs, or claims processing. They are for the purpose of meeting the particular needs of the private sector. These codes are also used by the Medicaid program, but they are not payable by Medicare.

S0012   **Butorphanol tartrate, nasal spray, 25 mg** ☑
Use this code for Stadol NS.

S0013   **Esketamine, nasal spray, 1 mg**
Use this code for Spravato.

S0014   **Tacrine HCl, 10 mg** ☑
Use this code for Cognex.

S0017   **Injection, aminocaproic acid, 5 g** ☑
Use this code for Amicar.

S0020   ~~Injection, bupivicaine HCl, 30 ml~~

S0021   **Injection, cefoperazone sodium, 1 g** ☑
Use this code for Cefobid.

S0023   **Injection, cimetidine HCl, 300 mg** ☑
Use this code for Tagamet HCl.

S0028   **Injection, famotidine, 20 mg** ☑
Use this code for Pepcid.

S0030   ~~Injection, metronidazole, 500 mg~~

S0032   **Injection, nafcillin sodium, 2 g** ☑
Use this code for Nallpen, Unipen.

S0034   **Injection, ofloxacin, 400 mg** ☑
Use this code for Floxin IV.

S0039   **Injection, sulfamethoxazole and trimethoprim, 10 ml** ☑
Use this code for Bactrim IV, Septra IV, SMZ-TMP, Sulfatrim.

S0040   **Injection, ticarcillin disodium and clavulanate potassium, 3.1 g** ☑
Use this code for Timentin.

S0073   ~~Injection, aztreonam, 500 mg~~

S0074   **Injection, cefotetan disodium, 500 mg** ☑
Use this code for Cefotan.

S0077   ~~Injection, clindamycin phosphate, 300 mg~~

S0078   **Injection, fosphenytoin sodium, 750 mg** ☑
Use this code for Cerebryx.

S0080   **Injection, pentamidine isethionate, 300 mg** ☑
Use this code for NebuPent, Pentam 300, Pentacarinat. See also code J2545.

S0081   **Injection, piperacillin sodium, 500 mg** ☑
Use this code for Pipracil.

S0088   **Imatinib, 100 mg** ☑
Use this code for Gleevec.

S0090   **Sildenafil citrate, 25 mg** Ⓐ☑
Use this code for Viagra.

S0091   **Granisetron HCl, 1 mg (for circumstances falling under the Medicare statute, use Q0166)** ☑
Use this code for Kytril.

S0092   **Injection, hydromorphone HCl, 250 mg (loading dose for infusion pump)** ☑
Use this code for Dilaudid, Hydromorphone. See also J1170.

S0093   **Injection, morphine sulfate, 500 mg (loading dose for infusion pump)** ☑
Use this code for Duramorph, MS Contin, Morphine Sulfate. See also J2270, J2271, J2275.

S0104   **Zidovudine, oral, 100 mg** ☑
See also J3485 for Retrovir.

S0106   **Bupropion HCl sustained release tablet, 150 mg, per bottle of 60 tablets** ☑
Use this code for Wellbutrin SR tablets.

S0108   **Mercaptopurine, oral, 50 mg** ☑
Use this code for Purinethol oral.

S0109   **Methadone, oral, 5 mg** ☑
Use this code for Dolophine.

S0117   **Tretinoin, topical, 5 g** ☑

S0119   **Ondansetron, oral, 4 mg (for circumstances falling under the Medicare statute, use HCPCS Q code)** ☑
Use this code for Zofran, Zuplenz.

S0122   **Injection, menotropins, 75 IU** ☑
Use this code for Humegon, Pergonal, Repronex.
CMS: 100-02,15,50.5

S0126   **Injection, follitropin alfa, 75 IU** ☑
Use this code for Gonal-F.
CMS: 100-02,15,50.5

S0128   **Injection, follitropin beta, 75 IU** ♀☑
Use this code for Follistim.
CMS: 100-02,15,50.5

S0132   **Injection, ganirelix acetate, 250 mcg** ♀☑
Use this code for Antagon.
CMS: 100-02,15,50.5

S0136   **Clozapine, 25 mg** ☑
Use this code for Clozaril.

S0137   **Didanosine (ddI), 25 mg** ☑
Use this code for Videx.

S0138   **Finasteride, 5 mg** ♂☑
Use this code for Propecia (oral), Proscar (oral).

S0139   **Minoxidil, 10 mg** ☑

S0140   **Saquinavir, 200 mg** ☑
Use this code for Fortovase (oral), Invirase (oral).

S0142   **Colistimethate sodium, inhalation solution administered through DME, concentrated form, per mg** ☑

S0145   **Injection, PEGylated interferon alfa-2A, 180 mcg per ml** ☑
Use this code for Pegasys.
CMS: 100-02,15,50.5

S0148   **Injection, PEGylated interferon alfa-2B, 10 mcg** ☑
CMS: 100-02,15,50.5

S0155   **Sterile dilutant for epoprostenol, 50 ml** ☑
Use this code for Flolan.

S0156   **Exemestane, 25 mg** ☑
Use this code for Aromasin.

S0157   **Becaplermin gel 0.01%, 0.5 gm** ☑
Use this code for Regranex Gel.

S0160   **Dextroamphetamine sulfate, 5 mg** ☑

S0164   **Injection, pantoprazole sodium, 40 mg** ☑
Use this code for Protonix IV.

S0166   ~~Injection, olanzapine, 2.5 mg~~

S0169   **Calcitriol, 0.25 mcg** ☑
Use this code for Calcijex.

S0170   **Anastrozole, oral, 1 mg** ☑
Use this code for Arimidex.

S0171   ~~Injection, bumetanide, 0.5 mg~~

☑ Special Coverage Instructions   Noncovered by Medicare   Carrier Discretion   ☑ Quantity Alert   ● New Code   ○ Recycled/Reinstated   ▲ Revised Code

S0172 Chlorambucil, oral, 2 mg ☑
Use this code for Leukeran.

S0174 Dolasetron mesylate, oral 50 mg (for circumstances falling under the Medicare statute, use Q0180) ☑
Use this code for Anzemet.

S0175 Flutamide, oral, 125 mg ☑
Use this code for Eulexin.

S0176 Hydroxyurea, oral, 500 mg ☑
Use this code for Droxia, Hydrea, Mylocel.

S0177 Levamisole HCl, oral, 50 mg ☑
Use this code for Ergamisol.

S0178 Lomustine, oral, 10 mg ☑
Use this code for Ceenu.

S0179 Megestrol acetate, oral, 20 mg ☑
Use this code for Megace.

S0182 Procarbazine HCl, oral, 50 mg ☑
Use this code for Matulane.

S0183 Prochlorperazine maleate, oral, 5 mg (for circumstances falling under the Medicare statute, use Q0164) ☑
Use this code for Compazine.

S0187 Tamoxifen citrate, oral, 10 mg ☑
Use this code for Nolvadex.

S0189 Testosterone pellet, 75 mg ☑

S0190 Mifepristone, oral, 200 mg ♀☑
Use this code for Mifoprex 200 mg oral.

S0191 Misoprostol, oral, 200 mcg ☑

S0194 Dialysis/stress vitamin supplement, oral, 100 capsules ☑

S0197 Prenatal vitamins, 30-day supply ♀☑

S0199 Medically induced abortion by oral ingestion of medication including all associated services and supplies (e.g., patient counseling, office visits, confirmation of pregnancy by HCG, ultrasound to confirm duration of pregnancy, ultrasound to confirm completion of abortion) except drugs ♀

S0201 Partial hospitalization services, less than 24 hours, per diem

S0207 Paramedic intercept, nonhospital-based ALS service (nonvoluntary), nontransport

S0208 Paramedic intercept, hospital-based ALS service (nonvoluntary), nontransport

S0209 Wheelchair van, mileage, per mile ☑

S0215 Nonemergency transportation; mileage, per mile ☑
See also codes A0021-A0999 for transportation.

S0220 Medical conference by a physician with interdisciplinary team of health professionals or representatives of community agencies to coordinate activities of patient care (patient is present); approximately 30 minutes ☑

S0221 Medical conference by a physician with interdisciplinary team of health professionals or representatives of community agencies to coordinate activities of patient care (patient is present); approximately 60 minutes ☑

S0250 Comprehensive geriatric assessment and treatment planning performed by assessment team Ⓐ

S0255 Hospice referral visit (advising patient and family of care options) performed by nurse, social worker, or other designated staff
CMS: 100-04,11,10

S0257 Counseling and discussion regarding advance directives or end of life care planning and decisions, with patient and/or surrogate (list separately in addition to code for appropriate evaluation and management service)

S0260 History and physical (outpatient or office) related to surgical procedure (list separately in addition to code for appropriate evaluation and management service)

S0265 Genetic counseling, under physician supervision, each 15 minutes ☑

S0270 Physician management of patient home care, standard monthly case rate (per 30 days) ☑

S0271 Physician management of patient home care, hospice monthly case rate (per 30 days) ☑

S0272 Physician management of patient home care, episodic care monthly case rate (per 30 days) ☑

S0273 Physician visit at member's home, outside of a capitation arrangement

S0274 Nurse practitioner visit at member's home, outside of a capitation arrangement

S0280 Medical home program, comprehensive care coordination and planning, initial plan

S0281 Medical home program, comprehensive care coordination and planning, maintenance of plan

S0285 Colonoscopy consultation performed prior to a screening colonoscopy procedure

S0302 Completed early periodic screening diagnosis and treatment (EPSDT) service (list in addition to code for appropriate evaluation and management service)

S0310 Hospitalist services (list separately in addition to code for appropriate evaluation and management service)

S0311 Comprehensive management and care coordination for advanced illness, per calendar month

S0315 Disease management program; initial assessment and initiation of the program

S0316 Disease management program, follow-up/reassessment

S0317 Disease management program; per diem ☑

S0320 Telephone calls by a registered nurse to a disease management program member for monitoring purposes; per month

S0340 Lifestyle modification program for management of coronary artery disease, including all supportive services; first quarter/stage

S0341 Lifestyle modification program for management of coronary artery disease, including all supportive services; second or third quarter/stage

S0342 Lifestyle modification program for management of coronary artery disease, including all supportive services; fourth quarter/stage

S0353 Treatment planning and care coordination management for cancer initial treatment

S0354 Treatment planning and care coordination management for cancer established patient with a change of regimen

S0390 Routine foot care; removal and/or trimming of corns, calluses and/or nails and preventive maintenance in specific medical conditions (e.g., diabetes), per visit

S0395 Impression casting of a foot performed by a practitioner other than the manufacturer of the orthotic

S0400 Global fee for extracorporeal shock wave lithotripsy treatment of kidney stone(s)

S0500 Disposable contact lens, per lens ☑

Special Coverage Instructions   Noncovered by Medicare   Carrier Discretion   ☑ Quantity Alert ● New Code   ○ Recycled/Reinstated ▲ Revised Code

174 — S Codes   Ⓐ Age Edit   Ⓜ Maternity Edit ♀ Female Only ♂ Male Only Ⓐ-Ⓨ OPPS Status Indicators   © 2023 Optum360, LLC

S0504   Single vision prescription lens (safety, athletic, or sunglass), per lens ☑

S0506   Bifocal vision prescription lens (safety, athletic, or sunglass), per lens ☑

S0508   Trifocal vision prescription lens (safety, athletic, or sunglass), per lens ☑

S0510   Nonprescription lens (safety, athletic, or sunglass), per lens ☑

S0512   Daily wear specialty contact lens, per lens ☑

S0514   Color contact lens, per lens ☑

S0515   Scleral lens, liquid bandage device, per lens

S0516   Safety eyeglass frames

S0518   Sunglasses frames

S0580   Polycarbonate lens (list this code in addition to the basic code for the lens)

S0581   Nonstandard lens (list this code in addition to the basic code for the lens)

S0590   Integral lens service, miscellaneous services reported separately

S0592   Comprehensive contact lens evaluation

S0595   Dispensing new spectacle lenses for patient supplied frame

S0596   Phakic intraocular lens for correction of refractive error ☑

S0601   Screening proctoscopy ♂

S0610   Annual gynecological examination, new patient 🅐 ♀

S0612   Annual gynecological examination, established patient 🅐 ♀

S0613   Annual gynecological examination; clinical breast examination without pelvic evaluation ♀

S0618   Audiometry for hearing aid evaluation to determine the level and degree of hearing loss

S0620   Routine ophthalmological examination including refraction; new patient

S0621   Routine ophthalmological examination including refraction; established patient

S0622   Physical exam for college, new or established patient (list separately in addition to appropriate evaluation and management code)

S0630   Removal of sutures; by a physician other than the physician who originally closed the wound

S0800   Laser in situ keratomileusis (LASIK)

S0810   Photorefractive keratectomy (PRK)

S0812   Phototherapeutic keratectomy (PTK)

S1001   Deluxe item, patient aware (list in addition to code for basic item)
CMS: 100-02,15,110

S1002   Customized item (list in addition to code for basic item)

S1015   IV tubing extension set

S1016   Non-PVC (polyvinyl chloride) intravenous administration set, for use with drugs that are not stable in PVC, e.g., Paclitaxel

S1030   Continuous noninvasive glucose monitoring device, purchase (for physician interpretation of data, use CPT code)

S1031   Continuous noninvasive glucose monitoring device, rental, including sensor, sensor replacement, and download to monitor (for physician interpretation of data, use CPT code)

S1034   Artificial pancreas device system (e.g., low glucose suspend [LGS] feature) including continuous glucose monitor, blood glucose device, insulin pump and computer algorithm that communicates with all of the devices

S1035   Sensor; invasive (e.g., subcutaneous), disposable, for use with artificial pancreas device system

S1036   Transmitter; external, for use with artificial pancreas device system

S1037   Receiver (monitor); external, for use with artificial pancreas device system

S1040   Cranial remolding orthotic, pediatric, rigid, with soft interface material, custom fabricated, includes fitting and adjustment(s)

S1091   Stent, noncoronary, temporary, with delivery system (Propel)

S2053   Transplantation of small intestine and liver allografts

S2054   Transplantation of multivisceral organs

S2055   Harvesting of donor multivisceral organs, with preparation and maintenance of allografts; from cadaver donor

S2060   Lobar lung transplantation

S2061   Donor lobectomy (lung) for transplantation, living donor

S2065   Simultaneous pancreas kidney transplantation

S2066   Breast reconstruction with gluteal artery perforator (GAP) flap, including harvesting of the flap, microvascular transfer, closure of donor site and shaping the flap into a breast, unilateral

S2067   Breast reconstruction of a single breast with "stacked" deep inferior epigastric perforator (DIEP) flap(s) and/or gluteal artery perforator (GAP) flap(s), including harvesting of the flap(s), microvascular transfer, closure of donor site(s) and shaping the flap into a breast, unilateral

S2068   Breast reconstruction with deep inferior epigastric perforator (DIEP) flap or superficial inferior epigastric artery (SIEA) flap, including harvesting of the flap, microvascular transfer, closure of donor site and shaping the flap into a breast, unilateral

S2070   Cystourethroscopy, with ureteroscopy and/or pyeloscopy; with endoscopic laser treatment of ureteral calculi (includes ureteral catheterization)

S2079   Laparoscopic esophagomyotomy (Heller type)

S2080   Laser-assisted uvulopalatoplasty (LAUP)
AHA: 2Q,22

S2083   Adjustment of gastric band diameter via subcutaneous port by injection or aspiration of saline

S2095   Transcatheter occlusion or embolization for tumor destruction, percutaneous, any method, using yttrium-90 microspheres

S2102   Islet cell tissue transplant from pancreas; allogeneic

S2103   Adrenal tissue transplant to brain

S2107   Adoptive immunotherapy i.e. development of specific antitumor reactivity (e.g., tumor-infiltrating lymphocyte therapy) per course of treatment

S2112   Arthroscopy, knee, surgical for harvesting of cartilage (chondrocyte cells)

S2115   Osteotomy, periacetabular, with internal fixation

S2117   Arthroereisis, subtalar

S2118   Metal-on-metal total hip resurfacing, including acetabular and femoral components

S2120   Low density lipoprotein (LDL) apheresis using heparin-induced extracorporeal LDL precipitation

S2140   Cord blood harvesting for transplantation, allogeneic

S2142   Cord blood-derived stem-cell transplantation, allogeneic

---

Special Coverage Instructions   Noncovered by Medicare   Carrier Discretion   ☑ Quantity Alert ● New Code ○ Recycled/Reinstated ▲ Revised Code

S2150 Bone marrow or blood-derived stem cells (peripheral or umbilical), allogeneic or autologous, harvesting, transplantation, and related complications; including: pheresis and cell preparation/storage; marrow ablative therapy; drugs, supplies, hospitalization with outpatient follow-up; medical/surgical, diagnostic, emergency, and rehabilitative services; and the number of days of pre- and posttransplant care in the global definition

S2152 Solid organ(s), complete or segmental, single organ or combination of organs; deceased or living donor(s), procurement, transplantation, and related complications; including: drugs; supplies; hospitalization with outpatient follow-up; medical/surgical, diagnostic, emergency, and rehabilitative services, and the number of days of pre- and posttransplant care in the global definition

S2202 Echosclerotherapy

S2205 Minimally invasive direct coronary artery bypass surgery involving mini-thoracotomy or mini-sternotomy surgery, performed under direct vision; using arterial graft(s), single coronary arterial graft

S2206 Minimally invasive direct coronary artery bypass surgery involving mini-thoracotomy or mini-sternotomy surgery, performed under direct vision; using arterial graft(s), two coronary arterial grafts

S2207 Minimally invasive direct coronary artery bypass surgery involving mini-thoracotomy or mini-sternotomy surgery, performed under direct vision; using venous graft only, single coronary venous graft

S2208 Minimally invasive direct coronary artery bypass surgery involving mini-thoracotomy or mini-sternotomy surgery, performed under direct vision; using single arterial and venous graft(s), single venous graft

S2209 Minimally invasive direct coronary artery bypass surgery involving mini-thoracotomy or mini-sternotomy surgery, performed under direct vision; using two arterial grafts and single venous graft

S2225 Myringotomy, laser-assisted

S2230 Implantation of magnetic component of semi-implantable hearing device on ossicles in middle ear

S2235 Implantation of auditory brain stem implant

S2260 Induced abortion, 17 to 24 weeks ⓜ ♀

S2265 Induced abortion, 25 to 28 weeks ⓜ ♀

S2266 Induced abortion, 29 to 31 weeks ⓜ ♀

S2267 Induced abortion, 32 weeks or greater ⓜ ♀

S2300 Arthroscopy, shoulder, surgical; with thermally-induced capsulorrhaphy

S2325 Hip core decompression

S2340 Chemodenervation of abductor muscle(s) of vocal cord

S2341 Chemodenervation of adductor muscle(s) of vocal cord

S2342 Nasal endoscopy for postoperative debridement following functional endoscopic sinus surgery, nasal and/or sinus cavity(s), unilateral or bilateral

S2348 Decompression procedure, percutaneous, of nucleus pulposus of intervertebral disc, using radiofrequency energy, single or multiple levels, lumbar

S2350 Diskectomy, anterior, with decompression of spinal cord and/or nerve root(s), including osteophytectomy; lumbar, single interspace

S2351 Diskectomy, anterior, with decompression of spinal cord and/or nerve root(s), including osteophytectomy; lumbar, each additional interspace (list separately in addition to code for primary procedure)

S2400 Repair, congenital diaphragmatic hernia in the fetus using temporary tracheal occlusion, procedure performed in utero ⓜ ♀

S2401 Repair, urinary tract obstruction in the fetus, procedure performed in utero ⓜ ♀

S2402 Repair, congenital cystic adenomatoid malformation in the fetus, procedure performed in utero ⓜ ♀

S2403 Repair, extralobar pulmonary sequestration in the fetus, procedure performed in utero ⓜ ♀

S2404 Repair, myelomeningocele in the fetus, procedure performed in utero ⓜ ♀

S2405 Repair of sacrococcygeal teratoma in the fetus, procedure performed in utero ⓜ ♀

S2409 Repair, congenital malformation of fetus, procedure performed in utero, not otherwise classified ⓜ ♀

S2411 Fetoscopic laser therapy for treatment of twin-to-twin transfusion syndrome ⓜ ♀

S2900 Surgical techniques requiring use of robotic surgical system (list separately in addition to code for primary procedure)

S3000 Diabetic indicator; retinal eye exam, dilated, bilateral

S3005 Performance measurement, evaluation of patient self assessment, depression

S3600 STAT laboratory request (situations other than S3601)

S3601 Emergency STAT laboratory charge for patient who is homebound or residing in a nursing facility

S3620 Newborn metabolic screening panel, includes test kit, postage and the laboratory tests specified by the state for inclusion in this panel (e.g., galactose; hemoglobin, electrophoresis; hydroxyprogesterone, 17-d; phenylalanine (PKU); and thyroxine, total) Ⓐ

S3630 Eosinophil count, blood, direct

S3645 HIV-1 antibody testing of oral mucosal transudate

S3650 Saliva test, hormone level; during menopause Ⓐ ♀

S3652 Saliva test, hormone level; to assess preterm labor risk ⓜ ♀

S3655 Antisperm antibodies test (immunobead) ⓜ ♀

S3708 Gastrointestinal fat absorption study

S3722 Dose optimization by area under the curve (AUC) analysis, for infusional 5-fluorouracil

S3800 Genetic testing for amyotrophic lateral sclerosis (ALS)

S3840 DNA analysis for germline mutations of the RET proto-oncogene for susceptibility to multiple endocrine neoplasia type 2

S3841 Genetic testing for retinoblastoma

S3842 Genetic testing for Von Hippel-Lindau disease

S3844 DNA analysis of the connexin 26 gene (GJB2) for susceptibility to congenital, profound deafness

S3845 Genetic testing for alpha-thalassemia

S3846 Genetic testing for hemoglobin E beta-thalassemia

S3849 Genetic testing for Niemann-Pick disease

S3850 Genetic testing for sickle cell anemia

S3852 DNA analysis for APOE epsilon 4 allele for susceptibility to Alzheimer's disease

S3853 Genetic testing for myotonic muscular dystrophy

Special Coverage Instructions   Noncovered by Medicare   Carrier Discretion   ☑ Quantity Alert ● New Code   ○ Recycled/Reinstated ▲ Revised Code

176 — S Codes   Ⓐ Age Edit   ⓜ Maternity Edit   ♀ Female Only   ♂ Male Only   Ⓐ-Ⓨ OPPS Status Indicators   © 2023 Optum360, LLC

S3854	Gene expression profiling panel for use in the management of breast cancer treatment	
S3861	Genetic testing, sodium channel, voltage-gated, type V, alpha subunit (SCN5A) and variants for suspected Brugada Syndrome	
S3865	Comprehensive gene sequence analysis for hypertrophic cardiomyopathy	
S3866	Genetic analysis for a specific gene mutation for hypertrophic cardiomyopathy (HCM) in an individual with a known HCM mutation in the family	
S3870	Comparative genomic hybridization (CGH) microarray testing for developmental delay, autism spectrum disorder and/or intellectual disability	
S3900	Surface electromyography (EMG)	
S3902	Ballistocardiogram	
S3904	Masters two step	
S4005	Interim labor facility global (labor occurring but not resulting in delivery)	M ♀
S4011	In vitro fertilization; including but not limited to identification and incubation of mature oocytes, fertilization with sperm, incubation of embryo(s), and subsequent visualization for determination of development	M ♀
S4013	Complete cycle, gamete intrafallopian transfer (GIFT), case rate	M ♀
S4014	Complete cycle, zygote intrafallopian transfer (ZIFT), case rate	M ♀
S4015	Complete in vitro fertilization cycle, not otherwise specified, case rate	M ♀
S4016	Frozen in vitro fertilization cycle, case rate	M ♀
S4017	Incomplete cycle, treatment cancelled prior to stimulation, case rate	M ♀
S4018	Frozen embryo transfer procedure cancelled before transfer, case rate	M ♀
S4020	In vitro fertilization procedure cancelled before aspiration, case rate	M ♀
S4021	In vitro fertilization procedure cancelled after aspiration, case rate	M ♀
S4022	Assisted oocyte fertilization, case rate	M ♀
S4023	Donor egg cycle, incomplete, case rate	M ♀
S4025	Donor services for in vitro fertilization (sperm or embryo), case rate	A ♀
S4026	Procurement of donor sperm from sperm bank	♂
S4027	Storage of previously frozen embryos	M ♀
S4028	Microsurgical epididymal sperm aspiration (MESA)	A ♂
S4030	Sperm procurement and cryopreservation services; initial visit	A ♂
S4031	Sperm procurement and cryopreservation services; subsequent visit	A ♂
S4035	Stimulated intrauterine insemination (IUI), case rate	M ♀
S4037	Cryopreserved embryo transfer, case rate	M ♀
S4040	Monitoring and storage of cryopreserved embryos, per 30 days	M ♀
S4042	Management of ovulation induction (interpretation of diagnostic tests and studies, nonface-to-face medical management of the patient), per cycle	

S4981	Insertion of levonorgestrel-releasing intrauterine system	♀
S4989	Contraceptive intrauterine device (e.g., Progestasert IUD), including implants and supplies	M ♀
S4990	Nicotine patches, legend	☑
S4991	Nicotine patches, nonlegend	☑
S4993	Contraceptive pills for birth control	M ♀ ☑
S4995	Smoking cessation gum	☑
S5000	Prescription drug, generic	☑
S5001	Prescription drug, brand name	☑
S5010	5% dextrose and 0.45% normal saline, 1000 ml	☑
S5012	5% dextrose with potassium chloride, 1000 ml	☑
S5013	5% dextrose/0.45% normal saline with potassium chloride and magnesium sulfate, 1000 ml	☑
S5014	5% dextrose/0.45% normal saline with potassium chloride and magnesium sulfate, 1500 ml	☑
S5035	Home infusion therapy, routine service of infusion device (e.g., pump maintenance)	
S5036	Home infusion therapy, repair of infusion device (e.g., pump repair)	
S5100	Day care services, adult; per 15 minutes	A ☑
S5101	Day care services, adult; per half day	A ☑
S5102	Day care services, adult; per diem	A ☑
S5105	Day care services, center based; services not included in program fee, per diem	☑
S5108	Home care training to home care client, per 15 minutes	☑
S5109	Home care training to home care client, per session	☑
S5110	Home care training, family; per 15 minutes	☑
S5111	Home care training, family; per session	
S5115	Home care training, nonfamily; per 15 minutes	☑
S5116	Home care training, nonfamily; per session	☑
S5120	Chore services; per 15 minutes	☑
S5121	Chore services; per diem	☑
S5125	Attendant care services; per 15 minutes	☑
S5126	Attendant care services; per diem	☑
S5130	Homemaker service, NOS; per 15 minutes	☑
S5131	Homemaker service, NOS; per diem	☑
S5135	Companion care, adult (e.g., IADL/ADL); per 15 minutes	A ☑
S5136	Companion care, adult (e.g., IADL/ADL); per diem	A ☑
S5140	Foster care, adult; per diem	A ☑
S5141	Foster care, adult; per month	A ☑
S5145	Foster care, therapeutic, child; per diem	A ☑
S5146	Foster care, therapeutic, child; per month	A ☑
S5150	Unskilled respite care, not hospice; per 15 minutes	☑
S5151	Unskilled respite care, not hospice; per diem	☑
S5160	Emergency response system; installation and testing	
S5161	Emergency response system; service fee, per month (excludes installation and testing)	☑
S5162	Emergency response system; purchase only	
S5165	Home modifications; per service	

Temporary National Codes (Non-Medicare)

S3854 — S5165

Special Coverage Instructions   Noncovered by Medicare   Carrier Discretion   ☑ Quantity Alert   ● New Code   ○ Recycled/Reinstated   ▲ Revised Code

Temporary National Codes (Non-Medicare)

S5170 — S8430

S5170	Home delivered meals, including preparation; per meal
S5175	Laundry service, external, professional; per order
S5180	Home health respiratory therapy, initial evaluation
S5181	Home health respiratory therapy, NOS, per diem
S5185	Medication reminder service, nonface-to-face; per month ☑
S5190	Wellness assessment, performed by nonphysician
S5199	Personal care item, NOS, each
S5497	Home infusion therapy, catheter care/maintenance, not otherwise classified; includes administrative services, professional pharmacy services, care coordination, and all necessary supplies and equipment (drugs and nursing visits coded separately), per diem ☑
S5498	Home infusion therapy, catheter care/maintenance, simple (single lumen), includes administrative services, professional pharmacy services, care coordination and all necessary supplies and equipment, (drugs and nursing visits coded separately), per diem ☑
S5501	Home infusion therapy, catheter care/maintenance, complex (more than one lumen), includes administrative services, professional pharmacy services, care coordination, and all necessary supplies and equipment (drugs and nursing visits coded separately), per diem ☑
S5502	Home infusion therapy, catheter care/maintenance, implanted access device, includes administrative services, professional pharmacy services, care coordination and all necessary supplies and equipment (drugs and nursing visits coded separately), per diem (use this code for interim maintenance of vascular access not currently in use) ☑
S5517	Home infusion therapy, all supplies necessary for restoration of catheter patency or declotting
S5518	Home infusion therapy, all supplies necessary for catheter repair
S5520	Home infusion therapy, all supplies (including catheter) necessary for a peripherally inserted central venous catheter (PICC) line insertion
S5521	Home infusion therapy, all supplies (including catheter) necessary for a midline catheter insertion
S5522	Home infusion therapy, insertion of peripherally inserted central venous catheter (PICC), nursing services only (no supplies or catheter included)
S5523	Home infusion therapy, insertion of midline venous catheter, nursing services only (no supplies or catheter included)
S5550	Insulin, rapid onset, 5 units ☑
S5551	Insulin, most rapid onset (Lispro or Aspart); 5 units ☑
S5552	Insulin, intermediate acting (NPH or LENTE); 5 units ☑
S5553	Insulin, long acting; 5 units ☑ CMS: 100-02,15,50.5
S5560	Insulin delivery device, reusable pen; 1.5 ml size ☑
S5561	Insulin delivery device, reusable pen; 3 ml size ☑
S5565	Insulin cartridge for use in insulin delivery device other than pump; 150 units ☑
S5566	Insulin cartridge for use in insulin delivery device other than pump; 300 units ☑
S5570	Insulin delivery device, disposable pen (including insulin); 1.5 ml size ☑ CMS: 100-02,15,50.5
S5571	Insulin delivery device, disposable pen (including insulin); 3 ml size ☑ CMS: 100-02,15,50.5
S8030	Scleral application of tantalum ring(s) for localization of lesions for proton beam therapy
S8035	Magnetic source imaging
S8037	Magnetic resonance cholangiopancreatography (MRCP)
S8040	Topographic brain mapping
S8042	Magnetic resonance imaging (MRI), low-field
S8055	Ultrasound guidance for multifetal pregnancy reduction(s), technical component (only to be used when the physician doing the reduction procedure does not perform the ultrasound, guidance is included in the CPT code for multifetal pregnancy reduction (59866) Ⓜ ♀
S8080	Scintimammography (radioimmunoscintigraphy of the breast), unilateral, including supply of radiopharmaceutical
S8085	Fluorine-18 fluorodeoxyglucose (F-18 FDG) imaging using dual-head coincidence detection system (nondedicated PET scan)
S8092	Electron beam computed tomography (also known as ultrafast CT, cine CT)
S8096	Portable peak flow meter
S8097	Asthma kit (including but not limited to portable peak expiratory flow meter, instructional video, brochure, and/or spacer) ☑
S8100	Holding chamber or spacer for use with an inhaler or nebulizer; without mask
S8101	Holding chamber or spacer for use with an inhaler or nebulizer; with mask
S8110	Peak expiratory flow rate (physician services)
S8120	Oxygen contents, gaseous, 1 unit equals 1 cubic foot ☑
S8121	Oxygen contents, liquid, 1 unit equals 1 pound ☑
S8130	Interferential current stimulator, 2 channel
S8131	Interferential current stimulator, 4 channel
S8185	Flutter device
S8186	Swivel adaptor
S8189	Tracheostomy supply, not otherwise classified
S8210	Mucus trap
S8265	Haberman feeder for cleft lip/palate
S8270	Enuresis alarm, using auditory buzzer and/or vibration device
S8301	Infection control supplies, not otherwise specified
S8415	Supplies for home delivery of infant Ⓜ ♀
S8420	Gradient pressure aid (sleeve and glove combination), custom made
S8421	Gradient pressure aid (sleeve and glove combination), ready made
S8422	Gradient pressure aid (sleeve), custom made, medium weight
S8423	Gradient pressure aid (sleeve), custom made, heavy weight
S8424	Gradient pressure aid (sleeve), ready made
S8425	Gradient pressure aid (glove), custom made, medium weight
S8426	Gradient pressure aid (glove), custom made, heavy weight
S8427	Gradient pressure aid (glove), ready made
S8428	Gradient pressure aid (gauntlet), ready made
S8429	Gradient pressure exterior wrap
S8430	Padding for compression bandage, roll ☑

Special Coverage Instructions   Noncovered by Medicare   Carrier Discretion   ☑ Quantity Alert   ● New Code   ○ Recycled/Reinstated   ▲ Revised Code

S8431   Compression bandage, roll ☑

S8450   Splint, prefabricated, digit (specify digit by use of modifier) ☑

Various types of digit splints (S8450)

Static finger splint

Mobile dorsal splint

Slip-on splint

S8451   Splint, prefabricated, wrist or ankle ☑

S8452   Splint, prefabricated, elbow ☑

S8460   Camisole, postmastectomy

S8490   Insulin syringes (100 syringes, any size) ☑

S8930   Electrical stimulation of auricular acupuncture points; each 15 minutes of personal one-on-one contact with patient ☑

S8940   Equestrian/hippotherapy, per session

S8948   Application of a modality (requiring constant provider attendance) to one or more areas; low-level laser; each 15 minutes ☑

S8950   Complex lymphedema therapy, each 15 minutes ☑

S8990   Physical or manipulative therapy performed for maintenance rather than restoration

S8999   Resuscitation bag (for use by patient on artificial respiration during power failure or other catastrophic event)

S9001   Home uterine monitor with or without associated nursing services Ⓜ ♀

S9007   Ultrafiltration monitor

S9024   Paranasal sinus ultrasound

S9025   Omnicardiogram/cardiointegram

S9034   Extracorporeal shockwave lithotripsy for gall stones (if performed with ERCP, use 43265)

S9055   Procuren or other growth factor preparation to promote wound healing

S9056   Coma stimulation per diem ☑

S9061   Home administration of aerosolized drug therapy (e.g., Pentamidine); administrative services, professional pharmacy services, care coordination, all necessary supplies and equipment (drugs and nursing visits coded separately), per diem ☑

S9083   Global fee urgent care centers

S9088   Services provided in an urgent care center (list in addition to code for service)

S9090   Vertebral axial decompression, per session ☑

S9097   Home visit for wound care

S9098   Home visit, phototherapy services (e.g., Bili-lite), including equipment rental, nursing services, blood draw, supplies, and other services, per diem ☑

S9110   Telemonitoring of patient in their home, including all necessary equipment; computer system, connections, and software; maintenance; patient education and support; per month

S9117   Back school, per visit ☑

S9122   Home health aide or certified nurse assistant, providing care in the home; per hour ☑

S9123   Nursing care, in the home; by registered nurse, per hour (use for general nursing care only, not to be used when CPT codes 99500-99602 can be used) ☑

S9124   Nursing care, in the home; by licensed practical nurse, per hour ☑

S9125   Respite care, in the home, per diem ☑

S9126   Hospice care, in the home, per diem ☑
       CMS: 100-04,11,10

S9127   Social work visit, in the home, per diem ☑

S9128   Speech therapy, in the home, per diem ☑

S9129   Occupational therapy, in the home, per diem ☑

S9131   Physical therapy; in the home, per diem ☑

S9140   Diabetic management program, follow-up visit to non-MD provider ☑

S9141   Diabetic management program, follow-up visit to MD provider ☑

S9145   Insulin pump initiation, instruction in initial use of pump (pump not included)

S9150   Evaluation by ocularist

S9152   Speech therapy, re-evaluation

S9208   Home management of preterm labor, including administrative services, professional pharmacy services, care coordination, and all necessary supplies or equipment (drugs and nursing visits coded separately), per diem (do not use this code with any home infusion per diem code) Ⓜ ♀ ☑

S9209   Home management of preterm premature rupture of membranes (PPROM), including administrative services, professional pharmacy services, care coordination, and all necessary supplies or equipment (drugs and nursing visits coded separately), per diem (do not use this code with any home infusion per diem code) Ⓜ ♀ ☑

S9211   Home management of gestational hypertension, includes administrative services, professional pharmacy services, care coordination and all necessary supplies and equipment (drugs and nursing visits coded separately); per diem (do not use this code with any home infusion per diem code) Ⓜ ♀ ☑

☐ Special Coverage Instructions   ☐ Noncovered by Medicare   ☐ Carrier Discretion   ☑ Quantity Alert   ● New Code   ○ Recycled/Reinstated   ▲ Revised Code

S9212 Home management of postpartum hypertension, includes administrative services, professional pharmacy services, care coordination, and all necessary supplies and equipment (drugs and nursing visits coded separately), per diem (do not use this code with any home infusion per diem code) ♀ ☑

S9213 Home management of preeclampsia, includes administrative services, professional pharmacy services, care coordination, and all necessary supplies and equipment (drugs and nursing services coded separately); per diem (do not use this code with any home infusion per diem code) Ⓜ ♀ ☑

S9214 Home management of gestational diabetes, includes administrative services, professional pharmacy services, care coordination, and all necessary supplies and equipment (drugs and nursing visits coded separately); per diem (do not use this code with any home infusion per diem code) Ⓜ ♀ ☑

S9325 Home infusion therapy, pain management infusion; administrative services, professional pharmacy services, care coordination, and all necessary supplies and equipment, (drugs and nursing visits coded separately), per diem (do not use this code with S9326, S9327 or S9328) ☑

S9326 Home infusion therapy, continuous (24 hours or more) pain management infusion; administrative services, professional pharmacy services, care coordination and all necessary supplies and equipment (drugs and nursing visits coded separately), per diem ☑

S9327 Home infusion therapy, intermittent (less than 24 hours) pain management infusion; administrative services, professional pharmacy services, care coordination, and all necessary supplies and equipment (drugs and nursing visits coded separately), per diem ☑

S9328 Home infusion therapy, implanted pump pain management infusion; administrative services, professional pharmacy services, care coordination, and all necessary supplies and equipment (drugs and nursing visits coded separately), per diem ☑

S9329 Home infusion therapy, chemotherapy infusion; administrative services, professional pharmacy services, care coordination, and all necessary supplies and equipment (drugs and nursing visits coded separately), per diem (do not use this code with S9330 or S9331) ☑

S9330 Home infusion therapy, continuous (24 hours or more) chemotherapy infusion; administrative services, professional pharmacy services, care coordination, and all necessary supplies and equipment (drugs and nursing visits coded separately), per diem ☑

S9331 Home infusion therapy, intermittent (less than 24 hours) chemotherapy infusion; administrative services, professional pharmacy services, care coordination, and all necessary supplies and equipment (drugs and nursing visits coded separately), per diem ☑

S9335 Home therapy, hemodialysis; administrative services, professional pharmacy services, care coordination, and all necessary supplies and equipment (drugs and nursing services coded separately), per diem ☑

S9336 Home infusion therapy, continuous anticoagulant infusion therapy (e.g., Heparin), administrative services, professional pharmacy services, care coordination and all necessary supplies and equipment (drugs and nursing visits coded separately), per diem ☑

S9338 Home infusion therapy, immunotherapy, administrative services, professional pharmacy services, care coordination, and all necessary supplies and equipment (drugs and nursing visits coded separately), per diem ☑

S9339 Home therapy; peritoneal dialysis, administrative services, professional pharmacy services, care coordination and all necessary supplies and equipment (drugs and nursing visits coded separately), per diem ☑

S9340 Home therapy; enteral nutrition; administrative services, professional pharmacy services, care coordination, and all necessary supplies and equipment (enteral formula and nursing visits coded separately), per diem ☑

S9341 Home therapy; enteral nutrition via gravity; administrative services, professional pharmacy services, care coordination, and all necessary supplies and equipment (enteral formula and nursing visits coded separately), per diem ☑

S9342 Home therapy; enteral nutrition via pump; administrative services, professional pharmacy services, care coordination, and all necessary supplies and equipment (enteral formula and nursing visits coded separately), per diem ☑

S9343 Home therapy; enteral nutrition via bolus; administrative services, professional pharmacy services, care coordination, and all necessary supplies and equipment (enteral formula and nursing visits coded separately), per diem ☑

S9345 Home infusion therapy, antihemophilic agent infusion therapy (e.g., Factor VIII); administrative services, professional pharmacy services, care coordination, and all necessary supplies and equipment (drugs and nursing visits coded separately), per diem ☑

S9346 Home infusion therapy, alpha-1-proteinase inhibitor (e.g., Prolastin); administrative services, professional pharmacy services, care coordination, and all necessary supplies and equipment (drugs and nursing visits coded separately), per diem ☑

S9347 Home infusion therapy, uninterrupted, long-term, controlled rate intravenous or subcutaneous infusion therapy (e.g., epoprostenol); administrative services, professional pharmacy services, care coordination, and all necessary supplies and equipment (drugs and nursing visits coded separately), per diem ☑

S9348 Home infusion therapy, sympathomimetic/inotropic agent infusion therapy (e.g., Dobutamine); administrative services, professional pharmacy services, care coordination, all necessary supplies and equipment (drugs and nursing visits coded separately), per diem ☑

S9349 Home infusion therapy, tocolytic infusion therapy; administrative services, professional pharmacy services, care coordination, and all necessary supplies and equipment (drugs and nursing visits coded separately), per diem Ⓜ ♀ ☑

S9351 Home infusion therapy, continuous or intermittent antiemetic infusion therapy; administrative services, professional pharmacy services, care coordination, and all necessary supplies and equipment (drugs and visits coded separately), per diem ☑

S9353 Home infusion therapy, continuous insulin infusion therapy; administrative services, professional pharmacy services, care coordination, and all necessary supplies and equipment (drugs and nursing visits coded separately), per diem ☑

S9355 Home infusion therapy, chelation therapy; administrative services, professional pharmacy services, care coordination, and all necessary supplies and equipment (drugs and nursing visits coded separately), per diem ☑

S9357 Home infusion therapy, enzyme replacement intravenous therapy; (e.g., Imiglucerase); administrative services, professional pharmacy services, care coordination, and all necessary supplies and equipment (drugs and nursing visits coded separately), per diem ☑

Special Coverage Instructions Noncovered by Medicare Carrier Discretion ☑ Quantity Alert ● New Code ○ Recycled/Reinstated ▲ Revised Code

180 — S Codes Ⓐ Age Edit Ⓜ Maternity Edit ♀ Female Only ♂ Male Only Ⓐ-Ⓨ OPPS Status Indicators © 2023 Optum360, LLC

S9359 Home infusion therapy, antitumor necrosis factor intravenous therapy; (e.g., Infliximab); administrative services, professional pharmacy services, care coordination, and all necessary supplies and equipment (drugs and nursing visits coded separately), per diem ☑

S9361 Home infusion therapy, diuretic intravenous therapy; administrative services, professional pharmacy services, care coordination, and all necessary supplies and equipment (drugs and nursing visits coded separately), per diem ☑

S9363 Home infusion therapy, antispasmotic therapy; administrative services, professional pharmacy services, care coordination, and all necessary supplies and equipment (drugs and nursing visits coded separately), per diem ☑

S9364 Home infusion therapy, total parenteral nutrition (TPN); administrative services, professional pharmacy services, care coordination, and all necessary supplies and equipment including standard TPN formula (lipids, specialty amino acid formulas, drugs other than in standard formula and nursing visits coded separately), per diem (do not use with home infusion codes S9365-S9368 using daily volume scales) ☑

S9365 Home infusion therapy, total parenteral nutrition (TPN); one liter per day, administrative services, professional pharmacy services, care coordination, and all necessary supplies and equipment including standard TPN formula (lipids, specialty amino acid formulas, drugs other than in standard formula and nursing visits coded separately), per diem ☑

S9366 Home infusion therapy, total parenteral nutrition (TPN); more than one liter but no more than two liters per day, administrative services, professional pharmacy services, care coordination, and all necessary supplies and equipment including standard TPN formula (lipids, specialty amino acid formulas, drugs other than in standard formula and nursing visits coded separately), per diem ☑

S9367 Home infusion therapy, total parenteral nutrition (TPN); more than two liters but no more than three liters per day, administrative services, professional pharmacy services, care coordination, and all necessary supplies and equipment including standard TPN formula (lipids, specialty amino acid formulas, drugs other than in standard formula and nursing visits coded separately), per diem ☑

S9368 Home infusion therapy, total parenteral nutrition (TPN); more than three liters per day, administrative services, professional pharmacy services, care coordination, and all necessary supplies and equipment including standard TPN formula (lipids, specialty amino acid formulas, drugs other than in standard formula and nursing visits coded separately), per diem ☑

S9370 Home therapy, intermittent antiemetic injection therapy; administrative services, professional pharmacy services, care coordination, and all necessary supplies and equipment (drugs and nursing visits coded separately), per diem ☑

S9372 Home therapy; intermittent anticoagulant injection therapy (e.g., Heparin); administrative services, professional pharmacy services, care coordination, and all necessary supplies and equipment (drugs and nursing visits coded separately), per diem (do not use this code for flushing of infusion devices with Heparin to maintain patency) ☑

S9373 Home infusion therapy, hydration therapy; administrative services, professional pharmacy services, care coordination, and all necessary supplies and equipment (drugs and nursing visits coded separately), per diem (do not use with hydration therapy codes S9374-S9377 using daily volume scales) ☑

S9374 Home infusion therapy, hydration therapy; 1 liter per day, administrative services, professional pharmacy services, care coordination, and all necessary supplies and equipment (drugs and nursing visits coded separately), per diem ☑

S9375 Home infusion therapy, hydration therapy; more than 1 liter but no more than 2 liters per day, administrative services, professional pharmacy services, care coordination, and all necessary supplies and equipment (drugs and nursing visits coded separately), per diem ☑

S9376 Home infusion therapy, hydration therapy; more than 2 liters but no more than 3 liters per day, administrative services, professional pharmacy services, care coordination, and all necessary supplies and equipment (drugs and nursing visits coded separately), per diem ☑

S9377 Home infusion therapy, hydration therapy; more than 3 liters per day, administrative services, professional pharmacy services, care coordination, and all necessary supplies (drugs and nursing visits coded separately), per diem ☑

S9379 Home infusion therapy, infusion therapy, not otherwise classified; administrative services, professional pharmacy services, care coordination, and all necessary supplies and equipment (drugs and nursing visits coded separately), per diem ☑

S9381 Delivery or service to high risk areas requiring escort or extra protection, per visit

S9401 Anticoagulation clinic, inclusive of all services except laboratory tests, per session

S9430 Pharmacy compounding and dispensing services

S9432 Medical foods for noninborn errors of metabolism

S9433 Medical food nutritionally complete, administered orally, providing 100% of nutritional intake

S9434 Modified solid food supplements for inborn errors of metabolism

S9435 Medical foods for inborn errors of metabolism

S9436 Childbirth preparation/Lamaze classes, nonphysician provider, per session Ⓜ ♀ ☑

S9437 Childbirth refresher classes, nonphysician provider, per session Ⓜ ♀

S9438 Cesarean birth classes, nonphysician provider, per session Ⓜ ♀ ☑

S9439 VBAC (vaginal birth after cesarean) classes, nonphysician provider, per session Ⓜ ♀ ☑

S9441 Asthma education, nonphysician provider, per session ☑

S9442 Birthing classes, nonphysician provider, per session Ⓜ ♀ ☑

S9443 Lactation classes, nonphysician provider, per session Ⓜ ♀ ☑

S9444 Parenting classes, nonphysician provider, per session ☑

S9445 Patient education, not otherwise classified, nonphysician provider, individual, per session ☑

S9446 Patient education, not otherwise classified, nonphysician provider, group, per session ☑

S9447 Infant safety (including CPR) classes, nonphysician provider, per session ☑

S9449 Weight management classes, nonphysician provider, per session ☑

S9451 Exercise classes, nonphysician provider, per session

S9452 Nutrition classes, nonphysician provider, per session

S9453 Smoking cessation classes, nonphysician provider, per session

---

Special Coverage Instructions   Noncovered by Medicare   Carrier Discretion   ☑ Quantity Alert   ● New Code   ○ Recycled/Reinstated   ▲ Revised Code

S9454	Stress management classes, nonphysician provider, per session
S9455	Diabetic management program, group session
S9460	Diabetic management program, nurse visit
S9465	Diabetic management program, dietitian visit
S9470	Nutritional counseling, dietitian visit
S9472	Cardiac rehabilitation program, nonphysician provider, per diem
S9473	Pulmonary rehabilitation program, nonphysician provider, per diem
S9474	Enterostomal therapy by a registered nurse certified in enterostomal therapy, per diem
S9475	Ambulatory setting substance abuse treatment or detoxification services, per diem
S9476	Vestibular rehabilitation program, nonphysician provider, per diem
S9480	Intensive outpatient psychiatric services, per diem
S9482	Family stabilization services, per 15 minutes ☑
S9484	Crisis intervention mental health services, per hour ☑
S9485	Crisis intervention mental health services, per diem
S9490	Home infusion therapy, corticosteroid infusion; administrative services, professional pharmacy services, care coordination, and all necessary supplies and equipment (drugs and nursing visits coded separately), per diem ☑
S9494	Home infusion therapy, antibiotic, antiviral, or antifungal therapy; administrative services, professional pharmacy services, care coordination, and all necessary supplies and equipment (drugs and nursing visits coded separately), per diem (do not use this code with home infusion codes for hourly dosing schedules S9497-S9504) ☑
S9497	Home infusion therapy, antibiotic, antiviral, or antifungal therapy; once every 3 hours; administrative services, professional pharmacy services, care coordination, and all necessary supplies and equipment (drugs and nursing visits coded separately), per diem ☑
S9500	Home infusion therapy, antibiotic, antiviral, or antifungal therapy; once every 24 hours; administrative services, professional pharmacy services, care coordination, and all necessary supplies and equipment (drugs and nursing visits coded separately), per diem ☑
S9501	Home infusion therapy, antibiotic, antiviral, or antifungal therapy; once every 12 hours; administrative services, professional pharmacy services, care coordination, and all necessary supplies and equipment (drugs and nursing visits coded separately), per diem ☑
S9502	Home infusion therapy, antibiotic, antiviral, or antifungal therapy; once every 8 hours, administrative services, professional pharmacy services, care coordination, and all necessary supplies and equipment (drugs and nursing visits coded separately), per diem ☑
S9503	Home infusion therapy, antibiotic, antiviral, or antifungal; once every 6 hours; administrative services, professional pharmacy services, care coordination, and all necessary supplies and equipment (drugs and nursing visits coded separately), per diem ☑
S9504	Home infusion therapy, antibiotic, antiviral, or antifungal; once every 4 hours; administrative services, professional pharmacy services, care coordination, and all necessary supplies and equipment (drugs and nursing visits coded separately), per diem ☑
S9529	Routine venipuncture for collection of specimen(s), single homebound, nursing home, or skilled nursing facility patient ☑
S9537	Home therapy; hematopoietic hormone injection therapy (e.g., erythropoietin, G-CSF, GM-CSF); administrative services, professional pharmacy services, care coordination, and all necessary supplies and equipment (drugs and nursing visits coded separately), per diem ☑
S9538	Home transfusion of blood product(s); administrative services, professional pharmacy services, care coordination and all necessary supplies and equipment (blood products, drugs, and nursing visits coded separately), per diem ☑
S9542	Home injectable therapy, not otherwise classified, including administrative services, professional pharmacy services, care coordination, and all necessary supplies and equipment (drugs and nursing visits coded separately), per diem ☑
S9558	Home injectable therapy; growth hormone, including administrative services, professional pharmacy services, care coordination, and all necessary supplies and equipment (drugs and nursing visits coded separately), per diem ☑
S9559	Home injectable therapy, interferon, including administrative services, professional pharmacy services, care coordination, and all necessary supplies and equipment (drugs and nursing visits coded separately), per diem ☑
S9560	Home injectable therapy; hormonal therapy (e.g., leuprolide, goserelin), including administrative services, professional pharmacy services, care coordination, and all necessary supplies and equipment (drugs and nursing visits coded separately), per diem ☑
▲ S9562	Home injectable therapy, palivizumab or other monoclonal antibody for RSV, including administrative services, professional pharmacy services, care coordination, and all necessary supplies and equipment (drugs and nursing visits coded separately), per diem ☑ AHA: 2Q,23
● S9563	Home injectable therapy, immunotherapy, including administrative services, professional pharmacy services, care coordination, and all necessary supplies and equipment (drugs and nursing visits coded separately), per diem AHA: 2Q,23
S9590	Home therapy, irrigation therapy (e.g., sterile irrigation of an organ or anatomical cavity); including administrative services, professional pharmacy services, care coordination, and all necessary supplies and equipment (drugs and nursing visits coded separately), per diem ☑
S9810	Home therapy; professional pharmacy services for provision of infusion, specialty drug administration, and/or disease state management, not otherwise classified, per hour (do not use this code with any per diem code) ☑
S9900	Services by a Journal-listed Christian Science practitioner for the purpose of healing, per diem
S9901	Services by a Journal-listed Christian Science nurse, per hour
S9960	Ambulance service, conventional air services, nonemergency transport, one way (fixed wing)
S9961	Ambulance service, conventional air service, nonemergency transport, one way (rotary wing)
S9970	Health club membership, annual
S9975	Transplant related lodging, meals and transportation, per diem
S9976	Lodging, per diem, not otherwise classified
S9977	Meals, per diem, not otherwise specified

Special Coverage Instructions   Noncovered by Medicare   Carrier Discretion   ☑ Quantity Alert ● New Code ○ Recycled/Reinstated ▲ Revised Code

182 — S Codes   A Age Edit   M Maternity Edit   ♀ Female Only   ♂ Male Only   A-Y OPPS Status Indicators   © 2023 Optum360, LLC

Code	Description	
S9981	Medical records copying fee, administrative	
S9982	Medical records copying fee, per page	☑
S9986	Not medically necessary service (patient is aware that service not medically necessary)	
S9988	Services provided as part of a Phase I clinical trial	
S9989	Services provided outside of the United States of America (list in addition to code(s) for services(s))	
S9990	Services provided as part of a Phase II clinical trial	
S9991	Services provided as part of a Phase III clinical trial	
S9992	Transportation costs to and from trial location and local transportation costs (e.g., fares for taxicab or bus) for clinical trial participant and one caregiver/companion	
S9994	Lodging costs (e.g., hotel charges) for clinical trial participant and one caregiver/companion	
S9996	Meals for clinical trial participant and one caregiver/companion	
S9999	Sales tax	

Special Coverage Instructions Noncovered by Medicare Carrier Discretion ☑ Quantity Alert ● New Code ○ Recycled/Reinstated ▲ Revised Code

© 2023 Optum360, LLC A2-Z3 ASC Pmt **CMS:** IOM **AHA:** Coding Clinic ♿ DMEPOS Paid ⊘ SNF Excluded **S Codes — 183**

National T Codes Established for State Medicaid Agencies
T1000-T5999

The T codes are designed for use by Medicaid state agencies to establish codes for items for which there are no permanent national codes but for which codes are necessary to administer the Medicaid program (T codes are not accepted by Medicare but can be used by private insurers). This range of codes describes nursing and home health-related services, substance abuse treatment, and certain training-related procedures.

T1000   Private duty/independent nursing service(s), licensed, up to 15 minutes ☑

T1001   Nursing assessment/evaluation

T1002   RN services, up to 15 minutes ☑

T1003   LPN/LVN services, up to 15 minutes ☑

T1004   Services of a qualified nursing aide, up to 15 minutes ☑

T1005   Respite care services, up to 15 minutes ☑

T1006   Alcohol and/or substance abuse services, family/couple counseling

T1007   Alcohol and/or substance abuse services, treatment plan development and/or modification

T1009   Child sitting services for children of the individual receiving alcohol and/or substance abuse services

T1010   Meals for individuals receiving alcohol and/or substance abuse services (when meals not included in the program)

T1012   Alcohol and/or substance abuse services, skills development

T1013   Sign language or oral interpretive services, per 15 minutes ☑

T1014   Telehealth transmission, per minute, professional services bill separately

T1015   Clinic visit/encounter, all-inclusive

T1016   Case management, each 15 minutes ▣

T1017   Targeted case management, each 15 minutes ☑

T1018   School-based individualized education program (IEP) services, bundled

T1019   Personal care services, per 15 minutes, not for an inpatient or resident of a hospital, nursing facility, ICF/MR or IMD, part of the individualized plan of treatment (code may not be used to identify services provided by home health aide or certified nurse assistant) ☑

T1020   Personal care services, per diem, not for an inpatient or resident of a hospital, nursing facility, ICF/MR or IMD, part of the individualized plan of treatment (code may not be used to identify services provided by home health aide or certified nurse assistant)

T1021   Home health aide or certified nurse assistant, per visit

T1022   Contracted home health agency services, all services provided under contract, per day

T1023   Screening to determine the appropriateness of consideration of an individual for participation in a specified program, project or treatment protocol, per encounter

T1024   Evaluation and treatment by an integrated, specialty team contracted to provide coordinated care to multiple or severely handicapped children, per encounter Ⓐ

T1025   Intensive, extended multidisciplinary services provided in a clinic setting to children with complex medical, physical, mental and psychosocial impairments, per diem Ⓐ

▲ T1026   Intensive, extended multidisciplinary services provided in a clinic setting to children with complex medical, physical, mental, and psychosocial impairments, per hour Ⓐ

T1027   Family training and counseling for child development, per 15 minutes ☑

T1028   Assessment of home, physical and family environment, to determine suitability to meet patient's medical needs

T1029   Comprehensive environmental lead investigation, not including laboratory analysis, per dwelling

T1030   Nursing care, in the home, by registered nurse, per diem ☑

T1031   Nursing care, in the home, by licensed practical nurse, per diem ☑

T1032   Services performed by a doula birth worker, per 15 minutes
AHA: 4Q,22

T1033   Services performed by a doula birth worker, per diem
AHA: 4Q,22

T1040   Medicaid certified community behavioral health clinic services, per diem

T1041   Medicaid certified community behavioral health clinic services, per month

T1502   Administration of oral, intramuscular and/or subcutaneous medication by health care agency/professional, per visit ☑

T1503   Administration of medication, other than oral and/or injectable, by a health care agency/professional, per visit ☑

T1505   Electronic medication compliance management device, includes all components and accessories, not otherwise classified

T1999   Miscellaneous therapeutic items and supplies, retail purchases, not otherwise classified; identify product in "remarks"

T2001   Nonemergency transportation; patient attendant/escort

T2002   Nonemergency transportation; per diem ☑

T2003   Nonemergency transportation; encounter/trip

T2004   Nonemergency transport; commercial carrier, multipass

T2005   Nonemergency transportation; stretcher van

T2007   Transportation waiting time, air ambulance and nonemergency vehicle, one-half (1/2) hour increments ☑

T2010   Preadmission screening and resident review (PASRR) Level I identification screening, per screen ☑

T2011   Preadmission screening and resident review (PASRR) Level II evaluation, per evaluation

T2012   Habilitation, educational; waiver, per diem ☑

T2013   Habilitation, educational, waiver; per hour ☑

T2014   Habilitation, prevocational, waiver; per diem ☑

T2015   Habilitation, prevocational, waiver; per hour ☑

T2016   Habilitation, residential, waiver; per diem ☑

T2017   Habilitation, residential, waiver; 15 minutes ☑

T2018   Habilitation, supported employment, waiver; per diem ☑

T2019   Habilitation, supported employment, waiver; per 15 minutes ☑

T2020   Day habilitation, waiver; per diem ☑

T2021   Day habilitation, waiver; per 15 minutes ☑

T2022   Case management, per month ☑

T2023   Targeted case management; per month ☑

T2024   Service assessment/plan of care development, waiver

T2025   Waiver services; not otherwise specified (NOS)

T2026   Specialized childcare, waiver; per diem ☑

T2027   Specialized childcare, waiver; per 15 minutes ☑

Special Coverage Instructions   Noncovered by Medicare   Carrier Discretion   ☑ Quantity Alert   ● New Code   ○ Recycled/Reinstated   ▲ Revised Code

© 2023 Optum360, LLC   A2-Z3 ASC Pmt   **CMS:** IOM   **AHA:** Coding Clinic   ♿ DMEPOS Paid   ⊘ SNF Excluded   **T Codes — 185**

National T Codes

T2028 — T5999

Code	Description	
T2028	Specialized supply, not otherwise specified, waiver	
T2029	Specialized medical equipment, not otherwise specified, waiver	
T2030	Assisted living, waiver; per month	☑
T2031	Assisted living; waiver, per diem	☑
T2032	Residential care, not otherwise specified (NOS), waiver; per month	☑
T2033	Residential care, not otherwise specified (NOS), waiver; per diem	☑
T2034	Crisis intervention, waiver; per diem	☑
T2035	Utility services to support medical equipment and assistive technology/devices, waiver	
T2036	Therapeutic camping, overnight, waiver; each session	☑
T2037	Therapeutic camping, day, waiver; each session	☑
T2038	Community transition, waiver; per service	☑
T2039	Vehicle modifications, waiver; per service	☑
T2040	Financial management, self-directed, waiver; per 15 minutes	☑
T2041	Supports brokerage, self-directed, waiver; per 15 minutes	☑
T2042	Hospice routine home care; per diem CMS: 100-04,11,10	☑
T2043	Hospice continuous home care; per hour CMS: 100-04,11,10	☑
T2044	Hospice inpatient respite care; per diem CMS: 100-04,11,10	☑
T2045	Hospice general inpatient care; per diem CMS: 100-04,11,10	☑
T2046	Hospice long-term care, room and board only; per diem CMS: 100-04,11,10	☑
T2047	Habilitation, prevocational, waiver; per 15 minutes	
T2048	Behavioral health; long-term care residential (nonacute care in a residential treatment program where stay is typically longer than 30 days), with room and board, per diem	☑
T2049	Nonemergency transportation; stretcher van, mileage; per mile	☑
T2050	Financial management, self-directed, waiver; per diem	
T2051	Supports brokerage, self-directed, waiver; per diem	
T2101	Human breast milk processing, storage and distribution only	♀
T4521	Adult sized disposable incontinence product, brief/diaper, small, each	☑
T4522	Adult sized disposable incontinence product, brief/diaper, medium, each	☑
T4523	Adult sized disposable incontinence product, brief/diaper, large, each	☑
T4524	Adult sized disposable incontinence product, brief/diaper, extra large, each	☑
T4525	Adult sized disposable incontinence product, protective underwear/pull-on, small size, each	☑
T4526	Adult sized disposable incontinence product, protective underwear/pull-on, medium size, each	☑
T4527	Adult sized disposable incontinence product, protective underwear/pull-on, large size, each	☑

Code	Description	
T4528	Adult sized disposable incontinence product, protective underwear/pull-on, extra large size, each	☑
T4529	Pediatric sized disposable incontinence product, brief/diaper, small/medium size, each	☑
T4530	Pediatric sized disposable incontinence product, brief/diaper, large size, each	☑
T4531	Pediatric sized disposable incontinence product, protective underwear/pull-on, small/medium size, each	☑
T4532	Pediatric sized disposable incontinence product, protective underwear/pull-on, large size, each	☑
T4533	Youth sized disposable incontinence product, brief/diaper, each	☑
T4534	Youth sized disposable incontinence product, protective underwear/pull-on, each	☑
T4535	Disposable liner/shield/guard/pad/undergarment, for incontinence, each	☑
T4536	Incontinence product, protective underwear/pull-on, reusable, any size, each	☑
T4537	Incontinence product, protective underpad, reusable, bed size, each	☑
T4538	Diaper service, reusable diaper, each diaper	☑
T4539	Incontinence product, diaper/brief, reusable, any size, each	☑
T4540	Incontinence product, protective underpad, reusable, chair size, each	☑
T4541	Incontinence product, disposable underpad, large, each	☑
T4542	Incontinence product, disposable underpad, small size, each	☑
T4543	Adult sized disposable incontinence product, protective brief/diaper, above extra large, each	☑
T4544	Adult sized disposable incontinence product, protective underwear/pull-on, above extra large, each	
T4545	Incontinence product, disposable, penile wrap, each	
T5001	Positioning seat for persons with special orthopedic needs	
T5999	Supply, not otherwise specified	

Special Coverage Instructions   Noncovered by Medicare   Carrier Discretion   ☑ Quantity Alert ● New Code   ○ Recycled/Reinstated   ▲ Revised Code

186 — T Codes   🅐 Age Edit   🅜 Maternity Edit   ♀ Female Only   ♂ Male Only   🅐-🅨 OPPS Status Indicators   © 2023 Optum360, LLC

Coronavirus Services U0001-U0005

U0001   **CDC 2019 Novel Coronavirus (2019-nCoV) Real-Time RT-PCR Diagnostic Panel**
Use this code for CDC created tests.
AHA: 2Q,20

U0002   **2019-nCoV coronavirus, SARS-CoV-2/2019-nCoV (COVID-19), any technique, multiple types or subtypes (includes all targets), non-CDC**
Use this code for non-CDC created tests.
AHA: 2Q,20

U0003   ~~Infectious agent detection by nucleic acid (DNA or RNA); severe acute respiratory syndrome coronavirus 2 (SARS-CoV-2) (coronavirus disease [COVID-19]), amplified probe technique, making use of high throughput technologies as described by CMS-2020-01-R~~

U0004   ~~2019-nCoV coronavirus, SARS-CoV-2/2019-nCoV (COVID-19), any technique, multiple types or subtypes (includes all targets), non-CDC, making use of high throughput technologies as described by CMS-2020-01-R~~

U0005   ~~Infectious agent detection by nucleic acid (DNA or RNA); severe acute respiratory syndrome coronavirus 2 (SARS-CoV-2) (coronavirus disease [COVID-19]), amplified probe technique, CDC or non-CDC, making use of high throughput technologies, completed within 2 calendar days from date of specimen collection (list separately in addition to either HCPCS code U0003 or U0004) as described by CMS-2020-01-R2~~

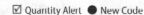

Vision Services V2020-V2799

These V codes include vision-related supplies, including spectacles, lenses, contact lenses, prostheses, intraocular lenses, and miscellaneous lenses.

Frames

V2020 Frames, purchases   A ♿

V2025 Deluxe frame   EI
     CMS: 100-04,1,30.3.5

Single Vision, Glass, or Plastic

V2100 Sphere, single vision, plano to plus or minus 4.00, per lens   A ☑ ♿

Monofocal spectacles
(V2100–V2114)

Trifocal spectacles
(V2300–V2314)

Low vision aids mounted
to spectacles (V2610)

Telescopic or other compound
lens fitted on spectacles
as a low vision aid (V2615)

V2101 Sphere, single vision, plus or minus 4.12 to plus or minus 7.00d, per lens   A ☑ ♿

V2102 Sphere, single vision, plus or minus 7.12 to plus or minus 20.00d, per lens   A ☑ ♿

V2103 Spherocylinder, single vision, plano to plus or minus 4.00d sphere, 0.12 to 2.00d cylinder, per lens   A ☑ ♿

V2104 Spherocylinder, single vision, plano to plus or minus 4.00d sphere, 2.12 to 4.00d cylinder, per lens   A ☑ ♿

V2105 Spherocylinder, single vision, plano to plus or minus 4.00d sphere, 4.25 to 6.00d cylinder, per lens   A ☑ ♿

V2106 Spherocylinder, single vision, plano to plus or minus 4.00d sphere, over 6.00d cylinder, per lens   A ☑ ♿

V2107 Spherocylinder, single vision, plus or minus 4.25 to plus or minus 7.00 sphere, 0.12 to 2.00d cylinder, per lens   A ☑ ♿

V2108 Spherocylinder, single vision, plus or minus 4.25d to plus or minus 7.00d sphere, 2.12 to 4.00d cylinder, per lens   A ☑ ♿

V2109 Spherocylinder, single vision, plus or minus 4.25 to plus or minus 7.00d sphere, 4.25 to 6.00d cylinder, per lens   A ☑ ♿

V2110 Spherocylinder, single vision, plus or minus 4.25 to 7.00d sphere, over 6.00d cylinder, per lens   A ☑ ♿

V2111 Spherocylinder, single vision, plus or minus 7.25 to plus or minus 12.00d sphere, 0.25 to 2.25d cylinder, per lens   A ☑ ♿

V2112 Spherocylinder, single vision, plus or minus 7.25 to plus or minus 12.00d sphere, 2.25 to 4.00d cylinder, per lens   A ☑ ♿

V2113 Spherocylinder, single vision, plus or minus 7.25 to plus or minus 12.00d sphere, 4.25 to 6.00d cylinder, per lens   A ☑ ♿

V2114 Spherocylinder, single vision, sphere over plus or minus 12.00d, per lens   A ☑ ♿

V2115 Lenticular (myodisc), per lens, single vision   A ☑ ♿

V2118 Aniseikonic lens, single vision   A ♿

V2121 Lenticular lens, per lens, single   A ☑ ♿

V2199 Not otherwise classified, single vision lens   A

Bifocal, Glass, or Plastic

V2200 Sphere, bifocal, plano to plus or minus 4.00d, per lens   A ☑ ♿

V2201 Sphere, bifocal, plus or minus 4.12 to plus or minus 7.00d, per lens   A ☑ ♿

V2202 Sphere, bifocal, plus or minus 7.12 to plus or minus 20.00d, per lens   A ☑ ♿

V2203 Spherocylinder, bifocal, plano to plus or minus 4.00d sphere, 0.12 to 2.00d cylinder, per lens   A ☑ ♿

V2204 Spherocylinder, bifocal, plano to plus or minus 4.00d sphere, 2.12 to 4.00d cylinder, per lens   A ☑ ♿

V2205 Spherocylinder, bifocal, plano to plus or minus 4.00d sphere, 4.25 to 6.00d cylinder, per lens   A ☑ ♿

V2206 Spherocylinder, bifocal, plano to plus or minus 4.00d sphere, over 6.00d cylinder, per lens   A ☑ ♿

V2207 Spherocylinder, bifocal, plus or minus 4.25 to plus or minus 7.00d sphere, 0.12 to 2.00d cylinder, per lens   A ☑ ♿

V2208 Spherocylinder, bifocal, plus or minus 4.25 to plus or minus 7.00d sphere, 2.12 to 4.00d cylinder, per lens   A ☑ ♿

V2209 Spherocylinder, bifocal, plus or minus 4.25 to plus or minus 7.00d sphere, 4.25 to 6.00d cylinder, per lens   A ☑ ♿

V2210 Spherocylinder, bifocal, plus or minus 4.25 to plus or minus 7.00d sphere, over 6.00d cylinder, per lens   A ☑ ♿

V2211 Spherocylinder, bifocal, plus or minus 7.25 to plus or minus 12.00d sphere, 0.25 to 2.25d cylinder, per lens   A ☑ ♿

V2212 Spherocylinder, bifocal, plus or minus 7.25 to plus or minus 12.00d sphere, 2.25 to 4.00d cylinder, per lens   A ☑ ♿

V2213 Spherocylinder, bifocal, plus or minus 7.25 to plus or minus 12.00d sphere, 4.25 to 6.00d cylinder, per lens   A ☑ ♿

V2214 Spherocylinder, bifocal, sphere over plus or minus 12.00d, per lens   A ☑ ♿

V2215 Lenticular (myodisc), per lens, bifocal   A ☑ ♿

V2218 Aniseikonic, per lens, bifocal   A ☑ ♿

V2219 Bifocal seg width over 28mm   A ☑ ♿

V2220 Bifocal add over 3.25d   A ☑ ♿

V2221 Lenticular lens, per lens, bifocal   A ♿

V2299 Specialty bifocal (by report)   A
     Pertinent documentation to evaluate medical appropriateness should be included when this code is reported.

Trifocal, Glass, or Plastic

V2300 Sphere, trifocal, plano to plus or minus 4.00d, per lens   A ☑ ♿

V2301 Sphere, trifocal, plus or minus 4.12 to plus or minus 7.00d per lens   A ☑ ♿

V2302 Sphere, trifocal, plus or minus 7.12 to plus or minus 20.00, per lens   A ☑ ♿

V2303 Spherocylinder, trifocal, plano to plus or minus 4.00d sphere, 0.12 to 2.00d cylinder, per lens   A ☑ ♿

V2304 Spherocylinder, trifocal, plano to plus or minus 4.00d sphere, 2.25 to 4.00d cylinder, per lens   A ☑ ♿

V2305 Spherocylinder, trifocal, plano to plus or minus 4.00d sphere, 4.25 to 6.00 cylinder, per lens   A ☑ ♿

Special Coverage Instructions   Noncovered by Medicare   Carrier Discretion   ☑ Quantity Alert   ● New Code   ○ Recycled/Reinstated   ▲ Revised Code

188 — V Codes   A Age Edit   M Maternity Edit   ♀ Female Only   ♂ Male Only   A-Y OPPS Status Indicators   © 2023 Optum360, LLC

V2306	Spherocylinder, trifocal, plano to plus or minus 4.00d sphere, over 6.00d cylinder, per lens	A ☑ ⅙
V2307	Spherocylinder, trifocal, plus or minus 4.25 to plus or minus 7.00d sphere, 0.12 to 2.00d cylinder, per lens	A ☑ ⅙
V2308	Spherocylinder, trifocal, plus or minus 4.25 to plus or minus 7.00d sphere, 2.12 to 4.00d cylinder, per lens	A ☑ ⅙
V2309	Spherocylinder, trifocal, plus or minus 4.25 to plus or minus 7.00d sphere, 4.25 to 6.00d cylinder, per lens	A ☑ ⅙
V2310	Spherocylinder, trifocal, plus or minus 4.25 to plus or minus 7.00d sphere, over 6.00d cylinder, per lens	A ☑ ⅙
V2311	Spherocylinder, trifocal, plus or minus 7.25 to plus or minus 12.00d sphere, 0.25 to 2.25d cylinder, per lens	A ☑ ⅙
V2312	Spherocylinder, trifocal, plus or minus 7.25 to plus or minus 12.00d sphere, 2.25 to 4.00d cylinder, per lens	A ☑ ⅙
V2313	Spherocylinder, trifocal, plus or minus 7.25 to plus or minus 12.00d sphere, 4.25 to 6.00d cylinder, per lens	A ☑ ⅙
V2314	Spherocylinder, trifocal, sphere over plus or minus 12.00d, per lens	A ☑ ⅙
V2315	Lenticular, (myodisc), per lens, trifocal	A ☑ ⅙
V2318	Aniseikonic lens, trifocal	A ⅙
V2319	Trifocal seg width over 28 mm	A ☑ ⅙
V2320	Trifocal add over 3.25d	A ☑ ⅙
V2321	Lenticular lens, per lens, trifocal	A ⅙
V2399	Specialty trifocal (by report)	A
	Pertinent documentation to evaluate medical appropriateness should be included when this code is reported.	

Variable Asphericity Lens, Glass, or Plastic

V2410	Variable asphericity lens, single vision, full field, glass or plastic, per lens	A ☑ ⅙
V2430	Variable asphericity lens, bifocal, full field, glass or plastic, per lens	A ☑ ⅙
V2499	Variable sphericity lens, other type	A

Contact Lens

V2500	Contact lens, PMMA, spherical, per lens	A ☑ ⅙
V2501	Contact lens, PMMA, toric or prism ballast, per lens	A ☑ ⅙
V2502	Contact lens PMMA, bifocal, per lens	A ☑ ⅙
V2503	Contact lens, PMMA, color vision deficiency, per lens	A ☑ ⅙
V2510	Contact lens, gas permeable, spherical, per lens	A ☑ ⅙
V2511	Contact lens, gas permeable, toric, prism ballast, per lens	A ☑ ⅙
V2512	Contact lens, gas permeable, bifocal, per lens	A ☑ ⅙
V2513	Contact lens, gas permeable, extended wear, per lens	A ☑ ⅙
V2520	Contact lens, hydrophilic, spherical, per lens	A ☑ ⅙
	Hydrophilic contact lenses are covered by Medicare only for aphakic patients. Local contractor if incident to physician services.	
V2521	Contact lens, hydrophilic, toric, or prism ballast, per lens	A ☑ ⅙
	Hydrophilic contact lenses are covered by Medicare only for aphakic patients. Local contractor if incident to physician services.	
V2522	Contact lens, hydrophilic, bifocal, per lens	A ☑ ⅙
	Hydrophilic contact lenses are covered by Medicare only for aphakic patients. Local contractor if incident to physician services.	

V2523	Contact lens, hydrophilic, extended wear, per lens	A ☑ ⅙
	Hydrophilic contact lenses are covered by Medicare only for aphakic patients.	
V2524	Contact lens, hydrophilic, spherical, photochromic additive, per lens	
V2525	Contact lens, hydrophilic, dual focus, per lens	
● **V2526**	Contact lens, hydrophilic, with blue-violet filter, per lens	
V2530	Contact lens, scleral, gas impermeable, per lens (for contact lens modification, see 92325)	A ☑ ⅙
V2531	Contact lens, scleral, gas permeable, per lens (for contact lens modification, see 92325)	A ☑ ⅙
V2599	Contact lens, other type	A
	Local contractor if incident to physician services.	

Vision Aids

V2600	Hand held low vision aids and other nonspectacle mounted aids	A
V2610	Single lens spectacle mounted low vision aids	A
V2615	Telescopic and other compound lens system, including distance vision telescopic, near vision telescopes and compound microscopic lens system	A

Prosthetic Eye

V2623	Prosthetic eye, plastic, custom	A ⅙

Implant

One type of eye implant

Reverse angle

Peg

Previously placed prosthetic receptacle

Implant

Peg

Peg hole drilled into prosthetic

Side view

V2624	Polishing/resurfacing of ocular prosthesis	A ⅙
V2625	Enlargement of ocular prosthesis	A ⅙
V2626	Reduction of ocular prosthesis	A ⅙
V2627	Scleral cover shell	A ⅙
	A scleral shell covers the cornea and the anterior sclera. Medicare covers a scleral shell when it is prescribed as an artificial support to a shrunken and sightless eye or as a barrier in the treatment of severe dry eye.	
V2628	Fabrication and fitting of ocular conformer	A ⅙
V2629	Prosthetic eye, other type	A

Special Coverage Instructions   Noncovered by Medicare   Carrier Discretion   ☑ Quantity Alert   ● New Code   ○ Recycled/Reinstated   ▲ Revised Code

© 2023 Optum360, LLC   A2-Z8 ASC Pmt   **CMS:** IOM   **AHA:** Coding Clinic   ⅙ DMEPOS Paid   ⊘ SNF Excluded   **V Codes — 189**

Hearing Services

V2630 — V5242

Intraocular Lenses

V2630 Anterior chamber intraocular lens N M &
The IOL must be FDA-approved for reimbursement. Medicare payment for an IOL is included in the payment for ASC facility services. Medicare jurisdiction: local contractor.

V2631 Iris supported intraocular lens N M &
The IOL must be FDA-approved for reimbursement. Medicare payment for an IOL is included in the payment for ASC facility services. Medicare jurisdiction: local contractor.

V2632 Posterior chamber intraocular lens N M &
The IOL must be FDA-approved for reimbursement. Medicare payment for an IOL is included in the payment for ASC facility services. Medicare jurisdiction: local contractor.
CMS: 100-04,32,120.2

Miscellaneous

V2700 Balance lens, per lens A ☑ &

V2702 Deluxe lens feature EI

V2710 Slab off prism, glass or plastic, per lens A ☑ &

V2715 Prism, per lens A ☑ &

V2718 Press-on lens, Fresnel prism, per lens A ☑ &

V2730 Special base curve, glass or plastic, per lens A ☑ &

V2744 Tint, photochromatic, per lens A ☑ &

V2745 Addition to lens; tint, any color, solid, gradient or equal, excludes photochromatic, any lens material, per lens A ☑ &

V2750 Antireflective coating, per lens A ☑ &

V2755 U-V lens, per lens A ☑ &

V2756 Eye glass case EI

V2760 Scratch resistant coating, per lens EI ☑ &

V2761 Mirror coating, any type, solid, gradient or equal, any lens material, per lens B ☑

V2762 Polarization, any lens material, per lens EI ☑ &

V2770 Occluder lens, per lens A ☑ &

V2780 Oversize lens, per lens A ☑ &

V2781 Progressive lens, per lens B ☑

V2782 Lens, index 1.54 to 1.65 plastic or 1.60 to 1.79 glass, excludes polycarbonate, per lens A ☑ &

V2783 Lens, index greater than or equal to 1.66 plastic or greater than or equal to 1.80 glass, excludes polycarbonate, per lens A ☑ &

V2784 Lens, polycarbonate or equal, any index, per lens A ☑ &

V2785 Processing, preserving and transporting corneal tissue F F4
Medicare jurisdiction: local contractor.
CMS: 100-04,4,200.1

V2786 Specialty occupational multifocal lens, per lens EI ☑ &

V2787 Astigmatism correcting function of intraocular lens EI
CMS: 100-04,32,120.1; 100-04,32,120.2

V2788 Presbyopia correcting function of intraocular lens EI
CMS: 100-04,32,120.1; 100-04,32,120.2

V2790 Amniotic membrane for surgical reconstruction, per procedure N M
Medicare jurisdiction: local contractor.
CMS: 100-04,4,200.4

V2797 Vision supply, accessory and/or service component of another HCPCS vision code EI

V2799 Vision item or service, miscellaneous A
Determine if an alternative HCPCS Level II or a CPT code better describes the service being reported. This code should be used only if a more specific code is unavailable.

Hearing Services V5008-V5364

This range of codes describes hearing tests and related supplies and equipment, speech-language pathology screenings, and repair of augmentative communicative system.

Hearing Services

V5008 Hearing screening EI

V5010 Assessment for hearing aid EI

V5011 Fitting/orientation/checking of hearing aid EI

V5014 Repair/modification of a hearing aid EI

V5020 Conformity evaluation EI

Monaural Hearing Aid

V5030 Hearing aid, monaural, body worn, air conduction EI

V5040 Hearing aid, monaural, body worn, bone conduction EI

V5050 Hearing aid, monaural, in the ear EI

V5060 Hearing aid, monaural, behind the ear EI

Other Hearing Services

V5070 Glasses, air conduction EI

V5080 Glasses, bone conduction EI

V5090 Dispensing fee, unspecified hearing aid EI

V5095 Semi-implantable middle ear hearing prosthesis EI

V5100 Hearing aid, bilateral, body worn EI

V5110 Dispensing fee, bilateral EI

Hearing Aids, Services, and Accessories

V5120 Binaural, body EI

V5130 Binaural, in the ear EI

V5140 Binaural, behind the ear EI

V5150 Binaural, glasses EI

V5160 Dispensing fee, binaural EI

V5171 Hearing aid, contralateral routing device, monaural, in the ear (ITE) EI

V5172 Hearing aid, contralateral routing device, monaural, in the canal (ITC) EI

V5181 Hearing aid, contralateral routing device, monaural, behind the ear (BTE) EI

V5190 Hearing aid, contralateral routing, monaural, glasses EI

V5200 Dispensing fee, contralateral, monaural EI

V5211 Hearing aid, contralateral routing system, binaural, ITE/ITE EI

V5212 Hearing aid, contralateral routing system, binaural, ITE/ITC EI

V5213 Hearing aid, contralateral routing system, binaural, ITE/BTE EI

V5214 Hearing aid, contralateral routing system, binaural, ITC/ITC EI

V5215 Hearing aid, contralateral routing system, binaural, ITC/BTE EI

V5221 Hearing aid, contralateral routing system, binaural, BTE/BTE EI

V5230 Hearing aid, contralateral routing system, binaural, glasses EI

V5240 Dispensing fee, contralateral routing system, binaural EI

V5241 Dispensing fee, monaural hearing aid, any type EI

V5242 Hearing aid, analog, monaural, CIC (completely in the ear canal) EI

Special Coverage Instructions   Noncovered by Medicare   Carrier Discretion   ☑ Quantity Alert   ● New Code   ○ Recycled/Reinstated   ▲ Revised Code

V5243	Hearing aid, analog, monaural, ITC (in the canal)	EI
V5244	Hearing aid, digitally programmable analog, monaural, CIC	EI
V5245	Hearing aid, digitally programmable, analog, monaural, ITC	FI
V5246	Hearing aid, digitally programmable analog, monaural, ITE (in the ear)	EI
V5247	Hearing aid, digitally programmable analog, monaural, BTE (behind the ear)	EI
V5248	Hearing aid, analog, binaural, CIC	EI
V5249	Hearing aid, analog, binaural, ITC	EI
V5250	Hearing aid, digitally programmable analog, binaural, CIC	EI
V5251	Hearing aid, digitally programmable analog, binaural, ITC	EI
V5252	Hearing aid, digitally programmable, binaural, ITE	EI
V5253	Hearing aid, digitally programmable, binaural, BTE	EI
V5254	Hearing aid, digital, monaural, CIC	EI
V5255	Hearing aid, digital, monaural, ITC	EI
V5256	Hearing aid, digital, monaural, ITE	EI
V5257	Hearing aid, digital, monaural, BTE	EI
V5258	Hearing aid, digital, binaural, CIC	EI
V5259	Hearing aid, digital, binaural, ITC	EI
V5260	Hearing aid, digital, binaural, ITE	EI
V5261	Hearing aid, digital, binaural, BTE	EI
V5262	Hearing aid, disposable, any type, monaural	EI
V5263	Hearing aid, disposable, any type, binaural	EI
V5264	Ear mold/insert, not disposable, any type	EI
V5265	Ear mold/insert, disposable, any type	EI
V5266	Battery for use in hearing device	FI
V5267	Hearing aid or assistive listening device/supplies/accessories, not otherwise specified	EI

Assistive Listening Device

V5268	Assistive listening device, telephone amplifier, any type	CI
V5269	Assistive listening device, alerting, any type	EI
V5270	Assistive listening device, television amplifier, any type	EI
V5271	Assistive listening device, television caption decoder	EI
V5272	Assistive listening device, TDD	EI
V5273	Assistive listening device, for use with cochlear implant	EI
V5274	Assistive listening device, not otherwise specified	EI

Miscellaneous Hearing Services

V5275	Ear impression, each	EI ☑
V5281	Assistive listening device, personal FM/DM system, monaural (1 receiver, transmitter, microphone), any type	EI
V5282	Assistive listening device, personal FM/DM system, binaural (2 receivers, transmitter, microphone), any type	EI
V5283	Assistive listening device, personal FM/DM neck, loop induction receiver	EI
V5284	Assistive listening device, personal FM/DM, ear level receiver	EI
V5285	Assistive listening device, personal FM/DM, direct audio input receiver	EI

V5286	Assistive listening device, personal blue tooth FM/DM receiver	EI
V5287	Assistive listening device, personal FM/DM receiver, not otherwise specified	EI
V5288	Assistive listening device, personal FM/DM transmitter assistive listening device	EI
V5289	Assistive listening device, personal FM/DM adapter/boot coupling device for receiver, any type	EI
V5290	Assistive listening device, transmitter microphone, any type	EI
V5298	Hearing aid, not otherwise classified	EI
V5299	Hearing service, miscellaneous	B ⊘

V5299 Determine if an alternative HCPCS Level II or a CPT code better describes the service being reported. This code should be used only if a more specific code is unavailable.

Speech-Language Pathology Services

V5336	Repair/modification of augmentative communicative system or device (excludes adaptive hearing aid)	EI

V5336 Medicare jurisdiction: DME regional contractor.

V5362	Speech screening	EI
V5363	Language screening	EI
V5364	Dysphagia screening	EI

Special Coverage Instructions   Noncovered by Medicare   Carrier Discretion   ☑ Quantity Alert   ● New Code   ○ Recycled/Reinstated   ▲ Revised Code

© 2023 Optum360, LLC   A2-Z3 ASC Pmt   **CMS:** IOM   **AHA:** Coding Clinic   & DMEPOS Paid   ⊘ SNF Excluded   **V Codes — 191**

Appendix 1 — Table of Drugs and Biologicals

INTRODUCTION AND DIRECTIONS

The HCPCS 2024 Table of Drugs and Biologicals is designed to quickly and easily direct the user to drug names and their corresponding codes. Both generic and brand or trade names are alphabetically listed in the "Drug Name" column of the table. The associated A, C, J, K, Q, or S code is given only for the generic name of the drug. While every effort is made to make the table comprehensive, it is not all-inclusive.

The "Unit Per" column lists the stated amount for the referenced generic drug as provided by CMS. "Up to" listings are inclusive of all quantities up to and including the listed amount. All other listings are for the amount of the drug as listed. The editors recognize that the availability of some drugs in the quantities listed is dependent on many variables beyond the control of the clinical ordering clerk. The availability in your area of regularly used drugs in the most cost-effective quantities should be relayed to your third-party payers.

The "Route of Administration" column addresses the most common methods of delivering the referenced generic drug as described in current pharmaceutical literature. The official definitions for Level II drug codes generally describe administration other than by oral method. Therefore, with a handful of exceptions, oral-delivered options for most drugs are omitted from the Route of Administration column.

Intravenous administration includes all methods, such as gravity infusion, injections, and timed pushes. When several routes of administration are listed, the first listing is simply the first, or most common, method as described in current reference literature. The "VAR" posting denotes various routes of administration and is used for drugs that are commonly administered into joints, cavities, tissues, or topical applications, in addition to other parenteral administrations. Listings posted with "OTH" alert the user to other administration methods, such as suppositories or catheter injections.

Please be reminded that the Table of Drugs and Biologicals, as well as all HCPCS Level II national definitions and listings, constitutes a post-treatment medical reference for billing purposes only. Although the editors have exercised all normal precautions to ensure the accuracy of the table and related material, the use of any of this information to select medical treatment is entirely inappropriate. Do not code directly from the table. Refer to the tabular section for complete information.

See Appendix 3 for abbreviations.

Drug Name	Units Per	Route	Code
10% LMD	500 ML	IV	J7100
5% DEXTROSE AND .45% NORMAL SALINE	1000 ML	IV	S5010
5% DEXTROSE IN LACTATED RINGERS	1000 CC	IV	J7121
5% DEXTROSE WITH POTASSIUM CHLORIDE	1000 ML	IV	S5012
5% DEXTROSE/.45% NS WITH KCL AND MAG SULFATE	1000ML	IV	S5013
5% DEXTROSE/.45% NS WITH KCL AND MAG SULFATE	1500 ML	IV	S5014
5% DEXTROSE/NORMAL SALINE	5%	VAR	J7042
5% DEXTROSE/WATER	500 ML	IV	J7060
A-HYDROCORT	100 MG	IV, IM, SC	J1720
A-METHAPRED	40 MG	IM, IV	J2920
A-METHAPRED	125 MG	IM, IV	J2930
ABATACEPT	10 MG	IV	J0129
ABCIXIMAB	10 MG	IV	J0130
ABECMA	UP TO 460 MILLION CELLS	IV	Q2055
ABELCET	10 MG	IV	J0287
ABILIFY	0.25 MG	IM	J0400
ABILIFY ASIMTUFII	1 MG	IM	C9152
ABILIFY ASIMTUFII	1 MG	IM	J0402
ABILIFY MAINTENA KIT	1 MG	IM	J0401
ABLAVAR	1 ML	IV	A9583
ABOBOTULINUMTOXINA	5 UNITS	IM	J0586

Drug Name	Units Per	Route	Code
ABRAXANE	1 MG	IV	J9264
ABRILADA	10 MG	SC	Q5132
AC5 ADVANCED WOUND SYSTEM (AC5)	SQ CM	OTH	A2020
ACCELULAR PERICARDIAL TISSUE MATRIX NONHUMAN	SQ CM	OTH	C9354
ACCUNEB NONCOMPOUNDED, CONCENTRATED	1 MG	INH	J7611
ACCUNEB NONCOMPOUNDED, UNIT DOSE	1 MG	INH	J7613
ACESSO DL	SQ CM	OTH	Q4293
ACESSO TL	SQ CM	OTH	Q4300
ACETADOTE	1 G	INH	J7608
ACETADOTE	100 MG	IV	J0132
ACETAMINOPHEN (B. BRAUN), NOT THERAPEUTICALLY EQUIVALENT TO J0131	10 MG	IV	J0136
ACETAMINOPHEN (FRESENIUS KABI), NOT THERAPEUTICALLY EQUIVALENT TO J0131	10 MG	IV	J0134
ACETAMINOPHEN (HIKMA) NOT THERAPEUTICALLY EQUIVALENT TO J0131	10 MG	IV	J0137
ACETAMINOPHEN NOS	10 MG	IV	J0131
ACETAZOLAMIDE SODIUM	500 MG	IM, IV	J1120
ACETYLCYSTEINE COMPOUNDED	PER G	INH	J7604
ACETYLCYSTEINE NONCOMPOUNDED	1 G	INH	J7608
ACTEMRA	1 MG	IV	J3262
ACTEMRA	1 MG	IV	Q0249
ACTHAR GEL	UP TO 40 UNITS	IM/SC	J0801
ACTHAR GEL (ANI)	UP TO 40 UNITS	IM/SC	J0802
ACTHREL	1 MCG	IV	J0795
ACTIMMUNE	3 MU	SC	J9216
ACTIVASE	1 MG	IV	J2997
ACTIVATE MATRIX	SQ CM	OTH	Q4301
ACUTECT	STUDY DOSE UP TO 20 MCI	IV	A9504
ACYCLOVIR	5 MG	IV	J0133
ADAGEN	25 IU	IM	J2504
ADAKVEO	5 MG	IV	J0791
ADALIMUMAB	20 MG	SC	J0135
ADALIMUMAB-AACF, BIOSIMILAR	20 MG	SC	Q5131
ADALIMUMAB-AFZB	10 MG	SC	Q5132
ADASUVE	1 MG	INH	J2062
ADCETRIS	1 MG	IV	J9042
ADENOCARD	1 MG	IV	J0153
ADENOSINE	1 MG	IV	J0153
ADENSOSCAN	1 MG	IV	J0153
ADO-TRASTUZUMAB EMTANSINE	1 MG	IV	J9354
ADRENALIN	0.1 MG	IM, IV, SC	J0171
ADRENOCORT	1 MG	IM, IV, OTH	J1100
ADRIAMYCIN	10 MG	IV	J9000
ADRUCIL	500 MG	IV	J9190
ADSTILADRIN	THERAPEUTIC DOSE	OTH	J9029
ADUCANUMAB-AVWA	2 MG	IV	J0172
ADUHELM	2 MG	IV	J0172
ADYNOVATE	1 IU	IV	J7207
AEROBID	1 MG	INH	J7641

Drug Name	Units Per	Route	Code
AFAMELANOTIDE IMPLANT	1 MG	OTH	J7352
AFFINITY	SQ CM	OTH	Q4159
AFINITOR	0.25 MG	ORAL	J7527
AFLIBERCEPT	1 MG	OTH	J0178
AFLIBERCEPT HD	1 MG	INJ	C9161
AFLURIA	EA	IM	Q2035
AFSTYLA	1 IU	IV	J7210
AGALSIDASE BETA	1 MG	IV	J0180
AGGRASTAT	12.5 MG	IM, IV	J3246
AGRIFLU	UNKNOWN	IM	Q2034
AJOVY	1 MG	SC	J3031
AKYNZEO	300 MG/0.5 MG	ORAL	J8655
AKYNZEO	235 MG/0.25 MG	IV	J1454
ALATROFLOXACIN MESYLATE	100 MG	IV	J0200
ALBUTEROL AND IPRATROPIUM BROMIDE NONCOMPOUNDED	2.5MG/0.5 MG	INH	J7620
ALBUTEROL COMPOUNDED, CONCENTRATED	1 MG	INH	J7610
ALBUTEROL COMPOUNDED, UNIT DOSE	1 MG	INH	J7609
ALBUTEROL NONCOMPOUNDED, UNIT DOSE	1 MG	INH	J7613
ALBUTEROL, NONCOMPOUNDED, CONCENTRATED FORM	1 MG	INH	J7611
ALDESLEUKIN	1 VIAL	IV	J9015
ALDURAZYME	0.1 MG	IV	J1931
ALEFACEPT	0.5 MG	IV, IM	J0215
ALEMTUZUMAB	1 MG	IV	J0202
ALFENTANIL HCL	500 MCG	IV	J0216
ALFERON N	250,000 IU	IM	J9215
ALGLUCERASE	10 U	IV	J0205
ALGLUCOSIDASE ALFA (LUMIZYME)	10 MG	IV	J0221
ALIQOPA	1 MG	IV	J9057
ALKERAN	2 MG	ORAL	J8600
ALLODERM	SQ CM	OTH	Q4116
ALLOGEN	1 CC	OTH	Q4212
ALLOGRAFT, CYMETRA	1 CC	INJ	Q4112
ALLOGRAFT, GRAFTJACKET EXPRESS	1 CC	INJ	Q4113
ALLOPATCHHD	SQ CM	OTH	Q4128
ALLOPURINOL SODIUM	1 MG	IV	J0206
ALLOSKIN	SQ CM	OTH	Q4115
ALLOSKIN AC	SQ CM	OTH	Q4141
ALLOSKIN RT	SQ CM	OTH	Q4123
ALLOWRAP DS OR DRY	SQ CM	OTH	Q4150
ALOXI	25 MCG	IV	J2469
ALPHA 1-PROTENIASE INHIBITOR (HUMAN) (GLASSIA)	10 MG	IV	J0257
ALPHANATE	FACTOR VIII IU	IV	J7186
ALPHANINE SD	1 IU	IV	J7193
ALPROLIX	IU	IV	J7201
ALPROSTADIL	1.25 MCG	IV	J0270
ALPROSTADIL	EA	OTH	J0275
ALTEPLASE RECOMBINANT	1 MG	IV	J2997
ALTIPLY	SQ CM	OTH	Q4235
ALTUVIIIO	IU	IV	J7214
ALUPENT, NONCOMPOUNDED, CONCENTRATED	10 MG	INH	J7668
ALUPENT, NONCOMPOUNDED, UNIT DOSE	10 MG	INH	J7669
ALYMSYS	10 MG	IV	Q5126

Drug Name	Units Per	Route	Code
AMANTADINE HCL (DEMONSTRATION PROJECT)	100 MG	ORAL	G9017
AMANTADINE HYDROCHLORIDE (BRAND NAME) (DEMONSTRTION PROJECT)	100 MG	ORAL	G9033
AMANTADINE HYDROCHLORIDE (GENERIC)	100 MG	ORAL	G9017
AMBISOME	10 MG	IV	J0289
AMCORT	5 MG	IM	J3302
AMELUZ	10 MG	OTH	J7345
AMERGAN	12.5 MG	ORAL	Q0169
AMEVIVE	0.5 MG	IV, IM	J0215
AMICAR	5 G	IV	S0017
AMIFOSTINE	500 MG	IV	J0207
AMIKACIN SULFATE	100 MG	IM, IV	J0278
AMINOCAPRIOC ACID	5 G	IV	S0017
AMINOLEVULINIC ACID HCL	354 MG	OTH	J7308
AMINOLEVULINIC ACID HCL	10 MG	OTH	J7345
AMINOPHYLLINE	250 MG	IV	J0280
AMIODARONE HCL	30 MG	IV	J0282
AMIODARONE HCL	30 MG	IV	J0283
AMISULPRIDE	~~1 MG~~	~~IV~~	~~C9153~~
AMISULPRIDE	1 MG	IV	J0184
AMITRIPTYLINE HCL	20 MG	IM	J1320
AMIVANTAMAB-VMJW	2 MG	IV	J9061
AMMONIA N-13	STUDY DOSE UP TO 40 MCI	IV	A9526
AMNICORE PRO	SQ CM	OTH	Q4298
AMNICORE PRO+	SQ CM	OTH	Q4299
AMNIO QUAD-CORE	SQ CM	OTH	Q4294
AMNIO TRI-CORE AMNIOTIC	SQ CM	OTH	Q4295
AMNIO-MAXX	SQ CM	OTH	Q4239
AMNIO-MAXX LITE	SQ CM	OTH	Q4239
AMNIOAMP-MP	SQ CM	OTH	Q4250
AMNIOARMOR	SQ CM	OTH	Q4188
AMNIOBAND	SQ CM	OTH	Q4151
AMNIOBAND	1 MG	OTH	Q4168
AMNIOBIND	SQ CM	OTH	Q4225
AMNIOCORE	SQ CM	OTH	Q4227
AMNIOCYTE PLUS	0.5 CC	OTH	Q4242
AMNIOEXCEL	SQ CM	OTH	Q4137
AMNIOEXCEL PLUS	SQ CM	OTH	Q4137
AMNIOMATRIX	1 CC	OTH	Q4139
AMNION BIO	SQ CM	OTH	Q4211
AMNIOREPAIR	SQ CM	OTH	Q4235
AMNIOTEXT	1 CC	OTH	Q4245
AMNIOTEXT PATCH	SQ CM	OTH	Q4247
AMNIOWOUND	SQ CM	OTH	Q4181
AMNIOWRAP2	SQ CM	OTH	Q4221
AMNIPLY	SQ CM	OTH	Q4249
AMOBARBITAL	125 MG	IM, IV	J0300
AMONDYS 45	10 MG	IV	J1426
AMPHOCIN	50 MG	IV	J0285
AMPHOTEC	10 MG	IV	J0287
AMPHOTERICIN B	50 MG	IV	J0285
AMPHOTERICIN B CHOLESTERYL SULFATE COMPLEX	10 MG	IV	J0288
AMPHOTERICIN B LIPID COMPLEX	10 MG	IV	J0287
AMPHOTERICIN B LIPOSOME	10 MG	IV	J0289
AMPICILLIN SODIUM	500 MG	IM, IV	J0290

Drug Name	Units Per	Route	Code
AMPICILLIN SODIUM/SULBACTAM SODIUM	1.5 G	IM, IV	J0295
AMVUTTRA	1 MG	SC	J0225
AMYGDALIN	VAR	INJ	J3570
AMYTAL	125 MG	IM, IV	J0300
AMYVID	UP TO 10 MILLICUIRES	IV	A9586
AN-DTPA DIAGNOSTIC	STUDY DOSE UP TO 25 MCI	IV	A9539
AN-DTPA THERAPEUTIC	STUDY DOSE UP TO 25 MCI	INH	A9567
ANACAULASE-BCDB, 8.8% GEL	1 G	OTH	J7353
ANASCORP	UP TO 120 MG	IV	J0716
ANASTROZOLE	1 MG	ORAL	S0170
ANAVIP	120 MG	IV	J0841
ANCEF	500 MG	IM, IV	J0690
ANDEXXA	10 MG	IV	J7169
ANECTINE	20 MG	IM, IV	J0330
ANGIOMAX	1 MG	IV	J0583
ANIDULAFUNGIN	1 MG	IV	J0348
ANIFROLUMAB-FNIA	1 MG	IV	J0491
ANISTREPLASE	30 U	IV	J0350
ANJESO	1 MG	IV	J1738
ANNOVERA VAGINAL RING	0.15 MG/0.013 MG	OTH	J7294
ANTAGON	250 MCG	SC	S0132
ANTI-INHIBITOR	1 IU	IV	J7198
ANTI-THYMOCYTE GLOBULIN,EQUINE	250 MG	OTH	J7504
ANTIEMETIC DRUG NOS	VAR	ORAL	J8597
ANTIHEMOPHILIC FACTOR (RECOMBINANT), FC-VWF-XTEN FUSION PROTEIN EIITL	IU	IV	J7214
ANTIHEMOPHILIC FACTOR PORCINE	1 IU	IV	J7191
ANTIHEMOPHILIC FACTOR VIII, XYNTHA, RECOMBINANT	1 IU	IV	J7185
ANTIHEMOPHILIC FACTOR VIII/VON WILLEBRAND FACTOR COMPLEX, HUMAN	FACTOR VIII IU	IV	J7186
ANTITHROMBIN RECOMBINANT	50 IU	IV	J7196
ANTIZOL	15 MG	IV	J1451
ANZEMET	10 MG	IV	J1260
ANZEMET	50 MG	ORAL	S0174
ANZEMET	100 MG	ORAL	Q0180
APIS	SQ CM	OTH	A2010
APLIGRAF	SQ CM	OTH	Q4101
APOKYN	1 MG	SC	J0364
APOMORPHINE HYDROCHLORIDE	1 MG	SC	J0364
APONVIE	1 MG	IV	C9145
APREPITANT	1 MG	IV	J0185
APREPITANT	1 MG	IV	C9145
APREPITANT	5 MG	ORAL	J8501
APRETUDE	1 MG	IM	J0739
APROTININ	10,000 KIU	IV	J0365
AQUAMEPHYTON	1 MG	IM, SC, IV	J3430
ARA-C	100 MG	SC, IV	J9100
ARALEN	UP TO 250 MG	IM, IV	J0390
ARAMINE	10 MG	IV, IM, SC	J0380
ARANESP, ESRD USE	1 MCG	SC, IV	J0882
ARANESP, NON-ESRD USE	1 MCG	SC, IV	J0881
ARBUTAMINE HCL	1 MG	IV	J0395
ARCALYST	1 MG	SC	J2793

Drug Name	Units Per	Route	Code
ARCHITECT EXTRACELLULAR MATRIX	SQ CM	OTH	Q4147
AREDIA	30 MG	IV	J2430
ARFORMOTEROL	15 MCG	INH	J7605
ARGATROBAN	1 MG	IV	J0883
ARGATROBAN	1 MG	IV	J0884
ARGATROBAN (ACCORD), NOT THERAPEUTICALLY EQUIVALENT TO J0883 (FOR NON-ESRD USE)	1 MG	IV	J0891
ARGATROBAN (ACCORD), NOT THERAPEUTICALLY EQUIVALENT TO J0884 (FOR ESRD ON DIALYSIS)	1 MG	IV	J0892
ARGATROBAN (AUROMEDICS), NOT THERAPEUTICALLY EQUIVALENT TO J0883 (FOR ESRD ON DIALYSIS)	1 MG	IV	J0899
ARGATROBAN (AUROMEDICS), NOT THERAPEUTICALLY EQUIVALENT TO J0883 (FOR NON-ESRD USE)	1 MG	IV	J0898
ARIDOL	5 MG	INH	J7665
ARIMIDEX	1 MG	ORAL	S0170
ARIPIPRAZOLE	0.25 MG	IM	J0400
ARIPIPRAZOLE	1 MG	IM	J0402
ARIPIPRAZOLE	1 MG	IM	C9152
ARIPIPRAZOLE LAUROXIL	1 MG	IM	J1943
ARIPIPRAZOLE LAUROXIL	1 MG	IM	J1944
ARIPIPRAZOLE, EXTENDED RELEASE	1 MG	IM	J0401
ARISTADA	1 MG	IM	J1944
ARISTADA INITIO	1 MG	IM	J1943
ARISTOCORT	5 MG	IM	J3302
ARISTOCORTE FORTE	5 MG	IM	J3302
ARISTOCORTE INTRALESIONAL	5 MG	OTH	J3302
ARISTOSPAN	5 MG	VAR	J3303
ARIXTRA	0.5 MG	SC	J1652
AROMASIN	25 MG	ORAL	S0156
ARRANON	50 MG	IV	J9261
ARRESTIN	200 MG	IM	J3250
ARSENIC TRIOXIDE	1 MG	IV	J9017
ARTACENT AC	1 MG	OTH	Q4189
ARTACENT AC	SQ CM	OTH	Q4190
ARTACENT CORD	SQ CM	OTH	Q4216
ARTACENT WOUND	SQ CM	OTH	Q4169
ARTESUNATE	1 MG	IV	J0391
ARTHROFLEX	SQ CM	OTH	Q4125
ARTISS FIBRIN SEALANT	2 ML	OTH	C9250
ARZERRA	10 MG	IV	J9302
ASCENIV	500 MG	IV	J1554
ASCENT	0.5 MG	OTH	Q4213
ASPARAGINASE	1,000 IU	IM,IV,SC	J9019
ASPARAGINASE, RECOMBINANT	0.1 MG	IM	J9021
ASPARLAS	10 UNITS	IV	J9118
ASTAGRAF XL	0.1 MG	ORAL	J7508
ASTRAMORPH PF	10 MG	OTH	J2274
ATEZOLIZUMAB	10 MG	INF	J9022
ATGAM	250 MG	OTH	J7504
ATIVAN	2 MG	IM, IV	J2060
ATOPICLAIR	ANY SIZE	OTH	A6250
ATROPEN	0.01 MG	IM	J0461
ATROPINE SULFATE	0.01 MG	IM, IV, SC	J0461
ATROPINE, COMPOUNDED, CONCENTRATED	1 MG	INH	J7635
ATROPINE, COMPOUNDED, UNIT DOSE	1 MG	INH	J7636

Drug Name	Units Per	Route	Code
ATROVENT, NONCOMPOUNDED, UNIT DOSE	1 MG	INH	J7644
ATRYN	50 IU	IV	J7196
AUROTHIOGLUCOSE	50 MG	IM	J2910
AUTOPLEX T	1 IU	IV	J7198
AVACINCAPTAD PEGOL	0.1 MG	INJ	C9162
AVALGLUCOSIDASE ALFA-NGPT	4 MG	IV	J0219
AVASTIN	0.25 MG	IV	C9257
AVASTIN	10 MG	IV	J9035
AVEED	1 MG	IM	J3145
AVELOX	100 MG	IV	J2280
AVELUMAB	10 MG	INF	J9023
AVONEX	30 MCG	IM	J1826
AVONEX	1 MCG	IM	Q3027
AVSOLA	10 MG	IV	Q5121
AVYCAZ	0.5 G/0.125 G	IV	J0714
AXICABTAGENE CILOLEUCEL	UP TO 200 MILLION CELLS	IV	Q2041
AXOBIOMEMBRANE	SQ CM	OTH	Q4211
AXOLOTL AMBIENT, AXOLOTL CRYO	0.1 MG	OTH	Q4215
AXOLOTL GRAFT, AXOLOTL DUALGRAFT	SQ CM	OTH	Q4210
AXUMIN	1 MCI	IV	A9588
AZACITIDINE	1 MG	SC	J9025
~~AZACTAM~~	~~500 MG~~	~~IV~~	~~S0073~~
AZACTAM	100 MG	IM/IV	J0457
AZASAN	50 MG	ORAL	J7500
AZATHIOPRINE	50 MG	ORAL	J7500
AZATHIOPRINE	100 MG	OTH	J7501
AZEDRA	1 MCI	IV	A9590
AZITHROMYCIN	1 G	ORAL	Q0144
AZITHROMYCIN	500 MG	IV	J0456
AZMACORT	1 MG	INH	J7684
AZMACORT CONCENTRATED	1 MG	INH	J7683
~~AZTREONAM~~	~~500 MG~~	~~IV, IM~~	~~S0073~~
AZTREONAM	100 MG	IM/IV	J0457
BACLOFEN	50 MCG	IT	J0476
BACLOFEN	10 MG	IT	J0475
BACTOCILL	250 MG	IM, IV	J2700
BACTRIM IV	10 ML	IV	S0039
BAL	100 MG	IM	J0470
BALFAXAR	IU	IV	C9159
BAMLANIVIMAB AND ETESEVIMAB	2100 MG	IV	Q0245
~~BARHEMSYS~~	~~1 MG~~	~~IV~~	~~C9153~~
BARHEMSYS	1 MG	IV	J0184
BARRERA SL OR BARRERA DL	SQ CM	OTH	Q4281
BASILIXIMAB	20 MG	IV	J0480
BAVENCIO	10 MG	INF	J9023
BAXDELA	1 MG	ORAL, IV	C9462
BCG LIVE INTRAVESICAL	1 MG	OTH	J9030
BEBTELOVIMAB	175 MG	IV	Q0222
BEBULIN VH	1 IU	IV	J7194
BECAPLERMIN GEL 0.01%	0.5 G	OTH	S0157
BECLOMETHASONE COMPOUNDED	1 MG	INH	J7622
BECLOVENT COMPOUNDED	1 MG	INH	J7622
BECONASE COMPOUNDED	1 MG	INH	J7622
BELANTAMAB MAFODOTIN-BLMF	0.5 MG	IV	J9037
BELATACEPT	1 MG	IV	J0485
BELEODAQ	10 MG	IV	J9032
BELIMUMAB	10 MG	IV	J0490
BELINOSTAT	10 MG	IV	J9032

Drug Name	Units Per	Route	Code
BELLACELL HD	SQ CM	OTH	Q4220
BELRAPZO	1 MG	IV	J9036
BENA-D 10	50 MG	IV, IM	J1200
BENA-D 50	50 MG	IV, IM	J1200
BENADRYL	50 MG	IV, IM	J1200
BENAHIST 10	50 MG	IV, IM	J1200
BENAHIST 50	50 MG	IV, IM	J1200
BENDAMUSTINE HCL	1 MG	IV	J9033
BENDAMUSTINE HCL	1 MG	IV	J9056
BENDAMUSTINE HCL	1 MG	IV	J9034
BENDAMUSTINE HCL (APOTEX)	1 MG	IV	J9058
BENDAMUSTINE HCL (BAXTER)	1 MG	IV	J9059
BENDAMUSTINE HYDROCHLORIDE	1 MG	IV	J9036
BENDEKA	1 MG	IV	J9034
BENLYSTA	10 MG	IV	J0490
BENOJECT-10	50 MG	IV, IM	J1200
BENOJECT-50	50 MG	IV, IM	J1200
BENRALIZUMAB	1 MG	SC	J0517
BENTYL	20 MG	IM	J0500
BENZTROPINE MESYLATE	1 MG	IM, IV	J0515
BEOVU	1 MG	INJ	J0179
BEREMAGENE GEPERPAVEC-SVDT	0.1 ML	OTH	J3401
BERINERT	10 U	IV	J0597
BERUBIGEN	1,000 MCG	SC, IM	J3420
BESPONSA	0.1 MG	IV	J9229
BETA-2	1 MG	INH	J7648
BETALIN 12	1,000 MCG	SC, IM	J3420
BETAMETHASONE ACETATE AND BETAMETHASONE SODIUM PHOSPHATE	3 MG/3 MG	IM	J0702
BETAMETHASONE COMPOUNDED, UNIT DOSE	1 MG	INH	J7624
BETASERON	0.25 MG	SC	J1830
BETHANECHOL CHLORIDE, MYOTONACHOL OR URECHOLINE	5 MG	SC	J0520
BEVACIZUMAB	10 MG	IV	J9035
BEVACIZUMAB	0.25 MG	IV	C9257
BEVACIZUMAB-ADCD	10 MG	IV	Q5129
BEVACIZUMAB-AWWB, BIOSIMILAR	10 MG	IV	Q5107
BEVACIZUMAB-BVZR, BIOSIMILAR	10 MG	IV	Q5118
BEVACIZUMAB-MALY, BIOSIMILAR, (ALYMSYS)	10 MG	IV	Q5126
BEZLOTOXUMAB	10 MG	INF	J0565
BICILLIN CR	100,000 UNITS	IM	J0558
BICILLIN CR 900/300	100,000 UNITS	IM	J0558
BICILLIN CR TUBEX	100,000 UNITS	IM	J0558
BICILLIN LA	100,000 U	IM	J0561
BICNU	100 MG	IV	J9050
BIMATOPROST, INTRACAMERAL IMPLANT	1 MCG	OTH	J7351
BIO-CONNEKT	SQ CM	OTH	Q4161
BIO-CONNEKT WOUND MATRIX	SQ CM	OTH	A2003
BIODEXCEL	SQ CM	OTH	Q4137
BIODFENCE	SQ CM	OTH	Q4140
BIODFENCE DRYFLEX	SQ CM	OTH	Q4138
BIODMATRIX	1 CC	OTH	Q4139
BIOSKIN	SQ CM	OTH	Q4163
BIOSKIN FLOW	SQ CM	OTH	Q4162
BIOTROPIN	1 MG	SC	J2941
BIOVANCE	SQ CM	OTH	Q4154

Drug Name	Units Per	Route	Code
BIOVANCE TRI-LAYER OR BIOVANCE 3L	SQ CM	OTH	Q4283
BIOWOUND, BIOWOUND PLUS, BIOWOUND XPLUS	SQ CM	OTH	Q4217
BIPERIDEN LACTATE	5 MG	IM, IV	J0190
BITOLTEROL MESYLATE, COMPOUNDED CONCENTRATED	1 MG	INH	J7628
BITOLTEROL MESYLATE, COMPOUNDED UNIT DOSE	MG	INH	J7629
BIVALIRUDIN	1 MG	IV	J0583
BIVIGAM	500 MG	IV	J1556
BLENOXANE	15 U	IM, IV, SC	J9040
BLENREP	0.5 MG	IV	J9037
BLEOMYCIN LYOPHILLIZED	15 U	IM, IV, SC	J9040
BLEOMYCIN SULFATE	15 U	IM, IV, SC	J9040
BLINATUMOMAB	1 MCG	IV	J9039
BLINCYTO	1 MCG	IV	J9039
BONIVA	1 MG	IV	J1740
BORTEZOMIB	0.1 MG	IV, SC	J9041
BORTEZOMIB (FRESENIUS KABI), NOT THERAPEUTICALLY EQUIVALENT TO J9041	0.1 MG	IV	J9048
BORTEZOMIB (HOSPIRA), NOT THERAPEUTICALLY EQUIVALENT TO J9041	0.1 MG	IV	J9049
BORTEZOMIB (MAIA), NOT THERAPEUTICALLY EQUIVALENT TO J9041	0.1 MG	IV	J9051
BORTEZOMIB, (DR. REDDY'S), NOT THERAPEUTICALLY EQUIVALENT TO J9041	0.1 MG	IV	J9046
BOTOX	1 UNIT	IM, OTH	J0585
BOTOX COSMETIC	1 UNIT	IM, OTH	J0585
BOTULINUM TOXIN TYPE A	1 UNIT	IM, OTH	J0585
BOTULINUM TOXIN TYPE B	100 U	OTH	J0587
BRACHYTHERAPY LINEAR SOURCE, NONSTRANDED, PALLADIUM-103	1 MM	OTH	C2636
BRACHYTHERAPY PLANAR SOURCE, PALLADIUM-103	SQ MM	OTH	C2645
BRACHYTHERAPY SOURCE, CESIUM-131 CHLORIDE SOLUTION	MCI	OTH	C2644
BRACHYTHERAPY SOURCE, NON-STRANDED, NOS	SOURCE	OTH	C2699
BRACHYTHERAPY SOURCE, NONSTRANDED, CESIUM-131	SOURCE	OTH	C2643
BRACHYTHERAPY SOURCE, NONSTRANDED, GOLD-198	SOURCE	OTH	C1716
BRACHYTHERAPY SOURCE, NONSTRANDED, HIGH ACTIVITY, IODINE-125, GREATER THAN 1.01 MCI (NIST)	SOURCE	OTH	C2634
BRACHYTHERAPY SOURCE, NONSTRANDED, HIGH ACTIVITY, PALLADIUM-103, GREATER THAN 2.2 MCI (NIST)	SOURCE	OTH	C2635
BRACHYTHERAPY SOURCE, NONSTRANDED, HIGH DOSE RATE IRIDIUM-192	SOURCE	OTH	C1717
BRACHYTHERAPY SOURCE, NONSTRANDED, IODINE-125	SOURCE	OTH	C2639
BRACHYTHERAPY SOURCE, NONSTRANDED, NONHIGH DOSE RATE IRIDIUM-192	SOURCE	OTH	C1719
BRACHYTHERAPY SOURCE, NONSTRANDED, NOS	SOURCE	OTH	C2699

Drug Name	Units Per	Route	Code
BRACHYTHERAPY SOURCE, NONSTRANDED, PALLADIUM-103	SOURCE	OTH	C2641
BRACHYTHERAPY SOURCE, NONSTRANDED, YTTERBIUM-169	SOURCE	OTH	C2637
BRACHYTHERAPY SOURCE, NONSTRANDED, YTTRIUM-90	SOURCE	OTH	C2616
BRACHYTHERAPY SOURCE, STRANDED, CESIUM-131	SOURCE	OTH	C2642
BRACHYTHERAPY SOURCE, STRANDED, IODINE-125	SOURCE	OTH	C2638
BRACHYTHERAPY SOURCE, STRANDED, NOS	SOURCE	OTH	C2698
BRACHYTHERAPY SOURCE, STRANDED, PALLADIUM-103	SOURCE	OTH	C2640
BRAVELLE	75 IU	SC, IM	J3355
BRENTUXIMAB VENDOTIN	1 MG	IV	J9042
BRETHINE	1 MG	INH	J7681
BRETHINE CONCENTRATED	1 MG	INH	J7680
BREXANOLONE	1 MG	IV	J1632
BREXUCABTAGENE AUTOLEUCEL	UP TO 200 MILLION CELLS	IV	Q2053
BREYANZI	UP TO 110 MILLION CELLS	IV	Q2054
BRICANYL	1 MG	INH	J7681
BRICANYL CONCENTRATED	1 MG	INH	J7680
BRINEURA	1 MG	OTH	J0567
BRIUMVI	1 MG	IV	J2329
BRIXADI	1M	SC	C9154
BRIXADI	1 MG	SC	J0576
BROLUCIZUMAB-DBLL	1 MG	INJ	J0179
BROM-A-COT	10 MG	IM, SC, IV	J0945
BROMPHENIRAMINE MALEATE	10 MG	IM, SC, IV	J0945
BUDESONIDE COMPOUNDED, CONCETRATED	0.25 MG	INH	J7634
BUDESONIDE, COMPOUNDED, UNIT DOSE	0.5 MG	INH	J7627
BUDESONIDE, NONCOMPOUNDED, CONCENTRATED	0.25 MG	INH	J7633
BUDESONIDE, NONCOMPOUNDED, UNIT DOSE	0.5 MG	INH	J7626
BUMETANIDE	0.5 MG	IM, IV	S0171
BUMETANIDE	0.5 MG	IM, IV	J1939
BUMEX	0.5 MG	IM, IV	J1939
BUNAVAIL	2.1 MG	ORAL	J0572
BUNAVAIL	6.3 MG	ORAL	J0574
BUNAVAIL	4.2 MG	ORAL	J0573
BUPIVACAINE	1 MG	INJ	C9144
BUPIVACAINE AND MELOXICAM	1 MG/0.03 MG	OTH	C9088
BUPIVACAINE HCL	30 ML	VAR	S0020
BUPIVACAINE LIPOSOME	1 MG	VAR	C9290
BUPIVACAINE, COLLAGEN-MATRIX IMPLANT	1 MG	OTH	C9089
BUPRENEX	0.1 MG	IM, IV	J0592
BUPRENORPHIN/NALOXONE	UP TO 3 MG	ORAL	J0572
BUPRENORPHIN/NALOXONE	> 10 MG	ORAL	J0575
BUPRENORPHINE EXTENDED-RELEASE	> 100 MG	SC	Q9992
BUPRENORPHINE EXTENDED-RELEASE	≤ 100 MG	SC	Q9991
BUPRENORPHINE EXTENDED-RELEASE	1 MG	SC	J0576
BUPRENORPHINE EXTENDED-RELEASE	1M	SC	C9154
BUPRENORPHINE HCL	0.1 MG	IM, IV	J0592

Drug Name	Units Per	Route	Code
BUPRENORPHINE IMPLANT	74.2 MG	OTH	J0570
BUPRENORPHINE ORAL	1 MG	ORAL	J0571
BUPRENORPHINE/NALOXONE	3.1 TO 6 MG	ORAL	J0573
BUPRENORPHINE/NALOXONE	6.1 TO 10 MG	ORAL	J0574
BUPROPION HCL	150 MG	ORAL	S0106
BUROSUMAB-TWZA	1 MG	SC	J0584
BUSULFAN	1 MG	IV	J0594
BUSULFAN	2 MG	ORAL	J8510
BUSULFEX	2 MG	ORAL	J8510
BUTORPHANOL TARTRATE	2 MG	IM, IV	J0595
BUTORPHANOL TARTRATE	25 MG	OTH	S0012
BYFAVO	1 MG	IV	J2249
BYOOVIZ	0.1 MG	INJ	Q5124
C-1 ESTERASE INHIBITOR (HUMAN)	10 UNITS	SC	J0599
C1 ESTERASE INHIBITOR (HUMAN) (BERINERT)	10 UNITS	IV	J0597
C1 ESTERASE INHIBITOR (HUMAN) (CINRYZE)	10 UNITS	IV	J0598
C1 ESTERASE INHIBITOR (RECOMBINANT)	10 UNITS	IV	J0596
CABAZITAXEL	1 MG	IV	J9043
CABAZITAXEL	1 MG	IV	J9064
CABENUVA	2 MG/3 MG	IM	J0741
CABERGOLINE	0.25 MG	ORAL	J8515
CABLIVI	1 MG	IV, SC	C9047
CABOTEGRAVIR	1 MG	IM	J0739
CABOTEGRAVIR AND RILPIVIRINE	2 MG/3 MG	IM	J0741
CAFCIT	5 MG	IV	J0706
CAFFEINE CITRATE	5 MG	IV	J0706
CALASPARGASE PEGOL-MKNL	10 UNITS	IV	J9118
CALCIJEX	0.25 MCG	INJ	S0169
CALCIJEX	0.1 MCG	IM	J0636
CALCIMAR	UP TO 400 U	SC, IM	J0630
CALCITONIN SALMON	400 U	SC, IM	J0630
CALCITRIOL	0.1 MCG	IM	J0636
CALCITRIOL	0.25 MCG	IM	S0169
CALCIUM DISODIUM VERSENATE	1,000 MG	IV, SC, IM	J0600
~~CALCIUM GLUCONATE (FRESENIUS KABI)~~	~~10 ML~~	~~IV~~	~~J0610~~
CALCIUM GLUCONATE (FRESENIUS KABI)	10 MG	IV	J0612
~~CALCIUM GLUCONATE (WG CRITICAL CARE)~~	~~10 ML~~	~~IV~~	~~J0611~~
CALCIUM GLUCONATE (WG CRITICAL CARE)	10 MG	IV	J0613
CALCIUM GLYCEROPHOSPHATE AND CALCIUM LACTATE	10 ML	IM, SC	J0620
CALDOLOR	100 MG	IV	J1741
CAMCEVI	1 MG	SC	J1952
CAMPTOSAR	20 MG	IV	J9206
CANAKINUMAB	1 MG	SC	J0638
CANCIDAS	5 MG	IV	J0637
CANTHARIDIN FOR TOPICAL ADMINISTRATION	3.2 MG	OTH	C9164
CAPECITABINE	150 MG	ORAL	J8520
CAPLACIZUMAB-YHDP	1 MG	IV, SC	C9047
CAPSAICIN 8% PATCH	1 SQ CM	OTH	J7336
CARBIDOPA/LEVODOPA	5 MG/20 MG	ORAL	J7340
CARBOCAINE	10 ML	VAR	J0670
CARBOPLATIN	50 MG	IV	J9045
CARBOXYDEXTRAN-COATED SUPERPARAMAGNETIC IRON OXIDE	STUDY DOSE	SC	A9697

Drug Name	Units Per	Route	Code
CARDENE IV	0.1 MG	IV	J2404
CARDIOGEN 82	STUDY DOSE UP TO 60 MCI	IV	A9555
CARDIOLITE	STUDY DOSE	IV	A9500
CAREPATCH	SQ CM	OTH	Q4236
CARFILZOMIB	1 MG	IV	J9047
CARMUSTINE	100 MG	IV	J9050
CARMUSTINE (ACCORD), NOT THERAPEUTICALLY EQUIVALENT TO J9050	100 MG	IV	J9052
CARNITOR	1 G	IV	J1955
CARTICEL		OTH	J7330
CARVYKTI	UP TO 100 MILLION CELLS	IV	Q2056
CASIMERSEN	10 MG	IV	J1426
CASIRIVIMAB AND IMDEVIMAB	2400 MG	IV	Q0243
CASIRIVIMAB AND IMDEVIMAB	600 MG	IV	Q0240
CASIRIVIMAB AND IMDEVIMAB	1200 MG	IV	Q0244
CASPOFUNGIN ACETATE	5 MG	IV	J0637
CATAPRES	1 MG	OTH	J0735
CATHFLO	1 MG	IV	J2997
CAVERJECT	1.25 MCG	VAR	J0270
CEA SCAN	STUDY DOSE UP TO 45 MCI	IV	A9568
CEENU	10 MG	ORAL	S0178
CEFAZOLIN SODIUM	500 MG	IM, IV	J0690
CEFAZOLIN SODIUM (BAXTER), NOT THERAPEUTICALLY EQUIVALENT TO J0690	500 MG	IV	J0689
CEFAZOLIN SODIUM (HIKMA), NOT THERAPEUTICALLY EQUIVALENT TO J0690	500 MG	IV	J0688
CEFEPIME HCL	500 MG	IV	J0692
CEFEPIME HCL (B. BRAUN), NOT THERAPEUTICALLY EQUIVALENT TO MAXIPIME	500 MG	IV	J0703
CEFEPIME HCL (BAXTER), NOT THERAPEUTICALLY EQUIVALENT TO MAXIPIME	500 MG	IV	J0701
CEFIDEROCOL	10 MG	IV	J0699
CEFIZOX	500 MG	IV, IM	J0715
CEFOBID	1 G	IV	S0021
CEFOPERAZONE SODIUM	1 G	IV	S0021
CEFOTAN	500 MG	IM, IV	S0074
CEFOTAXIME SODIUM	1 GM	IV, IM	J0698
CEFOTETAN DISODIUM	500 MG	IM. IV	S0074
CEFOXITIN SODIUM	1 GM	IV, IM	J0694
CEFTAROLINE FOSAMIL	10 MG	IV	J0712
CEFTAZIDIME	500 MG	IM, IV	J0713
CEFTAZIDIME AND AVIBACTAM	0.5 G/0.125 G	IV	J0714
CEFTIZOXIME SODIUM	500 MG	IV, IM	J0715
CEFTOLOZANE AND TAZOBACTAM	50 MG/25 MG	IV	J0695
CEFTRIAXONE SODIUM	250 MG	IV, IM	J0696
CEFUROXIME	750 MG	IM, IV	J0697
CEFUROXIME SODIUM STERILE	750 MG	IM, IV	J0697
CELERA DUAL LAYER/MEMBRANE	SQ CM	OTH	Q4259
CELESTONE SOLUSPAN	3 MG/3 MG	IM	J0702
CELLCEPT	250 MG	ORAL	J7517
CELLCEPT	10 MG	IV	J7519
CELLESTA CORD	SQ CM	OTH	Q4214
CELLESTA FLOWABLE AMNION	0.5 CC	OTH	Q4185
CELLESTA OR CELLESTA DUO	SQ CM	OTH	Q4184
CEMIPLIMAB-RWLC	1 MG	IV	J9119

Drug Name	Units Per	Route	Code
CENACORT FORTE	5 MG	IM	J3302
CENTRUROIDES (SCORPION) IMMUNE F(AB)2 (EQUINE)	UP TO 120 MG	IV	J0716
CEPHALOTHIN SODIUM	UP TO 1 G	INJ	J1890
CEPHAPIRIN SODIUM	1 G	IV	J0710
CEPTAZ	500 MG	IM, IV	J0713
CEREBRYX	50 MG	IM, IV	Q2009
CEREBRYX	750 MG	IM, IV	S0078
CEREDASE	10 U	IV	J0205
CERETEC	STUDY DOSE UP TO 25 MCI	IV	A9521
CEREZYME	10 U	IV	J1786
CERIANNA	1 MCI	IV	A9591
CERLIPONASE ALFA	1 MG	OTH	J0567
CERTOLIZUMAB PEGOL	1 MG	SC	J0717
CERUBIDINE	10 MG	IV	J9150
CESAMET	1 MG	ORAL	J8650
CETIRIZINE HCL	0.5 MG	IV	J1201
CETUXIMAB	10 MG	IV	J9055
CHEALAMIDE	150 MG	IV	J3520
CHLORAMBUCIL	2 MG	ORAL	S0172
CHLORAMPHENICOL SODIUM SUCCINATE	1 G	IV	J0720
CHLORDIAZEPOXIDE HCL	100 MG	IM, IV	J1990
CHLOROMYCETIN	1 G	IV	J0720
CHLOROPROCAINE HCL	1 MG	INJ	J2401
CHLOROPROCAINE HCL (CLOROTEKAL)	1 MG	INJ	J2402
CHLOROPROCAINE HCL OPHTHALMIC, 3% GEL	1 MG	OTH	J2403
CHLOROQUINE HCL	UP TO 250 MG	IM, IV	J0390
CHLOROTHIAZIDE SODIUM	500 MG	IV	J1205
CHLORPROMAZINE HCL	5 MG	ORAL	Q0161
CHLORPROMAZINE HCL	50 MG	IM, IV	J3230
CHOLETEC	STUDY DOSE UP TO 15 MCI	IV	A9537
CHOLINE C 11, DIAGNOSTIC, PER STUDY DOSE	UP TO 20 MCI	IV	A9515
CHOREX	1000 USP	IM	J0725
CHORIONIC GONADOTROPIN	1,000 USP U	IM	J0725
CHROMIC PHOSPHATE P32 (THERAPEUTIC)	1 MCI	IV	A9564
CHROMITOPE SODIUM	STUDY DOSE UP TO 250 UCI	IV	A9553
CHROMIUM CR-51 SODIUM IOTHALAMATE, DIAGNOSTIC	STUDY DOSE UP TO 250 UCI	IV	A9553
CIDOFOVIR	375 MG	IV	J0740
CILASTATIN SODIUM	250 MG	IV, IM	J0743
CILTACABTAGENE AUTOLEUCEL	UP TO 100 MILLION CELLS	IV	Q2056
CIMERLI	0.1 MG	INJ	Q5128
CIMETIDINE HCL	300 MG	IM, IV	S0023
CIMZIA	1 MG	SC	J0717
CINACALCET	1 MG	ORAL	J0604
CINQUAIR	1 MG	IV	J2786
CINRZYE	10 UNITS	IV	J0598
CINVANTI	1 MG	IV	J0185
CIPLA	1 MG	SC, INJ	J1932
CIPLA	7.5 MG	IM	J1954
CIPRO	200 MG	IV	J0744
CIPROFLOXACIN FOR INTRAVENOUS INFUSION	200 MG	IV	J0744
CIPROFLOXACIN OTIC SUSPENSION	6 MG	OTIC	J7342

Drug Name	Units Per	Route	Code
CIS-MDP	STUDY DOSE UP TO 30 MCI	IV	A9503
CIS-PYRO	STUDY DOSE UP TO 25 MCI	IV	A9538
CISPLATIN	10 MG	IV	J9060
CLADRIBINE	1 MG	IV	J9065
CLAFORAN	1 GM	IV, IM	J0698
CLARIX 100	SQ MC	OTH	Q4156
CLARIX CORD 1K	SQ CM	OTH	Q4148
CLARIXFLO	1 MG	OTH	Q4155
CLEOCIN PHOSPHATE	300 MG	IV	S0077
CLEVIDIPINE BUTYRATE	1 MG	IV	C9248
CLEVIPREX	1 MG	IV	C9248
CLINDAMYCIN PHOSPHATE	300 MG	IV	S0077
CLINDAMYCIN PHOSPHATE	300 MG	IV	J0736
CLINDAMYCIN PHOSPHATE (BAXTER) NOT THERAPEUTICALLY EQUIVALENT TO J0736	300 MG	IV	J0737
CLOFARABINE	1 MG	IV	J9027
CLOLAR	1 MG	IV	J9027
CLONIDINE HCL	1 MG	OTH	J0735
CLOZAPINE	25 MG	ORAL	S0136
CLOZARIL	25 MG	ORAL	S0136
COAGADEX	1 IU	IV	J7175
COAGULATION FACTOR IX (RECOMBINANT)	1 IU	IV	J7213
COAGULATION FACTOR XA (RECOMBINANT), INACTIVATED-ZHZO	10 MG	IV	J7169
COBAL	1,000 MCG	IM, SC	J3420
COBALT CO-57 CYNOCOBALAMIN, DIAGNOSTIC	STUDY DOSE UP TO 1 UCI	ORAL	A9559
COBATOPE 57	STUDY DOSE UP TO 1 UCI	ORAL	A9559
COBEX	1,000 MCG	SC, IM	J3420
COCAINE HYDROCHLORIDE NASAL SOLUTION	1 MG	OTH	C9046
COCAINE HYDROCHLORIDE NASAL SOLUTION (NUMBRINO)	1 MG	OTH	C9143
COCOON MEMBRANE	SQ CM	OTH	Q4264
CODEINE PHOSPHATE	30 MG	IM, IV, SC	J0745
COGENEX AMNIOTIC MEMBRANE	SQ CM	OTH	Q4229
COGENEX FLOWABLE AMNION	0.5 CC	OTH	Q4230
COGENTIN	1 MG	IM, IV	J0515
COGNEX	10 MG	ORAL	S0014
COLCHICINE	1 MG	IV	J0760
COLHIST	10 MG	IM, SC, IV	J0945
COLISTIMETHATE SODIUM	1 MG	INH	S0142
COLISTIMETHATE SODIUM	150 MG	IM, IV	J0770
COLL-E-DERM	SQ CM	OTH	Q4193
COLLAGEN BASED WOUND FILLER DRY FOAM	1 GM	OTH	A6010
COLLAGEN BASED WOUND FILLER, GEL/PASTE	1 GM	OTH	A6011
COLLAGEN MATRIX NERVE WRAP	0.5 CM	OTH	C9361
COLLAGEN NERVE CUFF	0.5 CM LENGTH	OTH	C9355
COLLAGEN WOUND DRESSING	SQ CM	OTH	Q4164
COLLAGENASE, CLOSTRIDIUM HISTOLYTICUM	0.01 MG	OTH	J0775
COLUMVI	2.5 MG	IV	J9286
COLY-MYCIN M	150 MG	IM, IV	J0770
COMPAZINE	10 MG	IM, IV	J0780
COMPAZINE	5 MG	ORAL	S0183

Drug Name	Units Per	Route	Code
COMPAZINE	5 MG	ORAL	Q0164
COMPLETE AA	SQ CM	OTH	Q4303
COMPLETE ACA	SQ CM	OTH	Q4302
COMPLETE FT	SQ CM	OTH	Q4271
COMPLETE SL	SQ CM	OTH	Q4270
CONIVAPTAN HYDROCHLORIDE	1 MG	INJ	C9488
CONTRACEPTIVE INTRAUTERINE DEVICE	EA	OTH	S4989
CONTRACEPTIVE SUPPLY, HORMONE CONTAINING PATCH	EACH	OTH	J7304
CONTRACEPTIVE SUPPLY, SPERMICIDE	EA	OTH	A4269
CONTRAST FOR ECHOCARDIOGRAM	STUDY	IV	A9700
COPANLISIB	1 MG	IV	J9057
COPAXONE	20 MG	SC	J1595
COPPER CU-64, DOTATATE, DIAGNOSTIC	1 MCI	IV	A9592
COPPER T MODEL TCU380A IUD COPPER WIRE/COPPER COLLAR	EA	OTH	J7300
CORDARONE	30 MG	IV	J0282
CORECYTE	0.5 CC	OTH	Q4240
CORETEXT	1 CC	OTH	Q4246
CORIFACT	1 IU	IV	J7180
CORPLEX	SQ CM	OTH	Q4232
CORPLEX P	1 CC	OTH	Q4231
CORTASTAT	1 MG	IM, IV, OTH	J1100
CORTASTAT LA	1 MG	IM	J1094
CORTICORELIN OVINE TRIFLUTATE	1 MCG	IV	J0795
CORTICOTROPIN	40 U	IV, IM, SC	J0800
CORTIMED	80 MG	IM	J1040
CORTROSYN	0.25 MG	IM, IV	J0834
CORVERT	1 MG	IV	J1742
COSELA	1 MG	IV	J1448
COSMEGEN	0.5 MG	IV	J9120
COSYNTROPIN	0.25 MG	IM, IV	J0834
COTOLONE	5 MG	ORAL	J7510
CRESEMBA	1 MG	IV	J1833
CRIZANLIZUMAB-TMCA	5 MG	IV	J0791
CROFAB	UP TO 1 GM	IV	J0840
CROMOLYN SODIUM COMPOUNDED	PER 10 MG	INH	J7632
CROMOLYN SODIUM NONCOMPOUNDED	10 MG	INH	J7631
CROTALIDAE IMMUNE F(AB')2 (EQUINE)	120 MG	IV	J0841
CROTALIDAE POLYVALENT IMMUNE FAB (OVINE)	UP TO 1 GM	IV	J0840
CRYO-CORD	SQ CM	OTH	Q4237
CRYSTAL B12	1,000 MCG	IM, SC	J3420
CRYSTICILLIN 300 A.S.	600,000 UNITS	IM, IV	J2510
CRYSTICILLIN 600 A.S.	600,000 UNITS	IM, IV	J2510
CRYSVITA	1 MG	SC	J0584
CUBICIN	1 MG	IV	J0878
CUTAQUIG	100 MG	IV	J1551
CUVITRU	100 MG	SC	J1555
CYANO	1,000 MCG	IM, SC	J3420
CYANOCOBALAMIN	1,000 MCG	IM, SC	J3420
CYANOCOBALAMIN COBALT 57/58	STUDY DOSE UP TO 1 UCI	IV	A9546
CYANOCOBALAMIN COBALT CO-57	STUDY DOSE UP TO 1 UCI	ORAL	A9559
CYCLOPHOSPHAMIDE	25 MG	ORAL	J8530
CYCLOPHOSPHAMIDE	100 MG	IV	J9070
CYCLOPHOSPHAMIDE, (AUROMEDICS)	5 MG	IV	J9071
CYCLOPHOSPHAMIDE, (DR. REDDY'S)	5 MG	IV	J9072
CYCLOSPORINE	25 MG	ORAL	J7515
CYCLOSPORINE	100 MG	ORAL	J7502
CYCLOSPORINE	250 MG	IV	J7516
CYGNUS	SQ CM	OTH	Q4170
CYGNUS DUAL	SQ CM	OTH	Q4282
CYGNUS MATRIX	SQ CM	OTH	Q4199
CYMETRA	1 CC	INJ	Q4112
CYRAMZA	5 MG	IV	J9308
CYSVIEW	STUDY DOSE	OTH	A9589
CYTAL	SQ CM	OTH	Q4166
CYTALUX	0.1 MG	IV	A9603
CYTARABINE	100 MG	SC, IV	J9100
CYTARABINE LIPOSOME	10 MG	IT	J9098
CYTOGAM	VIAL	IV	J0850
CYTOMEGALOVIRUS IMMUNE GLOB	VIAL	IV	J0850
CYTOSAR-U	100 MG	SC, IV	J9100
CYTOTEC	200 MCG	ORAL	S0191
CYTOVENE	500 MG	IV	J1570
CYTOXAN	25 MG	ORAL	J8530
CYTOXAN	100 MG	IV	J9070
D.H.E. 45	1 MG	IM, IV	J1110
DACARBAZINE	100 MG	IV	J9130
DACLIZUMAB	25 MG	OTH	J7513
DACOGEN	1 MG	IV	J0894
DACTINOMYCIN	0.5 MG	IV	J9120
DALALONE	1 MG	IM, IV, OTH	J1100
DALALONE LA	1 MG	IM	J1094
DALBAVANCIN	5 MG	IV	J0875
DALTEPARIN SODIUM	2,500 IU	SC	J1645
DALVANCE	5 MG	IV	J0875
DANYELZA	1 MG	IV	J9348
DAPRODUSTAT	1 MG	ORAL	J0889
DAPTOMYCIN	1 MG	IV	J0878
DAPTOMYCIN (HOSPIRA), NOT THERAPEUTICALLY EQUIVALENT TO J0878	1 MG	IV	J0877
DAPTOMYCIN (XELLIA), NOT THERAPEUTICALLY EQUIVALENT TO J0878	1 MG	IV	J0873
DAPTOMYCIN IN SODIUM CHLORIDE INJECTION	1 MG	IV	J0874
DARATUMUMAB	10 MG	IV	J9145
DARATUMUMAB AND HYALURONIDASE-FIHJ	10 MG	SC	J9144
DARBEPOETIN ALFA, ESRD USE	1 MCG	SC, IV	J0882
DARBEPOETIN ALFA, NON-ESRD USE	1 MCG	SC, IV	J0881
DARZALEX	10 MG	IV	J9145
DARZALEX FASPRO	10 MG	SC	J9144
DATSCAN	STUDY DOSE	IV	A9584
DAUNORUBICIN	10 MG	IV	J9150
DAUNORUBICIN CITRATE, LIPOOSOMAL FORMULATION	10 MG	IV	J9151
DAUNOXOME	10 MG	IV	J9151
DAXIBOTULINUMTOXINA-LANM	1 UNIT	IM	C9160
DAXXIFY	1 UNIT	IM	C9160
DDAVP	1 MCG	IV, SC	J2597
DECADRON	0.25 MG	ORAL	J8540
DECAJECT	1 MG	IM, IV, OTH	J1100

Drug Name	Units Per	Route	Code
DECITABINE	1 MG	IV	J0894
DECITABINE (SUN PHARMA), NOT THERAPEUTICALLY EQUIVALENT TO J0894	1 MG	IV	J0893
DECOLONE-50	50 MG	IM	J2320
DEFEROXAMINE MESYLATE	500 MG	IM, SC, IV	J0895
DEGARELIX	1 MG	SC	J9155
DELAFLOXACIN	1 MG	ORAL, IV	C9462
DELANDISTROGENE MOXEPARVOVEC-ROKL	THERAPEUTIC DOSE	IV	J1413
DELATESTRYL	1 MG	IM	J3121
DELESTROGEN	10 MG	IM	J1380
DELTA-CORTEF	5 MG	ORAL	J7510
DEMADEX	10 MG	IV	J3265
DEMEROL	100 MG	IM, IV, SC	J2175
DENILEUKIN DIFTITOX	300 MCG	IV	J9160
DENOSUMAB	1 MG	SC	J0897
DEOXYCHOLIC ACID	1 MG	SC	J0591
DEPGYNOGEN	UP TO 5 MG	IM	J1000
DEPHENACEN-50	50 MG	IM, IV	J1200
DEPMEDALONE	40 MG	IM	J1030
DEPMEDALONE	80 MG	IM	J1040
DEPO-ESTRADIOL CYPIONATE	UP TO 5 MG	IM	J1000
DEPO-MEDROL	40 MG	IM, OTH	J1030
DEPO-MEDROL	80 MG	IM, OTH	J1040
DEPO-MEDROL	20 MG	IM, OTH	J1020
DEPO-TESTOSTERONE	1 MG	IM	J1071
DEPOCYT	10 MG	IT	J9098
DEPOGEN	UP TO 5 MG	IM	J1000
DERM-MAXX	SQ CM	OTH	Q4238
DERMA-GIDE	SQ CM	OTH	Q4203
DERMABIND CH	SQ CM	OTH	Q4288
DERMABIND DL	SQ CM	OTH	Q4287
DERMABIND SL	SQ CM	OTH	Q4284
DERMABIND TL	SQ CM	OTH	Q4225
DERMACELL, DERMACELL AWM OR DERMACELL AWM POROUS	SQ CM	OTH	Q4122
DERMACYTE AMNIOTIC MEMBRANE ALLOGRAFT	SQ CM	OTH	Q4248
DERMAGRAFT	SQ CM	OTH	Q4106
DERMAL SUBSTITUTE, NATIVE, NONDENATURED COLLAGEN, FETAL	0.5 SQ CM	OTH	C9358
DERMAL SUBSTITUTE, NATIVE, NONDENATURED COLLAGEN, NEONATAL	0.5 SQ CM	OTH	C9360
DERMAPURE	SQ CM	OTH	Q4152
DERMAVEST AND PLURIVEST	SQ CM	OTH	Q4153
DESCOVY	200 MG/25 MG	ORAL	J0751
DESFERAL	500 MG	IM, SC, IV	J0895
DESMOPRESSIN ACETATE	1 MCG	IV, SC	J2597
DETECTNET	1 MCI	IV	A9592
DEXAMETHASONE	0.25 MG	ORAL	J8540
DEXAMETHASONE 9%	1 MCG	OTH	J1095
DEXAMETHASONE ACETATE	1 MG	IM	J1094
DEXAMETHASONE ACETATE ANHYDROUS	1 MG	IM	J1094
DEXAMETHASONE INTRAVITREAL IMPLANT	0.1 MG	OTH	J7312
DEXAMETHASONE SODIUM PHOSPHATE	1 MG	IM, IV, OTH	J1100
DEXAMETHASONE, COMPOUNDED, CONCENTRATED	1 MG	INH	J7637
DEXAMETHASONE, COMPOUNDED, UNIT DOSE	1 MG	INH	J7638
DEXAMETHASONE, LACRIMAL OPHTHALMIC INSERT	0.1 MG	OTH	J1096
DEXASONE	1 MG	IM, IV, OTH	J1100
DEXEDRINE	5 MG	ORAL	S0160
DEXIM	1 MG	IM, IV, OTH	J1100
DEXMEDETOMIDINE	1 MCG	ORAL	J1105
DEXONE	0.25 MG	ORAL	J8540
DEXONE	1 MG	IM, IV, OTH	J1100
DEXONE LA	1 MG	IM	J1094
DEXRAZOXANE HCL	250 MG	IV	J1190
DEXTENZA	0.1 MG	OTH	J1096
DEXTRAN 40	500 ML	IV	J7100
DEXTROAMPHETAMINE SULFATE	5 MG	ORAL	S0160
DEXTROSE	500 ML	IV	J7060
DEXTROSE, STERILE WATER, AND/OR DEXTROSE DILUENT/FLUSH	10 ML	VAR	A4216
DEXTROSE/SODIUM CHLORIDE	5%	VAR	J7042
DEXTROSE/THEOPHYLLINE	40 MG	IV	J2810
DEXTROSTAT	5 MG	ORAL	S0160
DEXYCU	1 MCG	OTH	J1095
DI-SPAZ	UP TO 20 MG	IM	J0500
DIALYSIS/STRESS VITAMINS	100 CAPS	ORAL	S0194
DIAMOX	500 MG	IM, IV	J1120
DIASTAT	5 MG	IV, IM	J3360
DIAZEPAM	5 MG	IV, IM	J3360
DIAZOXIDE	300 MG	IV	J1730
DIBENT	UP TO 20 MG	IM	J0500
DICLOFENAC SODIUM	0.5 MG	OTH	J1130
DICYCLOMINE HCL	20 MG	IM	J0500
DIDANOSINE (DDI)	25 MG	ORAL	S0137
DIDRONEL	300 MG	IV	J1436
DIETHYLSTILBESTROL DIPHOSPHATE	250 MG	INJ	J9165
DIFELIKEFALIN	0.1 MCG	IV	J0879
DIFLUCAN	200 MG	IV	J1450
DIGIBIND	VIAL	IV	J1162
DIGIFAB	VIAL	IV	J1162
DIGOXIN	0.5 MG	IM, IV	J1160
DIGOXIN IMMUNE FAB	VIAL	IV	J1162
DIHYDROERGOTAMINE MESYLATE	1 MG	IM, IV	J1110
DILANTIN	50 MG	IM, IV	J1165
DILAUDID	250 MG	OTH	S0092
DILAUDID	4 MG	SC, IM, IV	J1170
DIMENHYDRINATE	50 MG	IM, IV	J1240
DIMERCAPROL	100 MG	IM	J0470
DIMINE	50 MG	IV, IM	J1200
DINATE	50 MG	IM, IV	J1240
DINUTUXIMAB	0.1 MG	IV	J1246
DIOVAL	10 MG	IM	J1380
DIOVAL 40	10 MG	IM	J1380
DIOVAL XX	10 MG	IM	J1380
DIPHENHYDRAMINE HCL	50 MG	ORAL	Q0163
DIPHENHYDRAMINE HCL	50 MG	IV, IM	J1200
DIPRIVAN	10 MG	IV	J2704
DIPYRIDAMOLE	10 MG	IV	J1245
DISOTATE	150 MG	IV	J3520
DIURIL	500 MG	IV	J1205
DIURIL SODIUM	500 MG	IV	J1205
DIZAC	5 MG	IV, IM	J3360

Drug Name	Units Per	Route	Code
DMSO, DIMETHYL SULFOXIDE	50%, 50 ML	OTH	J1212
DOBUTAMINE HCL	250 MG	IV	J1250
DOBUTREX	250 MG	IV	J1250
DOCETAXEL	1 MG	IV	J9171
DOCETAXEL (INGENUS), NOT THERAPEUTICALLY EQUIVALENT TO J9171	1 MG	IV	J9172
DOLASETRON MESYLATE	100 MG	ORAL	Q0180
DOLASETRON MESYLATE	10 MG	IV	J1260
DOLASETRON MESYLATE	50 MG	ORAL	S0174
DOLOPHINE	5 MG	ORAL	S0109
DOLOPHINE HCL	10 MG	IM, SC	J1230
DOMMANATE	50 MG	IM, IV	J1240
DOPAMINE HCL	40 MG	IV	J1265
DORIBAX	10 MG	IV	J1267
DORIPENEM	10 MG	IV	J1267
DORNASE ALPHA, NONCOMPOUNDED, UNIT DOSE	1 MG	INH	J7639
DOSTARLIMAB-GXLY	10 MG	IV	J9272
DOSTINEX	0.25 MG	ORAL	J8515
DOTAREM	0.1 ML	IV	A9575
DOXERCALCIFEROL	1 MG	IV	J1270
DOXORUBICIN HCL	10 MG	IV	J9000
DOXORUBICIN HYDROCHLORIDE, LIPOSOMAL, IMPORTED LIPODOX	10 MG	IV	Q2049
DRAMAMINE	50 MG	IM, IV	J1240
DRAMANATE	50 MG	IM, IV	J1240
DRAMILIN	50 MG	IM, IV	J1240
DRAMOCEN	50 MG	IM, IV	J1240
DRAMOJECT	50 MG	IM, IV	J1240
DRAXIMAGE MDP-10	STUDY DOSE UP TO 30 MCI	IV	A9503
DRAXIMAGE MDP-25	STUDY DOSE UP TO 30 MCI	IV	A9503
DRONABINAL	2.5 MG	ORAL	Q0167
DROPERIDOL	5 MG	IM, IV	J1790
DROPERIDOL AND FENTANYL CITRATE	2 ML	IM, IV	J1810
DROXIA	500 MG	ORAL	S0176
DTIC-DOME	100 MG	IV	J9130
DTPA	STUDY DOSE UP TO 25 MCI	IV	A9539
DTPA	STUDY DOSE UP TO 25 MCI	INH	A9567
DUAL LAYER IMPAX MEMBRANE	SQ CM	OTH	Q4262
DUOPA	5 MG/20 MG	ORAL	J7340
DURACILLIN A.S.	600,000 UNITS	IM, IV	J2510
DURACLON	1 MG	OTH	J0735
DURAGEN-10	10 MG	IM	J1380
DURAGEN-20	10 MG	IM	J1380
DURAGEN-40	10 MG	IM	J1380
DURAMORPH	500 MG	OTH	S0093
DURAMORPH PF	10 MG	OTH	J2274
DURO CORT	80 MG	IM	J1040
DUROLANE	1 MG	INJ	J7318
DURVALUMAB	10 MG	IV	J9173
DURYSTA	1 MCG	OTH	J7351
DYLOJECT	0.5 MG	OTH	J1130
DYMENATE	50 MG	IM, IV	J1240
DYPHYLLINE	500 MG	IM	J1180
DYSPORT	5 UNITS	IM	J0586
E.D.T.A.	150 MG	IV	J3520

Drug Name	Units Per	Route	Code
ECALLANTIDE	1 MG	SC	J1290
ECHOCARDIOGRAM IMAGE ENHANCER OCTAFLUOROPROPANE	1 ML	IV	Q9956
ECHOCARDIOGRAM IMAGE ENHANCER PERFLEXANE	1 ML	IV	Q9955
ECULIZUMAB	10 MG	IV	J1300
EDARAVONE	1 MG	IV	J1301
EDETATE CALCIUM DISODIUM	1,000 MG	IV, SC, IM	J0600
EDETATE DISODIUM	150 MG	IV	J3520
EDEX	1.25 MCG	VAR	J0270
EFGARTIGIMOD ALFA-FCAB	2 MG	IV	J9332
EFGARTIGIMOD ALFA/ HYALURONIDASE-QVFC	2 MG	IV	J9334
~~ELAHERE~~	~~1 MG~~	~~IV~~	~~C9146~~
ELAHERE	1 MG	IV	J9063
ELAPRASE	1 MG	IV	J1743
ELAVIL	20 MG	IM	J1320
ELELYSO	10 U	IV	J3060
ELEVIDYS	THERAPEUTIC DOSE	IV	J1413
ELFABRIO	1 MG	IV	J2508
ELFLAPEGRASTIM-XNST	0.1 MG	SC	J1449
ELIGARD	7.5 MG	SC	J9217
ELITEK	0.5 MG	IM	J2783
ELLENCE	2 MG	IV	J9178
ELLIOTTS B SOLUTION	1 ML	IV, IT	J9175
ELOCTATE	IU	IV	J7205
ELOSULFASE ALFA	1 MG	IV	J1322
ELOTUZUMAB	1 MG	IV	J9176
ELOXATIN	0.5 MG	IV	J9263
ELRANATAMAB-BCMM	1 MG	SC	C9165
ELREXFIO	1 MG	SC	C9165
ELSPAR	1,000 IU	IM,IV, SC	J9019
ELUCIREM	1 ML	IV	A9573
ELZONRIS	10 MCG	IV	J9269
EMAPALUMAB-LZSG	1 MG	IV	J9210
EMEND	5 MG	ORAL	J8501
EMEND	1 MG	IV	J1453
EMERGE MATRIX	SQ CM	OTH	Q4297
EMICIZUMAB-KXWH	0.5 MG	SC	J7170
EMINASE	30 U	IV	J0350
~~EMPAVELI~~	~~1 MG~~	~~SC~~	~~C9151~~
EMPLICITI	1 MG	IV	J9176
EMTRICITABINE/TENOFOVIR ALAFENAMIDE	200 MG/25 MG	ORAL	J0751
EMTRICITABINE/TENOFOVIR DISOPROXIL FUMARATE	200 MG/300 MG	ORAL	J0750
ENBREL	25 MG	IM, IV	J1438
ENDOXAN-ASTA	100 MG	IV	J9070
ENDRATE	150 MG	IV	J3520
ENFORTUMAB VEDOTIN-EJFV	0.25 MG	IV	J9177
ENFUVIRTIDE	1 MG	SC	J1324
ENHERTU	1 MG	IV	J9358
ENJAYMO	10 MG	IV	J1302
ENOXAPARIN SODIUM	10 MG	SC	J1650
ENTYVIO	1 MG	IV	J3380
ENVARSUS XR	0.25 MG	ORAL	J7503
ENVERSE	SQ CM	OTH	Q4258
EOVIST	1 ML	IV	A9581
~~EPCORITAMAB-BYSP~~	~~0.16 MG~~	~~SC~~	~~C9155~~
EPCORITAMAB-BYSP	0.16 MG	SC	J9321

Drug Name	Units Per	Route	Code
EPICORD	SQ CM	OTH	Q4187
EPIEFFECT	SQ CM	OTH	Q4278
EPIFIX	SQ CM	OTH	Q4186
EPIFIX, INJECTABLE	1 MG	OTH	Q4145
EPINEPHRINE	0.1 MG	IM, IV, SC	J0171
EPINEPHRINE (BELCHER), NOT THERAPEUTICALLY EQUIVALENT TO J0171	0.1 MG	IV	J0173
EPIRUBICIN HCL	2 MG	IV	J9178
EPKINLY	0.16 MG	SC	C9155
EPKINLY	0.16 MG	SC	J9321
EPOETIN ALFA FOR ESRD DIALYSIS	100 U	INJ	Q4081
EPOETIN ALFA, BIOSIMILAR	100 UNITS	INJ, IV	Q5105
EPOETIN ALFA, BIOSIMILAR	1000 UNITS	INJ, IV	Q5106
EPOETIN ALFA, NON-ESRD USE	1,000 U	SC, IV	J0885
EPOETIN BETA FOR ESRD ON DIALYSIS	1 MCG	IV	J0887
EPOETIN BETA FOR NON-ESRD	1 MCG	IV, SC	J0888
EPOGEN/NON-ESRD	1,000 U	SC, IV	J0885
EPOPROSTENOL	0.5 MG	IV	J1325
EPOPROSTENOL STERILE DILUTANT	50 ML	IV	S0155
EPTIFIBATIDE	5 MG	IM, IV	J1327
EPTINEZUMAB-JJMR	1 MG	IV	J3032
ERAVACYCLINE	1 MG	IV	J0122
ERAXIS	1 MG	IV	J0348
ERBITUX	10 MG	IV	J9055
ERGAMISOL	50 MG	ORAL	S0177
ERGONOVINE MALEATE	0.2 MG	IM, IV	J1330
ERIBULIN MESYLATE	0.1 MG	IV	J9179
ERTAPENEM SODIUM	500 MG	IM, IV	J1335
ERYTHROCIN LACTOBIONATE	500 MG	IV	J1364
ESANO A	SQ CM	OTH	Q4272
ESANO AAA	SQ CM	OTH	Q4273
ESANO AC	SQ CM	OTH	Q4274
ESANO ACA	SQ CM	OTH	Q4275
ESKETAMINE, NASAL SPRAY	1 MG	OTH	S0013
ESMOLOL HCL	10 MG	IV	J1805
ESMOLOL HCL (WG CRITICAL CARE) NOT THERAPEUTICALLY EQUIVALENT TO J1805	10 MG	IV	J1806
ESPEROCT	1 IU	IV	J7204
ESTONE AQUEOUS	1 MG	IM, IV	J1435
ESTRA-L 20	10 MG	IM	J1380
ESTRA-L 40	10 MG	IM	J1380
ESTRADIOL CYPIONATE	UP TO 5 MG	IM	J1000
ESTRADIOL L.A.	10 MG	IM	J1380
ESTRADIOL L.A. 20	10 MG	IM	J1380
ESTRADIOL L.A. 40	10 MG	IM	J1380
ESTRADIOL VALERATE	10 MG	IM	J1380
ESTRAGYN	1 MG	IV, IM	J1435
ESTRO-A	1 MG	IV, IM	J1435
ESTROGEN CONJUGATED	25 MG	IV, IM	J1410
ESTRONE	1 MG	IV, IM	J1435
ESTRONOL	1 MG	IM, IV	J1435
ETANERCEPT	25 MG	IM, IV	J1438
ETELCALCETIDE	0.1 MG	IV	J0606
ETEPLIRSEN	10 MG	INF	J1428
ETHAMOLIN	100 MG	IV	J1430
ETHANOLAMINE OLEATE	100 MG	IV	J1430
ETHINYL ESTRADIOL AND ETONOGESTREL VAGINAL RING	0.015 MG/0.12 MG	OTH	J7295

Drug Name	Units Per	Route	Code
ETHYOL	500 MG	IV	J0207
ETIDRONATE DISODIUM	300 MG	IV	J1436
ETONOGESTREL	IMPLANT	OTH	J7307
ETOPOSIDE	50 MG	ORAL	J8560
ETOPOSIDE	10 MG	IV	J9181
ETRANACOGEN DEXAPARVOVEC-DRLB	THERAPEUTIC DOSE	IV	J1411
EUFLEXXA	DOSE	INJ	J7323
EULEXIN	125 MG	ORAL	S0175
EVENITY	1 MG	SC	J3111
EVEROLIMUS	0.25 MG	ORAL	J7527
EVINACUMAB-DGNB	5 MG	IV	J1305
EVKEEZA	5 MG	IV	J1305
EVOMELA	1 MG	IV	J9246
EVUSHELD	300 MG	IM	Q0220
EVUSHELD	600 MG	IM	Q0221
EXAMETAZIME LABELED AUTOLOGOUS WHITE BLOOD CELLS, TECHNETIUM TC-99M	STUDY DOSE	IV	A9569
EXCELLAGEN	0.1 CC	OTH	Q4149
EXMESTANE	25 MG	ORAL	S0156
EXONDYS 51	10 MG	INF	J1428
EXPAREL	1 MG	VAR	C9290
EYLEA HD	1 MG	INJ	C9161
EZ-DERM	SQ CM	OTH	Q4136
FABRAZYME	1 MG	IV	J0180
FACTOR IX (ANTIHEMOPHILIC FACTOR, RECOMBINANT), RIXIBUS, PER I.U.	IU	IV	J7200
FACTOR IX NON RECOMBINANT	1 IU	IV	J7193
FACTOR IX+ COMPLEX	1 IU	IV	J7194
FACTOR IX, (ANTIHEMOPHILIC FACTOR, RECOMBINANT), GLYCOPEGYLATED	1 IU	IV	J7203
FACTOR IX, ALBUMIN FUSION PROTEIN, (RECOMBINANT)	1 IU	IV	J7202
FACTOR IX, FC FUSION PROTEIN (ANTIHEMOPHILIC FACTOR, RECOMBINANT), ALPROLIX	IU	IV	J7201
FACTOR VIIA (ANTIHEMOPHILIC FACTOR, RECOMBINANT)-JNCW	1 MCG	IV	J7212
FACTOR VIIA RECOMBINANT	1 MCG	IV	J7189
FACTOR VIII (ANTIHEMOPHILIC FACTOR, RECOMBINANT)	1 IU	IV	J7209
FACTOR VIII (ANTIHEMOPHILIC FACTOR, RECOMBINANT)	IU	IV	J7188
FACTOR VIII (ANTIHEMOPHILIC FACTOR, RECOMBINANT) (NOVOEIGHT), PER IU	IU	IV	J7182
FACTOR VIII (ANTIHEMOPHILIC FACTOR, RECOMBINANT) PEGYLATED	1 IU	IV	J7207
FACTOR VIII FC FUSION (RECOMBINANT)	IU	IV	J7205
FACTOR VIII PORCINE	1 IU	IV	J7191
FACTOR VIII, (ANTIHEMOPHILIC FACTOR, RECOMBINANT) (AFSTYLA)	1 IU	IV	J7210
FACTOR VIII, (ANTIHEMOPHILIC FACTOR, RECOMBINANT) (KOVALTRY)	1 IU	IV	J7211
FACTOR VIII, (ANTIHEMOPHILIC FACTOR, RECOMBINANT), PEGYLATED-AUCL	1 IU	IV	J7208

Drug Name	Units Per	Route	Code
FACTOR VIII, ANTIHEMOPHILIC FACTOR (RECOMBINANT), GLYCOPEGYLATED-EXEI	1 IU	IV	J7204
FACTOR VIII, HUMAN	1 IU	IV	J7190
FACTOR X (HUMAN)	1 IU	IV	J7175
FACTOR XIII (ANTIHEMOPHILIC FACTOR, HUMAN)	1 IU	IV	J7180
FACTOR XIII A-SUBUNIT (RECOMBINANT)	10 IU	IV	J7181
FACTREL	100 MCG	SC, IV	J1620
FAM-TRASTUZUMAB DERUXTECAN-NXKI	1 MG	IV	J9358
FAMOTIDINE	20 MG	IV	S0028
FARICIMAB-SVOA	0.1 MG	INJ	J2777
FASENRA	1 MG	SC	J0517
FASLODEX	25 MG	IM	J9395
FDG	STUDY DOSE UP TO 45 MCI	IV	A9552
FECAL MICROBIOTA, LIVE-JSLM	1 ML	OTH	J1440
FEIBA-VH AICC	1 IU	IV	J7198
FENSOLVI	0.25 MG	SC	J1951
FENTANYL CITRATE	0.1 MG	IM, IV	J3010
FERAHEME (FOR ESRD)	1 MG	IV	Q0139
FERAHEME (NON-ESRD)	1 MG	IV	Q0138
FERIDEX IV	1 ML	IV	Q9953
FERRIC CARBOXYMALTOSE	1 MG	IV	J1439
FERRIC DERISOMALTOSE	10 MG	IV	J1437
FERRIC PYROPHOSPHATE CITRATE POWDER	0.1 MG	IV	J1444
FERRIC PYROPHOSPHATE CITRATE SOLUTION	0.1 MG	IV	J1443
FERRIC PYROPHOSPHATE CITRATE SOLUTION	0.1 MG	IV	J1445
FERRLECIT	12.5 MG	IV	J2916
FERTINEX	75 IU	SC	J3355
FERUMOXYTOL (FOR ESRD)	1 MG	IV	Q0139
FERUMOXYTOL (NON-ESRD)	1 MG	IV	Q0138
FETROJA	10 MG	IV	J0699
FIASP	5 U	SC, IV	J1812
FIASP	50 U	SC, IV	J1811
FIBRIN SEALANT (HUMAN)	2 ML	OTH	C9250
FIBRYGA	1 MG	IV	J7177
FILGRASTIM	1 MCG	SC, IV	J1442
FILGRASTIM-AAFI, BIOSIMILAR	1 MCG	INJ	Q5110
FILGRASTIM-AYOW, BIOSIMILAR	1 MCG	SC, IV	Q5125
FILGRASTIM-SNDZ, BIOSIMILAR	1 MCG	IV, SC	Q5101
FINASTERIDE	5 MG	ORAL	S0138
FIRAZYR	1 MG	SC	J1744
FIRMAGON	1 MG	SC	J9155
FISH OIL TRIGLYCERIDES	10 G	IV	B4187
FLAGYL	500 MG	IV	S0030
FLEBOGAMMA	500 MG	IV	J1572
FLEXHD	SQ CM	OTH	Q4128
FLEXON	60 MG	IV, IM	J2360
FLOLAN	0.5 MG	IV	J1325
FLORBETABEN F18, DIAGNOSTIC	STUDY DOSE UP TO 8.1 MCI	IV	Q9983
FLORTAUCIPIR F-18, DIAGNOSTIC	1 MCI	IV	A9601
FLOTUFOLASTAT F-18, DIAGNOSTIC	1 MCI	IV	C9156
FLOTUFOLASTAT F18, DIAGNOSTIC	1 MCI	IV	A9608
FLOWERAMNIOFLO	SQ CM	OTH	Q4177
FLOWERAMNIOPATCH	SQ CM	OTH	Q4178

Drug Name	Units Per	Route	Code
FLOWERDERM	SQ CM	OTH	Q4179
FLOXIN IV	400 MG	IV	S0034
FLOXURIDINE	500 MG	IV	J9200
FLUCICLOVINE F-18, DIAGNOSTIC	1 MCI	IV	A9588
FLUCONAZOLE	200 MG	IV	J1450
FLUDARA	50 MG	IV	J9185
FLUDARABINE PHOSPHATE	10 MG	ORAL	J8562
FLUDARABINE PHOSPHATE	50 MG	IV	J9185
FLUDEOXYGLUCOSE F18	STUDY DOSE UP TO 45 MCI	IV	A9552
FLUDEOXYGLUCOSE F18	UP TO 15 MCI	IV	A9609
FLUID FLOW, FLUID GF	1 CC	OTH	Q4206
FLULAVAL	EA	IM	Q2036
FLUMADINE (DEMONSTATION PROJECT)	100 MG	ORAL	G9036
FLUNISOLIDE, COMPOUNDED, UNIT DOSE	1 MG	INH	J7641
FLUOCINOLONE ACETONIDE INTRAVITREAL IMPLANT	IMPLANT	OTH	J7311
FLUOCINOLONE ACETONIDE, INTRAVITREAL IMPLANT	0.01 MG	OTH	J7313
FLUOCINOLONE ACETONIDE, INTRAVITREAL IMPLANT	0.01 MG	OTH	J7314
FLUORODEOXYGLUCOSE F-18 FDG, DIAGNOSTIC	STUDY DOSE UP TO 45 MCI	IV	A9552
FLUORODOPA F-18, DIAGNOSTIC	1 MCI	IV	A9602
FLUOROESTRADIOL F 18, DIAGNOSTIC	1 MCI	IV	A9591
FLUOROURACIL	500 MG	IV	J9190
FLUPHENAZINE DECANOATE	25 MG	SC, IM	J2680
FLUPHENAZINE HCL	1.25 MG	IM	J2679
FLUTAMIDE	125 MG	ORAL	S0175
FLUTEMETAMOL F18, DIAGNOSTIC	STUDY DOSE UP TO 5 MCI	IV	Q9982
FLUVIRIN	EA	IM	Q2037
FLUZONE	EA	IM	Q2038
FOLEX	5 MG	IV, IM, IT, IA	J9250
FOLEX	50 MG	IV, IM, IT, IA	J9260
FOLEX PFS	5 MG	IV, IM, IT, IA	J9250
FOLEX PFS	50 MG	IV, IM, IT, IA	J9260
FOLLISTIM	75 IU	SC, IM	S0128
FOLLITROPIN ALFA	75 IU	SC	S0126
FOLLITROPIN BETA	75 IU	SC, IM	S0128
FOLOTYN	1 MG	IV	J9307
FOMEPIZOLE	15 MG	IV	J1451
FOMIVIRSEN SODIUM	1.65 MG	OTH	J1452
FONDAPARINUX SODIUM	0.5 MG	SC	J1652
FORMOTEROL FUMERATE NONCOMPOUNDED UNIT DOSE FORM	20 MCG	INH	J7606
FORMOTEROL, COMPOUNDED, UNIT DOSE	12 MCG	INH	J7640
FORTAZ	500 MG	IM, IV	J0713
FORTEO	10 MCG	SC	J3110
FORTOVASE	200 MG	ORAL	S0140
FOSAPREPITANT	1 MG	IV	J1453
FOSAPREPITANT (TEVA), NOT THERAPEUTICALLY EQUIVALENT TO J1453	1 MG	IV	J1456
FOSCARNET SODIUM	1,000 MG	IV	J1455
FOSCAVIR	1,000 MG	IV	J1455
FOSNETUPITANT AND PALONOSETRON	235 MG/0.25 MG	IV	J1454

Drug Name	Units Per	Route	Code
FOSPHENYTOIN	50 MG	IM, IV	Q2009
FOSPHENYTOIN SODIUM	750 MG	IM, IV	S0078
FRAGMIN	2,500 IU	SC	J1645
FREMANEZUMAB-VFRM	1 MG	SC	J3031
FUDR	500 MG	IV	J9200
FULPHILA	0.5 MG	SC	Q5108
FULVESTRANT	25 MG	IM	J9395
FULVESTRANT (FRESENIUS KABI) NOT THERAPEUTICALLY EQUIVALENT TO J9395	25 MG	IM	J9394
FULVESTRANT (TEVA) NOT THERAPEUTICALLY EQUIVALENT TO J9395	25 MG	IM	J9393
FUNGIZONE	50 MG	IV	J0285
FUROSCIX	20 MG	SC	J1941
FUROSEMIDE	20 MG	IM, IV	J1940
FUROSEMIDE	20 MG	SC	J1941
FUZEON	1 MG	SC	J1324
FYARRO	1 MG	IV	J9331
FYLNETRA	0.5 MG	SC	Q5130
GABLOFEN	10 MG	IT	J0475
GABLOFEN	50 MCG	IT	J0476
GADAVIST	0.1 ML	IV	A9585
GADOBENATE DIMEGLUMINE (MULTIHANCE MULTIPACK)	1 ML	IV	A9577
GADOBUTROL	0.1 ML	IV	A9585
GADOFOSVESET TRISODIUM	1 ML	IV	A9583
GADOPICLENOL	1 ML	IV	A9573
GADOTERATE MEGLUMINE	0.1 ML	IV	A9575
GADOTERIDOL (PROHANCE MULTIPACK)	1 ML	IV	A9576
GADOXETATE DISODIUM	1 ML	IV	A9581
GALLIUM GA-67	1 MCI	IV	A9556
GALLIUM GA-68 GOZETOTIDE, DIAGNOSTIC	1 MCI	IV	A9596
GALLIUM GA-68 GOZETOTIDE, DIAGNOSTIC	1 MCI	IV	A9800
GALLIUM GA-68 PSMA-11, DIAGNOSTIC, (UCLA)	1 MCI	IV	A9594
GALLIUM GA-68 PSMA-11, DIAGNOSTIC, (UCSF)	1 MCI	IV	A9593
GALLIUM GA-68, DOTATATE, DIAGNOSTIC	0.1 MCI	IV	A9587
GALLIUM GA-68, DOTATOC, DIAGNOSTIC	0.01 MCI	IV	C9067
GALLIUM NITRATE	1 MG	IV	J1457
GALSULFASE	1 MG	IV	J1458
GAMASTAN	1 CC	IM	J1460
GAMASTAN	OVER 10 CC	IM	J1560
GAMASTAN SD	1 CC	IM	J1460
GAMASTAN SD	OVER 10 CC	IM	J1560
GAMIFANT	1 MG	IV	J9210
GAMMA GLOBULIN	1 CC	IM	J1460
GAMMA GLOBULIN	OVER 10 CC	IM	J1560
GAMMAGARD	500 MG	IV	J1569
GAMMAGRAFT	SQ CM	OTH	Q4111
GAMMAKED	500 MG	IV, SC	J1561
GAMMAPLEX	500 MG	IV	J1557
GAMUNEX	500 MG	IV, SQ	J1561
GAMUNEX-C	500 MG	IV, SC	J1561
GANCICLOVIR	4.5 MG	OTH	J7310
GANCICLOVIR SODIUM	500 MG	IV	J1570

Drug Name	Units Per	Route	Code
GANCICLOVIR SODIUM (EXELA) NOT THERAPEUTICALLY EQUIVALENT TO J1570	1 MG	IV	J1574
GANIRELIX ACETATE	250 MCG	SC	S0132
GANITE	1 MG	IV	J1457
GARAMYCIN	80 MG	IM, IV	J1580
GASTROCROM	10 MG	INH	J7631
GASTROMARK	1 ML	ORAL	Q9954
GATIFLOXACIN	10 MG	IV	J1590
GAZYVA	10 MG	IV	J9301
GEFITINIB	250 MG	ORAL	J8565
GEL-ONE	DOSE	INJ	J7326
GELSYN-3	0.1 MG	INJ	J7328
GEMCITABINE HCL (ACCORD), NOT THERAPEUTICALLY EQUIVALENT TO J9201	200 MG	IV	J9196
GEMCITABINE HYDROCHLORIDE	100 MG	IV	J9198
GEMTUZUMAB OZOGAMICIN	0.1 MG	INF	J9203
GENESIS AMNIOTIC MEMBRANE	SQ CM	OTH	Q4198
GENGRAF	25 MG	ORAL	J7515
GENGRAF	100 MG	ORAL	J7502
GENOTROPIN	1 MG	SC	J2941
GENOTROPIN MINIQUICK	1 MG	SC	J2941
GENOTROPIN NUTROPIN	1 MG	SC	J2941
GENTAMICIN	80 MG	IM, IV	J1580
GENTRAN	500 ML	IV	J7100
GENTRAN 75	500 ML	IV	J7110
GENVISC 850	1 MG	INJ	J7320
GEODON	10 MG	IM	J3486
GENEF	1 MCG	SC	Q0515
GIVLAARI	0.5 MG	SC	J0223
GIVOSIRAN	0.5 MG	SC	J0223
GLASSIA	10 MG	IV	J0257
GLATIRAMER ACETATE	20 MG	SC	J1595
GLEEVEC	100 MG	ORAL	S0088
GLOFIL-125	STUDY DOSE UP TO 10 UCI	IV	A9554
GLOFITAMAB-GXBM	2.5 MG	IV	J9286
GLUCAGEN	1 MG	SC, IM, IV	J1610
GLUCAGON	1 MG	SC, IM, IV	J1610
GLUCAGON HCL (FRESENIUS KABI), NOT THERAPEUTICALLY EQUIVALENT TO J1610	1 MG	INJ	J1611
GLUCOTOPE	STUDY DOSE UP TO 45 MCI	IV	A9552
GLYCOPYRROLATE	0.1 MG	IM, IV	J1596
GLYCOPYRROLATE, COMPOUNDED CONCENTRATED	1 MG	INH	J7642
GLYCOPYRROLATE, COMPOUNDED, UNIT DOSE	1 MG	INH	J7643
GOLD SODIUM THIOMALATE	50 MG	IM	J1600
GOLIMUMAB	1 MG	IV	J1602
GOLODIRSEN	10 MG	IV	J1429
GONADORELIN HCL	100 MCG	SC, IV	J1620
GONAL-F	75 IU	SC	S0126
GOPRELTO	1 MG	OTH	C9046
GOSERELIN ACETATE	3.6 MG	SC	J9202
GRAFIX CORE	SQ CM	OTH	Q4132
GRAFIX PLUS	SQ CM	OTH	Q4304
GRAFIX PRIME	SQ CM	OTH	Q4133
GRAFIXPL CORE	SQ CM	OTH	Q4132
GRAFIXPL PRIME	SQ CM	OTH	Q4133

Drug Name	Units Per	Route	Code
GRAFTJACKET	SQ CM	OTH	Q4107
GRAFTJACKET EXPRESS	1 CC	INJ	Q4113
GRANISETRON HCL	1 MG	ORAL	Q0166
GRANISETRON HCL	100 MCG	IV	J1626
GRANISETRON HCL	1 MG	IV	S0091
GRANISETRON, EXTENDED-RELEASE	0.1 MG	SC	J1627
GRANIX	1 MCG	IV	J1447
GUARDIAN	SQ CM	OTH	Q4151
GUSELKUMAB	1 MG	SC	J1628
GYNOGEN L.A. 10	10 MG	IM	J1380
GYNOGEN L.A. 20	10 MG	IM	J1380
GYNOGEN L.A. 40	10 MG	IM	J1380
H.P. ACTHAR GEL	UP TO 40 UNITS	OTH	J0800
HAEGARDA	10 UNITS	SC	J0599
HALAVEN	0.1 MG	IV	J9179
HALDOL	5 MG	IM, IV	J1630
HALDOL DECANOATE	50 MG	IM	J1631
HALOPERIDOL	5 MG	IM, IV	J1630
HECTOROL	1 MG	IV	J1270
HELICOLL	SQ CM	OTH	Q4164
HEMGENIX	THERAPEUTIC DOSE	IV	J1411
HEMIN	1 MG	IV	J1640
HEMLIBRA	0.5 MG	SC	J7170
HEMOFIL-M	1 IU	IV	J7190
HEMOSPRAY	UNKNOWN	OTH	C1052
HEMOSTATIC AGENT, GASTROINTESTINAL	UNKNOWN	OTH	C1052
HEP LOCK	10 U	IV	J1642
HEP-PAK	10 UNITS	IV	J1642
HEPAGAM B	0.5 ML	IM	J1571
HEPAGAM B	0.5 ML	IV	J1573
HEPARIN SODIUM	10 U	IV	J1642
HEPARIN SODIUM	1,000 U	IV, SC	J1644
HEPARIN SODIUM (PFIZER), NOT THERAPEUTICALLY EQUIVALENT TO J1644	1000 UNITS	INJ, IV, SC, OTH	J1643
HEPATITIS B IMMUNE GLOBULIN	0.5 ML	IV	J1573
HEPATOLITE	STUDY DOSE UP TO 15 MCI	IV	A9510
HERCEPTIN HYLECTA	10 MG	SC	J9356
HERCEPTIN, EXCLUDES BIOSIMILAR	10 MG	IV	J9355
HERZUMA	10 MG	IV	Q5113
HEXADROL	0.25 MG	ORAL	J8540
HEXAMINOLEVULINATE HYDROCHLORIDE	STUDY DOSE	OTH	A9589
HIGH OSMOLAR CONTRAST MATERIAL, UP TO 149 MG/ML IODINE CONCENTRATION	1 ML	IV	Q9958
HIGH OSMOLAR CONTRAST MATERIAL, UP TO 150-199 MG/ML IODINE CONCENTRATION	1 ML	IV	Q9959
HIGH OSMOLAR CONTRAST MATERIAL, UP TO 200-249 MG/ML IODINE CONCENTRATION	1 ML	IV	Q9960
HIGH OSMOLAR CONTRAST MATERIAL, UP TO 250-299 MG/ML IODINE CONCENTRATION	1 ML	IV	Q9961
HIGH OSMOLAR CONTRAST MATERIAL, UP TO 300-349 MG/ML IODINE CONCENTRATION	1 ML	IV	Q9962
HIGH OSMOLAR CONTRAST MATERIAL, UP TO 350-399 MG/ML IODINE CONCENTRATION	1 ML	IV	Q9963

Drug Name	Units Per	Route	Code
HIGH OSMOLAR CONTRAST MATERIAL, UP TO 400 OR GREATER MG/ML IODINE CONCENTRATION	1 ML	IV	Q9964
HISTERLIN IMPLANT (VANTAS)	50 MG	OTH	J9225
HISTRELIN ACETATE	10 MG	INJ	J1675
HISTRELIN IMPLANT (SUPPRELIN LA)	50 MG	OTH	J9226
HIZENTRA	100 MG	SC	J1559
HMATRIX	SQ CM	OTH	Q4134
HUMALOG	5 U	SC	J1815
HUMALOG	50 U	SC	J1817
HUMAN FIBRINOGEN CONCENTRATE	1 MG	IV	J7177
HUMAN HEALTH FACTOR 10 AMNIOTIC PATCH (HHF10-P)	SQ CM	OTH	Q4224
HUMATE-P	1 IU	IV	J7187
HUMATROPE	1 MG	SC	J2941
HUMIRA	20 MG	SC	J0135
HUMULIN	5 U	SC	J1815
HUMULIN	50 U	SC	J1817
HUMULIN R	5 U	SC	J1815
HUMULIN R U-500	5 U	SC	J1815
HYALGAN	DOSE	INJ	J7321
HYALOMATRIX	SQ CM	OTH	Q4117
HYALURONAN	0.1 MG	INJ	J7328
HYALURONAN	DOSE	INJ	J7327
HYALURONAN	DOSE	INJ	J7326
HYALURONAN	DOSE	INJ	J7323
HYALURONAN	DOSE	INJ	J7321
HYALURONAN	DOSE	INJ	J7324
HYALURONAN	1 MG	INJ	J7322
HYALURONAN	1 MG	INJ	J7325
HYALURONAN	1 MG	INJ	J7320
HYALURONAN	1 MG	INJ	J7332
HYALURONAN	1 MG	INJ	J7331
HYALURONAN	1 MG	INJ	J7329
HYALURONAN	1 MG	INJ	J7318
HYALURONIDASE	150 UNITS	VAR	J3470
HYALURONIDASE RECOMBINANT	1 USP UNIT	SC	J3473
HYALURONIDASE, OVINE, PRESERVATIVE FREE	1000 USP	OTH	J3472
HYALURONIDASE, OVINE, PRESERVATIVE FREE	1 USP	OTH	J3471
HYCAMTIN	0.1 MG	IV	J9351
HYCAMTIN	0.25 MG	ORAL	J8705
HYDRALAZINE HCL	20 MG	IV, IM	J0360
HYDRATE	50 MG	IM, IV	J1240
HYDREA	500 MG	ORAL	S0176
HYDROCORTISONE ACETATE	25 MG	IV, IM, SC	J1700
HYDROCORTISONE SODIUM PHOSPHATE	50 MG	IV, IM, SC	J1710
HYDROCORTISONE SODIUM SUCCINATE	100 MG	IV, IM, SC	J1720
HYDROCORTONE PHOSPHATE	50 MG	SC, IM, IV	J1710
HYDROMORPHONE HCL	250 MG	OTH	S0092
HYDROMORPHONE HCL	4 MG	SC, IM, IV	J1170
HYDROXOCOBALAMIN	1,000 MCG	IM, SC	J3420
HYDROXOCOBALAMIN	10 MCG	IM, SC	J3425
HYDROXYCOBAL	1,000 MCG	IM, SC	J3420
HYDROXYPROGESTERONE CAPROATE (MAKENA)	10 MG	IM	J1726
HYDROXYUREA	500 MG	ORAL	S0176

Drug Name	Units Per	Route	Code
HYDROXYZINE HCL	25 MG	IM	J3410
HYDROXYZINE PAMOATE	25 MG	ORAL	Q0177
HYMOVIS	1 MG	INJ	J7322
HYOSCYAMINE SULFATE	0.25 MG	SC, IM, IV	J1980
HYPERRHO S/D	300 MCG	IV	J2790
HYPERTET SD	UP TO 250 MG	IM	J1670
HYPERTONIC SALINE SOLUTION	1 ML	VAR	J7131
HYQVIA	100 MG	IV	J1575
HYREXIN	50 MG	IV, IM	J1200
HYZINE	25 MG	IM	J3410
HYZINE-50	25 MG	IM	J3410
IBALIZUMAB-UIYK	10 MG	IV	J1746
IBANDRONATE SODIUM	1 MG	IV	J1740
IBRITUMOMAB TUXETAN, DIAGNOSTIC	STUDY DOSE UP TO 5 MCI	IV	A9542
IBUPROFEN	100 MG	IV	J1741
IBUTILIDE FUMARATE	1 MG	IV	J1742
ICATIBANT	1 MG	SC	J1744
IDACIO, BIOSIMILAR	20 MG	SC	Q5131
IDAMYCIN	5 MG	IV	J9211
IDAMYCIN PFS	5 MG	IV	J9211
IDARUBICIN HCL	5 MG	IV	J9211
IDECABTAGENE VICLEUCEL	UP TO 460 MILLION CELLS	IV	Q2055
IDELVION	1 IU	IV	J7202
IDURSULFASE	1 MG	IV	J1743
IFEX	1 G	IV	J9208
IFOSFAMIDE	1 G	IV	J9208
IGALMI	1 MCG	ORAL	J1105
IHEEZO	1 MG	OTH	J2403
IL-2	1 VIAL	IV	J9015
ILARIS	1 MG	SC	J0638
ILETIN	5 UNITS	SC	J1815
ILETIN II NPH PORK	50 U	SC	J1817
ILETIN II REGULAR PORK	5 U	SC	J1815
ILLUCCIX	1 MCI	IV	A9596
ILOPROST INHALATION SOLUTION	DOSE UP TO 20 MCG	INH	Q4074
ILUMYA	1 MG	SC	J3245
ILUVIEN	0.01 MG	OTH	J7313
IMAGENT	1 ML	IV	Q9955
IMATINIB	100 MG	ORAL	S0088
IMFINZI	10 MG	IV	J9173
IMIGLUCERASE	10 U	IV	J1786
IMIPENEM, CILASTATIN, AND RELEBACTAM	4 MG/4 MG/2 MG	IV	J0742
IMITREX	6 MG	SC	J3030
IMJUDO	1 MG	IV	C9147
IMJUDO	1 MG	IV	J9347
IMLYGIC	1 MILLION	INTRALESIONAL	J9325
IMMUNE GLOBULIN	100 MG	IV	J1551
IMMUNE GLOBULIN (ASCENIV)	500 MG	IV	J1554
IMMUNE GLOBULIN (BIVIGAM)	500 MG	IV	J1556
IMMUNE GLOBULIN (CIVITRU)	100 MG	SC	J1555
IMMUNE GLOBULIN (FLEBOGAMMA, FLEBOGAMMA DIF)	500 MG	IV	J1572
IMMUNE GLOBULIN (GAMMAGARD LIQUID)	500 MG	IV	J1569
IMMUNE GLOBULIN (GAMMAPLEX)	500 MG	IV	J1557
IMMUNE GLOBULIN (GAMUNEX)	500 MG	IV	J1561

Drug Name	Units Per	Route	Code
IMMUNE GLOBULIN (HIZENTRA)	100 MG	SC	J1559
IMMUNE GLOBULIN (OCTAGAM)	500 MG	IV	J1568
IMMUNE GLOBULIN (PRIVIGEN) NONLYOPHILIZED	500 MG	IV	J1459
IMMUNE GLOBULIN (RHOPHYLAC)	100 IU	IM, IV	J2791
IMMUNE GLOBULIN (XEMBIFY)	100 MG	SC	J1558
IMMUNE GLOBULIN SUBCUTANEOUS	100 MG	SC	J1562
IMMUNE GLOBULIN, NON-LYOPHILIZED	500 MG	IV	J1576
IMMUNE GLOBULIN/ HYALURONIDASE	100 MG	IV	J1575
IMPLANON	IMPLANT	OTH	J7307
IMURAN	50 MG	ORAL	J7500
INAPSINE	5 MG	IM, IV	J1790
INCLISIRAN	1 MG	SC	J1306
INCOBUTULINUMTOXINA	1 UNIT	IM	J0588
INDERAL	1 MG	IV	J1800
INDIUM IN-111 CAPROMAB PENDETIDE, DIAGNOSTIC	STUDY DOSE UP TO 10 MCI	IV	A9507
INDIUM IN-111 IBRITUMOMAB TIUXETAN, DIAGNOSTIC	STUDY DOSE UP TO 5 MCI	IV	A9542
INDIUM IN-111 LABELED AUTOLOGOUS PLATELETS	STUDY DOSE	IV	A9571
INDIUM IN-111 LABELED AUTOLOGOUS WHITE BLOOD CELLS	STUDY DOSE	IV	A9570
INDIUM IN-111 OXYQUINOLINE, DIAGNOSTIC	0.5 MCI	IV	A9547
INDIUM IN-111 PENTETATE, DIAGNOSTIC	0.5 MCI	INJ	A9548
INDIUM IN-111 PENTETREOTIDE	STUDY DOSE UP TO 6 MCI	IV	A9572
INDIUM IN-111 SATUMOMAB PENDETIDE, DIAGNOSTIC	STUDY DOSE UP TO 6MCI	IV	A4642
INDURSALFASE	1 MG	IV	J1743
INEBILIZUMAB-CDON	1 MG	IV	J1823
INFED	50 MG	IM, IV	J1750
INFERGEN	1 MCG	SC	J9212
INFLECTRA	10 MG	IV	Q5103
INFLIXIMAB	10 MG	IV	J1745
INFLIXIMAB-ABDA, BIOSIMILAR	10 MG	IV	Q5104
INFLIXIMAB-AXXQ, BIOSIMILAR	10 MG	IV	Q5121
INFLIXIMAB-DYYB, BIOSIMILAR	10 MG	IV	Q5103
INFLIXIMAB-QBTX, BIOSIMILAR	10 MG	IV	Q5109
INFLUENZA VACCINE, AGRIFLU	UNKNOWN	IM	Q2034
INFLUENZA VIRUS VACCINE (AFLURIA)	EA	IM	Q2035
INFLUENZA VIRUS VACCINE (FLULAVAL)	EA	IM	Q2036
INFLUENZA VIRUS VACCINE (FLUVIRIN)	EA	IM	Q2037
INFLUENZA VIRUS VACCINE (FLUZONE)	EA	IM	Q2038
INFUGEM	100 MG	IV	J9198
INFUMORPH	10 MG	IM, IV, SC	J2270
INJECTAFER	1 MG	IV	J1439
INNOHEP	1,000 IU	SC	J1655
INNOVABURN OR INNOVAMATRIX XL	SQ CM	OTH	A2022
INNOVAMATRIX AC	SQ CM	OTH	A2001
INNOVAMATRIX FS	SQ CM	OTH	A2013
INNOVAMATRIX PD	SQ CM	OTH	A2023
INOTUZUMAB OZOGAMICIN	0.1 MG	IV	J9229
INSULIN	5 U	SC	J1815

Drug Name	Units Per	Route	Code
INSULIN	50 U	SC	J1817
INSULIN LISPRO	5 U	SC	S5551
INSULIN LISPRO	5 U	SC	J1815
INSULIN PURIFIED REGULAR PORK	5 U	SC	J1815
INTAL	10 MG	INH	J7631
INTEGRA BILAYER MATRIX DRESSING	SQ CM	OTH	Q4104
INTEGRA DERMAL REGENERATION TEMPLATE	SQ CM	OTH	Q4105
INTEGRA FLOWABLE WOUND MATRIX	1 CC	INJ	Q4114
INTEGRA MATRIX	SQ CM	OTH	Q4108
INTEGRA MESHED BILAYER WOUND MATRIX	SQ CM	OTH	C9363
INTEGRA MOZAIK OSTEOCONDUCTIVE SCAFFOLD PUTTY	0.5 CC	OTH	C9359
INTEGRA MOZAIK OSTEOCONDUCTIVE SCAFFOLD STRIP	0.5 CC	OTH	C9362
INTEGRA OMNIGRAFT DERMAL REGENERATION MATRIX	SQ CM	OTH	Q4105
INTEGRA OS OSTEOCONDUCTIVE SCAFFOLD PUTTY	0.5 CC	OTH	C9359
INTEGRILIN	5 MG	IM, IV	J1327
INTERFERON ALFA-2A	3,000,000 U	SC, IM	J9213
INTERFERON ALFA-2B	1,000,000 U	SC, IM	J9214
INTERFERON ALFA-N3	250,000 IU	IM	J9215
INTERFERON ALFACON-1	1 MCG	SC	J9212
INTERFERON BETA-1A	1 MCG	IM	Q3027
INTERFERON BETA-1A	30 MCG	IM, SC	J1826
INTERFERON BETA-1A	1 MCG	SC	Q3028
INTERFERON BETA-1B	0.25 MG	SC	J1830
INTERFERON, ALFA-2A, RECOMBINANT	3,000,000 U	SC, IM	J9213
INTERFERON, ALFA-2B, RECOMBINANT	1,000,000 U	SC, IM	J9214
INTERFERON, ALFA-N3, (HUMAN LEUKOCYTE DERIVED)	250,000 IU	IM	J9215
INTERFERON, GAMMA 1-B	3,000,000 U	SC	J9216
INTERFYL	1 MG	OTH	Q4171
INTERLUEKIN	1 VIAL	IV	J9015
INTRON A	1,000,000 U	SC, IM	J9214
INVANZ	500 MG	IM, IV	J1335
INVEGA HAFYERA	1 MG	IM	J2427
INVEGA SUSTENNA	1 MG	IM	J2426
INVEGA TRINZA	1 MG	IM	J2427
INVIRASE	200 MG	ORAL	S0140
IOBENGUANE SULFATE I-131	0.5 MCI	IV	A9508
IOBENGUANE, I-123, DIAGNOSTIC	STUDY DOSE UP TO 15 MCI	IV	A9582
IODINE I-123 IOBENGUANE, DIAGNOSTIC	STUDY DOSE UP TO 15 MCI	IV	A9582
IODINE I-123 IOFLUPANE	STUDY DOSE UP TO 5 MCI	IV	A9584
IODINE I-123 SODIUM IODIDE CAPSULE(S), DIAGNOSTIC	100-9999 UCI	ORAL	A9516
IODINE I-123 SODIUM IODIDE, DIAGNOSTIC	1 MCI	IV	A9509
IODINE I-125 SERUM ALBUMIN, DIAGNOSTIC	5 UCI	IV	A9532
IODINE I-125 SODIUM IOTHALAMATE, DIAGNOSTIC	STUDY DOSE UP TO 10 UCI	IV	A9554

Drug Name	Units Per	Route	Code
IODINE I-125, SODIUM IODIDE SOLUTION, THERAPEUTIC	1 MCI	OTH	A9527
IODINE I-131 IOBENGUANE SULFATE, DIAGNOSTIC	0.5 MCI	IV	A9508
IODINE I-131 IODINATED SERUM ALBUMIN, DIAGNOSTIC	PER 5 UCI	IV	A9524
IODINE I-131 SODIUM IODIDE CAPSULE(S), DIAGNOSTIC	1 MCI	ORAL	A9528
IODINE I-131 SODIUM IODIDE CAPSULE(S), THERAPEUTIC	1 MCI	ORAL	A9517
IODINE I-131 SODIUM IODIDE SOLUTION, DIAGNOSTIC	1 MCI	ORAL	A9529
IODINE I-131 SODIUM IODIDE SOLUTION, THERAPEUTIC	1 MCI	ORAL	A9530
IODINE I-131 SODIUM IODIDE, DIAGNOSTIC	UCI UP TO 100 UCI	IV	A9531
IODINE I-131, IOBENGUANE	1 MCI	IV	A9590
IODOTOPE THERAPEUTIC CAPSULE(S)	1 MCI	ORAL	A9517
IODOTOPE THERAPEUTIC SOLUTION	1 MCI	ORAL	A9530
IOFLUPANE	STUDY DOSE UP TO 5 MCI	IV	A9584
ION-BASED MAGNETIC RESONANCE CONTRAST AGENT	1 ML	IV	Q9953
IOTHALAMATE SODIUM I-125	STUDY DOSE UP TO 10 UCI	IV	A9554
IPILIMUMAB	1 MG	IV	J9228
IPLEX	1 MG	SC	J2170
IPRATROPIUM BROMIDE, NONCOMPOUNDED, UNIT DOSE	1 MG	INH	J7644
IPTRATROPIUM BROMIDE COMPOUNDED, UNIT DOSE	1 MG	INH	J7645
IRESSA	250 MG	ORAL	J8565
IRINOTECAN	20 MG	IV	J9206
IRINOTECAN LIPOSOME	1 MG	IV	J9205
IRON DEXTRAN, 50 MG	50 MG	IM, IV	J1750
IRON SUCROSE	1 MG	IV	J1756
ISATUXIMAB-IRFC	10 MG	IV	J9227
ISAVUCONAZONIUM	1 MG	IV	J1833
ISOCAINE	10 ML	VAR	J0670
ISOETHARINE HCL COMPOUNDED, CONCENTRATED	1 MG	INH	J7647
ISOETHARINE HCL COMPOUNDED, UNIT DOSE	1 MG	INH	J7650
ISOETHARINE HCL, NONCOMPOUNDED CONCENTRATED	1 MG	INH	J7648
ISOETHARINE HCL, NONCOMPOUNDED, UNIT DOSE	1 MG	INH	J7649
ISOJEX	5 UCI	IV	A9532
ISOPROTERENOL HCL COMPOUNDED, CONCENTRATED	1 MG	INH	J7657
ISOPROTERENOL HCL COMPOUNDED, UNIT DOSE	1 MG	INH	J7660
ISOPROTERENOL HCL, NONCOMPOUNDED CONCENTRATED	1 MG	INH	J7658
ISOPROTERNOL HCL, NONCOMPOUNDED, UNIT DOSE	1MG	INH	J7659
ISOSULFAN BLUE	1 MG	SC	Q9968
ISTODAX	0.1 MG	IV	J9319
ISUPREL	1 MG	INH	J7658
ISUPREL	1 MG	INH	J7659
ITRACONAZOLE	50 MG	IV	J1835
IXABEPILONE	1 MG	IV	J9207

Drug Name	Units Per	Route	Code
IXEMPRA	1 MG	IV	J9207
IXIFI	10 MG	IV	Q5109
IXINITY	1 IU	IV	J7213
IZERVAY	0.1 MG	INJ	C9162
JELMYTO	1 MG	OTH	J9281
JEMPERLI	10 MG	IV	J9272
JESDUVROQ	1 MG	ORAL	J0889
JETREA	0.125 MG	OTH	J7316
JEVTANA	1 MG	IV	J9043
JIVI	1 IU	IV	J7208
KADCYLA	1 MG	IV	J9354
KALBITOR	1 MG	SC	J1290
KANAMYCIN	500 MG	IM, IV	J1840
KANAMYCIN	75 MG	IM, IV	J1850
KANJINTI	10 MG	IV	Q5117
KANTREX	75 MG	IM, IV	J1850
KANTREX	500 MG	IM, IV	J1840
KANUMA	1 MG	IV	J2840
KCENTRA	1 IU	IV	J7168
KEFZOL	500 MG	IM, IV	J0690
KEPIVANCE	50 MCG	IV	J2425
KEPPRA	10 MG	IV	J1953
KERAMATRIX OR KERASORB	SQ CM	OTH	Q4165
KERECIS OMEGA3	SQ CM	OTH	Q4158
KERECIS OMEGA3 MARIGEN SHIELD	SQ CM	OTH	A2019
KEROXX	1 CC	OTH	Q4202
KESTRONE	1 MG	IV, IM	J1435
KETOROLAC TROMETHAMINE	15 MG	IM, IV	J1885
KEYTRUDA	1 MG	IV	J9271
KHAPZORY	0.5 MG	IV	J0642
KIMMTRAK	1 MCG	IV	J9274
KIMYRSA	10 MG	IV	J2406
KINEVAC	5 MCG	IV	J2805
KOATE-DVI	1 IU	IV	J7190
KONAKION	1 MG	SC, IM, IV	J3430
KONYNE 80	1 IU	IV	J7194
KORSUVA	0.1 MCG	IV	J0879
KOVALTRY	1 IU	IV	J7211
KRYSTEXXA	1 MG	IV	J2507
KYBELLA	1 MG	SC	J0591
KYLEENA	19.5 MG	OTH	J7296
KYMRIAH	UP TO 600 MILLION CELLS	IV	Q2042
KYPROLIS	1 MG	IV	J9047
KYTRIL	1 MG	IV	S0091
KYTRIL	1 MG	ORAL	Q0166
KYTRIL	100 MCG	IV	J1626
L.A.E. 20	10 MG	IM	J1380
LABETALOL HCL	5 MG	IV	J1920
LABETALOL HCL (HIKEMA)	5 MG	IV	J1921
LACOSAMIDE	1 MG	IV	C9254
LAETRILE	VAR	INJ	J3570
LAMELLAS	SQ CM	OTH	Q4292
LAMELLAS XT	SQ CM	OTH	Q4291
LAMZEDE	1 MG	IV	J0217
LANADELUMAB-FLYO	1 MG	SC	J0593
LANOXIN	0.5 MG	IM, IV	J1160
LANREOTIDE	1 MG	SC	J1930
LANREOTIDE	1 MG	SC, INJ	J1932
LANTUS	5 U	SC	J1815

Drug Name	Units Per	Route	Code
LARONIDASE	0.1 MG	IV	J1931
LARTRUVO	10 MG	INF	J9285
LASIX	20 MG	IM, IV	J1940
LECANEMAB-IRMB	1 MG	IV	J0174
LEFAMULIN	1 MG	IV	J0691
LEMTRADA	1 MG	IV	J0202
LENACAPAVIR	1 MG	SC	J1961
LENTE ILETIN I	5 U	SC	J1815
LEPIRUDIN	50 MG	IV	J1945
LEQEMBI	1 MG	IV	J0174
LEQVIO	1 MG	SC	J1306
LEUCOVORIN CALCIUM	50 MG	IM, IV	J0640
LEUKERAN	2 MG	ORAL	S0172
LEUKINE	50 MCG	IV	J2820
LEUPROLIDE	1 MG	SC	J1952
LEUPROLIDE ACETATE	7.5 MG	SC	J9217
LEUPROLIDE ACETATE	1 MG	IM	J9218
LEUPROLIDE ACETATE (FOR DEPOT SUSPENSION)	3.75 MG	IM	J1950
LEUPROLIDE ACETATE DEPOT	7.5 MG	SC	J9217
LEUPROLIDE ACETATE FOR DEPOT SUSPENSION	0.25 MG	SC	J1951
LEUPROLIDE ACETATE FOR DEPOT SUSPENSION	7.5 MG	IM	J1954
LEUPROLIDE ACETATE IMPLANT	65 MG	OTH	J9219
LEUSTATIN	1 MG	IV	J9065
LEVABUTEROL COMPOUNDED, UNIT DOSE	1 MG	INH	J7615
LEVABUTEROL, COMPOUNDED, CONCENTRATED	0.5 MG	INH	J7607
LEVALBUTEROL NONCOMPOUNDED, CONCENTRATED FORM	0.5 MG	INH	J7612
LEVALBUTEROL, NONCOMPOUNDED, UNIT DOSE	0.5 MG	INH	J7614
LEVAMISOLE HCL	50 MG	ORAL	S0177
LEVAQUIN	250 MG	IV	J1956
LEVEMIR	5 U	SC	J1815
LEVETIRACETAM	10 MG	IV	J1953
LEVO-DROMORAN	UP TO 2 MG	IV, IM	J1960
LEVOCARNITINE	1 G	IV	J1955
LEVOFLOXACIN	250 MG	IV	J1956
LEVOLEUCOVORIN	0.5 MG	IV	J0642
LEVONORGESTREL IMPLANT	IMPLANT	OTH	J7306
LEVONORGESTREL-RELEASING INTRAUTERINE CONTRACEPTIVE (MIRENA)	52 MG	OTH	J7298
LEVONORGESTREL-RELEASING INTRAUTERINE CONTRACEPTIVE (LILETTA)	52 MG	OTH	J7297
LEVONORGESTREL-RELEASING INTRAUTERINE CONTRACEPTIVE SYSTEM (KYLEENA)	19.5 MG	OTH	J7296
LEVONORGESTREL-RELEASING INTRAUTERINE CONTRACEPTIVE SYSTEM (SKYLA)	13.5 MG	OTH	J7301
LEVONORGESTREL-RELEASING INTRAUTERINE SYSTEM	EA	OTH	S4981
LEVORPHANOL TARTRATE	2 MG	SC, IV, IM	J1960
LEVSIN	0.25 MG	SC, IM, IV	J1980
LEVULAN KERASTICK	354 MG	OTH	J7308
LEXISCAN	0.1 MG	IV	J2785
LIBRIUM	100 MG	IM, IV	J1990
LIBTAYO	1 MG	IV	J9119

Drug Name	Units Per	Route	Code
LIDOCAINE 70 MG/TETRACAINE 70 MG	PATCH	OTH	C9285
LIDOCAINE HCL	10 MG	IV	J2001
LILETTA	52 MG	OTH	J7297
LINCOCIN HCL	300 MG	IV	J2010
LINCOMYCIN HCL	300 MG	IM, IV	J2010
LINEZOLID	200 MG	IV	J2020
LINEZOLID (HOSPIRA) NOT THERAPEUTICALLY EQUIVALENT TO J2020	200 MG	IV	J2021
LIORESAL	10 MG	IT	J0475
LIORESAL INTRATHECAL REFILL	50 MCG	IT	J0476
LIPODOX	10 MG	IV	Q2049
LIPOSOMAL, DAUNORUBICIN AND CYTARABINE	1 MG/2.27 MG	IV	J9153
LIQUAEMIN SODIUM	1,000 UNITS	SC, IV	J1644
LISOCABTAGENE MARALEUCEL	UP TO 110 MILLION CELLS	IV	Q2054
LISPRO-PFC	50 U	SC	J1817
LOCAMETZ	1 MCI	IV	A9800
LOK-PAK	10 UNITS	IV	J1642
LOMUSTINE	10 MG	ORAL	S0178
LONCASTUXIMAB TESIRINE-LPYL	1 MG	IV	J9359
LORAZEPAM	2 MG	IM, IV	J2060
LOVENOX	10 MG	SC	J1650
LOW OSMOLAR CONTRAST MATERIAL, 100-199 MG/ML IODINE CONCENTRATIONS	1 ML	IV	Q9965
LOW OSMOLAR CONTRAST MATERIAL, 200-299 MG/ML IODINE CONCENTRATION	1 ML	IV	Q9966
LOW OSMOLAR CONTRAST MATERIAL, 300-399 MG/ML IODINE CONCENTRATION	1 ML	IV	Q9967
LOW OSMOLAR CONTRAST MATERIAL, 400 OR GREATER MG/ML IODINE CONCENTRATION	1 ML	IV	Q9951
LOXAPINE	1 MG	INH	J2062
LUCENTIS	0.1 MG	IV	J2778
LUMASIRAN	0.5 MG	SC	J0224
LUMASON	1 ML	IV	Q9950
LUMIZYME	10 MG	IV	J0221
LUMOXITI	0.01 MG	IV	J9313
LUNSUMIO	1 MG	IV	J9350
LUPRON	1 MG	SC	J9218
LUPRON DEPOT	7.5 MG	SC	J9217
LUPRON DEPOT	3.75 MG	IM	J1950
LUPRON IMPLANT	65 MG	OTH	J9219
LURBINECTEDIN	0.1 MG	IV	J9223
LUSPATERCEPT-AAMT	0.25 MG	SC	J0896
LUTATHERA	1 MCI	IM	A9513
LUTETIUM LU 177 VIPIVOTIDE TETRAXETAN, THERAPEUTIC	1 MCI	IV	A9607
LUTETIUM LU 177, DOTATATE, THERAPEUTIC	1 MCI	IM	A9513
~~LUTRATE~~	~~7.5 MG~~	~~IM~~	~~J1954~~
LUTREPULSE	100 MCG	SC, IV	J1620
LUXTURNA	1 BILLION VECTOR GENOMES	OTH	J3398
LYMPHAZURIN	1 MG	SC	Q9968
LYMPHOCYTE IMMUNE GLOBULIN, ANTITHYMOCYTE GLOBULIN, EQUINE	250 MG	OTH	J7504

Drug Name	Units Per	Route	Code
LYMPHOCYTE IMMUNE GLOBULIN, ANTITHYMOCYTE GLOBULIN, RABBIT	25 MG	OTH	J7511
LYMPHOSEEK	0.5 MCI	SC, OTH	A9520
LYMUJEV	5 U	SC, IV	J1814
LYMUJEV	50 U	SC, IV	J1813
MACUGEN	0.3 MG	OTH	J2503
MAGNESIUM SULFATE	500 MG	IV	J3475
MAGNETIC RESONANCE CONTRAST AGENT	1 ML	ORAL	Q9954
MAGROTEC	STUDY DOSE UP TO 10 MCI	IV	A9540
MAGTRACE	STUDY DOSE	SC	A9697
MAKENA	10 MG	IM	J1726
MANNITOL	25% IN 50 ML	IV	J2150
MANNITOL	5 MG	INH	J7665
~~MARCAINE HCL~~	~~30 ML~~	~~VAR~~	~~S0020~~
MARGENZA	5 MG	IV	J9353
MARGETUXIMAB-CMKB	5 MG	IV	J9353
MARINOL	2.5 MG	ORAL	Q0167
MARMINE	50 MG	IM, IV	J1240
MARQIBO KIT	5 MG	IV	J9371
MATRION	SQ CM	OTH	Q4201
MATRISTEM MICROMATRIX	1 MG	OTH	Q4118
MATULANE	50 MG	ORAL	S0182
MAXIPIME	500 MG	IV	J0692
MDP-BRACCO	STUDY DOSE UP TO 30 MCI	IV	A9503
MECASERMIN	1 MG	SC	J2170
MECHLORETHAMINE HCL (NITROGEN MUSTARD)	10 MG	IV	J9230
MEDIDEX	1 MG	IM, IV, OTH	J1100
MEDISKIN	SQ CM	OTH	Q4135
MEDROL	4 MG	ORAL	J7509
MEDROXYPROGESTERONE ACETATE	1 MG	IM	J1050
MEFOXIN	1 G	IV	J0694
MEGACE	20 MG	ORAL	S0179
MEGESTROL ACETATE	20 MG	ORAL	S0179
MELOXICAM	1 MG	IV	J1738
MELPHALAN	1 MG	IV	J9246
MELPHALAN	2 MG	ORAL	J8600
MELPHALAN FLUFENAMIDE	1 MG	IV	J9247
MEMBRANE GRAFT OR MEMBRANE WRAP	SQ CM	OTH	Q4205
MEMBRANE WRAP-HYDRO	SQ CM	OTH	Q4290
MEMODERM	SQ CM	OTH	Q4126
MENADIONE	1 MG	IM, SC, IV	J3430
MENOTROPINS	75 IU	SC, IM, IV	S0122
MEPERGAN	50 MG	IM, IV	J2180
MEPERIDINE AND PROMETHAZINE HCL	50 MG	IM, IV	J2180
MEPERIDINE HCL	100 MG	IM, IV, SC	J2175
MEPIVACAINE HCL	10 ML	VAR	J0670
MEPOLIZUMAB	1 MG	SQ	J2182
MEPSEVII	1 MG	IV	J3397
MERCAPTOPURINE	50 MG	ORAL	S0108
MERITATE	150 MG	IV	J3520
MEROPENEM	100 MG	IV	J2185
MEROPENEM (B. BRAUN) NOT THERAPEUTICALLY EQUIVALENT TO J2185	100 MG	IV	J2184
MEROPENEM, VABORBACTAM	10 MG/10 MG	IV	J2186

Drug Name	Units Per	Route	Code
MERREM	100 MG	IV	J2185
MESNA	200 MG	IV	J9209
MESNEX	200 MG	IV	J9209
METAPROTERENOL SULFATE COMPOUNDED, UNIT DOSE	10 MG	INH	J7670
METAPROTERENOL SULFATE, NONCOMPOUNDED, CONCENTRATED	10 MG	INH	J7668
METAPROTERENOL SULFATE, NONCOMPOUNDED, UNIT DOSE	10 MG	INH	J7669
METARAMINOL BITARTRATE	10 MG	IV, IM, SC	J0380
METASTRON STRONTIUM 89 CHLORIDE	1 MCI	IV	A9600
METATRACE	STUDY DOSE UP TO 45 MCI	IV	A9552
METHACHOLINE CHLORIDE	1 MG	INH	J7674
METHADONE	5 MG	ORAL	S0109
METHADONE HCL	10 MG	IM, SC	J1230
METHAPREL, COMPOUNDED, UNIT DOSE	10 MG	INH	J7670
METHAPREL, NONCOMPOUNDED, CONCENTRATED	10 MG	INH	J7668
METHAPREL, NONCOMPOUNDED, UNIT DOSE	10 MG	INH	J7669
METHERGINE	0.2 MG	IM, IV	J2210
METHOTREXATE	2.5 MG	ORAL	J8610
METHOTREXATE	5 MG	IV, IM, IT, IA	J9250
METHOTREXATE	50 MG	IV, IM, IT, IA	J9260
METHOTREXATE (ACCORD), NOT THERAPEUTICALLY EQUIVALENT TO J9250 AND J9260	50 MG	IN I	J9255
METHOTREXATE LPF	5 MG	IV, IM, IT, IA	J9250
METHOTREXATE LPF	50 MG	IV, IM, IT, IA	J9260
METHYL AMINOLEVULINATE 16.8%	1 G	OTH	J7309
METHYLCOTOLONE	80 MG	IM	J1040
METHYLDOPA HCL	UP TO 250 MG	IV	J0210
METHYLDOPATE HCL	UP TO 250 MG	IV	J0210
METHYLENE BLUE	1 MG	SC	Q9968
METHYLERGONOVINE MALEATE	0.2 MG	IM, IV	J2210
METHYLNALTREXONE	0.1 MG	SC	J2212
METHYLPRED	4 MG	ORAL	J7509
METHYLPREDNISOLONE	4 MG	ORAL	J7509
METHYLPREDNISOLONE	125 MG	IM, IV	J2930
METHYLPREDNISOLONE	UP TO 40 MG	IM, IV	J2920
METHYLPREDNISOLONE ACETATE	20 MG	IM	J1020
METHYLPREDNISOLONE ACETATE	80 MG	IM	J1040
METHYLPREDNISOLONE ACETATE	40 MG	IM	J1030
METOCLOPRAMIDE	10 MG	IV	J2765
METRONIDAZOLE	500 MG	IV	S0030
METRONIDAZOLE	10 MG	IV	J1836
METVIXIA 16.8%	1 G	OTH	J7309
MIACALCIN	400 U	SC, IM	J0630
MIBG	0.5 MCI	IV	A9508
MICAFUNGIN SODIUM	1 MG	IV	J2248
MICAFUNGIN SODIUM (PAR PHARM) NOT THERAPEUTICALLY EQUIVALENT TO J2248	1 MG	IV	J2247
MICRHOGAM	50 MCG	IV	J2788
MICROLYTE MATRIX	SQ CM	OTH	A2005
MICROPOROUS COLLAGEN IMPLANTABLE SLIT TUBE	1 CM LENGTH	OTH	C9353
MICROPOROUS COLLAGEN IMPLANTABLE TUBE	1 CM LENGTH	OTH	C9352

Drug Name	Units Per	Route	Code
MIDAZOLAM HCI	1 MG	IM, IV	J2250
MIDAZOLAM HCL (WG CRITICAL CARE) NOT THERAPEUTICALLY EQUIVALENT TO J2250	1 MG	IV	J2251
MIFEPRISTONE	200 MG	ORAL	S0190
MILRINONE LACTATE	5 MG	IV	J2260
MINOCIN	1 MG	IV	J2265
MINOCYCLINE HCL	1 MG	IV	J2265
MINOXIDIL	10 MG	ORAL	S0139
MIRCERA	1 MCG	IV	J0887
MIRCERA	1 MCG	SC	J0888
MIRENA	52 MG	OTH	J7298
MIRO3D	CU CM	OTH	A2025
MIRODERM	SQ CM	OTH	Q4175
MIRRAGEN ADVANCED WOUND MATRIX	SQ CM	OTII	A2002
MIRVETUXIMAB SORAVTANSINE-GYNX	1 MG	IV	C9146
MIRVETUXIMAB SORAVTANSINE-GYNX	1 MG	IV	J9063
MISOPROSTOL	200 MG	ORAL	S0191
MITHRACIN	2.5 MG	IV	J9270
MITOMYCIN	5 MG	IV	J9280
MITOMYCIN	0.2 MG	OTH	J7315
MITOMYCIN PYELOCALYCEAL INSTILLATION	1 MG	OTH	J9281
MITOSOL	0.2 MG	OTH	J7315
MITOXANA	1 G	IV	J9208
MITOXANTRONE HCL	5 MG	IV	J9293
MLG-COMPLETE	SQ CM	OTH	Q4256
MOGAMULIZUMAB-KPKC	1 MG	IV	J9204
MOMETASONE FUROATE SINUS IMPLANT	10 MCG	OTH	J7402
MONARC-M	1 IU	IV	J7190
MONJUVI	2 MG	IV	J9349
MONOCLATE-P	1 IU	IV	J7190
MONOFERRIC	10 MG	IV	J1437
MONONINE	1 IU	IV	J7193
MONOPUR	75 IU	SC, IM	S0122
MONOVISC	DOSE	INJ	J7327
MORPHINE SULFATE	10 MG	IM, IV, SC	J2270
MORPHINE SULFATE	500 MG	OTH	S0093
MORPHINE SULFATE (FRESENIUS KABI) NOT THERAPEUTICALLY EQUIVALENT TO J2270	10 MG	INJ, IV, SC	J2272
MORPHINE SULFATE, PRESERVATIVE-FREE FOR EPIDURAL OR INTRATHECAL USE	10 MG	OTH	J2274
MOSUNETUZUMAB-AXGB	1 MG	IV	J9350
MOXETUMOMAB PASUDOTOX-TDFK	0.01 MG	IV	J9313
MOXIFLOXACIN	100 MG	IV	J2280
MOXIFLOXACIN (FRESENIUS KABI) NOT THERAPEUTICALLY EQUIVALENT TO J2280	100 MG	IV	J2281
MOZOBIL	1 MG	SC	J2562
MPI INDIUM DTPA	0.5 MCI	INJ	A9548
MS CONTIN	500 MG	OTH	S0093
MUCOMYST	1 G	INH	J7608
MUCOSIL	1 G	INH	J7608
MUGARD	1 ML	OTH	A9156
MULTIHANCE	1 ML	IV	A9577
MULTIHANCE MULTIPACK	1 ML	IV	A9578
MUROMONAB-CD3	5 MG	OTH	J7505

Drug Name	Units Per	Route	Code
MUSE	EA	OTH	J0275
MUSTARGEN	10 MG	IV	J9230
MUTAMYCIN	5 MG	IV	J9280
MVASI	10 MG	IV	Q5107
MYCAMINE	1 MG	IV	J2248
MYCOPHENOLATE	10 MG	IV	J7519
MYCOPHENOLATE MOFETIL	250 MG	ORAL	J7517
MYCOPHENOLIC ACID	180 MG	ORAL	J7518
MYFORTIC DELAYED RELEASE	180 MG	ORAL	J7518
MYLERAN	2 MG	ORAL	J8510
MYLOCEL	500 MG	ORAL	S0176
MYLOTARG	0.1 MG	INF	J9203
MYOBLOC	100 U	IM	J0587
MYOCHRYSINE	50 MG	IM	J1600
MYOWN SKIN	SQ CM	OTH	Q4226
MYOZYME	10 MG	IV	J0220
NABILONE	1 MG	ORAL	J8650
NADOFARAGENE FIRADENOVEC-VNCG	THERAPEUTIC DOSE	OTH	J9029
NAFCILLIN SODIUM	2 GM	IM, IV	S0032
NAGLAZYME	1 MG	IV	J1458
NALBUPHINE HCL	10 MG	IM, IV, SC	J2300
NALLPEN	2 GM	IM, IV	S0032
NALOXONE HCL	1 MG	IM, IV, SC	J2310
NALOXONE HCL (ZIMHI)	1 MG	SC	J2311
NALTREXONE, DEPOT FORM	1 MG	IM	J2315
NANDROLONE DECANOATE	50 MG	IM	J2320
NARCAN	1 MG	IM, IV, SC	J2310
NAROPIN	1 MG	VAR	J2795
NASALCROM	10 MG	INH	J7631
NATALIZUMAB	1 MG	IV	J2323
NATRECOR	0.1 MG	IV	J2325
NATURAL ESTROGENIC SUBSTANCE	1 MG	IM, IV	J1410
NAVELBINE	10 MG	IV	J9390
NAXITAMAB-GQGK	1 MG	IV	J9348
ND-STAT	10 MG	IM, SC, IV	J0945
NEBCIN	80 MG	IM, IV	J3260
NEBUPENT	300 MG	IM, IV	S0080
NEBUPENT	300 MG	INH	J2545
NECITUMUMAB	1 MG	IV	J9295
NELARABINE	50 MG	IV	J9261
NEMBUTAL SODIUM	50 MG	IM, IV, OTH	J2515
NEOMATRIX	SQ CM	OTH	A2021
NEOPATCH	SQ CM	OTH	Q4176
NEORAL	25 MG	ORAL	J7515
NEORAL	250 MG	ORAL	J7516
NEOSAR	100 MG	IV	J9070
NEOSCAN	1 MCI	IV	A9556
NEOSTIGMINE METHYLSULFATE	0.5 MG	IM, IV	J2710
NEOSTIM DL	SQ CM	OTH	Q4267
NEOSTIM MEMBRANE	SQ CM	OTH	Q4266
NEOSTIM TL	SQ CM	OTH	Q4265
NEOTECT	STUDY DOSE UP TO 35 MCI	IV	A9536
NEOX 100	SQ CM	OTH	Q4156
NEOX CORD 1K	SQ CM	OTH	Q4148
NEOX CORD RT	SQ EM	OTH	Q4148
NEOXFLO	1 MG	OTH	Q4155
NESIRITIDE	0.1 MG	IV	J2325
NETSPOT	0.1 MCI	IV	A9587

Drug Name	Units Per	Route	Code
NETUPITANT AND PALONOSETRON	300 MG/0.5 MG	ORAL	J8655
NEULASTA	0.5 MG	SC	J2506
NEUMEGA	5 MG	SC	J2355
NEUPOGEN	1 MCG	SC, IV	J1442
NEURAGEN NERVE GUIDE	1 CM LENGTH	OTH	C9352
NEUROLITE	STUDY DOSE UP TO 25 MCI	IV	A9557
NEUROMATRIX	0.5 CM LENGTH	OTH	C9355
NEUROMEND NERVE WRAP	0.5 CM	OTH	C9361
NEUROWRAP NERVE PROTECTOR	1 CM LENGTH	OTH	C9353
NEUTREXIN	25 MG	IV	J3305
NEUTROSPEC	STUDY DOSE UP TO 25 MCI	IV	A9566
NEXOBRID	1 G	OTH	J7353
NEXPLANON	IMPLANT	OTH	J7307
NEXTERONE	30 MG	IV	J0283
NEXVIAZYME	4 MG	IV	J0219
NICARDIPINE	0.1 MG	IV	J2404
NIPENT	10 MG	IV	J9268
NITROGEN MUSTARD	10 MG	IV	J9230
NITROGEN N-13 AMMONIA, DIAGNOSTIC	STUDY DOSE UP TO 40 MCI	INJ	A9526
NITROGLYCERIN	5 MG	IV	J2305
NIVESTYM	1 MCG	INJ	Q5110
NIVOLUMAB	1 MG	IV	J9299
NIVOLUMAB AND RELATLIMAB-RMBW	3 MG/1 MG	IV	J9298
NOLVADEX	10 MG	ORAL	S0187
NORDITROPIN	1 MG	SC	J2941
NORDYL	50 MG	IV, IM	J1200
NORFLEX	60 MG	IV, IM	J2360
NORMAL SALINE SOLUTION	1000 CC	IV	J7030
NORMAL SALINE SOLUTION	250 CC	IV	J7050
NORMAL SALINE SOLUTION	500 ML	IV	J7040
NOVACHOR	SQ CM	OTH	Q4194
NOVAFIX	SQ CM	OTH	Q4208
NOVAFIX DL	SQ CM	OTH	Q4254
NOVANTRONE	5 MG	IV	J9293
NOVAREL	1,000 USP U	IM	J0725
NOVOEIGHT	IU	IV	J7182
NOVOLIN	50 U	SC	J1817
NOVOLIN R	5 U	SC	J1815
NOVOLOG	50 U	SC	J1817
NOVOSEVEN	1 MCG	IV	J7189
NOVOSORB SYNPATH DERMAL MATRIX	SQ CM	OTH	A2006
NPH	5 UNITS	SC	J1815
NPLATE	10 MCG	SC	J2796
NUBAIN	10 MG	IM, IV, SC	J2300
NUCALA	1 MG	SQ	J2182
NUDYN	0.5 CC	OTH	Q4233
NUDYN DL, DL MESH	SQ CM	OTH	Q4285
NUDYN SL, SLW	SQ CM	OTH	Q4286
NULOJIX	1 MG	IV	J0485
NUMBRINO	1 MG	OTH	C9143
NUMORPHAN	1 MG	IV, SC, IM	J2410
NUSHIELD	SQ CM	OTH	Q4160
NUSINERSEN	0.1 MG	INJ	J2326
NUTRI-TWELVE	1,000 MCG	IM, SC	J3420
NUTROPIN	1 MG	SC	J2941
NUTROPIN A.Q.	1 MG	SC	J2941

Drug Name	Units Per	Route	Code
NUVARING VAGINAL RING	0.015 MG/0.12 MG	OTH	J7295
NUWIQ	1 IU	IV	J7209
NUZYRA	1 MG	IV	J0121
NYVEPRIA	0.5 MG	SC	Q5122
OASIS BURN MATRIX	SQ CM	OTH	Q4103
OASIS ULTRA TRI-LAYER WOUND MATRIX	SQ CM	OTH	Q4124
OASIS WOUND MATRIX	SQ CM	OTH	Q4102
OBINUTUZUMAB	10 MG	IV	J9301
OBIZUR	IU	IV	J7188
OCRELIZUMAB	1 MG	INJ	J2350
OCREVUS	1 MG	INJ	J2350
OCRIPLASMIN	0.125 MG	OTH	J7316
OCTAFLUOROPROPANE UCISPHERES	1 ML	IV	Q9956
OCTAGAM	500 MG	IV	J1568
OCTREOSCAN	STUDY DOSE UP TO 6 MCI	IV	A9572
OCTREOTIDE ACETATE DEPOT	1 MG	IM	J2353
OCTREOTIDE, NON-DEPOT FORM	25 MCG	SC, IV	J2354
OFATUMUMAB	10 MG	IV	J9302
OFIRMEV	10 MG	IV	J0131
OFLOXACIN	400 MG	IV	S0034
OFORTA	10 MG	ORAL	J8562
OGIVRI	10 MG	IV	Q5114
OLANZAPINE	0.5 MG	IM	J2359
OLANZAPINE	2.5 MG	IM	S0166
OLANZAPINE LONG ACTING	1 MG	IM	J2358
OLARATUMAB	10 MG	INF	J9285
OLICERIDINE	0.1 MG	IV	C9101
OLINVYK	0.1 MG	IV	C9101
OLIPUDASE ALFA-RPCP	1 MG	IV	J0218
OMACETAXINE MEPESUCCINATE	0.01 MG	SC	J9262
OMADACYCLINE	1 MG	IV	J0121
OMALIZUMAB	5 MG	SC	J2357
OMEGAVEN	10 G	IV	B4187
OMEZA COLLAGEN MATRIX	100 MG	OTH	A2014
OMIDRIA	1 ML	OTH	J1097
OMNIPAQUE 140	1 ML	IV	Q9965
OMNIPAQUE 180	1 ML	IV	Q9965
OMNIPAQUE 240	1 ML	IV	Q9966
OMNIPAQUE 300	1 ML	IV	Q9967
OMNIPAQUE 350	1 ML	IV	Q9967
OMONTYS (FOR ESRD ON DIALYSIS)	0.1 MG	SC, IV	J0890
ONABOTULINUMTOXINA	1 UNIT	IM, OTH	J0585
ONASEMNOGENE ABEPARVOVEC-XIOI	UP TO 5X10^{15} VECTOR GENOMES	IV	J3399
ONCASPAR	VIAL	IM, IV	J9266
ONCOSCINT CR/OV	STUDY DOSE UP TO 6 MCI	IV	A4642
ONDANSETRON	1 MG	ORAL	Q0162
ONDANSETRON	4 MG	ORAL	S0119
ONDANSETRON HYDROCHLORIDE	1 MG	IV	J2405
ONIVYDE	1 MG	IV	J9205
ONPATTRO	0.1 MG	IV	J0222
ONTAK	300 MCG	IV	J9160
ONTRUZANT	10 MG	IV	Q5112
OPDIVO	1 MG	IV	J9299
OPDUALAG	3 MG/1 MG	IV	J9298

Drug Name	Units Per	Route	Code
OPRELVEKIN	5 MG	SC	J2355
OPTIRAY	1 ML	IV	Q9967
OPTIRAY 160	1 ML	IV	Q9965
OPTIRAY 240	1 ML	IV	Q9966
OPTIRAY 300	1 ML	IV	Q9967
OPTIRAY 320	1 ML	IV	Q9967
OPTISON	1 ML	IV	Q9956
ORAL MAGNETIC RESONANCE CONTRAST AGENT, PER 100 ML	100 ML	ORAL	Q9954
ORAL MUCOADHESIVE, ANY TYPE	1 ML	OTH	A9156
ORBACTIV	10 MG	IV	J2407
ORENCIA	10 MG	IV	J0129
ORION	SQ CM	OTH	Q4276
ORITAVANCIN	10 MG	IV	J2407
ORITAVANCIN	10 MG	IV	J2406
ORPHENADRINE CITRATE	60 MG	IV, IM	J2360
ORTHADAPT BIOIMPLANT	SQ CM	OTH	C1781
ORTHOCLONE OKT3	5 MG	OTH	J7505
ORTHOVISC	DOSE	INJ	J7324
OSELTAMIVIR PHOSPHATE (BRAND NAME) (DEMONSTRATION PROJECT)	75 MG	ORAL	G9035
OSELTAMIVIR PHOSPHATE (GENERIC) (DEMONSTRATION PROJECT)	75 MG	ORAL	G9019
OSMITROL	25% IN 50 ML	IV	J2150
OTIPRIO	6 MG	OTIC	J7342
OXACILLIN SODIUM	250 MG	IM, IV	J2700
OXALIPLATIN	0.5 MG	IV	J9263
OXILAN 300	1 ML	IV	Q9967
OXILAN 350	1 ML	IV	Q9967
OXLUMO	0.5 MG	SC	J0224
OXYMORPHONE HCL	1 MG	IV, SC, IM	J2410
OXYTETRACYCLINE HCL	50 MG	IM	J2460
OXYTOCIN	10 U	IV, IM	J2590
OZURDEX	0.1 MG	OTH	J7312
PACIS BCG	1 MG	OTH	J9030
PACLITAXEL	1 MG	IV	J9267
PACLITAXEL PROTEIN-BOUND PARTICLES	1 MG	IV	J9264
PACLITAXEL PROTEIN-BOUND PARTICLES (AMERICAN REGENT)	1 MG	IV	J9259
PACLITAXEL PROTEIN-BOUND PARTICLES (TEVA), NOT THERAPEUTICALLY EQUIVALENT TO J9264	1 MG	IV	J9258
PADCEV	0.25 MG	IV	J9177
PAFOLACIANINE	0.1 MG	IV	A9603
PALIFERMIN	50 MCG	IV	J2425
PALINGEN OR PALINGEN XPLU	SQ CM	OTH	Q4173
PALINGEN OR PROMATRX	0.36 MG/0.25 CC	OTH	Q4174
PALIPERIDONE PALMITATE EXTENDED RELEASE	1 MG	IM	J2427
PALIPERIDONE PALMITATE EXTENDED RELEASE (INVEGA SUSTENNA)	1 MG	IM	J2426
PALONOSETRON HCL	25 MCG	IV	J2469
PAMIDRONATE DISODIUM	30 MG	IV	J2430
PANHEMATIN	1 MG	IV	J1640
PANITUMUMAB	10 MG	IV	J9303
PANTOPRAZOLE SODIUM	VIAL	IV	C9113
PANTOPRAZOLE SODIUM	40 MG	IV	S0164
PANZYGA	500 MG	IV	J1576
PAPAVERINE HCL	60 MG	IV, IM	J2440

Drug Name	Units Per	Route	Code
PARAGARD T380A	EA	OTH	J7300
PARAPLANTIN	50 MG	IV	J9045
PARICALCITOL	1 MCG	IV, IM	J2501
PARSABIV	0.1 MG	IV	J0606
PASIREOTIDE LONG ACTING	1 MG	IV	J2502
PATISIRAN	0.1 MG	IV	J0222
PEDIAPRED	5 MG	ORAL	J7510
PEDMARK	100 MG	IV	J0208
PEG-INTRON	180 MCG	SC	S0145
PEGADEMASE BOVINE	25 IU	IM	J2504
PEGAPTANIB SODIUM	0.3 MG	OTH	J2503
PEGASPARGASE	VIAL	IM, IV	J9266
PEGCETACOPLAN	1 MG	SC	C9151
PEGCETACOPLAN	1 MG	INJ	J2781
PEGFILGRASTIM, EXCLUDES BIOSIMILAR	0.5 MG	SC	J2506
PEGFILGRASTIM-APGF, BIOSIMILAR	0.5 MG	SC	Q5122
PEGFILGRASTIM-BMEZ, BIOSIMILAR	0.5 MG	SC	Q5120
PEGFILGRASTIM-CBQV, BIOSIMILAR	0.5 MG	SC	Q5111
PEGFILGRASTIM-FPGK, BIOSIMILAR	0.5 MG	SC	Q5127
PEGFILGRASTIM-JMDB, BIOSIMILAR	0.5 MG	SC	Q5108
PEGFILGRASTIM-PBBK	0.5 MG	SC	Q5130
PEGINESATIDE (FOR ESRD ON DIALYSIS)	0.1 MG	SC, IV	J0890
PEGINTERFERON ALFA-2A	180 MCG	SC	S0145
PEGLOTICASE	1 MG	IV	J2507
PEGUNIGALSIDASE ALFA-IWXJ	1 MG	IV	J2508
PEGYLATED INTERFERON ALFA-2A	180 MCG	SC	S0145
PEGYLATED INTERFERON ALFA-2B	10 MCG	SC	S0148
PEMBROLIZUMAB	1 MG	IV	J9271
PEMETREXED	10 MG	IV	J9304
PEMETREXED	10 MG	IV	J9324
PEMETREXED (ACCORD), NOT THERAPEUTICALLY EQUIVALENT TO J9305	10 MG	IV	J9296
PEMETREXED (BLUEPOINT) NOT THERAPEUTICALLY EQUIVALENT TO J9305	10 MG	IV	J9322
PEMETREXED (HOSPIRA), NOT THERAPEUTICALLY EQUIVALENT TO J9305	10 MG	IV	J9294
PEMETREXED (SANDOZ), NOT THERAPEUTICALLY EQUIVALENT TO J9305	10 MG	IV	J9297
PEMETREXED (TEVA) NOT THERAPEUTICALLY EQUIVALENT TO J9305	10 MG	IV	J9314
PEMETREXED DITROMETHAMINE	10 MG	IV	J9323
PEMFEXY	10 MG	IV	J9304
PEMRYDI RTU	10 MG	IV	J9324
PENICILLIN G BENZATHINE	100,000 U	IM	J0561
PENICILLIN G BENZATHINE AND PENICILLIN G PROCAINE	100,000 UNITS	IM	J0558
PENICILLIN G POTASSIUM	600,000 U	IM, IV	J2540
PENICILLIN G PROCAINE	600,000 U	IM, IV	J2510
PENTACARINAT	300 MG	INH	S0080
PENTAM	300 MG	IM, IV	J2545
PENTAM 300	300 MG	IM, IV	S0080
PENTAMIDINE ISETHIONATE	300 MG	IM, IV	S0080
PENTAMIDINE ISETHIONATE COMPOUNDED	300 MG	INH	J7676
PENTAMIDINE ISETHIONATE NONCOMPOUNDED	300 MG	INH	J2545

Drug Name	Units Per	Route	Code
PENTASPAN	100 ML	IV	J2513
PENTASTARCH 10% SOLUTION	100 ML	IV	J2513
PENTATE CALCIUM TRISODIUM	STUDY DOSE UP TO 75 MCI	INH	A9567
PENTATE CALCIUM TRISODIUM	STUDY DOSE UP TO 25 MCI	IV	A9539
PENTATE ZINC TRISODIUM	STUDY DOSE UP TO 25 MCI	IV	A9539
PENTATE ZINC TRISODIUM	STUDY DOSE UP TO 75 MCI	INH	A9567
PENTAZOCINE	30 MG	IM, SC, IV	J3070
PENTOBARBITAL SODIUM	50 MG	IM, IV, OTH	J2515
PENTOSTATIN	10 MG	IV	J9268
PEPAXTO	1 MG	IV	J9247
PEPCID	20 MG	IV	S0028
PERAMIVIR	1 MG	IV	J2547
PERFLEXANE LIPID MICROSPHERE	1 ML	IV	Q9955
PERFLUTREN LIPID MICROSPHERE	1 ML	IV	Q9957
PERFOROMIST	20 MCG	INH	J7606
PERJETA	1 MG	IV	J9306
PERMACOL	SQ CM	OTH	C9364
PERMEADERM B	SQ CM	OTH	A2016
PERMEADERM C	SQ CM	OTH	A2018
PERMEADERM GLOVE	EA	OTH	A2017
PERPHENAZINE	5 MG	IM, IV	J3310
PERPHENAZINE	4 MG	ORAL	Q0175
PERSANTINE	10 MG	IV	J1245
PERSERIS	0.5 MG	SC	J2798
PERTUZUMAB	1 MG	IV	J9306
PERTUZUMAB, TRASTUZUMAB, AND HYALURONIDASE-ZZXF	10 MG	SC	J9316
PFIZERPEN A.S.	600,000 U	IM, IV	J2510
PHENERGAN	50 MG	IM, IV	J2550
PHENERGAN	12.5 MG	ORAL	Q0169
PHENOBARBITAL SODIUM	120 MG	IM, IV	J2560
PHENOBARBITAL SODIUM	1 MG	IV	J2561
PHENTOLAMINE MESYLATE	5 MG	IM, IV	J2760
PHENYLEPHRINE 10.16 MG/ML AND KETOROLAC 2.88 MG/ML OPHTHALMIC IRRIGATION SOLUTION	1 ML	OTH	J1097
PHENYLEPHRINE HCL	1 ML	SC, IM, IV	J2370
PHENYLEPHRINE HCL	20 MCG	IV	J2371
PHENYLEPHRINE HCL (BIORPHEN)	20 MCG	IV	J2372
PHENYTOIN SODIUM	50 MG	IM, IV	J1165
PHESGO	10 MG	SC	J9316
PHOENIX WOUND MATRIX	SQ CM	OTH	A2015
PHOSPHOCOL	1 MCI	IV	A9563
PHOSPHOTEC	STUDY DOSE UP TO 25 MCI	IV	A9538
PHOTOFRIN	75 MG	IV	J9600
PHOTREXA VISCOUS	UP TO 3 ML	OTH	J2787
PHYTONADIONE	1 MG	IM, SC, IV	J3430
PIFLUFOLASTAT F-18, DIAGNOSTIC	1 MCI	IV	A9595
PIPERACILLIN SODIUM	500 MG	IM, IV	S0081
PIPERACILLIN SODIUM/ TAZOBACTAM SODIUM	1 G/1.125 GM	IV	J2543
PITOCIN	10 U	IV, IM	J2590
PLASMINOGEN, HUMAN-TVMH	1 MG	IV	J2998
PLATINOL AQ	10 MG	IV	J9060
PLAZOMICIN	5 MG	IV	J0291
PLERIXAFOR	1 MG	SC	J2562

Drug Name	Units Per	Route	Code
PLICAMYCIN	2.5 MG	IV	J9270
PLUVICTO	1 MCI	IV	A9607
PNEUMOCOCCAL CONJUGATE	EA	IM	S0195
PNEUMOVAX II	EA	IM	S0195
POLATUZUMAB VEDOTIN-PIIQ	1 MG	IV	J9309
POLIVY	1 MG	IV	J9309
POLOCAINE	10 ML	VAR	J0670
POLYCYTE	0.5 CC	OTH	Q4241
PORCINE IMPLANT, PERMACOL	SQ CM	OTH	C9364
PORFIMER SODIUM	75 MG	IV	J9600
PORK INSULIN	5 U	SC	J1815
POROUS PURIFIED COLLAGEN MATRIX BONE VOID FILLER	0.5 CC	OTH	C9362
POROUS PURIFIED COLLAGEN MATRIX BONE VOID FILLER, PUTTY	0.5 CC	OTH	C9359
PORTRAZZA.	1 MG	IV	J9295
POSIMIR	1 MG	INJ	C9144
POSLUMA	1 MCI	IV	C9156
POSLUMA	1 MCI	IV	A9608
POTASSIUM CHLORIDE	2 MEQ	IV	J3480
POTELIGEO	1 MG	IV	J9204
PRALATREXATE	1 MG	IV	J9307
PRALIDOXIME CHLORIDE	1 MG	IV, IM, SC	J2730
PREDNISOLONE	5 MG	ORAL	J7510
PREDNISOLONE ACETATE	1 ML	IM	J2650
PREDNISONE, IMMEDIATE RELEASE OR DELAYED RELEASE	1 MG	ORAL	J7512
PREDNORAL	5 MG	ORAL	J7510
PREGNYL	1,000 USP U	IM	J0725
PRELONE	5 MG	ORAL	J7510
PREMARIN	25 MG	IV, IM	J1410
PRENATAL VITAMINS	30 TABS	ORAL	S0197
PRI-METHYLATE	80 MG	IM	J1040
PRIALT	1 MCG	OTH	J2278
PRIMACOR	5 MG	IV	J2260
PRIMATRIX	SQ CM	OTH	Q4110
PRIMAXIN	250 MG	IV, IM	J0743
PRIMESTRIN AQUEOUS	1 MG	IM, IV	J1410
PRIMETHASONE	1 MG	IM, IV, OTH	J1100
PRIVIGEN	500 MG	IV	J1459
PROBUPHINE IMPLANT	74.2 MG	OTH	J0570
PROCAINAMIDE HCL	1 G	IM, IV	J2690
PROCARBAZINE HCL	50 MG	ORAL	S0182
PROCENTA	200 MG	OTH	Q4244
PROCHLOPERAZINE MALEATE	5 MG	ORAL	S0183
PROCHLORPERAZINE	10 MG	IM, IV	J0780
PROCHLORPERAZINE MALEATE	5 MG	ORAL	Q0164
PROCRIT, NON-ESRD USE	1,000 U	SC, IV	J0885
PROFILNINE HEAT-TREATED	1 IU	IV	J7194
PROFILNINE SD	1 IU	IV	J7194
PROFONIX	VIAL	INJ	C9113
PROGENAMATRIX	SQ CM	OTH	Q4222
PROGESTASERT IUD	EA	OTH	S4989
PROGESTERONE	50 MG	IM	J2675
PROGRAF	5 MG	OTH	J7525
PROGRAF	1 MG	ORAL	J7507
PROLEUKIN	1 VIAL	VAR	J9015
PROLIA	1 MG	SC	J0897
PROLIXIN DECANOATE	25 MG	SC, IM	J2680
PROMAZINE HCL	25 MG	IM	J2950
PROMETHAZINE HCL	12.5 MG	ORAL	Q0169

Drug Name	Units Per	Route	Code
PROMETHAZINE HCL	50 MG	IM, IV	J2550
PRONESTYL	1 G	IM, IV	J2690
PROPECIA	5 MG	ORAL	S0138
PROPLEX SX-T	1 IU	IV	J7194
PROPLEX T	1 IU	IV	J7194
PROPOFOL	10 MG	IV	J2704
PROPRANOLOL HCL	1 MG	IV	J1800
PROREX	50 MG	IM, IV	J2550
PROSCAR	5 MG	ORAL	S0138
PROSTASCINT	STUDY DOSE UP TO 10 MCI	IV	A9507
PROSTIGMIN	0.5 MG	IM, IV	J2710
PROSTIN VR	1.25 MCG	INJ	J0270
PROTAMINE SULFATE	10 MG	IV	J2720
PROTEIN C CONCENTRATE	10 IU	IV	J2724
PROTEXT	1 CC	OTH	Q4246
PROTHROMBIN COMPLEX CONCENTRATE (HUMAN)	IU	IV	C9159
PROTHROMBIN COMPLEX CONCENTRATE (HUMAN)	1 IU	IV	J7168
PROTIRELIN	250 MCG	IV	J2725
PROTONIX IV	40 MG	IV	S0164
PROTONIX IV	VIAL	IV	C9113
PROTOPAM CHLORIDE	1 G	SC, IM, IV	J2730
PROTROPIN	1 MG	SC, IM	J2940
PROVENGE	INFUSION	IV	Q2043
PROVENTIL NONCOMPOUNDED, CONCENTRATED	1 MG	INH	J7611
PROVENTIL NONCOMPOUNDED, UNIT DOSE	1 MG	INH	J7613
PROVOCHOLINE POWDER	1 MG	INH	J7674
PROZINE-50	25 MG	IM	J2950
PULMICORT	0.25 MG	INH	J7633
PULMICORT RESPULES	0.5 MG	INH	J7627
PULMICORT RESPULES NONCOMPOUNDED, CONCETRATED	0.25 MG	INH	J7626
PULMOZYME	1 MG	INH	J7639
PURAPLY	SQ CM	OTH	Q4195
PURAPLY AM	SQ CM	OTH	Q4196
PURAPLY XT	SQ CM	OTH	Q4197
PURINETHOL	50 MG	ORAL	S0108
PYLARIFY	1 MCI	IV	A9595
PYRIDOXINE HCL	100 MG	IM, IV	J3415
QALSODY	1 MG	INJ	C9157
QALSODY	1 MG	INJ	J1304
QUADRAMET	DOSE UP TO 150 MCI	IV	A9604
QUELICIN	20 MG	IM, IV	J0330
QUINUPRISTIN/DALFOPRISTIN	500 MG	IV	J2770
QUTENZA	1 SQ CM	OTH	J7336
QUZYTIIR	0.5 MG	IV	J1201
RADICAVA	1 MG	IV	J1301
RADIESSE	0.1 ML	OTH	Q2026
RADIOELEMENTS FOR BRACHYTHERAPY, ANY TYPE	EA	OTH	Q3001
RADIUM (RA) 223 DICHLORIDE THERAPEUTIC	MICROCURIE	IV	A9606
RAMUCIRUMAB	5 MG	IV	J9308
RANIBIZUMAB	0.1 MG	OTH	J2778
RANIBIZUMAB	0.1 MG	OTH	J2779
RANIBIZUMAB-EQRN	0.1 MG	INJ	Q5128
RANIBIZUMAB-NUNA	0.1 MG	INJ	Q5124

Appendix 1 — Table of Drugs and Biologicals

Drug Name	Units Per	Route	Code
RANITIDINE HCL	25 MG	INJ	J2780
RAPAMUNE	1 MG	ORAL	J7520
RAPIVAB	1 MG	IV	J2547
RASBURICASE	0.5 MG	IM	J2783
RAVULIZUMAB-CWVZ	10 MG	IV	J1303
REBETRON KIT	1,000,000 U	SC, IM	J9214
REBIF	30 MCG	SC	J1826
REBIF	1 MCG	SC	Q3028
REBINYN	1 IU	IV	J7203
REBLOZYL	0.25 MG	SC	J0896
REBOUND MATRIX	SQ CM	OTH	Q4296
REBYOTA	1 ML	OTH	J1440
RECARBRIO	4 MG/4 MG/2 MG	IV	J0742
RECLAST	1 MG	IV	J3489
REDISOL	1,000 MCG	SC. IM	J3420
REFLUDAN	50 MG	IM, IV	J1945
REGADENOSON	0.1 MG	IV	J2785
REGEN-COV	1200 MG	IV	Q0244
REGITINE	5 MG	IM, IV	J2760
REGLAN	10 MG	IV	J2765
REGRANEX GEL	0.5 G	OTH	S0157
REGUARD	SQ CM	OTH	Q4255
REGULAR INSULIN	5 UNITS	SC	J1815
RELAXIN	10 ML	IV, IM	J2800
RELENZA (DEMONSTRATION PROJECT)	10 MG	INH	G9034
RELESE	SQ CM	OTH	Q4257
RELEUKO	1 MCG	SC, IV	Q5125
RELION	5 U	SC	J1815
RELION NOVOLIN	50 U	SC	J1817
RELISTOR	0.1 MG	SC	J2212
REMDESIVIR	1 MG	IV	J0248
REMICADE	10 MG	IV	J1745
REMIMAZOLAM	1 MG	IV	J2249
REMODULIN	1 MG	SC	J3285
RENFLEXIS	10 MG	IV	Q5104
REODULIN	1 MG	SC	J3285
REOPRO	10 MG	IV	J0130
REPRIZA	SQ CM	OTH	Q4143
REPRONEX	75 IU	SC, IM, IV	S0122
RESLIZUMAB	1 MG	IV	J2786
RESOLVE MATRIX	SQ CM	OTH	A2024
RESPIROL NONCOMPOUNDED, CONCENTRATED	1 MG	INH	J7611
RESPIROL NONCOMPOUNDED, UNIT DOSE	1 MG	INH	J7613
RESTORIGIN	1 CC	INJ	Q4192
RESTORIGIN	SQ CM	OTH	Q4191
RESTRATA	SQ CM	OTH	A2007
RETACRIT	100 UNITS	INJ, IV	Q5105
RETACRIT	1000 UNITS	INJ, IV	Q5106
RETAVASE	18.1 MG	IV	J2993
RETEPLASE	18.1 MG	IV	J2993
RETIFANLIMAB-DLWR	1 MG	IV	J9345
RETISERT	IMPLANT	OTH	J7311
RETROVIR	10 MG	IV	J3485
RETROVIR	100 MG	ORAL	S0104
REVEFENACIN INHALATION	1 MCG	INH	J7677
REVITA	SQ CM	OTH	Q4180
REVITALON	SQ CM	OTH	Q4157
REVOSHIELD+ AMNIOTIC BARRIER	SQ CM	OTH	Q4289

Drug Name	Units Per	Route	Code
REZAFUNGIN	0.1 MG	IV	J0349
REZZAYO	0.1 MG	IV	J0349
RHEOMACRODEX	500 ML	IV	J7100
RHEUMATREX	2.5 MG	ORAL	J8610
RHEUMATREX DOSE PACK	2.5 MG	ORAL	J8610
RHO D IMMUNE GLOBULIN	300 MCG	IV	J2790
RHO D IMMUNE GLOBULIN (RHOPHYLAC)	100 IU	IM, IV	J2791
RHO D IMMUNE GLOBULIN MINIDOSE	50 MCG	IM	J2788
RHO D IMMUNE GLOBULIN SOLVENT DETERGENT	100 IU	IV	J2792
RHOGAM	50 MCG	IM	J2788
RHOGAM	300 MCG	IM	J2790
RHOPHYLAC	100 IU	IM, IV	J2791
RIABNI	10 MG	IV	Q5123
RIBOFLAVIN 5'-PHOSPHATE, OPHTHALMIC SOLUTION	UP TO 3 ML	OTH	J2787
RILONACEPT	1 MG	SC	J2793
RIMANTADINE HCL (DEMONSTRATION PROJECT)	100 MG	ORAL	G9020
RIMANTADINE HCL (DEMONSTRATION PROJECT)	100 MG	ORAL	G9036
RIMSO 50	50 ML	IV	J1212
RINGERS LACTATE INFUSION	UP TO 1000 CC	IV	J7120
RISANKIZUMAB-RZAA	1 MG	IV	J2327
RISPERDAL CONSTA	0.5 MG	IM	J2794
RISPERIDONE	0.5 MG	SC	J2798
RISPERIDONE	1 MG	SC	J2799
~~RISPERIDONE~~	~~1 MG~~	~~SC~~	~~C9158~~
RISPERIDONE	0.5 MG	IM	J2794
RITUXAN	10 MG	IV	J9312
RITUXAN HYCELA	10 MG	SC	J9311
RITUXIMAB	10 MG	IV	J9312
RITUXIMAB 10 MG AND HYALURONIDASE	10 MG	SC	J9311
RITUXIMAB-ABBS, BIOSIMILAR	10 MG	IV	Q5115
RITUXIMAB-ARRX, BIOSIMILAR	10 MG	IV	Q5123
RITUXIMAB-PVVR, BIOSIMILAR	10 MG	IV	Q5119
RIXUBIS	IU	IV	J7200
ROBAXIN	10 ML	IV, IM	J2800
ROCEPHIN	250 MG	IV, IM	J0696
ROCTAVIAN	1 ML	IV	J1412
ROFERON-A	3,000,000 U	SC, IM	J9213
ROLAPITANT	1 MG	ORAL	J8670
ROLAPITANT	0.5 MG	ORAL, IV	J2797
ROLVEDON	0.1 MG	SC	J1449
ROMIDEPSIN, LYOPHILIZED	0.1 MG	IV	J9319
ROMIDEPSIN, NONLYOPHILIZED	0.1 MG	IV	J9318
ROMIPLOSTIM	10 MCG	SC	J2796
ROMOSOZUMAB-AQQG	1 MG	SC	J3111
ROPIVACAINE HYDROCHLORIDE	1 MG	VAR	J2795
ROZANOLIXIZUMAB-NOLI	1 MG	SC	J9333
RUBEX	10 MG	IV	J9000
RUBIDIUM RB-82	STUDY DOSE UP TO 60 MCI	IV	A9555
RUBRAMIN PC	1,000 MCG	SC, IM	J3420
RUBRATOPE 57	STUDY DOSE UP TO 1 UCI	ORAL	A9559
RUCONEST	10 UNITS	IV	J0596
RUXIENCE	10 MG	IV	Q5119
RYBREVANT	2 MG	IV	J9061

Drug Name	Units Per	Route	Code
RYLAZE	0.1 MG	IM	J9021
RYPLAZIM	1 MG	IV	J2998
RYSTIGGO	1 MG	SC	J9333
SACITUZUMAB GOVITECAN-HZIY	2.5 MG	IV	J9317
SAIZEN	1 MG	SC	J2941
SAIZEN SOMATROPIN RDNA ORIGIN	1 MG	SC	J2941
SALINE OR STERILE WATER, METERED DOSE DISPENSER	10 ML	INH	A4218
SALINE, STERILE WATER, AND/OR DEXTROSE DILUENT/FLUSH	10 ML	VAR	A4216
SALINE/STERILE WATER	500 ML	VAR	A4217
SAMARIUM LEXIDRONAM	DOSE UP TO 150 MCI	IV	A9604
SANDIMMUNE	100 MG	ORAL	J7502
SANDIMMUNE	250 MG	IV	J7516
SANDIMMUNE	25 MG	ORAL	J7515
SANDOSTATIN	25 MCG	SC, IV	J2354
SANDOSTATIN LAR	1 MG	IM	J2353
SANGCYA	100 MG	ORAL	J7502
SANO-DROL	40 MG	IM	J1030
SANO-DROL	80 MG	IM	J1040
SAPHNELLO	1 MG	IV	J0491
SAQUINAVIR	200 MG	ORAL	S0140
SARCLISA	10 MG	IV	J9227
SARGRAMOSTIM (GM-CSF)	50 MCG	IV	J2820
SCANDONEST	10 ML	IV	J0670
SCENESSE	1 MG	OTH	J7352
SCULPTRA	0.5 ML	OTH	Q2028
SEBELIPASE ALFA	1 MG	IV	J2840
SECRETIN	1 MCG	IV	J2850
SECRETIN, SYNTHETIC, HUMAN	1 MCG	IV	J2850
SEGESTERONE ACETATE AND ETHINYL ESTRADIOL VAGINAL RING	0.15 MG/0.013 MG	OTH	J7294
SENSIPAR	1 MG	ORAL	J0604
SENSORCAINE	30 ML	VAR	S0020
SENTIMAG	STUDY DOSE	SC	A9697
SEPTRA IV	10 ML	IV	S0039
SERMORELIN ACETATE	1 MCG	IV	Q0515
SEROSTIM	1 MG	SC	J2941
SEROSTIM RDNA ORIGIN	1 MG	SC	J2941
SEVENFACT	1 MCG	IV	J7212
SEZABY	1 MG	IV	J2561
SIGNATURE APATCH	SQ CM	OTH	Q4260
SIGNIFOR LAR	1 MG	IV	J2502
SILDENAFIL CITRATE	25 MG	ORAL	S0090
SILTUXIMAB	10 MG	IV	J2860
SIMPONI	1 MG	IV	J1602
SIMULECT	20 MG	IV	J0480
SINCALIDE	5 MCG	IV	J2805
SINCALIDE (MAIA)	5 MCG	IV	J2806
SINUVA	10 MCG	OTH	J7402
SIPULEUCEL-T	INFUSION	IV	Q2043
SIROLIMUS	1 MG	ORAL	J7520
SIROLIMUS PROTEIN-BOUND PARTICLES	1 MG	IV	C9091
SIROLIMUS PROTEIN-BOUND PARTICLES	1 MG	IV	J9331
SIVEXTRO	1 MG	IV	J3090
SKINTE	SQ CM	OTH	Q4200
SKYLA	13.5 MG	OTH	J7301
SKYRIZI	1 MG	IV	J2327

Drug Name	Units Per	Route	Code
SMZ-TMP	10 ML	IV	S0039
SODIUM FERRIC GLUCONATE COMPLEX IN SUCROSE	12.5 MG	IV	J2916
SODIUM FLUORIDE F-18, DIAGNOSTIC	STUDY DOSE UP TO 30 MCI	IV	A9580
SODIUM IODIDE I-131 CAPSULE DIAGNOSTIC	1 MCI	ORAL	A9528
SODIUM IODIDE I-131 CAPSULE THERAPEUTIC	1 MCI	ORAL	A9517
SODIUM IODIDE I-131 SOLUTION THERAPEUTIC	1 MCI	ORAL	A9530
SODIUM PHOSPHATE P32	1 MCI	IV	A9563
SODIUM THIOSULFATE	100 MG	IV	J0208
SOLGANAL	50 MG	IM	J2910
SOLIRIS	10 MG	IV	J1300
SOLTAMOX	10 MG	ORAL	S0187
SOLU-CORTEF	100 MG	IV, IM, SC	J1720
SOLU-MEDROL	40 MG	IM, IV	J2920
SOLU-MEDROL	125 MG	IM, IV	J2930
SOLUREX	1 MG	IM, IV, OTH	J1100
SOMATREM	1 MG	SC, IM	J2940
SOMATROPIN	1 MG	SC	J2941
SOMATULINE	1 MG	SC	J1930
SOTALOL HYDROCHLORIDE	1 MG	IV	C9482
SOTROVIMAB	500 MG	IV	Q0247
SPECTINOMYCIN DIHYDROCHLORIDE	2 G	IM	J3320
SPECTRO-DEX	1 MG	IM, IV, OTH	J1100
SPESOLIMAB-SBZO	1 MG	IV	J1747
SPEVIGO	1 MG	IV	J1747
SPINRAZA	0.1 MG	INJ	J2326
SPORANOX	50 MG	IV	J1835
SPRAVATO	1 MG	OTH	S0013
STADOL	1 MG	IM, IV	J0595
STADOL NS	25 MG	OTH	S0012
STELARA	1 MG	SC	J3357
STELARA	1 MG	SC, IV	J3358
STERILE WATER OR SALINE, METERED DOSE DISPENSER	10 ML	INH	A4218
STERILE WATER, SALINE, AND/OR DEXTROSE DILUENT/FLUSH	10 ML	VAR	A4216
STERILE WATER/SALINE	500 ML	VAR	A4217
STIMUFEND	0.5 MG	SC	Q5127
STRATTICE TM	SQ CM	OTH	Q4130
STRAVIX	SQ CM	OTH	Q4133
STRAVIXPL	SQ CM	OTH	Q4133
STREPTASE	250,000 IU	IV	J2995
STREPTOKINASE	250,000 IU	IV	J2995
STREPTOMYCIN	1 G	IM	J3000
STREPTOZOCIN	1 G	IV	J9320
STRONTIUM 89 CHLORIDE	1 MCI	IV	A9600
SUBLIMAZE	0.1 MG	IM, IV	J3010
SUBLOCADE	> 100 MG	SC	Q9992
SUBLOCADE	≤ 100 MG	SC	Q9991
SUBOXONE	4 MG	ORAL	J0573
SUBOXONE	2 MG	ORAL	J0572
SUBOXONE	12 MG	ORAL	J0575
SUBOXONE	8 MG	ORAL	J0574
SUBUTEX	1 MG	ORAL	J0571
SUCCINYLCHOLINE CHLORIDE	20 MG	IM, IV	J0330
SULFAMETHOXAZOLE AND TRIMETHOPRIM	10 ML	IV	S0039

Drug Name	Units Per	Route	Code
SULFUR HEXAFLUORIDE LIPID MICROSPHERES	1 ML	IV	Q9950
SULFUTRIM	10 ML	IV	S0039
SUMATRIPTAN SUCCINATE	6 MG	SC	J3030
SUNLENCA	1 MG	SC	J1961
SUPARTZ	DOSE	INJ	J7321
SUPPRELIN LA	10 MCG	OTH	J1675
SUPRA SDRM	SQ CM	OTH	A2011
SUPRATHEL	SQ CM	OTH	A2012
SUREDERM	SQ CM	OTH	Q4220
SURFACTOR	0.5 CC	OTH	Q4233
SURGICORD	SQ CM	OTH	Q4218
SURGIGRAFT	SQ CM	OTH	Q4183
SURGIGRAFT-DUAL	SQ CM	OTH	Q4219
SURGIMEND COLLAGEN MATRIX, FETAL	0.5 SQ CM	OTH	C9358
SURGIMEND COLLAGEN MATRIX, NEONATAL	0.5 SQ CM	OTH	C9360
SURGRAFT	SQ CM	OTH	Q4209
SURGRAFT FT	SQ CM	OTH	Q4268
SURGRAFT TL	SQ CM	OTH	Q4263
SURGRAFT XT	SQ CM	OTH	Q4269
SUSTOL	0.1 MG	SC	J1627
SUSVIMO	0.1 MG	OTH	J2779
SUTIMLIMAB-JOME	10 MG	IV	J1302
SYFOVRE	1 MG	INJ	J2781
SYLVANT	10 MG	IV	J2860
SYMMETREL (DEMONSTRATION PROJECT)	100 MG	ORAL	G9033
SYMPHONY	SQ CM	OTH	A2009
SYNERA	70 MG/70 MG	OTH	C9285
SYNERCID	500 MG	IV	J2770
SYNOJOYNT	1 MG	INJ	J7331
SYNRIBO	0.01 MG	SC	J9262
SYNTOCINON	10 UNITS	IV	J2590
SYNVISC/SYNVISC-ONE	1 MG	INJ	J7325
SYTOBEX	1,000 MCG	SC, IM	J3420
T-GEN	250 MG	ORAL	Q0173
TACRINE HCL	10 MG	ORAL	S0014
TACROLIMUS	1 MG	ORAL	J7507
TACROLIMUS	5 MG	OTH	J7525
TACROLIMUS, EXTENDED RELEASE	0.25 MG	ORAL	J7503
TACROLIMUS, EXTENDED RELEASE	0.1 MG	ORAL	J7508
TAFASITAMAB-CXIX	2 MG	IV	J9349
TAG	SQ CM	OTH	Q4261
TAGAMET HCL	300 MG	IM, IV	S0023
TAGRAXOFUSP-ERZS	10 MCG	IV	J9269
TAKHZYRO	1 MG	SC	J0593
TALIGLUCERASE ALFA	10 U	IV	J3060
TALIMOGENE LAHERPAREPVEC	1 MILLION	INTRALESIONAL	J9325
TALQUETAMAB-TGVS	0.25 MG	SC	C9163
TALVEY	0.25 MG	SC	C9163
TALWIN	30 MG	IM, SC, IV	J3070
TALYMED	SQ CM	OTH	Q4127
TAMIFLU (DEMONSTRATION PROJECT)	75 MG	ORAL	G9019
TAMIFLU (DEMONSTRATION PROJECT)	75 MG	ORAL	G9035
TAMOXIFEN CITRATE	10 MG	ORAL	S0187
TAUVID	1 MCI	IV	A9601

Drug Name	Units Per	Route	Code
TAXOL	1 MG	IV	J9267
TAXOTERE	1 MG	IV	J9171
TAZICEF	500 MG	IM, IV	J0713
TBO-FILGRASTIM	1 MCG	IV	J1447
TC 99M TILOMANOCEPT	0.5 MCI	SC, OTH	A9520
TEBAMIDE	250 MG	ORAL	Q0173
TEBENTAFUSP-TEBN	1 MCG	IV	J9274
TEBOROXIME TECHNETIUM TC 99M	STUDY DOSE	IV	A9501
TEBOROXIME, TECHNETIUM	STUDY DOSE	IV	A9501
TECARTUS	UP TO 200 MILLION CELLS	IV	Q2053
TECENTRIQ	10 MG	INF	J9022
TECHNEPLEX	STUDY DOSE UP TO 25 MCI	IV	A9539
TECHNESCAN	STUDY DOSE UP TO 30 MCI	IV	A9561
TECHNESCAN FANOLESOMAB	STUDY DOSE UP TO 25 MCI	IV	A9566
TECHNESCAN MAA	STUDY DOSE UP TO 10 MCI	IV	A9540
TECHNESCAN MAG3	STUDY DOSE UP TO 15 MCI	IV	A9562
TECHNESCAN PYP	STUDY DOSE UP TO 25 MCI	IV	A9538
TECHNESCAN PYP KIT	STUDY DOSE UP TO 25 MCI	IV	A9538
TECHNETIUM SESTAMBI	STUDY DOSE	IV	A9500
TECHNETIUM TC 99M APCITIDE	STUDY DOSE UP TO 20 MCI	IV	A9504
TECHNETIUM TC 99M ARCITUMOMAB, DIAGNOSTIC	STUDY DOSE UP TO 45 MCI	IV	A9568
TECHNETIUM TC 99M BICISATE	STUDY DOSE UP TO 25 MCI	IV	A9557
TECHNETIUM TC 99M DEPREOTIDE	STUDY DOSE UP TO 35 MCI	IV	A9536
TECHNETIUM TC 99M EXAMETAZIME	STUDY DOSE UP TO 25 MCI	IV	A9521
TECHNETIUM TC 99M FANOLESOMAB	STUDY DOSE UP TO 25 MCI	IV	A9566
TECHNETIUM TC 99M LABELED RED BLOOD CELLS	STUDY DOSE UP TO 30 MCI	IV	A9560
TECHNETIUM TC 99M MACROAGGREGATED ALBUMIN	STUDY DOSE UP TO 10 MCI	IV	A9540
TECHNETIUM TC 99M MDI-MDP	STUDY DOSE UP TO 30 MCI	IV	A9503
TECHNETIUM TC 99M MEBROFENIN	STUDY DOSE UP TO 15 MCI	IV	A9537
TECHNETIUM TC 99M MEDRONATE	STUDY DOSE UP TO 30 MCI	IV	A9503
TECHNETIUM TC 99M MERTIATIDE	STUDY DOSE UP TO 15 MCI	IV	A9562
TECHNETIUM TC 99M OXIDRONATE	STUDY DOSE UP TO 30 MCI	IV	A9561
TECHNETIUM TC 99M PENTETATE	STUDY DOSE UP TO 25 MCI	IV	A9539
TECHNETIUM TC 99M PYROPHOSPHATE	STUDY DOSE UP TO 25 MCI	IV	A9538
TECHNETIUM TC 99M SODIUM GLUCEPTATE	STUDY DOSE UP TO 25 MCI	IV	A9550
TECHNETIUM TC 99M SUCCIMER	STUDY DOSE UP TO 10 MCI	IV	A9551
TECHNETIUM TC 99M SULFUR COLLOID	STUDY DOSE UP TO 20 MCI	IV	A9541
TECHNETIUM TC 99M TETROFOSMIN, DIAGNOSTIC	STUDY DOSE	IV	A9502

Drug Name	Units Per	Route	Code
TECHNETIUM TC-99M EXAMETAZIME LABELED AUTOLOGOUS WHITE BLOOD CELLS	STUDY DOSE	IV	A9569
TECHNETIUM TC-99M PERTECHNETATE, DIAGNOSTIC	1 MCI	IV	A9512
TECHNETIUM TC-99M TEBOROXIME	STUDY DOSE	IV	A9501
TECHNILITE	1 MCI	IV	A9512
~~TECLISTAMAB-CQYV~~	~~0.5 MG~~	~~SC~~	~~C9148~~
TECLISTAMAB-CQYV	0.5 MG	SC	J9380
~~TECVAYLI~~	~~0.5 MG~~	~~SC~~	~~C9148~~
TECVAYLI	0.5 MG	SC	J9380
TEDIZOLID PHOSPHATE	1 MG	IV	J3090
TEFLARO	10 MG	IV	J0712
TELAVANCIN	10 MG	IV	J3095
TEMODAR	5 MG	ORAL	J8700
TEMODAR	1 MG	IV	J9328
TEMOZOLOMIDE	5 MG	ORAL	J8700
TEMOZOLOMIDE	1 MG	IV	J9328
TEMSIROLIMUS	1 MG	IV	J9330
TENDON, POROUS MATRIX	SQ CM	OTH	C9356
TENDON, POROUS MATRIX CROSS-LINKED AND GLYCOSAMINOGLYCAN MATRIX	SQ CM	OTH	C9356
TENECTEPLASE	1 MG	IV	J3101
TENIPOSIDE	50 MG	IV	Q2017
TENOGLIDE TENDON PROTECTOR	SQ CM	OTH	C9356
TENOGLIDE TENDON PROTECTOR SHEET	SQ CM	OTH	C9356
TENSIX	SQ CM	OTH	Q4146
TEPEZZA	10 MG	IV	J3241
~~TEPLIZUMAB-MZWV~~	~~5 MCG~~	~~IV~~	~~C9149~~
TEPLIZUMAB-MZWV	5 MCG	IV	J9381
TEPROTUMUMAB-TRBW	10 MG	IV	J3241
TEQUIN	10 MG	IV	J1590
TERBUTALINE SULFATE	1 MG	SC, IV	J3105
TERBUTALINE SULFATE, COMPOUNDED, CONCENTRATED	1 MG	INH	J7680
TERBUTALINE SULFATE, COMPOUNDED, UNIT DOSE	1 MG	INH	J7681
TERIPARATIDE	10 MCG	SC	J3110
TERRAMYCIN	50 MG	IM	J2460
TESTOSTERONE CYPIONATE	1 MG	IM	J1071
TESTOSTERONE ENANTHATE	1 MG	IM	J3121
TESTOSTERONE PELLET	75 MG	OTH	S0189
TESTOSTERONE UNDECANOATE	1 MG	IM	J3145
TETANUS IMMUNE GLOBULIN	250 U	IM	J1670
TETRACYCLINE HCL	250 MG	IV	J0120
TEZEPELUMAB-EKKO	1 MG	SC	J2356
TEZSPIRE	1 MG	SC	J2356
THALLOUS CHLORIDE	1 MCI	IV	A9505
THALLOUS CHLORIDE TL-201	1 MCI	IV	A9505
THALLOUS CHLORIDE USP	1 MCI	IV	A9505
THEELIN AQUEOUS	1 MG	IM, IV	J1435
THEOPHYLLINE	40 MG	IV	J2810
THERAGENESIS	SQ CM	OTH	A2008
THERASKIN	SQ CM	OTH	Q4121
THERION	SQ CM	OTH	Q4176
THIAMINE HCL	100 MG	INJ	J3411
THIETHYLPERAZINE MALEATE	10 MG	IM	J3280
THIETHYLPERAZINE MALEATE	10 MG	ORAL	Q0174
THIMAZIDE	250 MG	ORAL	Q0173
THIOTEPA	15 MG	IV	J9340

Drug Name	Units Per	Route	Code
THORAZINE	50 MG	IM, IV	J3230
THROMBATE III	1 IU	IV	J7197
THYMOGLOBULIN	25 MG	OTH	J7511
THYROGEN	0.9 MG	IM, SC	J3240
THYROTROPIN ALPHA	0.9 MG	IM, SC	J3240
TICARCILLIN DISODIUM AND CLAVULANATE	3.1 G	IV	S0040
TICE BCG	1 MG	OTH	J9030
TICON	250 MG	IM	Q0173
TIGAN	200 MG	IM	J3250
TIGECYCLINE	1 MG	IV	J3243
TIGECYCLINE (ACCORD) NOT THERAPEUTICALLY EQUIVALENT TO J3243	1 MG	IV	J3244
TIJECT-20	200 MG	IM	J3250
TILDRAKIZUMAB	1 MG	SC	J3245
TIMENTIN	3.1 G	IV	S0040
TINZAPARIN	1,000 IU	SC	J1655
TIROFIBAN HCL	0.25 MG	IM, IV	J3246
TISAGENLECLEUCEL	UP TO 600 MILLION CELLS	IV	Q2042
TISOTUMAB VEDOTIN-TFTV	1 MG	IV	J9273
TIVDAK	1 MG	IV	J9273
TIXAGEVIMAB AND CILGAVIMAB	300 MG	IM	Q0220
TIXAGEVIMAB AND CILGAVIMAB	600 MG	IM	Q0221
TNKASE	1 MG	IV	J3101
TOBI	300 MG	INH	J7682
TOBRAMYCIN COMPOUNDED, UNIT DOSE	300 MG	INH	J7685
TOBRAMYCIN SULFATE	80 MG	IM, IV	J3260
TOBRAMYCIN, NONCOMPOUNDED, UNIT DOSE	300 MG	INH	J7682
TOCILIZUMAB	1 MG	IV	J3262
TOCILIZUMAB	1 MG	IV	Q0249
~~TOFERSEN~~	~~1 MG~~	~~INJ~~	~~C9157~~
TOFERSEN	1 MG	INJ	J1304
TOLAZOLINE HCL	25 MG	IV	J2670
TOPOSAR	10 MG	IV	J9181
TOPOTECAN	0.25 MG	ORAL	J8705
TOPOTECAN	0.1 MG	IV	J9351
TORADOL	15 MG	IV	J1885
TORISEL	1 MG	IV	J9330
TORNALATE	MG	INH	J7629
TORNALATE CONCENTRATE	1 MG	INH	J7628
TORSEMIDE	10 MG	IV	J3265
TOSITUMOMAB	450 MG	IV	G3001
TOTECT	250 MG	IV	J1190
TRABECTEDIN	0.1 MG	IV	J9352
TRANSCYTE	SQ CM	OTH	Q4182
TRASTUZUMAB AND HYALURONIDASE-OYSK	10 MG	SC	J9356
TRASTUZUMAB, EXCLUDES BIOSIMILAR	10 MG	IV	J9355
TRASTUZUMAB-ANNS, BIOSIMILAR	10 MG	IV	Q5117
TRASTUZUMAB-DKST, BIOSIMILAR	10 MG	IV	Q5114
TRASTUZUMAB-DTTB, BIOSIMILAR	10 MG	IV	Q5112
TRASTUZUMAB-PKRB, BIOSIMILAR	10 MG	IV	Q5113
TRASTUZUMAB-QYYP, BIOSIMILAR	10 MG	IV	Q5116
TRASYLOL	10,000 KIU	IV	J0365
TRAZIMERA	10 MG	IV	Q5116
TREANDA	1 MG	IV	J9033
TRELSTAR DEPOT	3.75 MG	IM	J3315

Drug Name	Units Per	Route	Code
TRELSTAR DEPOT PLUS DEBIOCLIP KIT	3.75 MG	IM	J3315
TRELSTAR LA	3.75 MG	IM	J3315
~~TREMELIMUMAB-ACTL~~	~~1 MG~~	~~IV~~	~~C9147~~
TREMELIMUMAB-ACTL	1 MG	IV	J9347
TREMFYA	1 MG	SC	J1628
TREPROSTINIL	1 MG	SC	J3285
TREPROSTINIL, INHALATION SOLUTION	1.74 MG	INH	J7686
TRETINOIN	5 G	OTH	S0117
TRETTEN	10 IU	IV	J7181
TRIAMCINOLONE ACETONIDE	1 MG	INJ	J3299
TRIAMCINOLONE ACETONIDE, PRESERVATIVE FREE	1 MG	INJ	J3300
TRIAMCINOLONE ACETONIDE, PRESERVATIVE-FREE, EXTENDED-RELEASE, MICROSPHERE FORMULATION	1 MG	OTH	J3304
TRIAMCINOLONE DIACETATE	5 MG	IM	J3302
TRIAMCINOLONE HEXACETONIDE	5 MG	VAR	J3303
TRIAMCINOLONE, COMPOUNDED, CONCENTRATED	1 MG	INH	J7683
TRIAMCINOLONE, COMPOUNDED, UNIT DOSE	1 MG	INH	J7684
TRIBAN	250 MG	ORAL	Q0173
TRIESENCE	1 MG	OTH	J3300
TRIFERIC AVNU	0.1 MG	IV	J1445
TRIFERIC POWDER	0.1 MG	IV	J1444
TRIFERIC SOLUTION	0.1 MG	IV	J1443
TRIFLUPROMAZINE HCL	UP TO 20 MG	INJ	J3400
TRILACICLIB	1 MG	IV	J1448
TRILIFON	4 MG	ORAL	Q0175
TRILONE	5 MG	IM	J3302
TRILURON	1 MG	INJ	J7332
TRIMETHOBENZAMIDE HCL	200 MG	IM	J3250
TRIMETHOBENZAMIDE HCL	250 MG	ORAL	Q0173
TRIMETREXATE GLUCURONATE	25 MG	IV	J3305
TRIPTODUR	3.75 MG	IM	J3316
TRIPTORELIN PAMOATE	3.75 MG	IM	J3315
TRIPTORELIN, EXTENDED-RELEASE	3.75 MG	IM	J3316
TRISENOX	1 MG	IV	J9017
TRIVARIS	1 MG	VAR	J3300
TRIVISC	1 MG	INJ	J7329
TROBICIN	2 G	IM	J3320
TRODELVY	2.5 MG	IV	J9317
TROGARZO	10 MG	IV	J1746
TRUSKIN	SQ CM	OTH	Q4167
TRUVADA	200 MG/300 MG	ORAL	J0750
TRUXADRYL	50 MG	IV, IM	J1200
TRUXIMA	10 MG	IV	Q5115
TYGACIL	1 MG	IV	J3243
TYPE A BOTOX	1 UNIT	IM, OTH	J0585
TYSABRI	1 MG	IV	J2323
TYVASO	1.74 MG	INH	J7686
~~TZIELD~~	~~5 MCG~~	~~IV~~	~~C9149~~
TZIELD	5 MCG	IV	J9381
UBLITUXIMAB-XIIY	1 MG	IV	J2329
UDENYCA	0.5 MG	SC	Q5111
ULTOMIRIS	10 MG	IV	J1303
ULTRA-TECHNEKOW	1 MCI	IV	A9512
ULTRALENTE	5 U	SC	J1815

Drug Name	Units Per	Route	Code
ULTRATAG	STUDY DOSE UP TO 30 MCI	IV	A9560
ULTRAVIST 150	1 ML	IV	Q9965
ULTRAVIST 240	1 ML	IV	Q9966
ULTRAVIST 300	1 ML	IV	Q9967
ULTRAVIST 370	1 ML	IV	Q9967
UNASYN	1.5 G	IM, IV	J0295
UNITUXIN	0.1 MG	IV	J1246
UPLIZNA	1 MG	IV	J1823
UREA	40 G	IV	J3350
URECHOLINE	UP TO 5 MG	SC	J0520
UROFOLLITROPIN	75 IU	SC, IM	J3355
UROKINASE	5,000 IU	IV	J3364
UROKINASE	250,000 IU	IV	J3365
USTEKINUMAB	1 MG	SC	J3357
USTEKINUMAB	1 MG	SC, IV	J3358
~~UZEDY~~	~~1 MG~~	~~SC~~	~~C9158~~
UZEDY	1 MG	SC	J2799
VABOMERE	10 MG/10 MG	IV	J2186
VABYSMO	0.1 MG	INJ	J2777
VALERGEN	10 MG	IM	J1380
VALIUM	5 MG	IV, IM	J3360
VALOCTOCOGENE ROXAPARVOVEC-RVOX	1 ML	IV	J1412
VALRUBICIN INTRAVESICAL	200 MG	OTH	J9357
VALSTAR	200 MG	OTH	J9357
VANCOCIN	500 MG	IM, IV	J3370
VANCOMYCIN HCL	500 MG	IV, IM	J3370
VANCOMYCIN HCL (MYLAN) NOT THERAPEUTICALLY EQUIVALENT TO J3370	500 MG	IV	J3371
VANCOMYCIN HCL (XELLIA) NOT THERAPEUTICALLY EQUIVALENT TO J3370	500 MG	IV	J3372
VANTAS	50 MG	OTH	J9225
VAPRISOL	1 MG	INJ	C9488
VARUBI	1 MG	ORAL	J8670
VARUBI	0.5 MG	ORAL, IV	J2797
VASOPRESSIN	1 U	IV	J2598
VASOPRESSIN (AMERICAN REGENT)	1 U	IV	J2599
VECTIBIX	10 MG	IV	J9303
VEDOLIZUMAB	1 MG	IV	J3380
VEGZELMA	10 MG	IV	Q5129
VEKLURY	1 MG	IV	J0248
VELAGLUCERASE ALFA	100 U	IV	J3385
VELBAN	I MG	IV	J9360
~~VELCADE~~	~~0.1 MG~~	~~IV, SC~~	~~J9041~~
VELETRI	0.5 MG	IV	J1325
VELMANASE ALFA-TYCV	1 MG	IV	J0217
VELOSULIN	5 U	SC	J1815
VELOSULIN BR	5 U	SC	J1815
VENDAJE	SQ CM	OTH	Q4252
VENDAJE AC	SQ CM	OTH	Q4279
VENOFER	1 MG	IV	J1756
VENTOLIN NONCOMPOUNDED, CONCENTRATED	1 MG	INH	J7611
VENTOLIN NONCOMPOUNDED, UNIT DOSE	1 MG	INH	J7613
VEPESID	50 MG	ORAL	J8560
VEPESID	10 MG	IV	J9181
VERITAS	SQ CM	OTH	C9354
VERSED	1 MG	IM, IV	J2250

Drug Name	Units Per	Route	Code
VERTEPORFIN	0.1 MG	IV	J3396
VESTRONIDASE ALFA-VJBK	1 MG	IV	J3397
VFEND	200 MG	IV	J3465
VIAGRA	25 MG	ORAL	S0090
VIBATIV	10 MG	IV	J3095
VIDAZA	1 MG	SC	J9025
VIDEX	25 MG	ORAL	S0137
VILTEPSO	10 MG	IV	J1427
VILTOLARSEN	10 MG	IV	J1427
VIM	SQ CM	OTH	Q4251
VIMIZIM	1 MG	IV	J1322
VIMPAT	1 MG	IV, ORAL	C9254
VINBLASTINE SULFATE	1 MG	IV	J9360
VINCASCAR	1 MG	IV	J9370
VINCRISTINE SULFATE	1 MG	IV	J9370
VINCRISTINE SULFATE LIPOSOME	5 MG	IV	J9371
VINORELBINE TARTRATE	10 MG	IV	J9390
VIRILON	1 CC, 200 MG	IM	J1080
VISCO-3	DOSE	INJ	J7321
VISTAJECT-25	25 MG	IM	J3410
VISTARIL	25 MG	IM	J3410
VISTARIL	25 MG	ORAL	Q0177
VISTIDE	375 MG	IV	J0740
VISUDYNE	0.1 MG	IV	J3396
VITAMIN B-12 CYANOCOBALAMIN	1,000 MCG	IM, SC	J3420
VITAMIN B-17	VAR	INJ	J3570
VITRASE	1 USP	OTH	J3471
VITRASE	1,000 USP	OTH	J3472
VITRASERT	4.5 MG	OTH	J7310
VITRAVENE	1.65 MG	OTH	J1452
VIVIMUSTA	1 MG	IV	J9056
VIVITROL	1 MG	IM	J2315
VOCABRIA	1 MG	IM	J0739
VON WILLEBRAND FACTOR (RECOMBINANT)	1 IU	IV	J7179
VON WILLEBRAND FACTOR COMPLEX (HUMAN) (WILATE)	1 IU	IV	J7183
VON WILLEBRAND FACTOR COMPLEX, HUMATE-P	1 IU	IV	J7187
VON WILLEBRAND FACTOR VIII COMPLEX, HUMAN	FACTOR VIII IU	IV	J7186
VONVENDI	1 IU	IV	J7179
VORAXAZE	10 UNITS	IV	C9293
VORETIGENE NEPARVOVEC-RZYL	1 BILLION VECTOR GENOMES	OTH	J3398
VORICONAZOLE	200 MG	IV	J3465
VPRIV	100 U	IV	J3385
VUEWAY	1 ML	IV	A9573
VUMON	50 MG	IV	Q2017
VUTRISIRAN	1 MG	SC	J0225
VYEPTI	1 MG	IV	J3032
VYJUVEK	0.1 ML	OTH	J3401
VYONDYS 53	10 MG	IV	J1429
VYVGART	2 MG	IV	J9332
VYVGART	2 MG	IV	J9334
VYXEOS	1 MG/2.27 MG	IV	J9153
WEHAMINE	50 MG	IM, IV	J1240
WEHDRYL	50 MG	IM, IV	J1200
WELBUTRIN SR	150 MG	ORAL	S0106
WILATE	1 IU	IV	J7183

Drug Name	Units Per	Route	Code
WINRHO SDF	100 IU	IV	J2792
WOUNDEX	SQ CM	OTH	Q4163
WOUNDEX FLOW	0.5 CC	OTH	Q4162
WOUNDFIX, WOUNDFIX PLUS, WOUNDFIX XPLUS	SQ CM	OTH	Q4217
WOUNDPLUS MEMBRANE OR E-GRAFT	SQ CM	OTH	Q4277
WYCILLIN	600,000 U	IM, IV	J2510
XARACOLL	1 MG	OTH	C9089
XCELL AMNIO MATRIX	SQ CM	OTH	Q4280
XCELLERATE	SQ CM	OTH	Q4234
XCELLISTEM	1 MG	OTH	A2004
XCM BIOLOGIC TISSUE MATRIX	SQ CM	OTH	Q4142
XELODA	150 MG	ORAL	J8520
XELODA	500 MG	ORAL	J8521
XEMBIFY	100 MG	SC	J1558
XENLETA	1 MG	IV	J0691
XENON XE-129 HYPERPOLARIZED GAS, DIAGNOSTIC	STUDY DOSE	INH	C9150
XENON XE-133	10 MCI	INH	A9558
XENOVIEW	STUDY DOSE	INH	C9150
XENPOZYME	1 MG	IV	J0218
XEOMIN	1 UNIT	IM	J0588
XERAVA	1 MG	IV	J0122
XGEVA	1 MG	SC	J0897
XIAFLEX	0.01 MG	OTH	J0775
XIPERE	1 MG	INJ	J3299
XOFIGO	MICROCURIE	IV	A9606
XOLAIR	5 MG	SC	J2357
XWRAP	SQ CM	OTH	Q4204
XYLOCAINE	10 MG	IV	J2001
XYNTHA	1 IU	IV	J7185
YCANTII	3.2 MG	OTH	C9164
YERVOY	1 MG	IV	J9228
YESCARTA	UP TO 200 MILLION CELLS	IV	Q2041
YONDELIS	0.1 MG	IV	J9352
YTTRIUM-90 IBRITUMOMAB TIUXETAN, THERAPEUTIC	TX DOSE UP TO 40 MCI	IV	A9543
YUPELRI	1 MCG	INH	J7677
YUTIQ	0.01 MG	OTH	J7314
ZALTRAP	1 MG	IV	J9400
ZANAMIVIR (BRAND) (DEMONSTRATION PROJECT)	10 MG	INH	G9034
ZANAMIVIR (GENERIC) (DEMONSTRATION PROJECT)	10 MG	INH	G9018
ZANOSAR	1 GM	IV	J9320
ZANTAC	25 MG	INJ	J2780
ZARXIO	1 MCG	IV, SC	Q5101
ZEMDRI	5 MG	IV	J0291
ZEMPLAR	1 MCG	IV, IM	J2501
ZENAPAX	25 MG	OTH	J7513
ZENITH AMNIOTIC MEMBRANE	SQ CM	OTH	Q4253
ZEPZELCA	0.1 MG	IV	J9223
ZERBAXA	50 MG/25 MG	IV	J0695
ZEVALIN, DIAGNOSTIC	STUDY DOSE UP TO 5 MCI	IV	A9542
ZEVALIN, THERAPEUTIC	TX DOSE UP TO 40 MCI	IV	A9543
ZICONOTIDE	1 MCG	IT	J2278
ZIDOVUDINE	100 MG	ORAL	S0104
ZIDOVUDINE	10 MG	IV	J3485

Drug Name	Units Per	Route	Code
ZIEXTENZO	0.5 MG	SC	Q5120
ZILRETTA	1 MG	OTH	J3304
ZIMHI	1 MG	SC	J2311
ZINACEFT	750 MG	IM, IV	J0697
ZINECARD	250 MG	IV	J1190
ZINPLAVA	10 MG	INF	J0565
ZIPRASIDONE MESYLATE	10 MG	IM	J3486
ZIRABEV	10 MG	IV	Q5118
ZITHROMAX	500 MG	IV	J0456
ZITHROMAX	1 G	ORAL	Q0144
ZIV-AFLIBERCEPT	1 MG	IV	J9400
ZOFRAN	1 MG	IV	J2405
ZOFRAN	4 MG	ORAL	S0119
ZOFRAN	1 MG	ORAL	Q0162
ZOLADEX	3.6 MG	SC	J9202
ZOLEDRONIC ACID	1 MG	IV	J3489
ZOLGENSMA	UP TO 5X10^{15} VECTOR GENOMES	IV	J3399
ZOMETA	1.MG	IV	J3489
ZORBTIVE	1 MG	SC	J2941
ZORTRESS	0.25 MG	ORAL	J7527
ZOSYN	1 G/1.125 GM	IV	J2543
ZOVIRAX	5 MG	IV	J0133
ZUBSOLV	1.4 MG	ORAL	J0572
ZUBSOLV	5.7 MG	ORAL	J0573
ZULRESSO	1 MG	IV	J1632
ZUPLENZ	4 MG	ORAL	S0119
ZUPLENZ	1 MG	ORAL	Q0162
ZYLONTA	1 MG	IV	J9359
ZYNRELEF	1 MG/0.03 MG	OTH	C9088
ZYNYZ	1 MG	IV	J9345
ZYPREXA	2.5 MG	IM	S0166
ZYPREXA RELPREVV	1 MG	IM	J2358
ZYVOX	200 MG	IV	J2020

NOT OTHERWISE CLASSIFIED DRUGS

Drug Name	Unit Per	Route	Code
ALGLUCOSIDASE ALFA NOS	10 MG	IV	J0220
ALPHA 1 - PROTEINASE INHIBITOR (HUMAN), NOS	10 MG	IV	J0256
ANTIEMETIC NOC	VAR	ORAL	Q0181
ANTIEMETIC DRUG, ORAL, NOS	VAR	ORAL	J8597
ANTIEMETIC DRUG, RECTAL/ SUPPOSITORY, NOS	1 EA	OTH	J8498
ASPARAGINASE, NOS	10,000 U	IM, IV, SC	J9020
BUPIVICAINE, NOS	0.5 MG	INJ	J0665
COMPOUNDED DRUG, NOC	VAR	VAR	J7999
DOXORUBICIN HCL, LIPOSOMAL, NOS	10 MG	IV	Q2050
DRUG OR BIOLOGICAL, NOC, PART B DRUG COMPETITIVE ACQUISITION PROGRAM (CAP)	VAR	VAR	Q4082
FACTOR IX (ANTIHEMOPHILIC FACTOR, RECOMBINANT), NOS	1 IU	IV	J7195
FACTOR VIII (ANTIHEMOPHILIC FACTOR, RECOMBINANT), NOS	1 IU	IV	J7192
FDA-APPROVED PRESCRIPTION DRUG, ONLY FOR USE AS HIV PRE-EXPOSURE PROPHYLAXIS	VAR	VAR	J0799
GADOLINIUM -BASED CONTRAST, NOS	1 ML	IV	A9579

Drug Name	Unit Per	Route	Code
GEMCITABINE HCL, NOS	200 MG	IV	J9201
HEMOPHILIA CLOTTING FACTOR, NOC	VAR	INJ	J7199
HUMAN FIBRINOGEN CONCENTRATE, NOS	1 MG	IV	J7178
HYDROXYPROGESTERONE CAPROATE, NOS	10 MG	IM	J1729
IMMUNE GLOBULIN LYOPHILIZED, NOS	500 MG	IV	J1566
IMMUNE GLOBULIN, NONLYOPHILIZED (NOS)	500 MG	IV	J1599
IMMUNOSUPPRESSIVE DRUG, NOC	VAR	VAR	J7599
INFLUENZA VIRUS VACCINE, NOS	EA	IM	Q2039
LEVOLEUCOVORIN, NOS	0.5 MG	IV	J0641
MELPHALAN HCL, NOS	50 MG	IV	J9245
MULTIPLE VITAMINS, WITH OR WITHOUT MINERALS AND TRACE ELEMENTS	VAR	ORAL	A9153
NOC DRUGS, INHALATION SOLUTION ADMINISTERED THROUGH DME	1 EA	OTH	J7699
NOC DRUGS, OTHER THAN INHALATION DRUGS, ADMINISTERED THROUGH DME	1 EA	OTH	J7799
NONRADIOACTIVE CONTRACT IMAGING MATERIAL	STUDY DOSE	IV	A9698
NOT OTHERWISE CLASSIFIED, ANTINEOPLASTIC DRUGS	VAR	VAR	J9999
PEMETREXED, NOS	10 MG	IV	J9305
POSITRON EMISSION TOMOGRAPHY RADIOPHARMACEUTICAL, DIAGNOSTIC, FOR NON-TUMOR IDENTIFICATION	STUDY DOSE	IV	A9598
POSITRON EMISSION TOMOGRAPHY RADIOPHARMACEUTICAL, DIAGNOSTIC, FOR TUMOR IDENTIFICATION	STUDY DOSE	IV	A9597
PRESCRIPTION DRUG, ORAL, CHEMOTHERAPEUTIC, NOS	VAR	ORAL	J8999
PRESCRIPTION DRUG, ORAL, NONCHEMOTHERAPEUTIC, NOS	VAR	ORAL	J8499
RADIOPHARMACEUTICAL, DIAGNOSTIC, NOC	VAR	VAR	A4641
RADIOPHARMACEUTICAL, THERAPEUTIC	STUDY DOSE	IV	A9699
SINGLE VITAMIN/MINERAL/TRACE ELEMENT	VAR	ORAL	A9152
SKIN SUBSTITUTE, FDA-CLEARED AS A DEVICE, NOS	SQ CM	OTH	A4100
SKIN SUBSTITUTE, NOS	VAR	OTH	Q4100
TRIAMCINOLONE ACETONIDE, NOS	10 MG	IM	J3301
UNCLASSIFIED BIOLOGICS	VAR	VAR	J3590
UNCLASSIFIED DRUG OR BIOLOGICAL USED FOR ESRD ON DIALYSIS	VAR	VAR	J3591
UNCLASSIFIED DRUGS	VAR	VAR	J3490
UNCLASSIFIED DRUGS OR BIOLOGICALS	VAR	VAR	C9399
WOUND FILLER, DRY FORM, PER G, NOS	1 G	OTH	A6262
WOUND FILLER, GEL/PASTE, PER FL OZ, NOS	1 OZ	OTH	A6261

Appendix 2 — Modifiers

A modifier is a two-position code that is added to the end of a code to clarify the services being billed. Modifiers provide a means by which a service can be altered without changing the procedure code. They add more information, such as the anatomical site, to the code. In addition, they help to eliminate the appearance of duplicate billing and unbundling. Modifiers are used to increase accuracy in reimbursement, coding consistency, editing, and to capture payment data.

A1 Dressing for one wound

A2 Dressing for two wounds

A3 Dressing for three wounds

A4 Dressing for four wounds

A5 Dressing for five wounds

A6 Dressing for six wounds

A7 Dressing for seven wounds

A8 Dressing for eight wounds

A9 Dressing for nine or more wounds

AA Anesthesia services performed personally by anesthesiologist

AB Audiology service furnished personally by an audiologist without a physician/NPP order for nonacute hearing assessment unrelated to disequilibrium, or hearing aids, or examinations for the purpose of prescribing, fitting, or changing hearing aids; service may be performed once every 12 months, per beneficiary

AD Medical supervision by a physician: more than four concurrent anesthesia procedures

AE Registered dietician

AF Specialty physician

AG Primary physician

AH Clinical psychologist

AI Principal physician of record

AJ Clinical social worker

AK Nonparticipating physician

AM Physician, team member service

AO Alternate payment method declined by provider of service

AP Determination of refractive state was not performed in the course of diagnostic ophthalmological examination

AQ Physician providing a service in an unlisted health professional shortage area (HPSA)

AR Physician provider services in a physician scarcity area

AS Physician assistant, nurse practitioner, or clinical nurse specialist services for assistant at surgery

AT Acute treatment (this modifier should be used when reporting service 98940, 98941, 98942)

AU Item furnished in conjunction with a urological, ostomy, or tracheostomy supply

AV Item furnished in conjunction with a prosthetic device, prosthetic or orthotic

AW Item furnished in conjunction with a surgical dressing

AX Item furnished in conjunction with dialysis services

AY Item or service furnished to an ESRD patient that is not for the treatment of ESRD

AZ Physician providing a service in a dental health professional shortage area for the purpose of an electronic health record incentive payment

BA Item furnished in conjunction with parenteral enteral nutrition (PEN) services

BL Special acquisition of blood and blood products

BO Orally administered nutrition, not by feeding tube

BP The beneficiary has been informed of the purchase and rental options and has elected to purchase the item

BR The beneficiary has been informed of the purchase and rental options and has elected to rent the item

BU The beneficiary has been informed of the purchase and rental options and after 30 days has not informed the supplier of his/her decision

CA Procedure payable only in the inpatient setting when performed emergently on an outpatient who expires prior to admission

CB Service ordered by a renal dialysis facility (RDF) physician as part of the ESRD beneficiary's dialysis benefit, is not part of the composite rate, and is separately reimbursable

CC Procedure code change (use CC when the procedure code submitted was changed either for administrative reasons or because an incorrect code was filed)

CD AMCC test has been ordered by an ESRD facility or MCP physician that is part of the composite rate and is not separately billable

CE AMCC test has been ordered by an ESRD facility or MCP physician that is a composite rate test but is beyond the normal frequency covered under the rate and is separately reimbursable based on medical necessity

CF AMCC test has been ordered by an ESRD facility or MCP physician that is not part of the composite rate and is separately billable

CG Policy criteria applied

CH Zero percent impaired, limited or restricted

CI At least 1 percent but less than 20 percent impaired, limited or restricted

CJ At least 20 percent but less than 40 percent impaired, limited or restricted

CK At least 40 percent but less than 60 percent impaired, limited or restricted

CL At least 60 percent but less than 80 percent impaired, limited or restricted

CM At least 80 percent but less than 100 percent impaired, limited or restricted

CN 100 percent impaired, limited or restricted

CO Outpatient occupational therapy services furnished in whole or in part by an occupational therapy assistant

CQ Outpatient physical therapy services furnished in whole or in part by a physical therapist assistant

CR Catastrophe/disaster related

CS Cost-sharing waived for specified COVID-19 testing-related services that result in an order for or administration of a COVID-19 test and/or used for cost-sharing waived preventive services furnished via telehealth in rural health clinics and federally qualified health centers during the COVID-19 public health emergency

CT Computed tomography services furnished using equipment that does not meet each of the attributes of the national electrical manufacturers association (NEMA) XR-29-2013 standard

DA Oral health assessment by a licensed health professional other than a dentist

E1 Upper left, eyelid

E2 Lower left, eyelid

E3 Upper right, eyelid

E4 Lower right, eyelid

EA Erythropoietic stimulating agent (ESA) administered to treat anemia due to anticancer chemotherapy

EB Erythropoietic stimulating agent (ESA) administered to treat anemia due to anticancer radiotherapy

EC Erythropoietic stimulating agent (ESA) administered to treat anemia not due to anticancer radiotherapy or anticancer chemotherapy

ED Hematocrit level has exceeded 39 percent (or hemoglobin level has exceeded 13.0 G/dl) for three or more consecutive billing cycles immediately prior to and including the current cycle

EE Hematocrit level has not exceeded 39 percent (or hemoglobin level has not exceeded 13.0 G/dl) for three or more consecutive billing cycles immediately prior to and including the current cycle

EJ Subsequent claims for a defined course of therapy, e.g., EPO, sodium hyaluronate, infliximab

EM Emergency reserve supply (for ESRD benefit only)

EP Service provided as part of Medicaid early periodic screening diagnosis and treatment (EPSDT) program

ER Items and services furnished by a provider-based, off-campus emergency department

ET Emergency services

EX Expatriate beneficiary

EY No physician or other licensed health care provider order for this item or service

F1 Left hand, second digit

F2 Left hand, third digit

F3 Left hand, fourth digit

F4 Left hand, fifth digit

F5 Right hand, thumb

F6 Right hand, second digit

F7 Right hand, third digit

F8 Right hand, fourth digit

F9 Right hand, fifth digit

FA Left hand, thumb

FB Item provided without cost to provider, supplier or practitioner, or full credit received for replaced device (examples, but not limited to, covered under warranty, replaced due to defect, free samples)

FC Partial credit received for replaced device

FP Service provided as part of family planning program

FQ The service was furnished using audio-only communication technology

FR The supervising practitioner was present through two-way, audio/video communication technology

FS Split (or shared) evaluation and management visit

FT Unrelated evaluation and management (E/M) visit on the same day as another E/M visit or during a global procedure (preoperative, postoperative period, or on the same day as the procedure, as applicable). (Report when an E/M visit is furnished within the global period but is unrelated, or when one or more additional E/M visits furnished on the same day are unrelated)

FX X-ray taken using film

FY X-ray taken using computed radiography technology/cassette-based imaging

G0 Telehealth services for diagnosis, evaluation, or treatment, of symptoms of an acute stroke

G1 Most recent URR reading of less than 60

G2 Most recent URR reading of 60 to 64.9

G3 Most recent URR reading of 65 to 69.9

G4 Most recent URR reading of 70 to 74.9

G5 Most recent URR reading of 75 or greater

G6 ESRD patient for whom less than six dialysis sessions have been provided in a month

G7 Pregnancy resulted from rape or incest or pregnancy certified by physician as life threatening

G8 Monitored anesthesia care (MAC) for deep complex, complicated, or markedly invasive surgical procedure

G9 Monitored anesthesia care for patient who has history of severe cardiopulmonary condition

GA Waiver of liability statement issued as required by payer policy, individual case

GB Claim being resubmitted for payment because it is no longer covered under a global payment demonstration

GC This service has been performed in part by a resident under the direction of a teaching physician

GE This service has been performed by a resident without the presence of a teaching physician under the primary care exception

GF Nonphysician (e.g., nurse practitioner (NP), certified registered nurse anesthetist (CRNA), certified registered nurse (CRN), clinical nurse specialist (CNS), physician assistant (PA)) services in a critical access hospital

GG Performance and payment of a screening mammogram and diagnostic mammogram on the same patient, same day

GH Diagnostic mammogram converted from screening mammogram on same day

GJ "Opt out" physician or practitioner emergency or urgent service

GK Reasonable and necessary item/service associated with a GA or GZ modifier

GL Medically unnecessary upgrade provided instead of nonupgraded item, no charge, no advance beneficiary notice (ABN)

GM Multiple patients on one ambulance trip

GN Services delivered under an outpatient speech language pathology plan of care

GO Services delivered under an outpatient occupational therapy plan of care

GP Services delivered under an outpatient physical therapy plan of care

GQ Via asynchronous telecommunications system

GR This service was performed in whole or in part by a resident in a Department of Veterans Affairs medical center or clinic, supervised in accordance with VA policy

GS Dosage of erythropoietin stimulating agent has been reduced and maintained in response to hematocrit or hemoglobin level

GT Via interactive audio and video telecommunication systems

GU Waiver of liability statement issued as required by payer policy, routine notice

GV Attending physician not employed or paid under arrangement by the patient's hospice provider

GW Service not related to the hospice patient's terminal condition

GX Notice of liability issued, voluntary under payer policy

GY Item or service statutorily excluded, does not meet the definition of any Medicare benefit or, for non-Medicare insurers, is not a contract benefit

GZ Item or service expected to be denied as not reasonable and necessary

H9 Court-ordered

HA Child/adolescent program

HB Adult program, nongeriatric

HC Adult program, geriatric

HD Pregnant/parenting women's program

HE Mental health program

HF Substance abuse program

HG Opioid addiction treatment program

HH Integrated mental health/substance abuse program

HI Integrated mental health and intellectual disability/developmental disabilities program

HJ Employee assistance program

HK Specialized mental health programs for high-risk populations

HL Intern

HM Less than bachelor degree level

HN Bachelors degree level

HO Masters degree level

HP Doctoral level

HQ Group setting

HR Family/couple with client present

HS Family/couple without client present

HT Multidisciplinary team

HU Funded by child welfare agency

HV Funded state addictions agency

HW Funded by state mental health agency

HX Funded by county/local agency

HY Funded by juvenile justice agency

HZ Funded by criminal justice agency

J1 Competitive acquisition program no-pay submission for a prescription number

J2 Competitive acquisition program, restocking of emergency drugs after emergency administration

J3 Competitive acquisition program (CAP), drug not available through CAP as written, reimbursed under average sales price methodology

J4 DMEPOS item subject to DMEPOS competitive bidding program that is furnished by a hospital upon discharge

J5 Off-the-shelf orthotic subject to DMEPOS competitive bidding program that is furnished as part of a physical therapist or occupational therapist professional service

JA Administered intravenously

JB Administered subcutaneously

JC Skin substitute used as a graft

JD Skin substitute not used as a graft

JE Administered via dialysate

JF Compounded drug

JG   Drug or biological acquired with 340B drug pricing program discount, reported for informational purposes

- **JK**   One month supply or less of drug or biological

- **JL**   Three month supply of drug or biological

JW   Drug amount discarded/not administered to any patient

JZ   Zero drug amount discarded/not administered to any patient

K0   Lower extremity prosthesis functional level 0 - does not have the ability or potential to ambulate or transfer safely with or without assistance and a prosthesis does not enhance their quality of life or mobility

K1   Lower extremity prosthesis functional level 1 - has the ability or potential to use a prosthesis for transfers or ambulation on level surfaces at fixed cadence, typical of the limited and unlimited household ambulator

K2   Lower extremity prosthesis functional level 2 - has the ability or potential for ambulation with the ability to traverse low level environmental barriers such as curbs, stairs or uneven surfaces, typical of the limited community ambulator

K3   Lower extremity prosthesis functional level 3 - has the ability or potential for ambulation with variable cadence, typical of the community ambulator who has the ability to transverse most environmental barriers and may have vocational, therapeutic, or exercise activity that demands prosthetic utilization beyond simple locomotion

K4   Lower extremity prosthesis functional level 4 - has the ability or potential for prosthetic ambulation that exceeds the basic ambulation skills, exhibiting high impact, stress, or energy levels, typical of the prosthetic demands of the child, active adult, or athlete

KA   Add on option/accessory for wheelchair

KB   Beneficiary requested upgrade for ABN, more than four modifiers identified on claim

KC   Replacement of special power wheelchair interface

KD   Drug or biological infused through DME

KE   Bid under round one of the DMEPOS competitive bidding program for use with noncompetitive bid base equipment

KF   Item designated by FDA as Class III device

KG   DMEPOS item subject to DMEPOS competitive bidding program number 1

KH   DMEPOS item, initial claim, purchase or first month rental

KI   DMEPOS item, second or third month rental

KJ   DMEPOS item, parenteral enteral nutrition (PEN) pump or capped rental, months four to fifteen

KK   DMEPOS item subject to DMEPOS competitive bidding program number 2

KL   DMEPOS item delivered via mail

KM   Replacement of facial prosthesis including new impression/moulage

KN   Replacement of facial prosthesis using previous master model

KO   Single drug unit dose formulation

KP   First drug of a multiple drug unit dose formulation

KQ   Second or subsequent drug of a multiple drug unit dose formulation

KR   Rental item, billing for partial month

KS   Glucose monitor supply for diabetic beneficiary not treated with insulin

KT   Beneficiary resides in a competitive bidding area and travels outside that competitive bidding area and receives a competitive bid item

KU   DMEPOS item subject to DMEPOS competitive bidding program number 3

KV   DMEPOS item subject to DMEPOS competitive bidding program that is furnished as part of a professional service

KW   DMEPOS item subject to DMEPOS competitive bidding program number 4

KX   Requirements specified in the medical policy have been met

KY   DMEPOS item subject to DMEPOS competitive bidding program number 5

KZ   New coverage not implemented by managed care

LC   Left circumflex coronary artery

LD   Left anterior descending coronary artery

LL   Lease/rental (use the LL modifier when DME equipment rental is to be applied against the purchase price)

LM   Left main coronary artery

LR   Laboratory round trip

LS   FDA-monitored intraocular lens implant

LT   Left side (used to identify procedures performed on the left side of the body)

▲ **LU**   Fractionated payment

M2   Medicare secondary payer (MSP)

MA   Ordering professional is not required to consult a Clinical Decision Support Mechanism due to service being rendered to a patient with a suspected or confirmed emergency medical condition

MB   Ordering professional is not required to consult a Clinical Decision Support Mechanism due to the significant hardship exception of insufficient internet access

MC   Ordering professional is not required to consult a Clinical Decision Support Mechanism due to the significant hardship exception of electronic health record or Clinical Decision Support Mechanism vendor issues

MD   Ordering professional is not required to consult a Clinical Decision Support Mechanism due to the significant hardship exception of extreme and uncontrollable circumstances

ME   The order for this service adheres to Appropriate Use Criteria in the Clinical Decision Support Mechanism consulted by the ordering professional

MF   The order for this service does not adhere to the Appropriate Use Criteria in the Clinical Decision Support Mechanism consulted by the ordering professional

MG   The order for this service does not have applicable Appropriate Use Criteria in the qualified Clinical Decision Support Mechanism consulted by the ordering professional

MH   Unknown if ordering professional consulted a Clinical Decision Support Mechanism for this service, related information was not provided to the furnishing professional or provider

MS   Six month maintenance and servicing fee for reasonable and necessary parts and labor which are not covered under any manufacturer or supplier warranty

- **N1**   Group 1 oxygen coverage criteria met

- **N2**   Group 2 oxygen coverage criteria met

- **N3**   Group 3 oxygen coverage criteria met

NB   Nebulizer system, any type, FDA-cleared for use with specific drug

NR   New when rented (use the NR modifier when DME which was new at the time of rental is subsequently purchased)

NU   New equipment

P1   A normal healthy patient

P2   A patient with mild systemic disease

P3   A patient with severe systemic disease

P4   A patient with severe systemic disease that is a constant threat to life

P5   A moribund patient who is not expected to survive without the operation

P6   A declared brain-dead patient whose organs are being removed for donor purposes

PA   Surgical or other invasive procedure on wrong body part

PB   Surgical or other invasive procedure on wrong patient

PC   Wrong surgery or other invasive procedure on patient

PD   Diagnostic or related nondiagnostic item or service provided in a wholly owned or operated entity to a patient who is admitted as an inpatient within three days

PI   Positron emission tomography (PET) or pet/computed tomography (CT) to inform the initial treatment strategy of tumors that are biopsy proven or strongly suspected of being cancerous based on other diagnostic testing

PL   Progressive addition lenses

PM   Post mortem

PN   Nonexcepted service provided at an off-campus, outpatient, provider-based department of a hospital

PO   Excepted service provided at an off-campus, outpatient, provider-based department of a hospital

PS   Positron emission tomography (PET) or pet/computed tomography (CT) to inform the subsequent treatment strategy of cancerous tumors when the beneficiary's treating physician determines that the PET study is needed to inform subsequent antitumor strategy

PT Colorectal cancer screening test; converted to diagnostic test or other procedure

Q0 Investigational clinical service provided in a clinical research study that is in an approved clinical research study

Q1 Routine clinical service provided in a clinical research study that is in an approved clinical research study

Q2 Demonstration procedure/service

Q3 Live kidney donor surgery and related services

Q4 Service for ordering/referring physician qualifies as a service exemption

Q5 Service furnished under a reciprocal billing arrangement by a substitute physician or by a substitute physical therapist furnishing outpatient physical therapy services in a health professional shortage area, a medically underserved area, or a rural area

Q6 Service furnished under a fee-for-time compensation arrangement by a substitute physician or by a substitute physical therapist furnishing outpatient physical therapy services in a health professional shortage area, a medically underserved area, or a rural area

Q7 One Class A finding

Q8 Two Class B findings

Q9 One Class B and two Class C findings

QA Prescribed amounts of stationary oxygen for daytime use while at rest and nighttime use differ and the average of the two amounts is less than 1 liter per minute (LPM)

QB Prescribed amounts of stationary oxygen for daytime use while at rest and nighttime use differ and the average of the two amounts exceeds 4 liters per minute (LPM) and portable oxygen is prescribed

QC Single channel monitoring

QD Recording and storage in solid state memory by a digital recorder

QE Prescribed amount of stationary oxygen while at rest is less than 1 liter per minute (LPM)

QF Prescribed amount of stationary oxygen while at rest exceeds 4 liters per minute (LPM) and portable oxygen is prescribed

QG Prescribed amount of stationary oxygen while at rest is greater than 4 liters per minute (LPM)

QH Oxygen conserving device is being used with an oxygen delivery system

QJ Services/items provided to a prisoner or patient in state or local custody; however, the state or local government, as applicable, meets the requirements in 42 CFR 411.4 (B)

QK Medical direction of two, three, or four concurrent anesthesia procedures involving qualified individuals

QL Patient pronounced dead after ambulance called

QM Ambulance service provided under arrangement by a provider of services

QN Ambulance service furnished directly by a provider of services

QP Documentation is on file showing that the laboratory test(s) was ordered individually or ordered as a CPT-recognized panel other than automated profile codes 80002-80019, G0058, G0059, and G0060.

QQ Ordering professional consulted a qualified clinical decision support mechanism for this service and the related data was provided to the furnishing professional

QR Prescribed amounts of stationary oxygen for daytime use while at rest and nighttime use differ and the average of the two amounts is greater than 4 liters per minute (LPM)

QS Monitored anesthesiology care service

QT Recording and storage on tape by an analog tape recorder

QW CLIA waived test

QX CRNA service: with medical direction by a physician

QY Medical direction of one certified registered nurse anesthetist (CRNA) by an anesthesiologist

QZ CRNA service: without medical direction by a physician

RA Replacement of a DME, orthotic or prosthetic item

RB Replacement of a part of a DME, orthotic or prosthetic item furnished as part of a repair

RC Right coronary artery

RD Drug provided to beneficiary, but not administered "incident-to"

RE Furnished in full compliance with FDA-mandated risk evaluation and mitigation strategy (REMS)

RI Ramus intermedius coronary artery

RR Rental (use the RR modifier when DME is to be rented)

RT Right side (used to identify procedures performed on the right side of the body)

SA Nurse practitioner rendering service in collaboration with a physician

SB Nurse midwife

SC Medically necessary service or supply

SD Services provided by registered nurse with specialized, highly technical home infusion training

SE State and/or federally-funded programs/services

SF Second opinion ordered by a professional review organization (PRO) per section 9401, p.l. 99-272 (100 percent reimbursement - no Medicare deductible or coinsurance)

SG Ambulatory surgical center (ASC) facility service

SH Second concurrently administered infusion therapy

SJ Third or more concurrently administered infusion therapy

SK Member of high risk population (use only with codes for immunization)

SL State supplied vaccine

SM Second surgical opinion

SN Third surgical opinion

SQ Item ordered by home health

SS Home infusion services provided in the infusion suite of the IV therapy provider

ST Related to trauma or injury

SU Procedure performed in physician's office (to denote use of facility and equipment)

SV Pharmaceuticals delivered to patient's home but not utilized

SW Services provided by a certified diabetic educator

SY Persons who are in close contact with member of high-risk population (use only with codes for immunization)

SZ Habilitative services

T1 Left foot, second digit

T2 Left foot, third digit

T3 Left foot, fourth digit

T4 Left foot, fifth digit

T5 Right foot, great toe

T6 Right foot, second digit

T7 Right foot, third digit

T8 Right foot, fourth digit

T9 Right foot, fifth digit

TA Left foot, great toe

TB Drug or biological acquired with 340B drug pricing program discount, reported for informational purposes for select entities

TC Technical component; under certain circumstances, a charge may be made for the technical component alone; under those circumstances the technical component charge is identified by adding modifier TC to the usual procedure number; technical component charges are institutional charges and not billed separately by physicians; however, portable x-ray suppliers only bill for technical component and should utilize modifier TC; the charge data from portable x-ray suppliers will then be used to build customary and prevailing profiles

TD RN

TE LPN/LVN

TF Intermediate level of care

TG Complex/high tech level of care

TH Obstetrical treatment/services, prenatal or postpartum

TJ Program group, child and/or adolescent

TK Extra patient or passenger, nonambulance

TL Early intervention/individualized family service plan (IFSP)

TM Individualized education program (IEP)

TN Rural/outside providers' customary service area

TP Medical transport, unloaded vehicle

TQ Basic life support transport by a volunteer ambulance provider

TR School-based individualized education program (IEP) services provided outside the public school district responsible for the student

TS Follow-up service

TT Individualized service provided to more than one patient in same setting

TU Special payment rate, overtime

TV Special payment rates, holidays/weekends

TW Back-up equipment

U1 Medicaid level of care 1, as defined by each state

U2 Medicaid level of care 2, as defined by each state

U3 Medicaid level of care 3, as defined by each state

U4 Medicaid level of care 4, as defined by each state

U5 Medicaid level of care 5, as defined by each state

U6 Medicaid level of care 6, as defined by each state

U7 Medicaid level of care 7, as defined by each state

U8 Medicaid level of care 8, as defined by each state

U9 Medicaid level of care 9, as defined by each state

UA Medicaid level of care 10, as defined by each state

UB Medicaid level of care 11, as defined by each state

UC Medicaid level of care 12, as defined by each state

UD Medicaid level of care 13, as defined by each state

UE Used durable medical equipment

UF Services provided in the morning

UG Services provided in the afternoon

UH Services provided in the evening

UJ Services provided at night

UK Services provided on behalf of the client to someone other than the client (collateral relationship)

UN Two patients served

UP Three patients served

UQ Four patients served

UR Five patients served

US Six or more patients served

V1 Demonstration modifier 1

V2 Demonstration modifier 2

V3 Demonstration modifier 3

V4 Demonstration modifier 4

V5 Vascular catheter (alone or with any other vascular access)

V6 Arteriovenous graft (or other vascular access not including a vascular catheter)

V7 Arteriovenous fistula only (in use with two needles)

V8 Infection present

V9 No infection present

VM Medicare Diabetes Prevention Program (MDPP) virtual make-up session

VP Aphakic patient

X1 Continuous/broad services: for reporting services by clinicians, who provide the principal care for a patient, with no planned endpoint of the relationship; services in this category represent comprehensive care, dealing with the entire scope of patient problems, either directly or in a care coordination role; reporting clinician service examples include, but are not limited to, primary care, and clinicians providing comprehensive care to patients in addition to specialty care

X2 Continuous/focused services: for reporting services by clinicians whose expertise is needed for the ongoing management of a chronic disease or a condition that needs to be managed and followed with no planned endpoint to the relationship; reporting clinician service examples include, but are not limited to, a rheumatologist taking care of the patient's rheumatoid arthritis longitudinally but not providing general primary care services

X3 Episodic/broad servies: for reporting services by clinicians who have broad responsibility for the comprehensive needs of the patient that is limited to a defined period and circumstance such as a hospitalization; reporting clinician service examples include, but are not limited to, the hospitalist's services rendered providing comprehensive and general care to a patient while admitted to the hospital

X4 Episodic/focused services: for reporting services by clinicians who provide focused care on particular types of treatment limited to a defined period and circumstance; the patient has a problem, acute or chronic, that will be treated with surgery, radiation, or some other type of generally time-limited intervention; reporting clinician service examples include, but are not limited to, the orthopedic surgeon performing a knee replacement and seeing the patient through the postoperative period

X5 Diagnostic services requested by another clinician: for reporting services by a clinician who furnishes care to the patient only as requested by another clinician or subsequent and related services requested by another clinician; this modifier is reported for patient relationships that may not be adequately captured by the above alternative categories; reporting clinician service examples include, but are not limited to, the radiologist's interpretation of an imaging study requested by another clinician

XE Separate encounter, a service that is distinct because it occurred during a separate encounter

XP Separate practitioner, a service that is distinct because it was performed by a different practitioner

XS Separate structure, a service that is distinct because it was performed on a separate organ/structure

XU Unusual nonoverlapping service, the use of a service that is distinct because it does not overlap usual components of the main service

Appendix 3 — Abbreviations and Acronyms

HCPCS Abbreviations and Acronyms

The following abbreviations and acronyms are used in the HCPCS descriptions:

/	or
<	less than
<=	less than equal to
>	greater than
>=	greater than equal to
AC	alternating current
ACE/ACEI	angiotensin-converting enzyme inhibitor
AFO	ankle-foot orthosis
AHI	apnea hypopnea index
AICC	anti-inhibitor coagulant complex
AK	above the knee
AKA	above knee amputation
ALS	advanced life support
AMP	ampule
AO	ankle orthosis
ARB	angiotensin receptor blocker
ART	artery
ART	arterial
ASC	ambulatory surgery center
ATT	attached
A-V	arteriovenous
AVF	arteriovenous fistula
BICROS	bilateral routing of signals
BK	below the knee
BLS	basic life support
BMI	body mass index
BP	blood pressure
BTE	behind the ear (hearing aid)
CAPD	continuous ambulatory peritoneal dialysis
Carb	carbohydrate
CBC	complete blood count
cc	cubic centimeter
CCPD	continuous cycling peritoneal analysis
CGM	continuous glucose monitoring
CHF	congestive heart failure
CIC	completely in the canal (hearing aid)
CIM	Coverage Issue Manual
CKD	chronic kidney disease
Clsd	closed
cm	centimeter
CMN	certificate of medical necessity
CMS	Centers for Medicare and Medicaid Services
CMV	cytomegalovirus
Conc	concentrate
Conc	concentrated
Cont	continuous
CP	clinical psychologist
CPAP	continuous positive airway pressure
CPT	Current Procedural Terminology
CRF	chronic renal failure
CRNA	certified registered nurse anesthetist
CROS	contralateral routing of signals
CSW	clinical social worker
CT	computed tomography
CTLSO	cervical-thoracic-lumbar-sacral orthosis
cu	cubic
DC	direct current
DI	diurnal rhythm
Dx	diagnosis
DLI	donor leukocyte infusion
DME	durable medical equipment
DME MAC	durable medical equipment Medicare administrative contractor
DMEPOS	durable medical equipment, prosthetics, orthotics and other supplies

DMERC	durable medical equipment regional carrier
DR	diagnostic radiology
DX	diagnostic
e.g.	for example
Ea	each
ECF	extended care facility
EEG	electroencephalogram
EGFR	estimated glomerular filtration rate
EKG	electrocardiogram
EMG	electromyography
EO	elbow orthosis
EP	electrophysiologic
EPO	epoetin alfa
EPSDT	early periodic screening, diagnosis and treatment
ERCP	endoscopic retrograde cholangiopancreatography
ESRD	end-stage renal disease
EWHO	elbow-wrist-hand orthotic
Ex	extended
Exper	experimental
Ext	external
F	french
FDA	Food and Drug Administration
FDG-PET	positron emission with tomography with 18 fluorodeoxyglucose
Fem	female
FO	finger orthosis
FPD	fixed partial denture
Fr	french
ft	foot
G-CSF	filgrastim (granulocyte colony-stimulating factor)
gm	gram (g)
H2O	water
HCl	hydrochloric acid, hydrochloride
HCPCS	Healthcare Common Procedural Coding System
HCT	hematocrit
HFO	hand-finger orthosis
HHA	home health agency
HI	high
HI-LO	high-low
HIT	home infusion therapy
HKAFO	hip-knee-ankle foot orthosis
HLA	human leukocyte antigen
HMES	heat and moisture exchange system
HNPCC	hereditary non-polyposis colorectal cancer
HO	hip orthosis
HPSA	health professional shortage area
HST	home sleep test
IA	intra-arterial administration
ip	interphalangeal
I-131	Iodine 131
ICF	intermediate care facility
ICU	intensive care unit
IM	intramuscular
in	inch
INF	infusion
INH	inhalation solution
INJ	injection
IOL	intraocular lens
IPD	intermittent peritoneal dialysis
IPPB	intermittent positive pressure breathing
IT	intrathecal administration
ITC	in the canal (hearing aid)
ITE	in the ear (hearing aid)
IU	international units
IV	intravenous
IVF	in vitro fertilization
KAFO	knee-ankle-foot orthosis
KO	knee orthosis

KOH	potassium hydroxide
L	left
LASIK	laser in situ keratomileusis
LAUP	laser assisted uvulopalatoplasty
lbs	pounds
LDL	low density lipoprotein
LDS	lipodystrophy syndrome
Lo	low
LO	lumbar orthosis
LPM	liters per minute
LPN/LVN	Licensed Practical Nurse/Licensed Vocational Nurse
LSO	lumbar-sacral orthosis
lvad	left ventricular assist device
lvef	left ventricular ejection fraction
MAC	Medicare administrative contractor
mp	metacarpophalangeal
mcg	microgram
mCi	millicurie
MCM	Medicare Carriers Manual
MCP	metacarparpophalangeal joint
MCP	monthly capitation payment
mEq	milliequivalent
MESA	microsurgical epididymal sperm aspiration
mg	milligram
mgs	milligrams
MHT	megahertz
ml	milliliter
mm	millimeter
mmHg	millimeters of Mercury
MRA	magnetic resonance angiography
MRI	magnetic resonance imaging
NA	sodium
NCI	National Cancer Institute
NEC	not elsewhere classified
NG	nasogastric
NH	nursing home
NMES	neuromuscular electrical stimulation
NOC	not otherwise classified
NOS	not otherwise specified
NRS	numeric rating scale
O2	oxygen
OBRA	Omnibus Budget Reconciliation Act
OMT	osteopathic manipulation therapy
OPPS	outpatient prospective payment system
ORAL	oral administration
OSA	obstructive sleep apnea
Ost	ostomy
OTH	other routes of administration
oz	ounce
PA	physician's assistant
PAR	parenteral
PCA	patient controlled analgesia
PCH	pouch
PEN	parenteral and enteral nutrition
PENS	percutaneous electrical nerve stimulation
PET	positron emission tomography
PHP	pre-paid health plan
PHP	physician hospital plan
PI	paramedic intercept
PICC	peripherally inserted central venous catheter
PKR	photorefractive keratotomy
Pow	powder
PRK	photoreactive keratectomy
PRO	peer review organization
PSA	prostate specific antigen
PTB	patellar tendon bearing
PTK	phototherapeutic keratectomy
PVC	polyvinyl chloride
QPP	Quality Payment Program
R	right

RDI	respiratory disturbance index
REI	respiratory event index
Repl	replace
RN	registered nurse
RP	retrograde pyelogram
Rx	prescription
SACH	solid ankle, cushion heel
SC	subcutaneous
SCT	specialty care transport
SEO	shoulder-elbow orthosis
SEWHO	shoulder-elbow-wrist-hand orthosis
SEXA	single energy x-ray absorptiometry
SGD	speech generating device
SGD	sinus rhythm
SM	samarium
SNCT	sensory nerve conduction test
SNF	skilled nursing facility
SO	sacroilliac othrosis
SO	shoulder orthosis
Sol	solution
SQ	square
SR	screen
ST	standard
ST	sustained release
Syr	syrup
TABS	tablets
Tc	technetium
Tc 99m	technetium isotope
TENS	transcutaneous electrical nerve stimulator
THKAO	thoracic-hip-knee-ankle orthosis
TLSO	thoracic-lumbar-sacral-orthosis
TM	temporomandibular
TMJ	temporomandibular joint
TPN	total parenteral nutrition
U	unit
UACR	urine albumin-creatinine ratio
uCi	microcurie
VAR	various routes of administration
VAS	visual analog scale
VRS	visual rating scale
w	with
w/	with
w/o	without
WAK	wearable artificial kidney
wc	wheelchair
WHFO	wrist-hand-finger orthotic
WHO	wrist-hand orthotic
Wk	week
w/o	without
Xe	xenon (isotope mass of xenon 133)

Appendix 4 — Medicare Internet-only Manuals (IOMs)

The Centers for Medicare and Medicaid Services (CMS) restructured its paper-based manual system as a web-based system on October 1, 2003. Called the online CMS manual system, it combines all of the various program instructions into Internet-only Manuals (IOMs), which are used by all CMS programs and contractors. In many instances, the references from the online manuals in appendix 4 contain a mention of the old paper manuals from which the current information was obtained when the manuals were converted. This information is shown in the header of the text, in the following format, when applicable, as A3-3101, HO-210, and B3-2049.

Effective with implementation of the IOMs, the former method of publishing program memoranda (PMs) to communicate program instructions was replaced by the following four templates:

- One-time notification
- Manual revisions
- Business requirements
- Confidential requirements

The web-based system has been organized by functional area (e.g., eligibility, entitlement, claims processing, benefit policy, program integrity) in an effort to eliminate redundancy within the manuals, simplify updating, and make CMS program instructions available more quickly. The web-based system contains the functional areas included below:

Pub. 100	Introduction
Pub. 100-01	Medicare General Information, Eligibility, and Entitlement Manual
Pub. 100-02	Medicare Benefit Policy Manual
Pub. 100-03	Medicare National Coverage Determinations (NCD) Manual
Pub. 100-04	Medicare Claims Processing Manual
Pub. 100-05	Medicare Secondary Payer Manual
Pub. 100-06	Medicare Financial Management Manual
Pub. 100-07	State Operations Manual
Pub. 100-08	Medicare Program Integrity Manual
Pub. 100-09	Medicare Contractor Beneficiary and Provider Communications Manual
Pub. 100-10	Quality Improvement Organization Manual
Pub. 100-11	Programs of All-Inclusive Care for the Elderly (PACE) Manual
Pub. 100-12	State Medicaid Manual (The new manual is under development. Please continue to use the Paper Based Manual to make your selection.)
Pub. 100-13	Medicaid State Children's Health Insurance Program (Under Development)
Pub. 100-15	Medicaid Program Integrity Manual
Pub. 100-16	Medicare Managed Care Manual
Pub. 100-17	CMS/Business Partners Systems Security Manual
Pub. 100-18	Medicare Prescription Drug Benefit Manual
Pub. 100-19	Demonstrations
Pub. 100-20	One-Time Notification
Pub. 100-21	Reserved
Pub. 100-22	Medicare Quality Reporting Incentive Programs Manual
Pub. 100-23	Payment Error Rate Measurement (Under Development)
Pub. 100-24	State Payment of Medicare Premiums
Pub. 100-25	Information Security Acceptable Risk Safeguards Manual

A brief description of the Medicare manuals primarily used for *HCPCS Level II* follows:

The *National Coverage Determinations Manual* (NCD), is organized according to categories such as diagnostic services, supplies, and medical procedures. The table of contents lists each category and subject within that category. Revision transmittals identify any new or background material, recap the changes, and provide an effective date for the change. The manual contains four sections and is organized in accordance with CPT category sequence and contains a list of HCPCS codes related to coverage determinations, where appropriate.

The *Medicare Benefit Policy Manual* contains Medicare general coverage instructions that are not national coverage determinations. As a general rule, in the past these instructions have been found in chapter II of the *Medicare Carriers Manual*, the *Medicare Intermediary Manual*, other provider manuals, and program memoranda.

The *Medicare Claims Processing Manual* contains instructions for processing claims for contractors and providers.

The *Medicare Program Integrity Manual* communicates the priorities and standards for the Medicare integrity programs.

Medicare IOM References

A printed version of the Medicare IOM references will no longer be published in Optum's *HCPCS Level II* product. Complete versions of all the manuals can be found online at https://www.cms.gov/medicare/regulations-guidance/manuals/internet-only-manuals-ioms.

Appendix 5 — New, Revised, and Deleted Codes for 2024

NEW CODES

A4287	Disposable collection and storage bag for breast milk, any size, any type, each
A4457	Enema tube, with or without adapter, any type, replacement only, each
A4468	Exsufflation belt, includes all supplies and accessories
A4540	Distal transcutaneous electrical nerve stimulator, stimulates peripheral nerves of the upper arm
A4541	Monthly supplies for use of device coded at E0733
A4542	Supplies and accessories for external upper limb tremor stimulator of the peripheral nerves of the wrist
A6520	Gradient compression garment, glove, padded, for nighttime use, each
A6521	Gradient compression garment, glove, padded, for nighttime use, custom, each
A6522	Gradient compression garment, arm, padded, for nighttime use, each
A6523	Gradient compression garment, arm, padded, for nighttime use, custom, each
A6524	Gradient compression garment, lower leg and foot, padded, for nighttime use, each
A6525	Gradient compression garment, lower leg and foot, padded, for nighttime use, custom, each
A6526	Gradient compression garment, full leg and foot, padded, for nighttime use, each
A6527	Gradient compression garment, full leg and foot, padded, for nighttime use, custom, each
A6528	Gradient compression garment, bra, for nighttime use, each
A6529	Gradient compression garment, bra, for nighttime use, custom, each
A6552	Gradient compression stocking, below knee, 30-40 mm Hg, each
A6553	Gradient compression stocking, below knee, 30-40 mm Hg, custom, each
A6554	Gradient compression stocking, below knee, 40 mm Hg or greater, each
A6555	Gradient compression stocking, below knee, 40 mm Hg or greater, custom, each
A6556	Gradient compression stocking, thigh length, 18-30 mm Hg, custom, each
A6557	Gradient compression stocking, thigh length, 30-40 mm Hg, custom, each
A6558	Gradient compression stocking, thigh length, 40 mm Hg or greater, custom, each
A6559	Gradient compression stocking, full length/chap style, 18-30 mm Hg, custom, each
A6560	Gradient compression stocking, full length/chap style, 30-40 mm Hg, custom, each
A6561	Gradient compression stocking, full length/chap style, 40 mm Hg or greater, custom, each
A6562	Gradient compression stocking, waist length, 18-30 mm Hg, custom, each
A6563	Gradient compression stocking, waist length, 30-40 mm Hg, custom, each
A6564	Gradient compression stocking, waist length, 40 mm Hg or greater, custom, each
A6565	Gradient compression gauntlet, custom, each
A6566	Gradient compression garment, neck/head, each
A6567	Gradient compression garment, neck/head, custom, each
A6568	Gradient compression garment, torso and shoulder, each
A6569	Gradient compression garment, torso/shoulder, custom, each
A6570	Gradient compression garment, genital region, each
A6571	Gradient compression garment, genital region, custom, each
A6572	Gradient compression garment, toe caps, each
A6573	Gradient compression garment, toe caps, custom, each
A6574	Gradient compression arm sleeve and glove combination, custom, each
A6575	Gradient compression arm sleeve and glove combination, each
A6576	Gradient compression arm sleeve, custom, medium weight, each
A6577	Gradient compression arm sleeve, custom, heavy weight, each
A6578	Gradient compression arm sleeve, each
A6579	Gradient compression glove, custom, medium weight, each
A6580	Gradient compression glove, custom, heavy weight, each
A6581	Gradient compression glove, each
A6582	Gradient compression gauntlet, each
A6583	Gradient compression wrap with adjustable straps, below knee, 30-50 mm Hg, each
A6584	Gradient compression wrap with adjustable straps, not otherwise specified
A6585	Gradient pressure wrap with adjustable straps, above knee, each
A6586	Gradient pressure wrap with adjustable straps, full leg, each
A6587	Gradient pressure wrap with adjustable straps, foot, each
A6588	Gradient pressure wrap with adjustable straps, arm, each
A6589	Gradient pressure wrap with adjustable straps, bra, each
A6593	Accessory for gradient compression garment or wrap with adjustable straps, not otherwise specified
A6594	Gradient compression bandaging supply, bandage liner, lower extremity, any size or length, each
A6595	Gradient compression bandaging supply, bandage liner, upper extremity, any size or length, each
A6596	Gradient compression bandaging supply, conforming gauze, per linear yd, any width, each
A6597	Gradient compression bandage roll, elastic long stretch, linear yd, any width, each
A6598	Gradient compression bandage roll, elastic medium stretch, per linear yd, any width, each
A6599	Gradient compression bandage roll, inelastic short stretch, per linear yd, any width, each
A6600	Gradient compression bandaging supply, high density foam sheet, per 250 sq cm, each
A6601	Gradient compression bandaging supply, high density foam pad, any size or shape, each
A6602	Gradient compression bandaging supply, high density foam roll for bandage, per linear yd, any width, each
A6603	Gradient compression bandaging supply, low density channel foam sheet, per 250 sq cm, each
A6604	Gradient compression bandaging supply, low density flat foam sheet, per 250 sq cm, each
A6605	Gradient compression bandaging supply, padded foam, per linear yd, any width, each
A6606	Gradient compression bandaging supply, padded textile, per linear yd, any width, each
A6607	Gradient compression bandaging supply, tubular protective absorption layer, per linear yd, any width, each
A6608	Gradient compression bandaging supply, tubular protective absorption padded layer, per linear yd, any width, each
A6609	Gradient compression bandaging supply, not otherwise specified
A6610	Gradient compression stocking, below knee, 18-30 mm Hg, custom, each
A7023	Mechanical allergen particle barrier/inhalation filter, cream, nasal, topical
A9608	Flotufolastat F18, diagnostic, 1 mCi
A9609	Fludeoxyglucose F18, up to 15 mCi
C1600	Catheter, transluminal intravascular lesion preparation device, bladed, sheathed (insertable)
C1601	Endoscope, single-use (i.e., disposable), pulmonary, imaging/illumination device (insertable)
C1602	Orthopedic/device/drug matrix/absorbable bone void filler, antimicrobial-eluting (implantable)
C1603	Retrieval device, insertable, laser (used to retrieve intravascular inferior vena cava filter)
C1604	Graft, transmural transvenous arterial bypass (implantable), with all delivery system components

NEW CODES (continued)

C7556 Bronchoscopy, rigid or flexible, with bronchial alveolar lavage and transendoscopic endobronchial ultrasound (EBUS) during bronchoscopic diagnostic or therapeutic intervention(s) for peripheral lesion(s), including fluoroscopic guidance, when performed

C7557 Catheter placement in coronary artery(s) for coronary angiography, including intraprocedural injection(s) for coronary angiography, imaging supervision and interpretation with left heart catheterization including intraprocedural injection(s) for left ventriculography, when performed and intraprocedural coronary fractional flow reserve (FFR) with 3D functional mapping of color-coded FFR values for the coronary tree, derived from coronary angiogram data, for real-time review and interpretation of possible atherosclerotic stenosis(es) intervention

C7558 Catheter placement in coronary artery(s) for coronary angiography, including intraprocedural injection(s) for coronary angiography, imaging supervision and interpretation with right and left heart catheterization including intraprocedural injection(s) for left ventriculography, when performed, catheter placement(s) in bypass graft(s) (internal mammary, free arterial, venous grafts) with bypass graft angiography with pharmacologic agent administration (eg, inhaled nitric oxide, intravenous infusion of nitroprusside, dobutamine, milrinone, or other agent) including assessing hemodynamic measurements before, during, after and repeat pharmacologic agent administration, when performed

C7560 Endoscopic retrograde cholangiopancreatography (ERCP) with removal of foreign body(ies) or stent(s) from biliary/pancreatic duct(s) and endoscopic cannulation of papilla with direct visualization of pancreatic/common bile duct(s)

C7561 Debridement, bone (includes epidermis, dermis, subcutaneous tissue, muscle and/or fascia, if performed); first 20 sq cm or less with manual preparation and insertion of drug-delivery device(s), deep (e.g., subfascial)

C7903 Group psychotherapy service for diagnosis, evaluation, or treatment of a mental health or substance use disorder provided remotely by hospital staff who are licensed to provide mental health services under applicable state law(s), when the patient is in their home, and there is no associated professional service

C9159 Injection, prothrombin complex concentrate (human), Balfaxar, per IU of Factor IX activity

C9160 Injection, daxibotulinumtoxina-lanm, 1 unit

C9161 Injection, aflibercept HD, 1 mg

C9162 Injection, avacincaptad pegol, 0.1 mg

C9163 Injection, talquetamab-tgvs, 0.25 mg

C9164 Cantharidin for topical administration, 0.7%, single unit dose applicator (3.2 mg)

C9165 Injection, elranatamab-bcmm, 1 mg

C9793 3D predictive model generation for preplanning of a cardiac procedure, using data from cardiac computed tomographic angiography with report

C9794 Therapeutic radiology simulation-aided field setting; complex, including acquisition of PET and CT imaging data required for radiopharmaceutical-directed radiation therapy treatment planning (i.e., modeling)

C9795 Stereotactic body radiation therapy, treatment delivery, per fraction to 1 or more lesions, including image guidance and real-time positron emissions-based delivery adjustments to 1 or more lesions, entire course not to exceed 5 fractions

E0492 Power source and control electronics unit for oral device/appliance for neuromuscular electrical stimulation of the tongue muscle, controlled by phone application

E0493 Oral device/appliance for neuromuscular electrical stimulation of the tongue muscle, used in conjunction with the power source and control electronics unit, controlled by phone application, 90-day supply

E0530 Electronic positional obstructive sleep apnea treatment, with sensor, includes all components and accessories, any type

E0678 Nonpneumatic sequential compression garment, full leg

E0679 Nonpneumatic sequential compression garment, half leg

E0680 Nonpneumatic compression controller with sequential calibrated gradient pressure

E0681 Nonpneumatic compression controller without calibrated gradient pressure

E0682 Nonpneumatic sequential compression garment, full arm

E0732 Cranial electrotherapy stimulation (CES) system, any type

E0733 Transcutaneous electrical nerve stimulator for electrical stimulation of the trigeminal nerve

E0734 External upper limb tremor stimulator of the peripheral nerves of the wrist

E0735 Noninvasive vagus nerve stimulator

E1301 Whirlpool tub, walk-in, portable

E2001 Suction pump, home model, portable or stationary, electric, any type, for use with external urine management system

E3000 Speech volume modulation system, any type, including all components and accessories

G0011 Individual counseling for pre-exposure prophylaxis (PrEP) by physician or qualified health care professional (QHP) to prevent human immunodeficiency virus (HIV), includes HIV risk assessment (initial or continued assessment of risk HIV risk reduction and medication adherence, 15 to 30 minutes

G0012 Injection of pre-exposure prophylaxis (PrEP) drug for HIV prevention, under skin or into muscle

G0013 Individual counseling for pre-exposure prophylaxis (PrEP) by clinical staff to prevent human immunodeficiency virus (HIV), includes: HIV risk assessment (initial or continued assessment of risk), HIV risk reduction and medication adherence

G0017 Psychotherapy for crisis furnished in an applicable site of service (any place of service at which the nonfacility rate for psychotherapy for crisis services applies, other than the office setting); first 60 minutes

G0018 Psychotherapy for crisis furnished in an applicable site of service (any place of service at which the nonfacility rate for psychotherapy for crisis services applies, other than the office setting); each additional 30 minutes (list separately in addition to code for primary service)

G0019 Community health integration services performed by certified or trained auxiliary personnel, including a community health worker, under the direction of a physician or other practitioner, 60 minutes per calendar month, in the following activities to address social determinants of health (SDOH) need(s) that are significantly limiting the ability to diagnose or treat problem(s) addressed in an initiating visit:

G0022 Community health integration services, each additional 30 minutes per calendar month (list separately in addition to G0019)

G0023 Principal illness navigation services by certified or trained auxiliary personnel under the direction of a physician or other practitioner, including a patient navigator, 60 minutes per calendar month, in the following activities:

G0024 Principal illness navigation services, additional 30 minutes per calendar month (list separately in addition to G0023)

G0136 Administration of a standardized, evidence-based social determinants of health risk assessment tool, 5 to 15 minutes

G0137 Intensive outpatient services, weekly bundle, minimum of 9 services over a 7 contiguous day period, which can include:

G0140 Principal illness navigation-peer support by certified or trained auxiliary personnel under the direction of a physician or other practitioner, including a certified peer specialist, 60 minutes per calendar month, in the following activities:

G0146 Principal illness navigation-peer support, additional 30 minutes per calendar month (list separately in addition to G0140)

J0184 Injection, amisulpride, 1 mg

J0217 Injection, velmanase alfa-tycv, 1 mg

J0391 Injection, artesunate, 1 mg

J0402 Injection, aripiprazole (Abilify Asimtufii), 1 mg

J0576 Injection, buprenorphine extended-release (Brixadi), 1 mg

J0688 Injection, cefazolin sodium (Hikma), not therapeutically equivalent to J0690, 500 mg

J0750 Emtricitabine 200 mg and tenofovir disoproxil fumarate 300 mg, oral, FDA-approved prescription, only for use as HIV pre-exposure prophylaxis (not for use as treatment of HIV)

J0751 Emtricitabine 200 mg and tenofovir alafenamide 25 mg, oral, FDA-approved prescription, only for use as HIV pre-exposure prophylaxis (not for use as treatment of HIV)

J0799 FDA-approved prescription drug, only for use as HIV pre-exposure prophylaxis (not for use as treatment of HIV), not otherwise classified

J0873 Injection, daptomycin (Xellia), not therapeutically equivalent to J0878, 1 mg

J1105 Dexmedetomidine, oral, 1 mcg

NEW CODES (continued)

Code	Description
J1246	Injection, dinutuximab, 0.1 mg
J1304	Injection, tofersen, 1 mg
J1412	Injection, valoctocogene roxaparvovec-rvox, per ml, containing nominal 2×10^{13} vector genomes
J1413	Injection, delandistrogene moxeparvovec-rokl, per therapeutic dose
J1596	Injection, glycopyrrolate, 0.1 mg
J1939	Injection, bumetanide, 0.5 mg
J2404	Injection, nicardipine, 0.1 mg
J2508	Injection, pegunigalsidase alfa-iwxj, 1 mg
J2679	Injection, fluphenazine HCl, 1.25 mg
J2799	Injection, risperidone (Uzedy), 1 mg
J3401	Beremagene geperpavec-svdt for topical administration, containing nominal 5×10^{9} PFU/ml vector genomes, per 0.1 ml
J3425	Injection, hydroxocobalamin, 10 mcg
J9052	Injection, carmustine (Accord), not therapeutically equivalent to J9050, 100 mg
J9072	Injection, cyclophosphamide, (Dr. Reddy's), 5 mg
J9172	Injection, docetaxel (Ingenus), not therapeutically equivalent to J9171, 1 mg
J9255	Injection, methotrexate (Accord), not therapeutically equivalent to J9250 and J9260, 50 mg
J9258	Injection, paclitaxel protein-bound particles (Teva), not therapeutically equivalent to J9264, 1 mg
J9286	Injection, glofitamab-gxbm, 2.5 mg
J9321	Injection, epcoritamab-bysp, 0.16 mg
J9324	Injection, pemetrexed (Pemrydi RTU), 10 mg
J9333	Injection, rozanolixizumab-noli, 1 mg
J9334	Injection, efgartigimod alfa, 2 mg and hyaluronidase-qvfc
L3161	Foot, adductus positioning device, adjustable
L5615	Addition, endoskeletal knee-shin system, 4 bar linkage or multiaxial, fluid swing and stance phase control
L5926	Addition to lower extremity prosthesis, endoskeletal, knee disarticulation, above knee, hip disarticulation, positional rotation unit, any type
M1211	Most recent hemoglobin A1c level > 9.0%
M1212	Hemoglobin A1c level is missing, or was not performed during the measurement period (12 months)
M1213	No history of spirometry results with confirmed airflow obstruction (FEV1/FVC < 70%) and present spirometry is >= 70%
M1214	Spirometry results with confirmed airflow obstruction (FEV1/FVC < 70%) documented and reviewed
M1215	Documentation of medical reason(s) for not documenting and reviewing spirometry results (e.g., patients with dementia or tracheostomy)
M1216	No spirometry results with confirmed airflow obstruction FEV1/FVC < 70%) documented and/or no spirometry performed with results documented during the encounter
M1217	Documentation of system reason(s) for not documenting and reviewing spirometry results (e.g., spirometry equipment not available at the time of the encounter)
M1218	Patient has COPD symptoms (e.g., dyspnea, cough/sputum, wheezing)
M1219	Anaphylaxis due to the vaccine on or before the date of the encounter
M1220	Dilated retinal eye exam with interpretation by an ophthalmologist or optometrist or artificial intelligence (AI) interpretation documented and reviewed; with evidence of retinopathy
M1221	Dilated retinal eye exam with interpretation by an ophthalmologist or optometrist or artificial intelligence (AI) interpretation documented and reviewed; without evidence of retinopathy
M1222	Glaucoma plan of care not documented, reason not otherwise specified
M1223	Glaucoma plan of care documented
M1224	Intraocular pressure (IOP) reduced by a value less than 20% from the pre-intervention level
M1225	Intraocular pressure (IOP) reduced by a value of greater than or equal to 20% from the pre-intervention level
M1226	IOP measurement not documented, reason not otherwise specified
M1227	Evidence-based therapy was prescribed
M1228	Patient, who has a reactive HCV antibody test, and has a follow up HCV viral test that detected HCV viremia, has HCV treatment initiated within 3 months of the reactive HCV antibody test
M1229	Patient, who has a reactive HCV antibody test, and has a follow up HCV viral test that detected HCV viremia, is referred within 1 month of the reactive HCV antibody test to a clinician who treats HCV infection
M1230	Patient has a reactive HCV antibody test and does not have a follow-up HCV viral test, or patient has a reactive HCV antibody test and has a follow-up HCV viral test that detects HCV viremia and is not referred to a clinician who treats HCV infection within 1 month and does not have HCV treatment initiated within 3 months of the reactive HCV antibody test, reason not given
M1231	Patient receives HCV antibody test with nonreactive result
M1232	Patient receives HCV antibody test with reactive result
M1233	Patient does not receive HCV antibody test or patient does receive HCV antibody test but results not documented, reason not given
M1234	Patient has a reactive HCV antibody test, and has a follow-up HCV viral test that does not detect HCV viremia
M1235	Documentation or patient report of HCV antibody test or HCV RNA test which occurred prior to the performance period
M1236	Baseline MRS > 2
M1237	Patient reason for not screening for food insecurity, housing instability, transportation needs, utility difficulties, and interpersonal safety (e.g., patient declined or other patient reasons)
M1238	Documentation that administration of second recombinant zoster vaccine could not occur during the performance period due to the recommended 2 to 6 month interval between doses (i.e, first dose received after October 31)
M1239	Patient did not respond to the question of "Patient felt heard and understood by this provider and team"
M1240	Patient did not respond to the question of "Patient felt this provider and team put my best interests first when making recommendations about my care"
M1241	Patient did not respond to the question of "Patient felt this provider and team saw me as a person, not just someone with a medical problem"
M1242	Patient did not respond to the question of "Patient felt this provider and team understood what is important to me in my life"
M1243	Patient provided a response other than "completely true" for the question of "Patient felt heard and understood by this provider and team"
M1244	Patient provided a response other than "completely true" for the question of "Patient felt this provider and team put my best interests first when making recommendations about my care"
M1245	Patient provided a response other than "completely true" for the question of "Patient felt this provider and team saw me as a person, not just someone with a medical problem"
M1246	Patient provided a response other than "completely true" for the question of "Patient felt this provider and team understood what is important to me in my life"
M1247	Patient responded "completely true" for the question of "Patient felt this provider and team put my best interests first when making recommendations about my care"
M1248	Patient responded "completely true" for the question of "Patient felt this provider and team saw me as a person, not just someone with a medical problem"
M1249	Patient responded "completely true" for the question of "Patient felt this provider and team understood what is important to me in my life"
M1250	Patient responded as "completely true" for the question of "Patient felt heard and understood by this provider and team"
M1251	Patients for whom a proxy completed the entire HU survey on their behalf for any reason (no patient involvement)
M1252	Patients who did not complete at least one of the four patient experience HU survey items and return the HU survey within 60 days of the ambulatory palliative care visit
M1253	Patients who respond on the patient experience HU survey that they did not receive care by the listed ambulatory palliative care provider in the last 60 days (disavowal)
M1254	Patients who were deceased when the HU survey reached them
M1255	Patients who have another reason for visiting the clinic [not prenatal or postpartum care] and have a positive pregnancy test but have not established the clinic as an OB provider (e.g., plan to terminate the pregnancy or seek prenatal services elsewhere)

NEW CODES (continued)

M1256 Prior history of known CVD

M1257 CVD risk assessment not performed or incomplete (e.g., CVD risk assessment was not documented), reason not otherwise specified

M1258 CVD risk assessment performed, have a documented calculated risk score

M1259 Patients listed on the kidney-pancreas transplant waitlist or who received a living donor transplant within the first year following initiation of dialysis

M1260 Patients who were not listed on the kidney-pancreas transplant waitlist or patients who did not receive a living donor transplant within the first year following initiation of dialysis

M1261 Patients who were on the kidney or kidney-pancreas waitlist prior to initiation of dialysis

M1262 Patients who had a transplant prior to initiation of dialysis

M1263 Patients in hospice on their initiation of dialysis date or during the month of evaluation

M1264 Patients age 75 or older on their initiation of dialysis date

M1265 CMS Medical Evidence Form 2728 for dialysis patients: initial form completed

M1266 Patients admitted to a skilled nursing facility (SNF)

M1267 Patients not on any kidney or kidney-pancreas transplant waitlist or is not in active status on any kidney or kidney-pancreas transplant waitlist as of the last day of each month during the measurement period

M1268 Patients on active status on any kidney or kidney-pancreas transplant waitlist as of the last day of each month during the measurement period

M1269 Receiving ESRD MCP dialysis services by the provider on the last day of the reporting month

M1270 Patients not on any kidney or kidney-pancreas transplant waitlist as of the last day of each month during the measurement period

M1271 Patients with dementia at any time prior to or during the month

M1272 Patients on any kidney or kidney-pancreas transplant waitlist as of the last day of each month during the measurement period

M1273 Patients who were admitted to a skilled nursing facility (SNF) within 1 year of dialysis initiation according to the CMS-2728 Form

M1274 Patients who were admitted to a skilled nursing facility (SNF) during the month of evaluation were excluded from that month

M1275 Patients determined to be in hospice were excluded from month of evaluation and the remainder of reporting period

M1276 BMI documented outside normal parameters, no follow-up plan documented, no reason given

M1277 Colorectal cancer screening results documented and reviewed

M1278 Elevated or hypertensive blood pressure reading documented, and the indicated follow-up is documented

M1279 Elevated or hypertensive blood pressure reading documented, indicated follow-up not documented, reason not given

M1280 Women who had a bilateral mastectomy or who have a history of a bilateral mastectomy or for whom there is evidence of a right and a left unilateral mastectomy

M1281 Blood pressure reading not documented, reason not given

M1282 Patient screened for tobacco use and identified as a tobacco non-user

M1283 Patient screened for tobacco use and identified as a tobacco user

M1284 Patients age 66 or older in institutional special needs plans (SNP) or residing in long-term care with POS code 32, 33, 34, 54, or 56 for more than 90 consecutive days during the measurement period

M1285 Screening, diagnostic, film, digital or digital breast tomosynthesis (3D) mammography results were not documented and reviewed, reason not otherwise specified

M1286 BMI is documented as being outside of normal parameters, follow-up plan is not completed for documented medical reason

M1287 BMI is documented below normal parameters and a follow-up plan is documented

M1288 Documented reason for not screening or recommending a follow-up for high blood pressure

M1289 Patient identified as tobacco user did not receive tobacco cessation intervention during the measurement period or in the 6 months prior to the measurement period (counseling and/or pharmacotherapy)

M1290 Patient not eligible due to active diagnosis of hypertension

M1291 Patients 66 years of age and older with at least one claim/encounter for frailty during the measurement period and a dispensed medication for dementia during the measurement period or the year prior to the measurement period

M1292 Patients 66 years of age and older with at least one claim/encounter for frailty during the measurement period and either one acute inpatient encounter with a diagnosis of advanced illness or two outpatient, observation, ED or nonacute inpatient encounters on different dates of service with an advanced illness diagnosis during the measurement period or the year prior to the measurement period

M1293 BMI is documented above normal parameters and a follow-up plan is documented

M1294 Normal blood pressure reading documented, follow-up not required

M1295 Patients with a diagnosis or past history of total colectomy or colorectal cancer

M1296 BMI is documented within normal parameters and no follow-up plan is required

M1297 BMI not documented due to medical reason or patient refusal of height or weight measurement

M1298 Documentation of patient pregnancy anytime during the measurement period prior to and including the current encounter

M1299 Influenza immunization administered or previously received

M1300 Influenza immunization was not administered for reasons documented by clinician (e.g., patient allergy or other medical reasons, patient declined or other patient reasons, vaccine not available or other system reasons)

M1301 Patient identified as a tobacco user received tobacco cessation intervention during the measurement period or in the 6 months prior to the measurement period (counseling and/or pharmacotherapy)

M1302 Screening, diagnostic, film digital or digital breast tomosynthesis (3D) mammography results documented and reviewed

M1303 Hospice services provided to patient any time during the measurement period

M1304 Patient did not receive any pneumococcal conjugate or polysaccharide vaccine on or after their 19th birthday and before the end of the measurement period

M1305 Patient received any pneumococcal conjugate or polysaccharide vaccine on or after their 19th birthday and before the end of the measurement period

M1306 Patient had anaphylaxis due to the pneumococcal vaccine any time during or before the measurement period

M1307 Documentation stating the patient has received or is currently receiving palliative or hospice care

M1308 Influenza immunization was not administered, reason not given

M1309 Palliative care services provided to patient any time during the measurement period

M1310 Patient screened for tobacco use and received tobacco cessation intervention during the measurement period or in the 6 months prior to the measurement period (counseling, pharmacotherapy, or both), if identified as a tobacco user

M1311 Anaphylaxis due to the vaccine on or before the date of the encounter

M1312 Patient not screened for tobacco use

M1313 Tobacco screening not performed or tobacco cessation intervention not provided during the measurement period or in the 6 months prior to the measurement period

M1314 BMI not documented and no reason is given

M1315 Colorectal cancer screening results were not documented and reviewed; reason not otherwise specified

M1316 Current tobacco non-user

M1317 Patients who are counseled on connection with a CSP and explicitly opt out

M1318 Patients who did not have documented contact with a CSP for at least one of their screened positive HRSNS within 60 days after screening or documentation that there was no contact with a CSP

M1319 Patients who had documented contact with a CSP for at least one of their screened positive HRSNS within 60 days after screening

M1320 Patients who screened positive for at least 1 of the 5 HRSNS

M1321 Patients who were not seen within 7 weeks following the date of injection for follow-up or who did not have a documented IOP or no plan of care documented if the IOP was >25 mm Hg

NEW CODES (continued)

M1322   Patients seen within 7 weeks following the date of injection and are screened for elevated intraocular pressure (IOP) with tonometry with documented IOP =<25 mm Hg for injected eye

M1323   Patients seen within 7 weeks following the date of injection and are screened for elevated intraocular pressure (IOP) with tonometry with documented IOP >25 mm Hg and a plan of care was documented

M1324   Patients who had an intravitreal or periocular corticosteroid injection (e.g., triamcinolone, preservative-free triamcinolone, dexamethasone, dexamethasone intravitreal implant, or fluocinolone intravitreal implant)

M1325   Patients who were not seen for reasons documented by clinician for patient or medical reasons (e.g., inadequate time for follow-up, patients who received a prior intravitreal or periocular steroid injection within the last 6 months and had a subsequent IOP evaluation with IOP <25mm Hg within 7 weeks of treatment)

M1326   Patients with a diagnosis of hypotony

M1327   Patients who were not appropriately evaluated during the initial exam and/or who were not re-evaluated within 8 weeks

M1328   Patients with a diagnosis of acute vitreous hemorrhage

M1329   Patients with a post-operative encounter of the eye with the acute PVD within 2 weeks before the initial encounter or 8 weeks after initial acute PVD encounter

M1330   Documentation of patient reason(s) for not having a follow-up exam (e.g., inadequate time for follow-up)

M1331   Patients who were appropriately evaluated during the initial exam and were re-evaluated no later than 8 weeks from initial exam

M1332   Patients who were not appropriately evaluated during the initial exam and/or who were not re-evaluated within 2 weeks

M1333   Acute vitreous hemorrhage

M1334   Patients with a post-operative encounter of the eye with the acute PVD within 2 weeks before the initial encounter or 2 weeks after initial acute PVD encounter

M1335   Documentation of patient reason(s) for not having a follow-up exam (e.g., inadequate time for follow-up)

M1336   Patients who were appropriately evaluated during the initial exam and were re-evaluated no later than 2 weeks

M1337   Acute PVD

M1338   Patients who had follow-up assessment 30 to 180 days after the index assessment who did not demonstrate positive improvement or maintenance of functioning scores during the performance period

M1339   Patients who had follow-up assessment 30 to 180 days after the index assessment who demonstrated positive improvement or maintenance of functioning scores during the performance period

M1340   Index assessment completed using the 12-item WHODAS 2.0 or SDS during the denominator identification period

M1341   Patients who did not have a follow-up assessment or did not have an assessment within 30 to 180 days after the index assessment during the performance period

M1342   Patients who died during the performance period

M1343   Patients who are at PAM level 4 at baseline or patients who are flagged with extreme straight line response sets on the PAM

M1344   Patients who did not have a baseline PAM score and/or a second score within 6 to 12 month of baseline PAM score

M1345   Patients who had a baseline PAM score and a second score within 6 to 12 month of baseline PAM score

M1346   Patients who did not have a net increase in PAM score of at least 6 points within a 6 to 12 month period

M1347   Patients who achieved a net increase in PAM score of at least 3 points in a 6 to 12 month period (passing)

M1348   Patients who achieved a net increase in PAM score of at least 6 points in a 6 to 12 month period (excellent)

M1349   Patients who did not have a net increase in PAM score of at least 3 points within 6 to 12 month period

M1350   Patients who had a completed suicide safety plan initiated, reviewed, or updated in collaboration with their clinician (concurrent or within 24 hours of the index clinical encounter)

M1351   Patients who had a suicide safety plan initiated, reviewed, or updated and reviewed and updated in collaboration with the patient and their clinician (concurrent or within 24 hours of clinical encounter and within 120 days after initiation)

M1352   Suicidal ideation and/or behavior symptoms based on the C-SSRS or equivalent assessment

M1353   Patients who did not have a completed suicide safety plan initiated, reviewed, or updated in collaboration with their clinician (concurrent or within 24 hours of the index clinical encounter)

M1354   Patients who did not have a suicide safety plan initiated, reviewed, or updated or reviewed and updated in collaboration with the patient and their clinician (concurrent or within 24 hours of clinical encounter and within 120 days after initiation)

M1355   Suicide risk based on their clinician's evaluation or a clinician-rated tool

M1356   Patients who died during the measurement period

M1357   Patients who had a reduction in suicidal ideation and/or behavior upon follow-up assessment within 120 days of index assessment

M1358   Patients who did not have a reduction in suicidal ideation and/or behavior upon follow-up assessment within 120 days of index assessment

M1359   Index assessment during the denominator period when the suicidal ideation and/or behavior symptoms or increased suicide risk by clinician determination occurs and a non-zero C-SSRS score is obtained

M1360   Suicidal ideation and/or behavior symptoms based on the C-SSRS

M1361   Suicide risk based on their clinician's evaluation or a clinician-rated tool

M1362   Patients who died during the measurement period

M1363   Patients who did not have a follow-up assessment within 120 days of the index assessment

M1364   Calculated 10-year ASCVD risk score of >=20 percent during the performance period

M1365   Patient encounter during the performance period with hospice and palliative care specialty code 17

M1366   Focusing on women's health MIPS value pathway

M1367   Quality care for the treatment of ear, nose, and throat disorders MIPS value pathway

M1368   Prevention and treatment of infectious disorders including hepatitis C and HIV MIPS value pathway

M1369   Quality care in mental health and substance use disorders MIPS value pathway

M1370   Rehabilitative support for musculoskeletal care MIPS value pathway

Q0516   Pharmacy supplying fee for HIV pre-exposure prophylaxis FDA-approved prescription drug, per 30-days

Q0517   Pharmacy supplying fee for HIV pre-exposure prophylaxis FDA-approved prescription drug, per 60-days

Q0518   Pharmacy supplying fee for HIV pre-exposure prophylaxis FDA-approved prescription drug, per 90-days

Q4279   Vendaje AC, per sq cm

Q4287   DermaBind DL, per sq cm

Q4288   DermaBind CH, per sq cm

Q4289   RevoShield+ Amniotic Barrier, per sq cm

Q4290   Membrane Wrap-Hydro™, per sq cm

Q4291   Lamellas XT, per sq cm

Q4292   Lamellas, per sq cm

Q4293   Acesso DL, per sq cm

Q4294   Amnio Quad-Core, per sq cm

Q4295   Amnio Tri-Core Amniotic, per sq cm

Q4296   Rebound Matrix, per sq cm

Q4297   Emerge Matrix, per sq cm

Q4298   AmniCore Pro, per sq cm

Q4299   AmniCore Pro+, per sq cm

Q4300   Acesso TL, per sq cm

Q4301   Activate Matrix, per sq cm

Q4302   Complete ACA, per sq cm

Q4303   Complete AA, per sq cm

Q4304   GRAFIX PLUS, per sq cm

Q5132   Injection, adalimumab-afzb (Abrilada), biosimilar, 10 mg

REVISED CODES

A6531 Gradient compression stocking, below knee, 30-40 mm Hg, used as a surgical dressing, each

A6532 Gradient compression stocking, below knee, 40-50 mm Hg, used as a surgical dressing, each

A6535 Gradient compression stocking, thigh length, 40 mm Hg or greater, each

A6538 Gradient compression stocking, full length/chap style, 40 mm Hg or greater, each

A6541 Gradient compression stocking, waist length, 40 mm Hg or greater, each

A6545 Gradient compression wrap, nonelastic, below knee, 30-50 mm Hg, used as a surgical dressing, each

A6549 Gradient compression garment, not otherwise specified

G0129 Occupational therapy services requiring the skills of a qualified occupational therapist, furnished as a component of a partial hospitalization or intensive outpatient treatment program, per session (45 minutes or more)

G0410 Group psychotherapy other than of a multiple-family group, in a partial hospitalization or intensive outpatient setting, approximately 45 to 50 minutes

G0411 Interactive group psychotherapy, in a partial hospitalization or intensive outpatient setting, approximately 45 to 50 minutes

G2137 Back pain measured by the visual analog scale (VAS) or numeric pain scale at 3 months (6 to 20 weeks) postoperatively was greater than 3.0 and back pain measured by the visual analog scale (VAS) or numeric pain scale within 3 months preoperatively and at 3 months (6 to 20 weeks) postoperatively demonstrated improvement of less than 5.0 points

G2139 Back pain measured by the visual analog scale (VAS) or numeric pain scale at 1 year (9 to 15 months) postoperatively was greater than 3.0 and back pain measured by the visual analog scale (VAS) or numeric pain scale within 3 months preoperatively and at 1 year (9 to 15 months) postoperatively demonstrated improvement of less than 5.0 points

G2141 Leg pain measured by the visual analog scale (VAS) or numeric pain scale at 3 months (6 to 20 weeks) postoperatively was greater than 3.0 and leg pain measured by the visual analog scale (VAS) or numeric pain scale within 3 months preoperatively and at 3 months (6 to 20 weeks) postoperatively demonstrated improvement of less than 5.0 points

G2147 Leg pain measured by the visual analog scale (VAS) or numeric pain scale at 1 year (9 to 15 months) postoperatively was greater than 3.0 and leg pain measured by the visual analog scale (VAS) or numeric pain scale within 3 months preoperatively and at 1 year (9 to 15 months) postoperatively demonstrated improvement of less than 5.0 points

G2174 URI episodes where the patient is taking antibiotics (Table 1) in the 30 days prior to the episode date

G8474 Angiotensin converting enzyme (ACE) inhibitor or angiotensin receptor blocker (ARB) therapy not prescribed for reasons documented by the clinician (e.g., allergy, intolerance, pregnancy, renal failure due to ACE inhibitor, diseases of the aortic or mitral valve, other medical reasons) or (e.g., patient declined, other patient reasons)

G8535 Elder maltreatment screen not documented; documentation that patient is not eligible for the elder maltreatment screen at the time of the encounter related to one of the following reasons: (1) patient refuses to participate in the screening and has reasonable decisional capacity for self-protection, or (2) patient is in an urgent or emergent situation where time is of the essence and to delay treatment to perform the screening would jeopardize the patient's health status

G8601 IV thrombolytic therapy not initiated within 4.5 hours (<= 270 minutes) of time last known well for reasons documented by clinician (e.g., patient enrolled in clinical trial for stroke, patient admitted for elective carotid intervention)

G8807 Transabdominal or transvaginal ultrasound not performed for reasons documented by clinician (e.g., patient has a documented intrauterine pregnancy [IUP])

G8851 Adherence to therapy was assessed at least annually through an objective informatics system or through self-reporting (if objective reporting is not available, documented)

G8854 Documentation of reason(s) for not objectively reporting adherence to evidence-based therapy (e.g., patients who have been diagnosed with a terminal or advanced disease with an expected life span of less than 6 months, patients who decline therapy, patients who do not return for follow-up at least annually, patients unable to access/afford therapy, patient's insurance will not cover therapy)

G8855 Adherence to therapy was not assessed at least annually through an objective informatics system or through self-reporting (if objective reporting is not available), reason not given

G8924 Spirometry results documented (FEV1/FVC < 70%)

G8936 Clinician documented that patient was not an eligible candidate for angiotensin converting enzyme (ACE) inhibitor or angiotensin receptor blocker (ARB) therapy (e.g., allergy, intolerance, pregnancy, renal failure due to ACE inhibitor, diseases of the aortic or mitral valve, other medical reasons) or (e.g., patient declined, other patient reasons)

G8942 Functional outcome assessment using a standardized tool is documented within the previous 30 days and a care plan, based on identified deficiencies is documented within 2 days of the functional outcome assessment

G8968 Documentation of medical reason(s) for not prescribing an FDA-approved anticoagulant (e.g., present or planned atrial appendage occlusion or ligation or patient being currently enrolled in a clinical trial related to AF/atrial flutter treatment)

G9380 Patient offered assistance with end of life issues or existing end of life plan was reviewed or updated during the measurement period

G9382 Patient not offered assistance with end of life issues or existing end of life plan was not reviewed or updated during the measurement period

G9452 Documentation of medical reason(s) for not receiving HCV antibody test due to limited life expectancy

G9696 Documentation of medical reason(s) for not prescribing a long-acting inhaled bronchodilator (e.g., patient intolerance or history of side effects)

G9698 Documentation of system reason(s) for not prescribing a long-acting inhaled bronchodilator (e.g., cost of treatment or lack of insurance)

G9703 Episodes where the patient is taking antibiotics (Table 1) in the 30 days prior to the episode date

G9717 Documentation stating the patient has had a diagnosis of bipolar disorder

G9771 At least one body temperature measurement equal to or greater than 35.5 degrees Celsius (or 95.9 degrees Fahrenheit) achieved within the 30 minutes immediately before or 15 minutes immediately after anesthesia end time

G9772 Documentation of medical reason(s) for not achieving at least one body temperature measurement equal to or greater than 35.5 degrees Celsius (or 95.9 degrees Fahrenheit) within the 30 minutes immediately before or 15 minutes immediately after anesthesia end time (e.g., emergency cases, intentional hypothermia, etc.)

G9773 At least one body temperature measurement equal to or greater than 35.5 degrees Celsius (or 95.9 degrees Fahrenheit) not achieved within the 30 minutes immediately before or 15 minutes immediately after anesthesia end time, reason not given

G9779 Patients who are breastfeeding at any time during the performance period

G9780 Patients who have a diagnosis of rhabdomyolysis at any time during the performance period

G9914 Patient initiated an anti-TNF agent

G9938 Patients aged 66 or older in institutional special needs plans (SNP) or residing in long-term care with POS code 32, 33, 34, 54, or 56 for more than 90 consecutive days during the 6 months prior to the measurement period through December 31 of the measurement period

G9990 Patient did not receive any pneumococcal conjugate or polysaccharide vaccine on or after their 19th birthday and before the end of the measurement period

G9991 Patient received any pneumococcal conjugate or polysaccharide vaccine on or after their 19th birthday and before the end of the measurement period

G9998 Documentation of medical reason(s) for an interval of less than 3 years since the last colonoscopy (e.g., last colonoscopy incomplete, last colonoscopy had inadequate prep, piecemeal removal of adenomas, or sessile serrated polyps >= 20 mm in size, last colonoscopy found greater than 10 adenomas, lower gastrointestinal bleeding, or patient at high risk for colon cancer due to underlying medical history [i.e., Crohn's disease, ulcerative colitis, personal or family history of colon cancer, hereditary colorectal cancer syndromes])

J0739 Injection, cabotegravir, 1 mg, FDA-approved prescription, only for use as HIV pre-exposure prophylaxis (not for use as treatment for HIV)

M0005 Value in primary care MIPS value pathway

REVISED CODES (continued)

M0201   Administration of pneumococcal, influenza, hepatitis B, and/or COVID-19 vaccine inside a patient's home; reported only once per individual home per date of service when such vaccine administration(s) are performed at the patient's home

M1174   Patient received at least two doses of the herpes zoster recombinant vaccine (at least 28 days apart) anytime on or after the patient's 50th birthday before or during the measurement period

M1176   Patient did not receive at least two doses of the herpes zoster recombinant vaccine (at least 28 days apart) anytime on or after the patient's 50th birthday before or during the measurement period

M1197   Itch severity assessment score is reduced by three or more points from the initial (index) assessment score to the follow-up visit score

M1198   Itch severity assessment score was not reduced by at least three points from initial (index) score to the follow-up visit score or assessment was not completed during the follow-up encounter

M1205   Itch severity assessment score is reduced by three or more points from the initial (index) assessment score to the follow-up visit score

M1206   Itch severity assessment score was not reduced by at least three points from initial (index) score to the follow-up visit score or assessment was not completed during the follow-up encounter

M1207   Patient is screened for food insecurity, housing instability, transportation needs, utility difficulties, and interpersonal safety

M1208   Patient is not screened for food insecurity, housing instability, transportation needs, utility difficulties, and interpersonal safety

Q4225   AmnioBind or DermaBind TL, per sq cm

T1026   Intensive, extended multidisciplinary services provided in a clinic setting to children with complex medical, physical, mental, and psychosocial impairments, per hour

DELETED CODES

C9152	C9153	C9154	C9155	C9156	C9157	C9158
C9770	C9771	C9788	C9803	G0056	G2066	G2108
G2109	G2110	G8506	G8818	G8825	G8852	G8883
G8884	G8885	G8941	G8963	G8964	G9192	G9229
G9451	G9453	G9454	G9596	G9612	G9613	G9614
G9697	G9715	G9725	G9852	G9853	G9854	G9927
G9995	J9160	K1001	K1002	K1003	K1005	K1006
K1009	K1013	K1014	K1015	K1016	K1017	K1018
K1019	K1020	K1021	K1022	K1023	K1024	K1025
K1026	K1028	K1029	K1031	K1032	K1033	M1156
M1157	M1158	S0166	S0171			

Appendix 6 — Place of Service and Type of Service

Place-of-Service Codes for Professional Claims

Listed below are place of service codes and descriptions. These codes should be used on professional claims to specify the entity where service(s) were rendered. Check with individual payers (e.g., Medicare, Medicaid, other private insurance) for reimbursement policies regarding these codes. To comment on a code(s) or description(s), please send your request to posinfo@cms.gov.

01	Pharmacy	A facility or location where drugs and other medically related items and services are sold, dispensed, or otherwise provided directly to patients.
02	Telehealth Provided Other than in Patient's Home	The location where health services and health related services are provided or received, through telecommunication technology. Patient is not located in their home when receiving health services or health related services through telecommunication technology.
03	School	A facility whose primary purpose is education.
04	Homeless Shelter	A facility or location whose primary purpose is to provide temporary housing to homeless individuals (e.g., emergency shelters, individual or family shelters).
05	Indian Health Service Free-standing Facility	A facility or location, owned and operated by the Indian Health Service, which provides diagnostic, therapeutic (surgical and non-surgical), and rehabilitation services to American Indians and Alaska Natives who do not require hospitalization.
06	Indian Health Service Provider-based Facility	A facility or location, owned and operated by the Indian Health Service, which provides diagnostic, therapeutic (surgical and non-surgical), and rehabilitation services rendered by, or under the supervision of, physicians to American Indians and Alaska Natives admitted as inpatients or outpatients.
07	Tribal 638 Free-standing Facility	A facility or location owned and operated by a federally recognized American Indian or Alaska Native tribe or tribal organization under a 638 agreement, which provides diagnostic, therapeutic (surgical and non-surgical), and rehabilitation services to tribal members who do not require hospitalization.
08	Tribal 638 Provider-based Facility	A facility or location owned and operated by a federally recognized American Indian or Alaska Native tribe or tribal organization under a 638 agreement, which provides diagnostic, therapeutic (surgical and non-surgical), and rehabilitation services to tribal members admitted as inpatients or outpatients.
09	Prison/Correctional Facility	A prison, jail, reformatory, work farm, detention center, or any other similar facility maintained by either Federal, State or local authorities for the purpose of confinement or rehabilitation of adult or juvenile criminal offenders.
10	Telehealth Provided in Patient's Home	The location where health services and health related services are provided or received, through telecommunication technology. Patient is located in their home (which is a location other than a hospital or other facility where the patient receives care in a private residence) when receiving health services or health related services through telecommunication technology.
11	Office	Location, other than a hospital, skilled nursing facility (SNF), military treatment facility, community health center, State or local public health clinic, or intermediate care facility (ICF), where the health professional routinely provides health examinations, diagnosis, and treatment of illness or injury on an ambulatory basis.
12	Home	Location, other than a hospital or other facility, where the patient receives care in a private residence.
13	Assisted Living Facility	Congregate residential facility with self-contained living units providing assessment of each resident's needs and on-site support 24 hours a day, 7 days a week, with the capacity to deliver or arrange for services including some health care and other services.
14	Group home	A residence, with shared living areas, where clients receive supervision and other services such as social and/or behavioral services, custodial service, and minimal services (e.g., medication administration).
15	Mobile Unit	A facility/unit that moves from place-to-place equipped to provide preventive, screening, diagnostic, and/or treatment services.
16	Temporary Lodging	A short term accommodation such as a hotel, campground, hostel, cruise ship or resort where the patient receives care, and which is not identified by any other POS code.
17	Walk-in Retail Health Clinic	A walk-in health clinic, other than an office, urgent care facility, pharmacy, or independent clinic and not described by any other Place of Service code, that is located within a retail operation and provides, on an ambulatory basis, preventive and primary care services.
18	Place of Employment Worksite	A location, not described by any other POS code, owned or operated by a public or private entity where the patient is employed, and where a health professional provides on-going or episodic occupational medical, therapeutic or rehabilitative services to the individual.
19	Off Campus-Outpatient Hospital	A portion of an off-campus hospital provider based department which provides diagnostic, therapeutic (both surgical and nonsurgical), and rehabilitation services to sick or injured persons who do not require hospitalization or institutionalization.
20	Urgent Care Facility	Location, distinct from a hospital emergency room, an office, or a clinic, whose purpose is to diagnose and treat illness or injury for unscheduled, ambulatory patients seeking immediate medical attention.
21	Inpatient Hospital	A facility, other than psychiatric, which primarily provides diagnostic, therapeutic (both surgical and nonsurgical), and rehabilitation services by, or under, the supervision of physicians to patients admitted for a variety of medical conditions.
22	On Campus-Outpatient Hospital	A portion of a hospital's main campus which provides diagnostic, therapeutic (both surgical and nonsurgical), and rehabilitation services to sick or injured persons who do not require hospitalization or institutionalization.
23	Emergency Room-Hospital	A portion of a hospital where emergency diagnosis and treatment of illness or injury is provided.
24	Ambulatory Surgical Center	A freestanding facility, other than a physician's office, where surgical and diagnostic services are provided on an ambulatory basis.
25	Birthing center	A facility, other than a hospital's maternity facilities or a physician's office, which provides a setting for labor, delivery, and immediate post-partum care as well as immediate care of new born infants.

26	Military Treatment Facility	A medical facility operated by one or more of the Uniformed services. Military Treatment Facility (MTF) also refers to certain former US Public Health Service (USPHS) facilities now designated as Uniformed Service Treatment Facilities (USTF).
27	Outreach Site/Street	A non-permanent location on the street or found environment, not described by any other POS code, where health professionals provide preventive, screening, diagnostic, and/or treatment services to unsheltered homeless individuals.
28-30	Unassigned	N/A
31	Skilled Nursing Facility	A facility which primarily provides inpatient skilled nursing care and related services to patients who require medical, nursing, or rehabilitative services but does not provide the level of care or treatment available in a hospital.
32	Nursing Facility	A facility which primarily provides to residents skilled nursing care and related services for the rehabilitation of injured, disabled, or sick persons, or, on a regular basis, health-related care services above the level of custodial care to individuals other than those with intellectual disabilities.
33	Custodial Care Facility	A facility which provides room, board, and other personal assistance services, generally on a long-term basis, and which does not include a medical component.
34	Hospice	A facility, other than a patient's home, in which palliative and supportive care for terminally ill patients and their families are provided.
35-40	Unassigned	N/A
41	Ambulance-Land	A land vehicle specifically designed, equipped and staffed for lifesaving and transporting the sick or injured.
42	Ambulance-Air or Water	An air or water vehicle specifically designed, equipped and staffed for lifesaving and transporting the sick or injured.
43-48	Unassigned	N/A
49	Independent Clinic	A location, not part of a hospital and not described by any other Place-of-Service code, that is organized and operated to provide preventive, diagnostic, therapeutic, rehabilitative, or palliative services to outpatients only.
50	Federally Qualified Health Center	A facility located in a medically underserved area that provides Medicare beneficiaries preventive primary medical care under the general direction of a physician.
51	Inpatient Psychiatric Facility	A facility that provides inpatient psychiatric services for the diagnosis and treatment of mental illness on a 24-hour basis, by or under the supervision of a physician.
52	Psychiatric Facility-Partial Hospitalization	A facility for the diagnosis and treatment of mental illness that provides a planned therapeutic program for patients who do not require full time hospitalization, but who need broader programs than are possible from outpatient visits to a hospital-based or hospital-affiliated facility.

53	Community Mental Health Center	A facility that provides the following services: outpatient services, including specialized outpatient services for children, the elderly, individuals who are chronically ill, and residents of the CMHC's mental health services area who have been discharged from inpatient treatment at a mental health facility; 24 hour a day emergency care services; day treatment, other partial hospitalization services, or psychosocial rehabilitation services; screening for patients being considered for admission to State mental health facilities to determine the appropriateness of such admission; and consultation and education services.
54	Intermediate Care Facility/Individuals with Intellectual Disabilities	A facility which primarily provides health-related care and services above the level of custodial care to individuals but does not provide the level of care or treatment available in a hospital or SNF.
55	Residential Substance Abuse Treatment Facility	A facility which provides treatment for substance (alcohol and drug) abuse to live-in residents who do not require acute medical care. Services include individual and group therapy and counseling, family counseling, laboratory tests, drugs and supplies, psychological testing, and room and board.
56	Psychiatric Residential Treatment Center	A facility or distinct part of a facility for psychiatric care which provides a total 24-hour therapeutically planned and professionally staffed group living and learning environment.
57	Non-residential Substance Abuse Treatment Facility	A location which provides treatment for substance (alcohol and drug) abuse on an ambulatory basis. Services include individual and group therapy and counseling, family counseling, laboratory tests, drugs and supplies, and psychological testing.
58	Non-residential Opioid Treatment Facility	A location that provides treatment for opioid use disorder on an ambulatory basis. Services include methadone and other forms of Medication Assisted Treatment (MAT).
59	Unassigned	N/A
60	Mass Immunization Center	A location where providers administer pneumococcal pneumonia and influenza virus vaccinations and submit these services as electronic media claims, paper claims, or using the roster billing method. This generally takes place in a mass immunization setting, such as, a public health center, pharmacy, or mall but may include a physician office setting.
61	Comprehensive Inpatient Rehabilitation Facility	A facility that provides comprehensive rehabilitation services under the supervision of a physician to inpatients with physical disabilities. Services include physical therapy, occupational therapy, speech pathology, social or psychological services, and orthotics and prosthetics services.
62	Comprehensive Outpatient Rehabilitation Facility	A facility that provides comprehensive rehabilitation services under the supervision of a physician to outpatients with physical disabilities. Services include physical therapy, occupational therapy, and speech pathology services.
63-64	Unassigned	N/A
65	End-Stage Renal Disease Treatment Facility	A facility other than a hospital, which provides dialysis treatment, maintenance, and/or training to patients or caregivers on an ambulatory or home-care basis.
66-70	Unassigned	N/A
71	Public Health Clinic	A facility maintained by either State or local health departments that provides ambulatory primary medical care under the general direction of a physician.

72	Rural Health Clinic	A certified facility which is located in a rural medically underserved area that provides ambulatory primary medical care under the general direction of a physician.
73-80	Unassigned	N/A
81	Independent Laboratory	A laboratory certified to perform diagnostic and/or clinical tests independent of an institution or a physician's office.
82-98	Unassigned	N/A
99	Other Place of Service	Other place of service not identified above.

Type of Service

Common Working File Type of Service (TOS) Indicators

For submitting a claim to the Common Working File (CWF), use the following table to assign the proper TOS. Some procedures may have more than one applicable TOS. CWF will reject codes with incorrect TOS designations. CWF will produce alerts on codes with incorrect TOS designations.

The only exceptions to this annual update are:

- Surgical services billed for dates of service through December 31, 2007, containing the ASC facility service modifier SG must be reported as TOS F. Effective for services on or after January 1, 2008, the SG modifier is no longer applicable for Medicare services. ASC providers should discontinue applying the SG modifier on ASC facility claims. The indicator F does not appear in the TOS table because its use depends upon claims submitted with POS 24 (ASC facility) from an ASC (specialty 49). This became effective for dates of service January 1, 2008, or after.

- Surgical services billed with an assistant-at-surgery modifier (80-82, AS,) must be reported with TOS 8. The 8 indicator does not appear on the TOS table because its use is dependent upon the use of the appropriate modifier. (See Pub. 100-04 *Medicare Claims Processing Manual,* chapter 12, "Physician/Practitioner Billing," for instructions on when assistant-at-surgery is allowable.)

  TOS H appears in the list of descriptors. However, it does not appear in the table. In CWF, "H" is used only as an indicator for hospice. The contractor should not submit TOS H to CWF at this time.

- For outpatient services, when a transfusion medicine code appears on a claim that also contains a blood product, the service is paid under reasonable charge at 80 percent; coinsurance and deductible apply. When transfusion medicine codes are paid under the clinical laboratory fee schedule they are paid at 100 percent; coinsurance and deductible do not apply.

Note: For injection codes with more than one possible TOS designation, use the following guidelines when assigning the TOS:

When the choice is L or 1:

- Use TOS L when the drug is used related to ESRD; or
- Use TOS 1 when the drug is not related to ESRD and is administered in the office.

When the choice is G or 1:

- Use TOS G when the drug is an immunosuppressive drug; or
- Use TOS 1 when the drug is used for other than immunosuppression.

When the choice is P or 1:

- Use TOS P if the drug is administered through durable medical equipment (DME); or
- Use TOS 1 if the drug is administered in the office.

The place of service or diagnosis may be considered when determining the appropriate TOS. The descriptors for each of the TOS codes listed in the annual HCPCS update are:

0	Whole blood only
1	Medical care
2	Surgery
3	Consultation
4	Diagnostic radiology
5	Diagnostic laboratory
6	Therapeutic radiology
7	Anesthesia
8	Assistant at surgery
9	Other medical items or services
A	Used durable medical equipment (DME)
D	Ambulance
E	Enteral/parenteral nutrients/supplies
F	Ambulatory surgical center (facility usage for surgical services)
G	Immunosuppressive drugs
J	Diabetic shoes
K	Hearing items and services
L	ESRD supplies
M	Monthly capitation payment for dialysis
N	Kidney donor
P	Lump sum purchase of DME, prosthetics, orthotics
Q	Vision items or services
R	Rental of DME
S	Surgical dressings or other medical supplies
T	Outpatient mental health limitation
U	Occupational therapy
V	Pneumococcal/flu vaccine
W	Physical therapy

Appendix 7 — Deleted Code Crosswalk

Code	Cross Reference
C9151	To report, see ~J2781
C9152	To report, see ~J0402
C9153	To report, see ~J0184
C9154	To report, see ~J0576
C9155	To report, see ~J9321
C9156	To report, see ~A9608
C9157	To report, see ~J1304
C9158	To report, see ~J2799
K1001	To report, see ~E0530
K1002	To report, see ~E0732
K1003	To report, see ~E1301
K1005	To report, see ~A4287
K1006	To report, see ~E2001
K1009	To report, see ~E3000
K1013	To report, see ~A4457
K1014	To report, see ~L5615
K1015	To report, see ~L3161
K1016	To report, see ~E0733
K1017	To report, see ~A4541
K1018	To report, see ~E0734
K1019	To report, see ~A4542
K1020	To report, see ~E0735
K1021	To report, see ~A4468
K1022	To report, see ~L5926
K1023	To report, see ~A4540
K1024	To report, see ~E0680-E0681
K1025	To report, see ~E0682
K1026	To report, see ~A7023
K1028	To report, see ~E0492-E0493
K1029	To report, see ~E0492-E0493
K1031	To report, see ~E0680-E0681
K1032	To report, see ~E0678
K1033	To report, see ~E0679

Appendix 8 — Glossary

accession. Process of identifying a specimen and entering a unique specimen identifier into laboratory records.

alveoplasty. Procedure in which the physician alters the contours of the alveolus by removing sharp areas or undercuts of alveolar bone.

angiography. Radiographic imaging of the arteries. Imaging may be performed to study the vasculature of any given organ, body system, or area of circulation such as the brain, heart, chest, kidneys, limbs, gastrointestinal tract, aorta, and pulmonary circulation to visualize the formation and the function of the blood vessels to detect problems such as a blockage or stricture. A catheter is inserted through an accessible blood vessel and the artery is injected with a radiopaque contrast material after which x-rays are taken.

apnea. Absence of breathing or breath.

apnea monitor. Device used to monitor breathing during sleep that sounds an alarm if breathing stops for more than the specified amount of time.

aqueous shunt. Silicone tube inserted into the anterior chamber of the eye and connected to a reservoir plate behind the pars plana to enhance drainage in the eye's anterior chamber and improve aqueous flow.

arthroscopy. Use of an endoscope to examine the interior of a joint (diagnostic) or to perform surgery on joint structures (therapeutic).

auditory osseointegrated implant. Surgically placed titanium bone-anchored implant that delivers sound to the inner ear via direct bone conduction.

ballistocardiogram. Graphic recording of the movements of the body caused by cardiac contractions and blood flow, used to evaluate cardiac function.

BMI. Body mass index. Tool for calculating weight appropriateness in adults. The Centers for Disease Control and Prevention places adult BMIs in the following categories: below 18.5, underweight; 18.5 to 24.9, normal; 25.0 to 29.9 overweight; 30.0 and above, obese. BMI may be a factor in determining medical necessity for bariatric procedures.

brace. Orthotic device that supports, in correct position, any moveable body part, and allows for limited movement. Medicare has a strict definition of a brace that includes only rigid or semirigid devices.

brachytherapy. Form of radiation therapy in which radioactive pellets or seeds are implanted directly into the tissue being treated to deliver their dose of radiation in a more directed fashion. Brachytherapy provides radiation to the prescribed body area while minimizing exposure to normal tissue.

cardiointegram. Experimental, noninvasive analysis of electrical signals of the heart. Cardiointegram converts analog EKG signals to digital and performs a computer analysis that considers the time element.

cardiokymography. Noninvasive test that measures left anterior ventricle segmental wall motion.

cardioverter-defibrillator. Device that uses both low energy cardioversion or defibrillating shocks and antitachycardia pacing to treat ventricular tachycardia or ventricular fibrillation.

cast. 1) Rigid encasement or dressing molded to the body from a substance that hardens upon drying to hold a body part immobile during the healing period; a model or reproduction made from an impression or mold. Generally, the supply of a cast is included in the codes describing the reduction. **2)** In dentistry and some other specialties, model or reproduction made from taking an impression or mold.

catheter. Flexible tube inserted into an area of the body for introducing or withdrawing fluid.

cervical cap. Contraceptive device similar in form and function to the diaphragm but that can be left in place for 48 hours.

chemotherapy. Treatment of disease, especially cancerous conditions, using chemical agents.

CMS. Centers for Medicare and Medicaid Services. Federal agency that administers the public health programs.

CMV. 1) Controlled mechanical ventilation. **2)** Cytomegalovirus.

collagen. Protein based substance of strength and flexibility that is the major component of connective tissue, found in cartilage, bone, tendons, and skin.

colorectal cancer screening test. One of the following procedures performed for the purpose of detecting colorectal cancer: screening barium enema, screening fecal-occult blood test, screening flexible sigmoidoscopy, screening colonography, and screening colonoscopy.

compression sleeve. Fitted wrap that accelerates recovery in patients with vein disease, lymphedema, or diabetes. Compression sleeves increase circulation and decrease swelling and fluid buildup following surgery.

contrast material. Radiopaque substance placed into the body to enable a system or body structure to be visualized, such as nonionic and low osmolar contrast media (LOCM), ionic and high osmolar contrast media (HOCM), barium, and gadolinium.

covered osteoporosis drug. Injectable drug approved for treating post-menopausal osteoporosis provided to an individual that has suffered a bone fracture related to post-menopausal osteoporosis.

dermis. Skin layer found under the epidermis that contains a papillary upper layer and the deep reticular layer of collagen, vascular bed, and nerves.

dermis graft. Skin graft that has been separated from the epidermal tissue and the underlying subcutaneous fat, used primarily as a substitute for fascia grafts in plastic surgery.

dialysis. Artificial filtering of the blood to remove contaminating waste elements and restore normal balance.

disarticulation. Removal of a limb through a joint.

diskectomy. Surgical excision of an intervertebral disk.

DME MAC. Durable medical equipment Medicare administrative contractor. Entity where claims for specific DMEPOS must be submitted for processing and reimbursement.

DME PDAC. Durable Medical Equipment Pricing Data Analysis and Coding. Medicare contractor responsible for maintaining the durable medical equipment classification system (DMECS), including HCPCS coding determinations, and providing durable medical equipment, prosthetics, orthotics, and supplies (DMEPOS) allowables.

drug eluting stent. Specialized device placed inside blood vessels for intraluminal support that is coated with a controlled time-release drug that enters the surrounding tissue and helps prevent or slow the growth of plaque or stenotic tissue.

drug formulary. List of prescription medications preferred for use by a health plan and dispensed through participating pharmacies to covered persons.

drugs and biologicals. Drugs and biologicals included - or approved for inclusion - in the United States Pharmacopoeia, the National Formulary, the United States Homeopathic Pharmacopoeia, in New Drugs or Accepted Dental Remedies, or approved by the pharmacy and drug therapeutics committee of the medical staff of the hospital. Also included are medically accepted and FDA approved drugs used in an anticancer chemotherapeutic regimen. The carrier determines medical acceptance based on supportive clinical evidence.

dual-lead device. Implantable cardiac device (pacemaker or implantable cardioverter-defibrillator [ICD]) in which pacing and sensing components are placed in only two chambers of the heart.

durable medical equipment. Medical equipment that can withstand repeated use, is not disposable, is used to serve a medical purpose, is generally not useful to a person in the absence of a sickness or injury, and is appropriate for use in the home. Examples of durable medical equipment include hospital beds, wheelchairs, and oxygen equipment.

Dx. Diagnosis.

electrocardiogram. Recording of the electrical activity of the heart on a moving strip of paper that detects and records the electrical potential of the heart during contraction.

electroencephalography. Testing involving amplification, recording, and analysis of the electrical activity of the brain.

electromyography. Test that measures muscle response to nerve stimulation determining if muscle weakness is present and if it is related to the muscles themselves or a problem with the nerves that supply the muscles.

enteral. Pertaining to the intestines; enteral is often used in the context of nutrition management: formulas, jejunostomy tubes, nasogastric devices, etc.

epidermis. Outermost, nonvascular layer of skin that contains four to five differentiated layers depending on its body location: stratum corneum, lucidum, granulosum, spinosum, and basale.

EPO. *1)* Epoetin alpha. *2)* Exclusive provider organization. In health care contracting, an organization similar to an HMO, but the member must remain within the provider network to receive benefits. EPOs are regulated under insurance statutes rather than HMO legislation.

ESRD. End stage renal disease. Progression of chronic renal failure to lasting and irreparable kidney damage that requires dialysis or renal transplant for survival.

EVAR. Endovascular aortic repair. Deployment of a prosthetic stent via a catheter into the site of an abdominal aortic aneurysm (AAA). The stent provides a safe conduit for blood flow to relieve pressure on the aneurysm as the blood flows through the stent instead of continuing to bulge the sac formed by the aorta wall dilation.

event recorder. Portable, ambulatory heart monitor worn by the patient that makes electrocardiographic recordings of the length and frequency of aberrant cardiac rhythm to help diagnose heart conditions and to assess pacemaker functioning or programming.

fecal microbiota transplant (FMT). Procedure in which healthy bacteria (microbiota) is extracted from the feces of a screened donor and transferred to the colon of the recipient via colonoscopy or upper endoscopy, most often to treat persistent *C. difficile* infections.

Food and Drug Administration (FDA). Federal agency responsible for protecting public health by substantiating the safety, efficacy, and security of human and veterinary drugs, biological products, medical devices, national food supply, cosmetics, and items that give off radiation.

FOTO. Focus on therapeutic outcomes.

gait. Manner in which a person walks.

gene. Basic unit of heredity that contains nucleic acid. Genes are arranged in different and unique sequences or strings that determine the gene's function. Human genes usually include multiple protein coding regions such as exons separated by introns which are nonprotein coding sections.

genetic test. Test that is able to detect a gene mutation, either inherited or caused by the environment.

gingivoplasty. Repair or reconstruction of the gum tissue, altering the gingival contours by excising areas of gum tissue or making incisions through the gingiva to create a gingival flap.

glaucoma. Rise in intraocular pressure, restricting blood flow and decreasing vision.

habilitative services. Procedures or services provided to assist a patient in learning, keeping, and improving new skills needed to perform daily living activities. Habilitative services assist patients in acquiring a skill for the first time.

halo. Tool for stabilizing the head and spine.

health care provider. Entity that administers diagnostic and therapeutic services.

hemodialysis. Cleansing of wastes and contaminating elements from the blood by virtue of different diffusion rates through a semipermeable membrane, which separates blood from a filtration solution that diffuses other elements out of the blood.

home health services. Services furnished to patients in their homes under the care of physicians. These services include part-time or intermittent skilled nursing care, physical therapy, medical social services, medical supplies, and some rehabilitation equipment. Home health supplies and services must be prescribed by a physician, and the beneficiary must be confined at home in order for Medicare to pay the benefits in full.

hospice. Organization that furnishes inpatient, outpatient, and home health care for the terminally ill. Hospices emphasize support and counseling services for terminally ill people and their families, pain relief, and symptom management. When the Medicare beneficiary chooses hospice benefits, all other Medicare benefits are discontinued, except physician services and treatment of conditions not related to the terminal illness.

hypertrophic. Enlarged or overgrown from an increase in cell size of the affected tissue.

implant. Material or device inserted or placed within the body for therapeutic, reconstructive, or diagnostic purposes.

implantable cardioverter-defibrillator. Implantable electronic cardiac device used to control rhythm abnormalities such as tachycardia, fibrillation, or bradycardia by producing high- or low-energy stimulation and pacemaker functions. It may also have the capability to provide the functions of an implantable loop recorder or implantable cardiovascular monitor.

in situ. Located in the natural position or contained within the origin site, not spread into neighboring tissue.

incontinence. Inability to control urination or defecation.

infusion. Introduction of a therapeutic fluid, other than blood, into the bloodstream.

infusion pump. Device that delivers a measured amount of drug or intravenous solution through injection over a period of time.

intra-arterial. Within an artery or arteries.

intramuscular. Within a muscle.

intraocular lens. Artificial lens implanted into the eye to replace a damaged natural lens or cataract.

intravenous. Within a vein or veins.

introducer. Instrument, such as a catheter, needle, or tube, through which another instrument or device is introduced into the body.

keratoprosthesis. Surgical procedure in which the physician creates a new anterior chamber with a plastic optical implant to replace a severely damaged cornea that cannot be repaired.

LDS. Lipodystrophy syndrome. Syndrome which involves the partial or total absence of fat and/or the abnormal deposition and distribution of fat in the body due to a disturbance of the lipid metabolism.

magnetic resonance angiography. Diagnostic technique utilizing magnetic fields and radio waves rather than radiation to produce detailed, cross-sectional images of internal body structures.

multiple-lead device. Implantable cardiac device (pacemaker or implantable cardioverter-defibrillator [ICD]) in which pacing and sensing components are placed in at least three chambers of the heart.

mutation. Alteration in gene function that results in changes to a gene or chromosome. Can cause deficits or disease that can be inherited, can have beneficial effects, or result in no noticeable change.

nasogastric tube. Long, hollow, cylindrical catheter made of soft rubber or plastic that is inserted through the nose down into the stomach, and is used for feeding, instilling medication, or withdrawing gastric contents.

nebulizer. Latin for mist, a device that converts liquid into a fine spray and is commonly used to deliver medicine to the upper respiratory, bronchial, and lung areas.

negative pressure dressing. Adjunctive therapy used to speed wound healing in skin grafts or large wounds. It has been shown to increase blood flow, decrease bacterial count, and increase formation of granulation tissues. A foam pad is placed on the defect and covered with an occlusive drape. A small tube that is non-collapsible is placed into the foam and attached to a disposable pump that provides negative pressure up to -125 mmHg.

NMES. Neuromuscular electrical stimulation. Technology that uses percutaneous stimulation to deliver electrical impulses for muscle flexion to trigger action. NMES can, in some cases, create an ability to ambulate among paraplegic patients.

obturator. Prosthesis used to close an acquired or congenital opening in the palate that aids in speech and chewing.

occult blood test. Chemical or microscopic test to determine the presence of blood in a specimen.

occupational therapy. Training, education, and assistance intended to assist a person who is recovering from a serious illness or injury perform the activities of daily life.

ocular implant. Implant inside muscular cone.

omnicardiogram. Method of mathematically interpreting the usual linear form of the electrocardiogram in a different, roughly circular shape. This interpretation is then compared to a normal template and an analysis is performed on two randomly selected cycles from leads I, II, V4, V, and/or V6.

oral. Pertaining to the mouth.

ordering physician. Physician who orders nonphysician services (e.g., laboratory services, pharmaceutical services, imaging services, or durable medical equipment) for a patient.

orphan drugs. Drugs that treat diseases that affect fewer than 200,000 people in the United States, as designated by the FDA. Orphan drugs follow a varied process from other drugs regulated by the FDA.

orthosis. Derived from a Greek word meaning "to make straight," it is an artificial appliance that supports, aligns, or corrects an anatomical deformity or improves the use of a moveable body part. Unlike a prosthesis, an orthotic device is always functional in nature.

orthotic. Associated with the making and fitting of an orthosis(es).

osteo-. Having to do with bone.

osteogenesis stimulator. Device used to stimulate the growth of bone by electrical impulses or ultrasound.

ostomy. Artificial (surgical) opening in the body used for drainage or for delivery of medications or nutrients.

pacemaker. Implantable cardiac device that controls the heart's rhythm and maintains regular beats by artificial electric discharges. This device consists of the pulse generator with a battery and the electrodes, or leads, which are placed in single or dual chambers of the heart, usually transvenously.

parenteral. Other than the alimentary canal and is usually used in a method of delivery context: total parenteral nutrition (TPN) and parenteral nutrition therapy (PNT) formulas, kits, and devices.

parenteral nutrition. Nutrients provided subcutaneously, intravenously, intramuscularly, or intradermally for patients during the postoperative period and in other conditions, such as shock, coma, and renal failure.

partial hospitalization. Situation in which the patient only stays part of each day over a long period. Cardiac, rehabilitation, and chronic pain patients, for example, could use this service.

passive mobilization. Pressure, movement, or pulling of a limb or body part utilizing an apparatus or device.

periradicular. Surrounding part of the tooth's root.

peritoneal. Space between the lining of the abdominal wall, or parietal peritoneum, and the surface layer of the abdominal organs, or visceral peritoneum. It contains a thin, watery fluid that keeps the peritoneal surfaces moist.

peritoneal dialysis. Dialysis that filters waste from blood inside the body using the peritoneum, the natural lining of the abdomen, as the semipermeable membrane across which ultrafiltration is accomplished. A special catheter is inserted into the abdomen and a dialysis solution is drained into the abdomen. This solution extracts fluids and wastes, which are then discarded when the fluid is drained. Various forms of peritoneal dialysis include CAPD, CCPD, and NIDP.

peritoneal effusion. Persistent escape of fluid within the peritoneal cavity.

pessary. Device placed in the vagina to support and reposition a prolapsing or retropositioned uterus, rectum, or vagina.

photocoagulation. Application of an intense laser beam of light to disrupt tissue and condense protein material to a residual mass, used especially for treating ocular conditions.

physician. Legally authorized practitioners including a doctor of medicine or osteopathy, a doctor of dental surgery or of dental medicine, a doctor of podiatric medicine, a doctor of optometry, and a chiropractor only with respect to treatment by means of manual manipulation of the spine (to correct a subluxation).

PICC. Peripherally inserted central catheter. PICC is inserted into one of the large veins of the arm and threaded through the vein until the tip sits in a large vein just above the heart.

prehensile. Ability to grasp, seize, or hold.

prodrug. Inactive drug that goes through a metabolic process when given resulting in a chemical conversion that changes the drug into an active pharmacological agent.

prophylaxis. Intervention or protective therapy intended to prevent a disease.

prostate cancer screening tests. Test that consists of any (or all) of the procedures provided for the early detection of prostate cancer to a man 50 years of age or older who has not had a test during the preceding year. The procedures are as follows: A digital rectal examination; A prostate-specific antigen blood test. After 2002, the list of procedures may be expanded as appropriate for the early detection of prostate cancer, taking into account changes in technology and standards of medical practice, availability, effectiveness, costs, and other factors.

prosthetic. Device that replaces all or part of an internal body organ or body part, or that replaces part of the function of a permanently inoperable or malfunctioning internal body organ or body part.

pulse generator. Component of a pacemaker or an implantable cardioverter defibrillator that contains the battery and the electronics for producing the electrical discharge sent to the heart to control cardiac rhythm. Insertion or replacement of the pulse generator may be done alone, not in conjunction with insertion or replacement of the entire pacemaker system.

qualitative. To determine the nature or characteristics of the components of a substance.

quantitative. To determine the number or amount of the components of a substance.

rehabilitation services. Therapy services provided primarily for assisting in a rehabilitation program of evaluation and service including cardiac rehabilitation, medical social services, occupational therapy, physical therapy, respiratory therapy, skilled nursing, speech therapy, psychiatric rehabilitation, and alcohol and substance abuse rehabilitation.

residual limb. Portion of an arm or leg that remains attached to the body after an amputation.

screening mammography. Radiologic images taken of the female breast for the early detection of breast cancer.

screening pap smear. Diagnostic laboratory test consisting of a routine exfoliative cytology test (Papanicolaou test) provided to a woman for the early detection of cervical or vaginal cancer. The exam includes a clinical breast examination and a physician's interpretation of the results.

sialodochoplasty. Surgical repair of a salivary gland duct.

single-lead device. Implantable cardiac device (pacemaker or implantable cardioverter-defibrillator [ICD]) in which pacing and sensing components are placed in only one chamber of the heart.

skin substitute. Non-autologous human or non-human skin that forms a base for skin growth, often considered a graft dressing.

speech prosthetic. Electronic speech aid device for patient who has had a laryngectomy. One operates by placing a vibrating head against the throat; the other amplifies sound waves through a tube which is inserted into the user's mouth.

splint. Brace or support. *1)* dynamic splint: brace that permits movement of an anatomical structure such as a hand, wrist, foot, or other part of the body after surgery or injury. *2)* static splint: brace that prevents movement and maintains support and position for an anatomical structure after surgery or injury.

stent. Tube to provide support in a body cavity or lumen.

stereotactic radiosurgery. Delivery of externally-generated ionizing radiation to specific targets for destruction or inactivation. Most often utilized in the treatment of brain or spinal tumors, high-resolution stereotactic imaging is used to identify the target and then deliver the treatment. Computer-assisted planning may also be employed. Simple and complex cranial lesions and spinal lesions are typically treated in a single planning and treatment session, although a maximum of five sessions may be required. No incision is made for stereotactic radiosurgery procedures.

subcutaneous. Below the skin.

TENS. Transcutaneous electrical nerve stimulator. TENS is applied by placing electrode pads over the area to be stimulated and connecting the electrodes to a transmitter box, which sends a current through the skin to sensory nerve fibers to help decrease pain in that nerve distribution.

terminal device. Addition to an upper limb prosthesis that replaces the function and/or appearance of a missing hand.

tracheostomy. Formation of a tracheal opening on the neck surface with tube insertion to allow for respiration in cases of obstruction or decreased patency. A tracheostomy may be planned or performed on an emergency basis for temporary or long-term use.

traction. Drawing out or holding tension on an area by applying a direct therapeutic pulling force.

transcutaneous electrical nerve stimulator. Device that delivers a controlled amount of electricity to an area of the body to stimulate healing and/or to mitigate post-surgical or post-traumatic pain.

transesophageal echocardiography. Guidance of a small probe into the esophagus under sedation to closely evaluate the heart and blood vessels within the chest.

type A emergency department. Emergency department licensed and advertised to be available to provide emergent care 24 hours a day, seven days a week. Type A emergency departments must meet both the CPT book definition of an emergency department and the EMTALA definition of a dedicated emergency department.

type B emergency department. Emergency department licensed and advertised to provide emergent care less than 24 hours a day, seven days a week. Type B emergency departments must meet the EMTALA definition of a dedicated emergency department.

vascular closure device. vascular closure devices seal femoral artery punctures caused by invasive or interventional procedures. The closure or seal is achieved by percutaneous delivery of the device's two primary structures, which are usually an anchor and a suture, clip or biologic substance (e.g., collagen, bioabsorbable polymer) or suture through the tissue tract.

Appendix 9 — Quality Payment Program

In 2015, Congress passed the Medicare Access and CHIP Reauthorization Act (MACRA), which included sweeping changes for practitioners who provide services reimbursed under the Medicare physician fee schedule (MPFS). The act focused on repealing the faulty Medicare sustainable growth rate, focusing on quality of patient outcomes, and controlling Medicare spending.

A MACRA final rule in October 2016 established the Quality Payment Program (QPP), which was effective January 1, 2017. This value-based payment model rewards eligible clinicians (ECs) who provide high-quality care and reduce the payments for those who fail to meet specific performance standards.

ECs can receive incentives under the QPP. Once the performance threshold is established, all ECs who score above that threshold are eligible to receive a positive payment adjustment. Keep in mind that the key requirement is that an EC **submit data** to avoid the negative payment adjustment and receive the incentives. The Centers for Medicare and Medicaid Services (CMS) has redesigned the scoring so that clinicians are able to know how well they are doing in the program, as benchmarks are known in advance of participating.

The QPP consists of two tracks that clinicians may choose from based on their practice size, location, specialty, or patient population:

- The merit-based incentive payment system (MIPS)

- Alternative payment models (APMs)

The 2017 QPP final rule established regulations for MIPS and APMs as well as related policies applicable to eligible clinicians who participate in the Shared Savings Program. These policies included requirements for Shared Savings Program accountable care organizations (ACOs) regarding reporting for the MIPS Quality performance category and a policy that gave ACOs full credit for the MIPS Improvement Activities performance category based on their participation in the Shared Savings Program. Since that time, revisions and modifications have been made to allow more focus on measurement efforts and to reduce barriers to entry into advanced APMs. Refinements will continue in order to reduce reporting burden and focus on patient outcomes.

MIPS provides specified performance categories under which payment adjustments may be earned for Part B covered professional services. Eligible clinicians can obtain a composite performance score (CPS) of up to 100 points from these weighted performance categories, which focus on patient care quality and cost, improvements in patient engagement and clinical care processes, and use of certified electronic health record technology (CEHRT). This performance score then defines the payment adjustments in the second calendar year after the year the score is obtained. For instance, the score obtained for the 2022 performance year is linked to payment for Medicare Part B services in 2024.

ECs currently have three available reporting frameworks, depending on individual needs and eligibility—traditional MIPS, MIPS Value Pathways (MVPs), and the alternative payment model (APM) performance pathway (APP).

Traditional MIPS currently consists of the following performance categories:

- Quality

- Improvement Activities

- Promoting Interoperability (PI)

- Cost

MVPs, which were added as a result of complaints by some physicians of confusing quality measures, allow clinicians to report only on those measures that apply to their specialty. The CY 2024 proposed rule continues refinement and focus on subgroups for MVP reporting that will provide more granularity in reporting and improve patient care. Additional MVPs will gradually be implemented for more specialties and subspecialties that participate in the program.

The APP is intended for MIPS-eligible ECs who also participate in MIPS APMs. Performance is measured across three areas (Quality, Improvement Activities, and Promoting Interoperability) in this reporting and scoring pathway, which aims to decrease reporting burden, encourage APM participation, and create new opportunities for scoring for existing MIPS APM participants. For performance year 2023, the APP Quality performance category accounted for 50 percent of the MIPS final score; the PI performance category weight was 30 percent; and the Improvement Activities performance category weight was 20 percent.

Proposed 2024 Changes

As noted earlier, the majority of the updates for CY 2023 focus on MVP refinement. Proposals in the CY 2024 proposed rule include:

- Changes in the APM that continue to move ACOs toward digital measurement of quality and align with the QPP

- Expanded period of time to identify beneficiary requirement for primary care service from ACO professional

- Changes in how assignable beneficiaries are identified in certain Shared Savings Program calculations

- Updated definition of primary care services for beneficiary assignment to remain consistent with billing and coding guidelines

- Refined financial benchmarking methodology for ACOs to cap the risk score growth in an ACOs regional service area

- Use of CMS-HCC risk adjustment methodology in calculating risk scores for Medicare fee for service (FFS) beneficiaries

- Adoption of measures to mitigate negative impacts to ACOs caring for medically complex, high-cost beneficiaries

Evaluation continues regarding an incremental timeline to transition to mandatory MVP reporting that will coincide with the sunset of traditional MIPS. The timeline currently being considered is the end of the CY 2027 performance period/2029 MIPS payment year, although this is not an official proposal at this time.

Detailed information regarding the Quality Payment Program may be found at https://qpp.cms.gov/. This website will also announce the final CMS determinations of MVPs, advanced APMs, and MIPS APMs for the 2024 performance period.